Kelly's Dimensions of Professional Nursing

Notice

Medicine is an ever-changing science. As new research and clinical experience broaden our knowledge, changes in treatment and drug therapy are required. The author and the publisher of this work have checked with sources believed to be reliable in their efforts to provide information that is complete and generally in accord with the standards accepted at the time of publication. However, in view of the possibility of human error or changes in medical sciences, neither the author nor the publisher nor any other party who has been involved in the preparation or publication of this work warrants that the information contained herein is in every respect accurate or complete, and they disclaim all responsibility for any errors or omissions or for the results obtained from use of the information contained in this work. Readers are encouraged to confirm the information contained herein with other sources. For example and in particular, readers are advised to check the product information sheet included in the package of each drug they plan to administer to be certain that the information contained in this work is accurate and that changes have not been made in the recommended dose or in the contraindications for administration. This recommendation is of particular importance in connection with new or infrequently used drugs.

Kelly's Dimensions of Professional Nursing

Tenth Edition

LUCILLE A. JOEL, RN, EdD, FAAN
Professor, College of Nursing
Rutgers, The State University of New Jersey
Newark, New Jersey

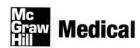

New York   Chicago   San Francisco   Lisbon   London   Madrid   Mexico City
Milan   New Delhi   San Juan   Seoul   Singapore   Sydney   Toronto

Kelly's Dimensions of Professional Nursing, *Tenth Edition*

Copyright © 2011, 2003 by The **McGraw-Hill Companies,** Inc. All rights reserved. Printed in the United States of America. Except as permitted under the United States Copyright Act of 1976, no part of this publication may be reproduced or distributed in any form or by any means, or stored in a data base or retrieval system, without the prior written permission of the publisher.

Copyright © 1999, 1995, 1991, 1985 by Lucie Young Kelly. Earlier editions, entitled *Dimensions of Professional Nursing,* copyright © 1962 by Cordelia W. Kelly and copyright © 1968, 1975, 1981 by Thomas M. Kelly.

1 2 3 4 5 6 7 8 9 0   DOC/DOC   14 13 12 11

ISBN 978-0-07-174099-9
MHID 0-07-174099-6

This book was set in Minion by Glyph International.
The editors were Joseph Morita and Peter J. Boyle.
The production supervisor was Phil Galea.
The designer was Mary McKeon.
Project management by Vastavikta Sharma, Glyph International.
RR Donnelley was the printer and binder.

This book is printed on acid-free paper.

Library of Congress Cataloging-in-Publication Data

Joel, Lucille A.
　　Kelly's dimensions of professional nursing / Lucille A. Joel. —10th ed.
　　　　p. ; cm.
　　Dimensions of professional nursing
　　Includes bibliographical references and indexes.
　　ISBN-13: 978-0-07-174099-9 (pbk. : alk. paper)
　　ISBN-10: 0-07-174099-6 (pbk. : alk. paper)   1. Nursing.   2. Nursing—United States.
　　I. Kelly, Lucie Young.   II. Title.   III. Title: Dimensions of professional nursing.
　　[DNLM: 1. Nursing.   WY 16]
　　RT82.J635   2011
　　610.73—dc22

　　　　　　　　　　　　　　　　　　　　　　　　　　　　2010036817

McGraw-Hill books are available at special quantity discounts to use as premiums and sales promotions, or for use in corporate training programs. To contact a representative please e-mail us at bulksales@mcgraw-hill.com.

Contents

Preface

As *Dimensions of Professional Nursing* enters the new millennium, it is most evident that the past has indeed been prologue. *Dimensions'* proud history began in 1962 with Cordelia Kelly's original work. After her untimely death in 1966, Edith (Pat) Lewis completed the second edition, and in 1975 Lucie Kelly picked up the torch, becoming the sole author of every edition until 1995. *Dimensions* has been synonymous with the name of Lucie Kelly. For the seventh edition (1995), Dr. Kelly invited Lucille Joel to join her as coauthor, and the eighth edition followed with that partnership. The ninth and tenth editions find Lucille Joel carrying forward the tradition of *Dimensions*. *Dimensions* has served the nursing profession for almost 50 years, chronicling its history, issues, and trends with unflinching honesty and detail. This standard has prompted many readers to make *Dimensions* a permanent part of their professional library, continually returning to its pages as a reference after their course work is completed.

Dimensions has held true to its original intent, expressed by Cordelia Kelly as ". . . an overview of the non-clinical aspects of nursing in sufficient detail to be adaptable for use at all stages in all types of ... programs in professional nursing." That description is still valid, and *Dimensions* continues as a virtual compendium of the non-clinical aspects of nursing. In fact, a collection of the sequential editions provides an encyclopedic view of the changing scene in nursing: how it has developed, what it has become, and where it is going.

This tenth edition of *Kelly's Dimensions of Professional Nursing* is a most accurate representation of its times, introducing new and creative use of Internet capabilities. It is presumptuous to think that any bibliography will be adequate for the 4-year life of a book, which is the usual period of time between editions. Responding to that fact, and realizing that both students and faculty value direction to the best of supplementary readings, a bibliography is linked to the McGraw-Hill website and will be updated periodically by the author. Websites that are particularly useful for the reader are noted at the end of each section. Additional websites are included chapter by chapter online, as is PowerPoint—to complement class presentations, and study questions along with a rubric for the teacher to use in grading (specific to the teacher's edition). We are a product of our life and times, and nursing has had a proud life. Chapters 1 through 4 chronicle that history, providing the backdrop for our study of contemporary trends and issues. Part of historical reality is that the nursing profession has been the focus of perpetual study. These studies have exerted significant influence on what nursing has been and will become. They are summarized in Chapter 5. Chapters 6, 7, and 8 describe the environment in which nurses learn and practice, including the trends and public sentiment that are decisively reshaping today's health care system. Chapters 12 and 13 focus on our systems of education for practice, the issues that continue to frustrate, and those that have been successfully resolved over the years. There is justifiable pride in the fact that the profession has honored a commitment to the educational mobility of its members and has changed with the times to accommodate an exceedingly diverse constituency.

Chapter 10 on ethics should be read along with Chapter 21 on the law and Chapter 22 on the rights of people, because it is almost impossible today to draw the line between ethics and related law with the rights of people providing the vividly human background for your discussions. Chapter 10 includes pertinent information on the ethics of managed care, whistle-blowing, and the ethical environment, as well as consideration of new and evolving ethical dilemmas. In Chapter 22, newer dimensions of informed refusal and informed consent are discussed. The nurse's role in the controversial issue of professional assisted suicide is examined, as well as other aspects of the patient's right to die. Similarly, Chapter 21 explores the trends in litigation involving nurses, citing the most pertinent cases.

Nursing has achieved distinction as a scholarly discipline, and much of that status is reflected in Chapter 14 on nursing research. The nature of science, a general overview of research, and exposure to the variations in thinking among major nursing theorists make Chapter 14 particularly strategic and timely. Chapter 15 provides depth on career opportunities, including advanced practice. The material on supply and demand is analytic and characterizes the current employment scene accurately.

Nursing and health care have both experienced profound change since the ninth edition of *Dimensions*, and the most provocative changes are associated with legislation and credentialing. Chapters 19 and 20 reflect these dynamics.

While responding to changing times, nursing has maintained a degree of stability that is comforting both to the profession and the public it serves. A classic model of professionalism is presented in Chapters 9 and 11, while challenged by some newer perspectives. These sensitivities to professionalism combined with the content, references, and bibliography of Chapter 16 create a superb orientation to leadership for uncertain times.

Ultimately students will play out their career life in the workplace (for some this takes the form of a variety of entrepreneurial choices). Chapter 30 highlights the rights and responsibilities that come with transition to the role of graduate, and then to RN: workplace hazards, legal rights of employees, workplace representation, collective bargaining, maintaining competency, and career mapping. Material from earlier editions about professional writing has been retained because no other text includes this basic guidance for sharing your ideas and experiences through publication. In the spirit of transition to practice, the section on Nursing Organizations offers vital information for the new graduate. These organizations are your peer support systems, and their presence and publications are invaluable in developing your practice, socializing you into nursing, and helping you to maintain your competence.

Because cross-referencing from chapter to chapter has always been helpful to readers—enabling them both to get a more complete picture of a topic or issue and to see interrelationships—I have continued this tradition. I believe that the kinds of nurses who will strengthen the profession, change health care for the better, and take influential roles in the nursing community need and want the kind of in-depth analysis as well as the key information presented here.

Nursing is in a period of renaissance. Opportunities abound for nurses with the proper knowledge, courage, confidence, and determination. My hope is that this book will contribute to their armamentarium and allow them to be leaders in their profession and in their times.

LUCILLE A. JOEL

Acknowledgments

Consistent with the rapid changes in health care, *Kelly's Dimensions of Professional Nursing* requires a considerable number of changes with each edition. To be as up to date and accurate as possible, it has been my practice to reach out to a number of colleagues to share their information and expertise. All of them are highly respected, extremely busy, and remarkably generous. Therefore, I would like to acknowledge their valuable contributions.

Special thanks are deserving of Rita Munley-Gallagher of the ANA, who updated Chapter 25 with her usual precision and giving nature. In like fashion, Diane Mancino revisited material on the NSNA. So many others would have been willing, but the magic of the Internet has been able to fill-in innumerable gaps in information.

I owe a great deal to the teachers, students, and colleagues who over the years have used earlier editions of *Dimensions* and have commented so helpfully. They, like myself, agree that nurses, more than ever, need to know about their past as well as their present, to influence their future and the future of the profession that continues to endow their lives so richly.

Most especially and sincerely, my gratitude goes to Lucie Young Kelly whose genius, literary ability, and wisdom have kept *Dimensions* alive and well for all these years. She has provided the nursing community with an invaluable resource, and the modeling to continue this work in perpetuity.

LUCILLE A. JOEL

PART I

Development of Modern Nursing

Early Historical Influences

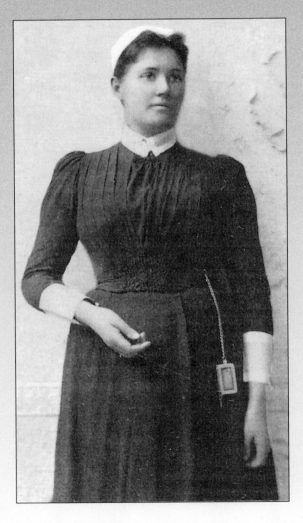

Isabel Hampton Robb, President of the Associated Alumnae of Trained Nurses of the United States. (The American Nurses Association, from the private collection of Lucie Young Kelly)

Care of the Sick: An Historical Overview

The clinical practice of nursing is quite rightly the major focus of most of its practitioners and the prime concern of students. Therefore, there is a tendency to greet nursing history with a "What good is it to me?" attitude.

Undoubtedly, nurses can give good nursing care even if they have never heard of Florence Nightingale, Isabel Hampton Robb, Lavinia Dock, or Lillian Wald. But one of the major differences between an occupation and a profession is its practitioners' long-term commitment to the profession, which includes working toward its development. To do so without some understanding of its past is possibly to repeat errors.

Nursing today was formed by its historical antecedents. Its development since ancient times, within the social contexts of those times, explains many things: its power or lack of power, its educational confusion, and the makeup of its practitioners. The changing relationships between nursing and other health care professions, nursing and other disciplines, and nursing and the public can be traced and better understood with the knowledge of past history. The impact of social and scientific changes on nursing and nursing's impact on society are ongoing processes that need to be studied; nursing does not exist in a vacuum. Sometimes there is a repetition of history, with the answer to the problems apparently not much clearer now than at the beginning of professional nursing. Certain issues with historical derivatives affect the practice of every nurse; in some cases, they are a factor in determining whether the nurse even chooses to stay in the profession. An understanding of the past can bring additional clarity to the decisions that shape the future.

The chapters in Part I are not intended in any way as a substitute for the many fine texts that are available on nursing history. Instead, they provide an overview to set the stage for the more detailed study of nursing history an individual may undertake for professional reasons or personal satisfaction.

■ PRIMITIVE SOCIETIES

Although historians sometimes advance theories and cite an occasional archaeological discovery to prove that prehistoric civilization practiced crude medicine and nursing, the supporting evidence about nursing is somewhat inconclusive. It must be assumed, however, that in most tribes there were some individuals who were more adept than others at caring for the sick and injured and helping the medicine men or witch doctors. It seems reasonable to assume further that some of these men and women taught their sons and daughters and certain members of the tribes to give this care, for these people were able to communicate. They wanted to survive; they were human beings with some ability to think, recall, and teach by example, if not by coherent explanation.

Indirect evidence of some of the beliefs and practices of ancient humans concerning illness has evolved from recent studies of primitive cultures. Apparently, many concepts of health and illness were related to belief in the supernatural. Everything in nature was seen as being alive, with invisible forces and supernatural powers. There were good and evil spirits that must be placated. Primitive humans believed that a person became sick (1) when an evil spirit entered the body; (2) when a good spirit within the body that was ordinarily able to fend off diseases left, either because someone or something had taken it away or of its own accord; and (3) because witchcraft had been performed on the affected part of the body, either directly or through some object that had been given to the person.

Thus, although it was probably recognized how heat, cold, certain foods, wounds, and strains were related to health, and empirical treatments developed for them, serious illness called for the services of a medicine man (witch doctor, shaman, root doctor). This mysterious figure, sometimes a woman but usually a man, functioned through a ritualistic mystique, frequently a shock or fright technique that was intended to induce evil spirits to leave the body. Included were the use of frightening masks and noises, incantations, vile odors, charms, spells, sacrifices, and fetishes. In a primitive version of modern trephining, the medicine man cut a hole in the skull to let the evil spirit out. Purgatives, emetics, deodorants, applied hot and cold substances, cauterization, massage, cupping, and blistering were frequently used.

A woman in abnormal labor was treated by similarly drastic measures, such as placing a lighted fire between her outstretched legs to hasten delivery. Needless to say, patients did not always survive this treatment, and if they did, there is no evidence that any daily ongoing care was given by the shaman. Probably a relative gave this "nursing" care. Women generally assisted other women in childbearing. But whether treatment of illness and injury through the use of herbs and other natural means was carried out by all men and women or by specially designated individuals is not known.

■ EARLY CIVILIZATIONS

In the written records of the early civilizations (500 BC to AD 476), there is very little reference to nursing as such. However, if there is evidence of a high standard of living, a good sanitation system, architectural achievement, interest in education and culture and scientific medicine, or even two or three of these, it is reasonably certain that the health of the inhabitants was of paramount importance and that nurses were not only present but were trained in some fashion to prepare them for the work they did.

The Babylonians

Babylonia was the center of ancient Mesopotamian culture, which was in ruins by the time the Christian era began. Located between the eastern Mediterranean Sea and the Persian Gulf and nourished by the Tigris and Euphrates rivers, this land was very fertile, offering a good life to its settlers. Coveted by many people, for thousands of years it came under the rule of one master and then another who took possession by force. Each influenced the others' development intellectually, socially, and scientifically. Their many wars brought misery and suffering, and, even in that abundant country, there must have been many illnesses and injuries in the normal course of life.

There is evidence that a legalized medical service was instituted and that some type of lay nurses cared for patients. They may have been men, but if they were women, their status was probably quite low, and they must have been subservient to physicians; men dominated the women of Babylonia and controlled their every action.

Herodotus, a Greek historian called the "Father of History," recorded that it was customary in Babylon for the sick to go to the marketplace where passersby could see them and stop to inquire into the "nature of their distemper." Those who had knowledge (acquired principally through experience) of how to treat a condition advised the ill on therapy that had helped them. This was hardly a scientific method of treatment, but it no doubt was effective in many instances.

Excavations made in 1849 of 700 medical tablets show that the Babylonian physician-priest allowed his patients to choose whether they wanted to be treated with medicine or charms. If they selected medicine, the physician had many vegetable and mineral preparations to employ. If they selected charms, the doctor told them which ones to wear for their particular illness and probably uttered a few incantations to accompany the charms, for it was still believed that disease was caused by sin and displeasure of the gods.

However, some of the treatments indicate a realistic attitude toward illness; they included diet, rest, enemas, bandaging, and massaging, plus emphasis on the importance of good personal hygiene. Family or a "nurse" might give this care.

King Hammurabi, who developed a code of laws for the whole empire, founded the first Babylonian Empire. The code is engraved on a huge stone, unearthed in 1902, and shows Hammurabi worshipping a sun god from whom he is receiving instructions about the laws. Included are laws concerning the fees that a physician was allowed to charge for his services and also punishment for the physician who committed "malpractice." Payments were to be made in *shekels* of silver—usually 2, 5, or 10, depending on whether the patient was a master or a slave. Punishment for causing a patient to lose his life or an eye was to "cut off the physician's hands if the patient was a noble man." (This kind of punishment was reserved for surgeons, not physician-priests.)

Wet nurses were also regulated as to remuneration and responsibility.

The Ancient Hebrews

Much of the story of the ancient Hebrews is told in the Talmud and the Old Testament. The Hebrews, alone of their contemporaries, believed in one god, Yahweh, not many.

They attributed their misfortunes and illnesses to God's wrath, and they depended on Him more than on fellow humans to restore them to health when they were sick. One facet of their religion was that it was their duty to be hospitable to strangers as well as to their own people, and they were obliged to give a tithe to augment their personal service in visiting the sick and needy.

The Hebrews brought many hygienic practices from Babylonia, where they had been in captivity, but under the leadership of Moses they also developed principles and practices of hygiene and sanitation. Moses decreed that all meat must be inspected, the selection and preparation of all foods must be carefully supervised, and cleanliness in all areas of living was absolutely essential. This has been called the first sanitary legislation. It represents one of the first public health movements on record.

Their people were taught to help prevent the spread of communicable diseases by burning infected people's garments and sometimes even their houses, and by scrubbing the room in which they were ill and the utensils they used. They were often able to diagnose and control the spread of leprosy and gonorrhea. They performed trephining operations skillfully and humanely, giving the patient a sleeping potion before surgery to dull the pain. They also performed cesarean sections, splenectomies, amputations, and circumcisions, and set fractures. They dressed wounds with oil, wine, and balsam, and used sutures and bandages. From these operations and careful examination of animals, they developed a body of knowledge about anatomy and physiology, although we know now that some of their information was understandably superficial and inaccurate.

The nurse is mentioned occasionally in the Old Testament and the Talmud, but in what capacity she served, except as wet nurse, is not entirely clear. It does appear that the nurse visited and possibly cared for the sick in their homes. She probably also had a role in health teaching.

The Persian Contribution

Between circa 550 and 500 BC, Cyrus the Great, king of Persia, and his son, Cambyses, acquired a vast empire in the Near East. They adopted many of the medical practices and much of the culture from the great lands they conquered—Asia Minor, Babylonia, Syria, Mesopotamia, Egypt, and several others.

In Egypt, the Emperor Darius, successor of Cambyses, restored a school for training priest-physicians and, in effect, established a government-controlled medical center, the first of its kind recorded in history. It is also known that there were practitioners who healed with holy words, herbs, and the knife—in decreasing order of practice.

The Art of Medicine in Egypt

There are references to nurses in accounts of Egyptian medicine as it was practiced in the pre-Christian era. The medical papyri discovered during excavations contain descriptions of such nursing procedures as feeding a tetanus patient and dressing wounds. The extent of the nurse's duties is not clear, however.

Graven inscriptions, the papyri, and other literature reveal Egyptian medicine, on the other hand, as having been rather advanced. In spite of the Egyptians' ideas about the origin of life, the journey that humans took after death, the causes of disease, and the catastrophic effects of incurring the wrath of the gods, they also practiced some very good medicine, although it may not have been based on scientific principles. Priests and physicians were identical in early Egyptian civilization. In healing temples, rest, rituals, and prayer were part of the treatment. Later, there emerged physicians who were concerned only with matters of health and hygiene.

Medical specialization became so common that a physician usually spent his entire career in caring for diseases of one particular part of the body. Members of the profession were organized to protect their medical secrets.

It was in ancient Egypt that the great physician Imhotep lived in about 2980 BC. Skilled in architecture, magic, and priestcraft as well as medicine, he became so famous that he was never forgotten. More than two and a half centuries after his death, he became the god of medicine, identified by the Greeks with their famous god of healing, Asclepios (Latin, *Aesculapius*).

In Egypt, as in most countries, one area of concern was the health of the people. The Egyptians formulated regulations about diet, baths, purgatives, and other matters of personal hygiene. They initiated laws of health suited to Egypt's climate and terrain. They developed diagnostic procedures (which differed in some respects from those of other ancient civilizations) for the common illnesses of their people. Examinations of mummies indicate that the Egyptians suffered many bone diseases and injuries. Osteoarthritis was apparently very common, and there must also have been ailments all humans are subject to such as abdominal, gynecologic, and genitourinary conditions.

There were medical schools and at least one school of midwifery for women, the graduates of which taught physicians about "women's conditions." They became quite well informed about some aspects of anatomy and physiology. For example, the papyri reveal that Egyptian physicians may have had reasonably accurate knowledge of the circulatory system, which was not described accurately and completely by modern people until the sixteenth century AD, when William Harvey studied it. Taking the pulse was a common practice, and the quality of both the heartbeat and the pulse was considered important in understanding a patient's condition. Treatments included the use of a kind of adhesive plaster for closing small wounds; swabs, bandages, and tampons made from linen ravelings; sutures; and molded splints. The papyri also contain records of the preparation of pills, ointments, snuffs, gargles, and emollients that have continued, at least in name, to modern times. Drugs included opium, castor oil, hemlock, salts of copper, and many others.

Dentistry was practiced skillfully, if the gold-filled teeth of mummies of wealthy citizens are to be accepted as evidence. Egyptians developed the art of embalming the body to provide a home for the soul as it went on its journey after death.

The Ancient Hindus

The history of pre-Christian India reports the establishment of hospitals, probably the first in the world, and also the first special nursing group of which we have accurate information. These male attendants staffed the hospitals to which surgeons with remarkable skills sent their patients for care. The Indian philosophy that assigned women to an inferior role in society would not allow them to work outside the home environment. The qualifications of these "nurses" were stated as follows in the *Charaka Samhita*, a medical manuscript.

> ... there should be secured a body of attendants of good behavior, distinguished for purity or cleanliness of habits, attached to the person for whose services they are engaged, possessed of cleverness and skill, endowed with kindness, skilled in every kind of service that a patient may require ... clever in bathing or washing a patient ... well skilled in making or cleaning beds ... and skillful in waiting upon one that is ailing, and never unwilling to do any act that they be commanded to do.

No one knows who did the "commanding" of these workers—patients, doctors, or both. The nurse's status is also unclear (it appears that he might have become a physician after training), but we at least know that he performed some nursing functions.

Knowledge of Indian medicine derives principally from several of their books and writings (in contrast to the reliance on archaeological discoveries for data about the Mesopotamian, Egyptian, and other civilizations). Of these, the sacred writings called the *Vedas,* a compendium of surgical works (*Susruta Samhita*), and another of medical works (*Charaka Samhita*) are most informative.

From the *Vedas,* which are the oldest scriptures of Hinduism, it is learned that the Indian people of ancient times were highly religious and believed in divine control of health and disease. They worshipped many gods, especially the sun god Brahma, until Buddhism originated in the sixth century BC. They used charms, invocations, and other primitive methods to quell the wrath of the gods, but from about 800 BC to AD 1000, all of India flourished and progressed; medicine also advanced. It was during this period that the hospitals mentioned earlier were built.

The two outstanding physicians of ancient times were Susruta and Charaka, who in their writings revealed that physicians were members of the upper castes and were required to be pure of mind and body and to be ethical in every respect. Their knowledge of anatomy and physiology was often inaccurate, but they evolved some theories that persisted for centuries. Among these was the belief that disease might be caused by impurities in the body fluids or humors. They used bloodletting procedures to rid the body of the impure fluids. The theory of humoral pathology was subsequently accepted by Greek physicians and became a basic concept of European medicine. The Indian physician had a great many drugs and other pharmaceutical preparations to help him in his work.

The surgery practiced in India was particularly outstanding for the time. With instruments they designed themselves, under the cleanest conditions possible, and without the aid of effective antiseptics or the benefits of anesthesia, the surgeons performed tonsillectomies, herniorrhaphies, tumor excisions, cataract operations, and other forms of surgery.

To help prevent disease, the Hindus formulated religious laws particularly covering matters of hygiene and diet suitable to the tropical climate.

Scientific medicine in India eventually lost its momentum, and during the Mohammedan era (beginning about

AD 622), it began to decline and became almost completely extinguished, a genuine loss to the world of medicine.

Ceylon (Sri Lanka), an island off India's southeast coast, had an advanced standard of living during the period of India's greatest achievement. History has recorded the establishment of many hospitals in which well-prepared physicians and nurses attended the sick. Hospitals for animals were also founded in India and Ceylon.

The Chinese

As in other ancient cultures, magic, demons, and evil spirits were part of Chinese medical beliefs. The beginning of a more modern medicine is credited to the emperor Shen Nung (circa 2700 BC), who apparently originated drug therapy and acupuncture. These were incorporated into the theory of yang and yin, which still exists. Yang, the male principle, is light, positive, and full of life; yin, the female principle, is dark, cold, and lifeless. When the two are in harmony, the patient is in good health. Originally, acupuncture consisted of inserting needles into areas called meridians, which controlled the flow of yang and yin. (With new interest in acupuncture, American medicine is trying to determine its anatomic and physiologic basis.)

Other Chinese contributions include the use of many still-pertinent drugs and further refinement of ancient measures of hydrotherapy, massage, cupping (bloodletting), *moxa* (a form of counterirritation), cautery, and the promotion of systematic exercise to maintain physical and mental well-being.

Sources of information include a book on medicine written by Shen Nung and later works, notably the classic *Canon of Medicine,* which is a complete discussion of anatomy and physiology with many details about blood circulation and pulse. Another outstanding book was the *Essay on Typhoid,* written in the first century AD by Chang Chung Ching, often regarded as China's greatest physician.

There is little mention of any type of hospital, perhaps because of strong family traditions that would naturally include giving care to the sick within the family circle. Thus, nursing care was probably given in the home.

The Great Achievement of Greece

Whenever ancient Greece is mentioned, one immediately thinks of education, philosophy, and democracy. But Plato, Aristotle, Socrates, Herodotus, Homer, Sophocles, Pericles, Euripides, and other great names of Greece were not typical of its earliest times, for this country too began under primitive conditions in about 2000 BC.

The ancient Greeks represented many peoples, principally the Achean, Dorian, Aegean, Ionian, Arcadian, and Aeolian, who came from the mountains, from fertile valleys where they had engaged in agriculture, and from the coast where seafaring was their occupation. Collectively they called themselves the Hellenes (after their ancestor Hellen, a legendary king of Phthia).

They were barbaric people at first, with the superstitions and practices of primitive people, but gradually there emerged the well-known Grecian character with a thirst for truth and knowledge. Because of their geographical location and the ease of maritime travel, they were able to visit such comparatively advanced countries as Crete and Mesopotamia and to borrow or usurp these countries' cultures.

They were also eager to expand their geographical borders and were so successful that within a few centuries their culture extended from Greece to India. Gradually they developed their own Hellenic civilization, and by 500 BC, if not before, they displayed the keen intellect, independence of thought, and democratic action for which they are famous. They also enjoyed religious freedom. Their great center of civilization was Athens, which was at its peak in the fourth century BC. Athenian culture spread to other beautiful cities, principally along the Mediterranean coast, some of which eventually surpassed Athens in brilliance.

In such a vital society, the art of medicine naturally kept pace with advances in other fields. But, like other ancient cultures, Greece went through centuries of belief in demons and spirits as causes of human ills, but with an element of greater complexity because of its acquisition of other cultures and a divergence of beliefs and practices among them. Here, too, the Greeks gradually evolved their own ideas about the relationships of the gods to health and illness. The famous Greek myths told in story and poem show a mixture of common sense and mysticism in their medical attitudes.

Asclepius, the classical god of medicine, is part of one such myth. Whether he actually lived or not seems uncertain, for his origin is obscure, but it is generally conceded that he did exist in person and that the mystery that surrounds him stems largely from his deification. A parallel is seen in the deification of Imhotep by the Egyptians. Hygieia, the goddess of health, is reputed to have been the daughter of Asclepios. (There are also some theories that it was *women* goddesses who were most important in the healing function.)[1]

His contributions, real or imagined, were further recognized by the founding of temples in his honor in localities suitable for rest and restoration to health. Sometimes referred to as hospitals, they were much more like the spas and health resorts of modern times, with mineral springs, baths, gymnasiums, athletic fields, and treatment and consultation rooms.

They differed from modern resorts, however, in that they were controlled by priests and were essentially religious institutions. Prayers, sacrifices, rituals, and offerings of thanks were part of every patient's regimen in one of these sanatoria. (However, pregnant women and individuals with incurable diseases were not admitted.) The therapeutic effects of these facilities were considerable, however, and knowledge of them was significant in later medical practice. Priestesses served as attendants and waited on the sick, but they could not be considered nurses. The best known of these temples was Epidauros, about 30 miles from Athens, the ruins of which can still be seen.

To Asclepius can also be traced the origin of the symbol of the medical profession—a serpent entwined on a staff—known as the caduceus. The staff was the staff of Asclepios; the serpent since primitive times had represented wisdom and knowledge.

The greatest name in Greek medicine—and possibly in all medicine—is Hippocrates. Born in Cos in 460 BC, he is frequently seen as the epitome of the ideal physician, both personally and professionally. Humane, brilliant, progressive, and a great physician, teacher, and leader, he is often known as the "Father of Medicine."

Hippocrates' medical achievements can be grouped into four major areas.

1. *Rejection of all beliefs in the supernatural origin of disease.* He divorced medicine from religion, philosophy, and the remaining traces of magic and taught that illness was caused by a breach of natural laws. He did not accept the theories of others who preceded him, but made his diagnosis on the basis of symptoms he observed in his patients. His emphasis was on the whole patient, and he advocated constant and continuous bedside care.

2. *Development of thorough patient assessment and recording.* He thoroughly examined his patients and then made a systematic recording of his findings: general appearance, temperature, pulse, respiration, sputum, excreta, ability to move about, and so on. Never before had physicians prepared good clinical records.

3. *Establishment of the highest ethical standards in medicine.* Hippocrates considered medicine one of the noblest arts and believed that the conduct of the physician should be above reproach. He must be loyal to his profession and never bring dishonor on it. He must be equally loyal to his patients and never injure them in any way. The Hippocratic Oath (probably written after his death) is cited in part in Chapter 10 and presumably encompasses some of his convictions.

4. *Author of medical books.* Although it is thought that much of the writing was actually done by contemporaries or possibly his students, the information is supposed to be based on Hippocrates' teachings. The works include his case histories, descriptions of techniques such as bathing and bandaging, and treatises on fractures and dislocations, diet in acute diseases, ulcers, epidemic diseases, and others. He reported on treatments that did not work, as well as those that did, to avoid repetition of errors.

Little is known of nursing as an occupation in pre-Christian Greece. In spite of advances in surgery, Greek physicians did not use the assistance of nurses to the degree that the surgeons of India did. Neither did the Greeks establish hospitals, and that may have been an important factor in the presence or absence of nursing. Through the ages, the development of nursing seems to have been greatly influenced by the physician's need for assistance, the quality of help that he wanted, and the amount of responsibility he was willing to delegate to others. If there were nurses who worked outside the home in Greece, they must have all been men because women held a very inferior position and were denied education as well as participation in community activities, both civil and humanitarian, except for the few instances in which women became midwives or physicians.

Advances in Alexandria

After Alexander the Great conquered Greece in about 338 BC, he spread Greek civilization throughout the known world. It reached a particularly high point in Alexandria, an Egyptian city on the Mediterranean Sea. Here the arts and sciences, including medicine, flourished for about 300 years.

In about 300 BC, the first great medical school of this period was established in Alexandria with clinics, laboratories, and a huge library of 500,000 volumes. The physicians were supported by the state and did not have to depend on their practice to make a living. Dissections were permitted, and this resulted in tremendous advances in the knowledge of anatomy and physiology. The studies made by the Alexandrian physicians are considered the first medical research worthy of the name. After the Romans defeated Cleopatra in 30 BC, Alexandria's place in the sun dimmed considerably, and the art of and interest in research declined.

Roman Hospitals and Sanitation

When the Etruscans conquered Rome in about 750 BC, they brought new arts to this farming community, particularly the use of bronze, skill in building stone edifices, and a written language. In about 500 BC, the Romans overthrew the Etruscans and became powerful masters of the Western world. Rome soon became a thriving commercial center and, through later conquests, a vast empire. Much emphasis was placed on government administration and related activities; on pleasures for the well-to-do, sometimes at the expense of the less fortunate; and on beautifully constructed public buildings, aqueducts, and roads.

Gradually Rome assimilated what it wanted of the Greek culture, and in some fields that was considerable. Although a temple of Asclepius was built, Romans were somewhat wary of the Greek methods of treating disease, believing that their own deities, folklore, and magic were functioning well enough. Moreover, they were reluctant to accept advice and direction from the Greek physicians who, they thought, might poison or assassinate them in the name of medicine. They considered them social inferiors and thought them mercenary because they charged fees for their services.

Nevertheless, Greek medicine gradually replaced or supplemented Roman practices, and medicine was soon considered part of the necessary education of upper-class Roman men. Celsus (first century AD), in his lay work *De Medicina,* reported on, among other things, dietetics, pharmacy, medical conditions (particularly dermatologic), surgical conditions (including cataract surgery and the use of ligatures), and mental illness. It might be added that physicians of ancient times had little interest in the care of childbearing women. Soranus, another Greek of this period, did write some treatises on obstetrics and gynecology, which is the first indication of a male physician's interest in these matters. Galen later referred to some of the techniques used by the midwives in delivery and care of the newborn, and it can be assumed that midwives were the key figures in the care of women. Galen (AD 130 to 201), considered one of the greatest Greek physicians, practiced in Rome after receiving an education in many cities, including Alexandria. He wrote some 100 treatises on medicine, so comprehensive that for 200 years they remained unchallenged. He is seen as the greatest scientific experimentalist before the seventeenth century and perhaps the originator of scientific medicine.

Major Roman contributions to health were in public health sanitation and law. Their aqueducts, sewage systems, and baths were unequaled for centuries, and their city planning included the appointment of both a water commissioner and a public health official. In addition, they may be credited with the development of hospitals. *Valetudinaria* were detached buildings or just a large room designated for the care of valuable slaves on Roman estates. Apparently attendants watched over the sick, possibly with the attention of a physician. There is some indication that, at a later time, individuals other than slaves might have been cared for in *valetudinaria*. Given even more attention was the care of sick and injured soldiers. Originally, they were billeted with local Roman families, who tried to outdo each other in the quality of care. But as the Roman wars expanded to new frontiers, permanent convalescent camps succeeded temporary mobile hospitals. Modern excavations along the Rhine and Danube show the remains of hospitals that could accommodate 200 patients, with wards, recreation areas, baths, pharmacies, and rooms for attendants. Roman historians report that military discipline prevailed and, although the patients received good care, they were also required to conduct themselves "quietly." It appears that the Romans took Greek medicine an additional step to the care of the sick by both male and female attendants.

■ THE FIRST FIVE CENTURIES OF CHRISTIANITY

After centuries of vilification, Christianity became the official religion of Rome in AD 335. The early Christian era brought another dimension to the care of the sick. Christian charity, based to a great extent on the Hebrew model as well as on the teachings of Christ, was reinforced by the persecution suffered by the early followers. Their beliefs included a strong emphasis on the sanctity of human life, and infanticide and abortion were considered murder. In the institutionalization of these ideals, bishops were given responsibility for the sick, the poor, widows, and children, but deacons and deaconesses were designated to carry out the services. (Deaconesses, found almost entirely in the Eastern Church until the eighth century and always fewer in number, had almost disappeared in the East by the eleventh century.)

The duties were not the same in all churches, but a deaconess usually assisted with such church services as the baptism of women, visiting sick women of the church in their homes, acting as ushers for women attending church, carrying messages for the clergy, and visiting prisoners when they could be helped through counseling. Not all were ordained by the church fathers, who resisted giving women too much recognition or freedom. Nor were they permitted to form orders with rules until somewhat later in history. The role of women was seen as marriage and the begetting of children. Young widows were encouraged to remarry. Widows over 60 (which in those days of early death must have restricted the number considerably) were designated to, among other things, watch over the sick. Some virgins also chose to take vows of service. It is not certain to what extent the early deaconesses were involved in such care, but it is clear that a group of specially designated women, whether deaconesses, widows, virgins, or matrons, cared for the sick.

Noted Women

Among the fabled women who made noted contributions to the care of the sick were the following:

- *Phoebe* (spelled *Phebe* in the Bible) of Cenchrea in southern Italy, who lived about AD 60, was the first deaconess who performed nursing functions that were referred to in records of such early times; St. Paul, in Romans 16: 1–2 (King James version), commends her to authorities in Rome—to which she traveled—as a "succorer of many and to myself, also."
- The *Empress Helena*, mother of Constantine the Great of Rome, lived circa AD 248 to 328. In circa AD 312, she converted to Christianity and made a pilgrimage to Jerusalem, reportedly to expiate the sins of her son. In the Holy Land, she built two churches and a Christian hospital. An influential personage, she won support for the Christian church and especially for its humanitarian aspects.
- *Olympias,* an aristocratic and beautiful young woman of Constantinople, was born in 368. Widowed at 19, she became a deaconess and devoted the rest of her life to work among the sick and poor. She was an excellent organizer, and the 40 deaconesses who worked under

her accomplished a great deal in alleviating suffering, caring for orphans and the aged, and converting others to Christianity. Perhaps unfortunately, Olympias is remembered in history chiefly for her extreme asceticism. She denied herself the luxury of a bath, dressed as the lowliest of beggars, and refused to observe any other rules of hygienic living. Fabiola, Paula, and others (both men and women) of the early Christian era had ascetic tendencies, but none to the degree that Olympias demonstrated. Largely because of her personal neglect, she contracted many illnesses and thus lessened the effectiveness of her work.
- *Fabiola*, a beautiful and wealthy matron of Rome, founded the first free hospital in that city in circa 390. Twice married and twice divorced, she embraced Christianity and spent her fortune and the rest of her life in service to the poor and sick. She personally nursed the sickest and filthiest people who came to her hospital, and was so gentle and kind that she was beloved by all Romans. Following her death, St. Jerome wrote a letter about her, sometimes called "the first literary document in the history of nursing."
- *Paula*, a friend of Fabiola, widowed at 23, learned and wealthy, also became a Christian. In about 385, she sailed from Rome to Palestine, where she built hospitals and inns for pilgrims and travelers along the route to Jerusalem, a monastery in Bethlehem, and a convent for women in Jerusalem. She, like Fabiola, performed nursing duties.

Hospitals

Following the closing of the temple of Asclepius, in those same early centuries, another form of hospital emerged, the *diakonia*, providing a combination of outpatient and welfare service, managed by the deacons and supervised by the bishop. This was replaced in time by "a house for the sick," as there was a house for the poor and a house for the old. Generally, only the poor, the destitute, or the traveler—those who could not be cared for in their own homes—chose this alternative, an attitude that persisted to a great extent into the eighteenth and nineteenth centuries.

One of these hospitals may have been the Basilias outside Caesarea, built in the third century by St. Basil, one of the Four Fathers of the Greek Church, and his sister Macrina. Huge and apparently magnificent, it had special rooms or areas for patients with different conditions, a separate building for lepers, and a special area where the physically handicapped could learn a new trade. There were homes for physicians and nurses, convalescent patients, and the elderly, as well as schools and workshops for foundlings. Presumably, some kind of attendant had to be present. Some of these were the women cited earlier, who probably came from their homes to give care. A brotherhood known as *parabolani*, organized in the third century during a great plague in Alexandria, gave care to the sick and buried the dead.

The most regrettable fact in the history of this period is the negative attitude of the Christians toward science and education—an attitude that stultified progress in all intellectual pursuits, including medicine, and permeated the so-called Dark Ages, which continued for another 500 years.

■ THE MIDDLE AGES

The term *Middle Ages* usually is applied to the years from approximately AD 500 to 1500, of which roughly the first half has been called the Dark Ages, to distinguish it from the periods of classical civilization preceding and following it. Some historians acknowledge that the Dark Ages may have been more enlightened than was formerly believed. Certainly there were many areas allied to nursing in which the era might have been termed "light gray" rather than "dark," for progress was made that influenced the later development of nursing as a profession for both women and men.

Politically, the world changed greatly during the Middle Ages. The early centuries brought invasions against the Roman Empire by "barbarians" (to the Roman, anyone outside the pale of the Empire), which resulted in the formation of many smaller kingdoms within the empire. By the twelfth century, many kingdoms existed, chiefly England, Scotland, France, Denmark, Poland, Hungary, Sicily, and several in Spain. In the meantime, the Vikings had settled in Scandinavia and parts of Russia and expanded rapidly. Trade routes were established between principal cities, and new occupations developed to meet the needs of a rapidly increasing population and changing economies and goals.

The barbarians were all pagans, and not until the thirteenth and fourteenth centuries were they converted to Christianity. Most of the work of conversion was carried out under the direction of the pope, and Roman Catholicism quite naturally was the principal religion of Europe at that time.

Also significant in the general picture of the known world during medieval times was the rise and fall of feudalism in Central Europe, with its devastating effects on the welfare of the common people. It was a time of famine and pestilence, with accompanying miseries and serious illnesses. Medical and nursing care was needed, but unfortunately was not available in either sufficient quality or quantity. Beginning in the thirteenth century, feudalism gradually disappeared.

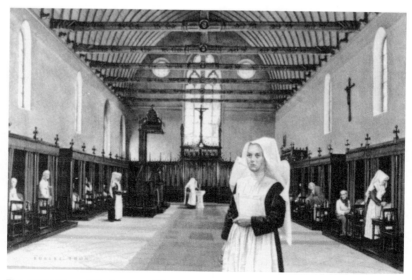

The Hotel Dieu of Paris, one of the earliest hospitals founded in the Middle Ages. (Courtesy of Parke, Davis and Company)

During the Middle Ages, the deaconesses, suppressed by the Western churches in particular, gradually declined and became almost extinct. However, a small spark remained that was fanned into a flame every now and then during history, resulting in the formation of a new order of deaconesses, the most important of which are mentioned later.

As the deaconesses declined, the religious orders grew stronger. Known as *monastic orders* and composed of monks and nuns (although not in the same orders), they controlled the hospitals, running them as institutions concerned more with the patients' religious problems than with their physical ailments. However, monks and some nuns were better educated than most people in those times, and their education may well have included some of the medical writings of Celsus and Galen.

Later, with the coming of the Renaissance in the fourteenth century, separation of hospital and church began, effecting spectacular improvement in the scientific and skillful treatment of the sick and injured. It was within the monasteries, however, that education in general progressed significantly during this earlier period.

Lay citizens banded together to form secular orders. Their work was similar to that of the monastic orders in that it was concerned with the sick and needy, but they lived in their own homes, were allowed to marry, and took no vows of the church. They usually adopted a uniform, or habit. Nursing was often their main work.

The military nursing orders, known as the *Knights Hospitallers*, were the outcome of the Crusades, the military expeditions undertaken by Christians in the eleventh, twelfth, and thirteenth centuries to recover the Holy Land from the Moslems. The most prominent of these three types of orders—religious, military, and secular—during the Middle Ages are described in the following paragraphs.

St. Benedict of Nursia (circa 480 to 543) founded the *Order of St. Benedict*, the foremost religious order, on the beautiful mountain Monte Cassino, about halfway between Rome and Naples. It became a great and powerful center that sent workers throughout Europe, raising standards of education and culture and providing better care for the sick and poor. St. Benedict's rule placed the care of the sick (in which bathing was stressed, a departure from the ascetic practices of some other orders) above and before every other duty of the monks. He established infirmaries within the monasteries primarily for the care of sick members of the order, but also to help centralize and organize the care of pilgrims, wayfarers, and "refugees."

With war, famine, and pestilence common occurrences, such service was sorely needed.

The Knights Hospitallers, an outgrowth of the Crusades, was the first military order of nurses. The first Crusade (there were nine in all) originated in 1095 when disorganized hordes of men and women of every age, type, and description answered Pope Urban II's call to march to Jerusalem and recover the Holy Land from the Moslems, who had taken it by force from the Byzantine Empire in the seventh century AD. Ill prepared physically and psychologically for such a journey, disorganized and inadequately equipped, the crusaders (whose symbol was an eight-pointed cross) died by the thousands along the way.

The later Crusades were essentially expeditions to assist the earlier crusaders in the Holy Land. It was during the first Crusade that the military order, the Knights Hospitallers, was established for the original purpose of bringing the wounded from the battlefield to the hospitals and caring for them there, which explains the name of the order. Later, two other branches of the Knights were formed, one to defend the wounded from the enemy while they were being brought to the hospital, and the other to defend the pilgrims when they were attacked.

There were three principal orders of the Knights Hospitallers: St. John of Jerusalem, the Teutonic Knights, and the Knights of St. Lazarus, whose principal mission was to care for victims of leprosy, one of the major health problems from the eleventh to the mid-thirteenth century. Women had their own branches of the Knights Hospitallers. They performed their services principally in hospitals to which only women patients were admitted.

The story of the Knights Hospitallers is both colorful and interesting. Wealthy and influential, these orders had their successes and failures for approximately seven centuries.

The *Hospital Brothers of St. Anthony* was a secular order founded about 1095 by a grateful man who had been miraculously cured of St. Anthony's fire, which was probably erysipelas. The men and women who joined the order cared only for patients with this disease in special hospitals to which no other patients were admitted. Thus, they succeeded in curtailing the spread of erysipelas and no doubt became specialists of a sort in the treatment of this disease.

The *Antonines* later became a religious order and, when these orders were suppressed, the character of their contribution to nursing changed. They took care of patients with other illnesses, the special hospitals for St. Anthony's fire closed, and erysipelas became a major problem for several centuries, especially among surgical and obstetric patients in general hospitals.

The *Beguines of Flanders*, believed to have been founded in about 1184 by a priest, was one of the most important secular orders. The widows and unmarried women who comprised its membership (at one time numbering 200,000) devoted their lives to helping others. Their nursing duties included the care of the sick in their homes and hospitals, serving soldiers and civilians during the Battle of Waterloo, caring for victims of cholera during the dreadful epidemics of the nineteenth century, and responding to calls for assistance in times of disastrous fires, floods, and famines. These sisterhoods spread to Germany, Switzerland, and France and became so numerous, strong, and popular that they were able to resist attempts to abolish them by monastic orders and religious leaders.

The *Third Order of St. Francis* is one of three orders founded by St. Francis of Assisi (1182 to 1226), probably the best known of the saints connected with nursing. A compassionate young man who loved people, birds, and animals, he was also a fanatic and ascetic with marked qualities of leadership, attracting the influential and learned as well as the humble and lowly to his orders.

The Third Order of St. Francis, also called the *Franciscan Tertiaries*, worked principally among the lepers. They were assisted by the women of the Order of Poor Clares, the second order formed by St. Francis, whose members were largely young women who had left their noble families for a life of service.

After the death of St. Francis at the age of 44, the ideals of the Franciscan friars changed considerably, improving in some respects and degenerating in others. But the friars extended their work to the sick and poor, particularly in the slum areas of Europe's large cities, and rendered remarkable service.

The *Order of Poor Clares* became an enclosed order, which greatly changed the lives of the sisters. They continued their work in some ways, however. It was the Franciscan sisters who helped Dr. W. W. Mayo, a civil war surgeon, to found the famous St. Mary's Hospital in Rochester, Minnesota, in 1889.

The *Order of the Holy Ghost* (Santo Spirito), a secular order, was founded in Montpellier, France, in the late twelfth century. Initiated by a knight known as Guy de Montpellier, its members included both men and women. They nursed the poor in the community and assumed responsibility for all of the nursing at the Santo Spirito Hospital in Rome in 1204. They later extended their service to other large hospitals in Italy, France, and Germany. They cared for lepers in shelters outside the hospitals and for persons with other infectious diseases. The order later became monastic and eventually almost disappeared.

Guy de Montpellier established this order in connection with a medical school that had existed in Montpellier since the eighth century, and that became famous as a center of medical education, reaching its period of greatest achievement in the thirteenth and fourteenth centuries. Patients flocked to Montpellier seeking cures under the care of renowned physicians, one of the most outstanding being the surgeon Guy de Chauliac (1298 to 1368).

The *Grey Sisters*, an order of uncloistered nuns that originated in about 1222, ministered to the poor and the sick in homes and hospitals for many years. In the fourteenth and fifteenth centuries when the plague invaded Europe, they worked closely with the Alexian Orders in meeting nursing needs.

The *Alexian Brotherhood* came into being in about 1348 in the Netherlands when the Black Death was sweeping Europe. The brothers took no vows and adopted no rule at the time, bending all their efforts to caring for the stricken and burying the victims of plague. Nearly a century later, in 1431, they organized as a religious order, taking vows of obedience, poverty, and chastity and choosing as their patron saint Alexus, a man of noble birth who in the fifth century had worked in a hospital in Syria. They were among the pioneers of organized nursing in Europe.

There were several outstanding personalities of the Middle Ages who were not members of orders, but who nonetheless made significant contributions to the health and welfare of the masses. Some of these were canonized, notably Elizabeth of Hungary, Catherine of Siena, and Hildegard of Bingen. The most prominent women were abbesses or members of royalty who nursed the sick, established educational programs for nurses, and sometimes wrote books and treatises. *Hildegarde of Bingen* (1098 to 1178) was educated in a Benedictine monastery and years later became its abbess. Several of her writings were related to medicine and the care of the sick, including general diseases of the body and their causes, symptoms, and treatment; aspects of anatomy and physiology; and human behavior. Many of these things were unknown to physicians of the time.

Medicine

The Dark Ages on the Continent halted the promising progress of medicine, and except for Galen, who died in

AD 200, no great physician practiced medicine in Europe during this period. The Christian church, obsessed with its belief that man's main purpose on earth was to prepare for a future life, saw little need for the science and philosophy of the Greeks or the hygienic teachings and sanitation systems of the Romans. Plagues swept Europe periodically for centuries. Medical knowledge survived and developed in only three areas.

In the eastern Roman Empire, Byzantine physicians nourished the teachings of Hippocrates and Galen, refusing to let them become obsolete; in Salerno in southern Italy, an educational ideal was fostered for medicine as well as for other areas of learning, a medical school was established, and laymen in Salerno translated many Greek manuscripts of importance in medical history; and vigorous medical activity was carried on in the Moslem Empires. Although there was warfare there, as in Europe, the conquerors preserved rather than destroyed the culture they found and encouraged further development. Within 100 years they had achieved a standard of culture that took the Germanic tribes who invaded the Roman Empire 10 times as long to develop.

The Arabs translated the works of Hippocrates, Galen, Aristotle, and others. Physicians adopted the Hippocratic method of careful observation of patients. One of the outstanding physicians was *Rhazes* (850 to 932) of Baghdad, who was especially interested in communicable diseases and gave an accurate account of smallpox.

Another and far more prominent physician was *Avicenna* (980 to 1037), a Persian whose *Canon of Medicine* was studied in the medical schools of Europe from the twelfth to the seventeenth centuries. *Moses ben Maimon* (*Maimonides*), born in Moslem-controlled Spain to a Jewish family descended from King David, was an excellent clinician who became the court physician to Sultan Saladin.

Medical centers that included hospitals were founded in Cairo, Alexandria, Damascus, and Baghdad. There the Arabs made advances in physiology, hygiene, chemistry, and particularly pharmacy. Because their religion prohibited human dissection, their knowledge of anatomy changed little during this time. Men probably gave care in these hospitals, because women were kept in seclusion.

Hospitals and Hospital Care

Hospitals in which the sick received care were established as the need increased and the wherewithal became available. At the close of the Middle Ages, there were hospitals all over Europe, particularly in larger cities such as Paris and Rome, and in England, where several hundred had been established. Most of these have long since been eliminated or abandoned, but a few have remained. The oldest of these is the Hotel Dieu of Lyons (House of God's Charity), built in 542, in which both men and women nursed the patients.

The Hotel Dieu of Paris, founded around 650, has a less favorable record as far as nursing is concerned. Staffed by Augustinian nuns who did the cooking and laundry as well as the nursing, and who had neither intellectual nor professional stimulation, the hospital was not distinguished for its care of patients. In 1908 the nuns were expelled from the Hotel Dieu. The records of nursing kept by this hospital were well done, however, and have been a source of enlightenment for historians. Still in existence in Rome is the Santo Spirito Hospital, established in 717 by order of the pope, to care only for the sick.

Hospitals in England during the Middle Ages differed from those on the Continent in that they were never completely church controlled, although they were founded on Christian principles and accepted responsibility for the sick and injured. The oldest and best-known English hospitals from a historical point of view are St. Bartholomew's, founded in 1123; St. Thomas's, founded in 1213; and Bethlehem Hospital, founded in 1247, originally a general hospital that later became famous as a mental institution, referred to frequently as Bedlam.

An interesting sidelight here is the treatment of the mentally ill. In Bedlam, as in similar institutions, the inmates were treated with inhumane cruelty. Beatings and starvation were not uncommon. However, in Gheel, Belgium, reports of miraculous cures at the tomb of St. Dymphna, an Irish princess murdered by her mad father, brought the mentally ill hope of healing. The people of Gheel took in the pilgrims as foster families and gave them care and affection.

The nursing care in most early hospitals was essentially basic: bathing, feeding, giving medicines, making beds, and so on. It was rarely of high quality, however, largely because of the lack of progress of nearly all civilization and the shortsighted attitude toward women that was typical of the Dark Ages.

■ THE RENAISSANCE

The word *renaissance* as used in history refers to both a movement and a period of time. In years, it is generally conceded to have lasted from 1400 to 1550, the years during which there was a transitional movement toward revival of the arts and sciences in Europe, culminating in the modern age. Also during this period great explorations were made, including the discovery of America. New impetus was given to literature, art, book-binding, and the founding of libraries, universities, and medical schools—but not nursing schools. These came more than three centuries later. Merchants made huge fortunes in trade. Bankers likewise became wealthy by making loans, especially to kings and princes.

The Age of Discovery, 1450 to 1550, a part of this period, brought a great increase in geographical knowledge. People became excited about the world around them and about the prospect of finding gold in other lands, particularly America. New passageways to old countries were sought, and the acquisition of new colonies and territories became extremely important to the established kingdoms and empires.

The Renaissance saw the birth and death of Leonardo da Vinci, Michelangelo, and other great artists. And to medicine it gave Paracelsus, Vesalius, and Paré.

- *Theophrastus Paracelsus* (1493 to 1541), a Swiss physician and exceptional chemist, made contributions chiefly in the area of pharmaceutical chemistry.
- *Andreas Vesalius* (1514 to 1564), a Belgian, made detailed anatomic studies in universities and hospitals, disproving by his practical methods some of the classical theories of Galen and others. One of his many published works was a voluminous illustrated book, *De Corporis Humani Fabrica Libri Septem* (*Seven Books on the Structure of the Human Body*), in which he displayed his great fund of knowledge and also criticized and corrected Galen. For this, advocates of Galen berated him. He gradually lost his tremendous energy and initiative and settled down to a routine physician's life.
- *Ambroise Paré* (1510 to 1590), a Frenchman, served as an apprentice to a barber-surgeon and later became the first surgeon of the Renaissance. A student of Vesalius, he became a great military surgeon who reintroduced the use of the ligature instead of the cautery to occlude blood vessels during surgery, adopted a simple technique of wound dressing to replace the oil-boiling method in wide use, improved obstetrical techniques, designed artificial limbs, and wrote books on surgery.

Barber-surgeons were men in France who not only did barbering but also performed such procedures as bleeding, cupping, leeching, giving enemas, and extracting teeth—procedures that the physicians of medieval times prescribed for their patients but considered undignified to perform. The barber-surgeon was required to wear a short robe, whereas the regular surgeons, of whom there were very few, were entitled to wear a long one.

There was understandable friction among the three groups—physicians, barber-surgeons, and surgeons—and the problems were not completely resolved until the practice of surgery improved greatly and the Royal College of Surgeons was established in 1800. The striped barber pole, symbol of the present-day barber, dates from the time when the patient being bled clung to a staff; the red stripe on the barber's pole represents the bloody bandage that covered his wound.

Nursing apparently continued in a way similar to that established in the earlier Middle Ages. The charter of St. Bartholomew's Hospital called for a matron and 12 other women to make beds, wash, and attend the poor patients. They were to receive about 2 pounds a year and room and board, with the matron receiving more. All slept in one room at the hospital. They cared for about 100 patients. However, whether this arrangement was typical is not known.

■ FROM REFORMATION TO NIGHTINGALE

The Reformation was a religious movement beginning early in the sixteenth century that resulted in the formation of various Protestant churches under leaders who revolted against the supremacy of the pope. Monasteries were closed and religious orders were dispersed, even in Catholic countries. Because many of these orders were involved in the care of the sick, nursing and hospital care suffered a severe setback. A startling effect was the almost total disappearance of male nurses. Almost all Catholic nursing orders after 1500 were made up of women. In Protestant countries too, women and nursing became almost synonymous, for Protestant leaders recognized the vacuum in care of the sick and urged the hiring of nurse deaconesses and elderly women to nurse the sick. Also out of this era came noted Catholic orders devoted to care of the sick.

The *Sisters of Charity* were founded by St. Vincent de Paul (1576 to 1660) of France, a Catholic priest. Mlle. Louise La Gras, a woman of noble birth greatly interested in nursing and social work, ably assisted him.

Once a prisoner himself, having been captured by pirates, St. Vincent de Paul became vitally interested in lessening the suffering of all slaves and prisoners. This interest expanded to include the sick and poor in his small county parish, and to help him in his work, he organized a society of women. This small group was so successful that similar groups were formed in other localities in France. The most famous of all, the Sisters of Charity, was organized in Paris under the direction of Mlle. La Gras. A younger group, the *Daughters of Charity*, was formed later. A noncloistered order, the Sisters were free to go wherever they were needed.

The Sisters of Charity were always carefully selected, and from the beginning their ideals and standards were very high. Members of this order took over the nursing service in many European hospitals, and came to Canada and the United States to give similar service during the early history of these countries.

In Spain, a man who gave care to the sick, with special attention to the mentally ill, founded the *Brothers Hospitallers of St. John of God*. The order spread throughout the world, and its members opened and staffed hospitals wherever they went, including the Americas. The care given in their hospitals in Goa, as described by a sixteenth-century traveler, seemed to be a model of its time, perhaps even ahead of its time.

In Italy, *Camillus*, also to be canonized, trained and supplied nurses (men) for hospital care and founded an order dedicated to the care of the sick and dying.

In the New World, *Cortez* founded the first hospital (in Mexico City); within 20 years, most major Spanish towns had one. It was 100 years later that a Hotel Dieu was founded in Sillery (Canada) and another in Montreal. In the latter, care was given by a young lay woman and three nursing sisters who came from France, but perhaps the first "nurse" in Canada was *Marie Herbert Hobau* in Nova Scotia, the widow of the surgeon and apothecary who accompanied Champlain.[2]

Records in Jamestown, Virginia, also tell of the selection of certain men and women to care for the sick. There were numerous health problems in the early American colonies, in part the result of the difficult living conditions. Hospitals of some type existed; one was described as accommodating 50 patients—if they slept two in a bed (not uncommon in Europe either).

The seventeenth and eighteenth centuries were periods of continuing change in Europe, and scientific advances had an enduring influence on medicine and health. Of the creative scientists of those times, the following are key figures:

- *William Harvey* (1578 to 1657), an English physician generally regarded as the father of modern medicine, was the first to describe completely (except for the capillary system) and accurately the circulatory system, replacing the earlier explanations that, although remarkable at the time, actually were at least partially incorrect.
- *Thomas Sydenham* (1624 to 1689), an Englishman educated at Oxford and Montpellier, revived the Hippocratic methods of observation and reasoning and in other ways "restored" clinical medicine to a sound basis.
- *Antonj van Leeuwenhoek* (1632 to 1723), of Holland, improved on Galileo's microscope and produced one that permitted the examination of body cells and bacteria.
- *William Hunter* (1718 to 1783) and his brother *John* (1728 to 1793), of Scotland, obstetrician and surgeon, respectively, conducted meticulous anatomical research and thus founded the science of pathology.
- *William Tuke* (1732 to 1822), an English merchant and philanthropist, instituted long overdue reforms in the care of the mentally ill. Chief founder of the York Retreat (1796), he had important influence on the subsequent treatment of the mentally ill.
- *Edward Jenner* (1749 to 1823), an English physician and friend and pupil of John Hunter, in 1796 originated vaccination against smallpox.
- *René Laennec* (1781 to 1826), of France, invented the stethoscope in 1819. Before this, the physician had listened to the patient's heartbeat by placing his ear against the patient's chest wall.

Even with these advances, medical education was still sketchy. Some practicing physicians had no medical education. An MD degree required apprenticeship with a physician, surgeon, or apothecary; some university classes; some dissecting at an anatomic school or hospital—or any variation of these. There were a few noted schools in Italy, Germany, and Scotland; the English colonies had one until 1765. A practical apothecary school started earlier, but most often pharmacists were also physicians.

By the end of the eighteenth century, nurses of some kind functioned in hospitals. Conditions were not attractive, and much has been written about drunken, thieving women who tended patients. However, some hospitals made real efforts to set standards. One set of criteria included such attributes as good health, good sight and hearing (to make pertinent observations), nimbleness, quietness, good temper, diligence, temperance, and "to have no children, or other to come much after her."[3] Already a hierarchy of nursing personnel had begun, with helpers and watchers assigned to help the sisters, as the early English nurses were called.

In other parts of Europe, nursing was becoming recognized as an important service. *Diderot*, whose *Encyclopedia* attempted to sum up all human knowledge, said that nursing "is as important for humanity as its functions are low and repugnant." Urging care in selection, because "all persons are not adapted to it," he described the nurse as "patient, mild, and compassionate. She should console the sick, foresee their needs, and relieve their tedium."[4] Another progressive step was the first nursing textbook, which was published in Vienna early in the eighteenth century.

Midwifery, too, was gaining new attention. In England in 1739, a small lying-in infirmary was started for the education of medical students and midwives, and soon other lying-in hospitals began to appear. In London, poor women also benefited from home deliveries when a famous physician began to teach medical students midwifery and also taught women to become nurse-midwives at the bedside. (His students had to contribute funds to the care and support of these women.) Nevertheless, it should be remembered that even with the tremendous increase in hospital building at that time, most care was still given in the home by wives and mothers.

The advent of the Industrial Revolution in England saw the development of power-driven machinery to do the spinning, weaving, and metal work that had previously been done manually in the home. Improvement in the steam engine as a source of power improved mining procedures and resulted in the development of factories, which the English called *mills*. The cotton, wool, and iron industries grew rapidly, and there was a corresponding improvement in agriculture.

The industrialization of Europe did not begin until the mid-nineteenth century, when England had already assumed international leadership; its empire was growing; and British trade was the center of world marketing.

People of means lived a most luxurious life. Graciousness and elegance prevailed, and a woman's mission in life was to carry on these traditions. For this she was educated and carefully prepared by her parents.

Common women worked largely as servants in private homes or not at all. With the coming of factories,

men, women, and children worked under cruel conditions. Caring for the sick in hospitals and homes were the "uncommon" women—prisoners and prostitutes—who were unkempt, unsavory, and disinterested. Health conditions were still dreadful, with epidemics such as cholera sweeping whole countries. Children orphaned in these epidemics were finally put in almshouses, which provided no improvement in their lot. The situation was no different in America, but was probably the worst in England, and a number of social reformers began to work for change.

Culturally, great progress was made, particularly on the Continent. The demand for intellectual liberty brought marked advancement in educational facilities for men, but not for women. This was also true in the United States where, for example, Harvard University, established in Cambridge, Massachusetts, in 1636, admitted only men, a policy it steadfastly maintained into the twentieth century. Columbia University in New York City, founded in 1754, followed a similar policy, but removed its ban on women with the founding of Barnard College in 1889. Teachers College was founded as a coeducational institution in 1888.

Out of this confused century came scientists and physicians who made dramatic breakthroughs in medical science.

Oliver Wendell Holmes (1809 to 1894), a Boston physician, furthered safe obstetric practice, pointing out the dangers of infection. He is the author of the famous treatise "The Contagiousness of Puerperal Fever," published in 1843.

Crawford W. Long (1815 to 1878), an American physician, excised a tumor of the neck under ether anesthesia in 1832, but did not make his discovery public until after Dr. William T. Morton announced his in 1846. This led to one of medicine's most enduring controversies: Who should receive credit for discovering the anesthetic properties of ether?

Ignaz P. Semmelweis (1818 to 1865) of Vienna is famous for his advances in the safe practice of obstetrics.

Louis Pasteur (1822 to 1895), of France, chemist and bacteriologist, became famous for his germ theory of disease, the development of the process known as pasteurization, and the discovery of a treatment for rabies. His work overlapped that of Robert Koch.

Lord Joseph Lister (1827 to 1912), English surgeon, in 1865 developed and proved his theory of the bacterial infection of wounds, on which modern aseptic surgery is based.

Robert Koch (1843 to 1910) of Germany founded modern bacteriology. He originated the drying and staining method of examining bacteria. His most important discovery was the identification of the tubercle bacillus, which eventually led to tremendous reductions in loss of life from tuberculosis.

Wilhelm Röntgen (1845 to 1923), a German physicist, discovered x-rays in 1895 and laid the foundation for the science of roentgenology and radiology.

Sir William Osler (1849 to 1919), a renowned Canadian teacher and medical historian, was associated with McGill University, the University of Pennsylvania, Johns Hopkins University, and Oxford University, England. He was knighted in 1911.

Pierre Curie (1859 to 1906), a French chemist, and his Polish wife, *Marie* (1867 to 1934), discovered radium in 1898.

■ NURSING IN THE NINETEENTH CENTURY

The dreary picture of secular nursing is not totally unexpected, given the times. Because proper young women did not work outside the home, nursing had no acceptance, much less prestige. Even those nurses not in the Dickens' Sairy Gamp mold or those desiring to nurse found themselves in competition with workhouse inmates, who were cheaper workers for hospital administrations.

It was acceptable to nurse as a member of a religious order, when the motivation was, of course, religious and the cost to the hospital was little or none. During the nineteenth century, several nursing orders were revived or originated that had substantial influence on modern nursing. In most instances, these orders cared for patients in hospitals that were already established, in contrast to the orders of earlier times, which had founded the hospitals in which they worked. The most influential are the following:

Theodor Fliedner (1800 to 1864), the pastor of a small parish in Kaiserswerth, Germany, revived the *Church Order of Deaconesses*, an ancient order, to care for the patients in a hospital he opened in 1836. At first he had only one deaconess, whom he trained in nursing. Although the training was quite superficial, the work expanded, more deaconesses joined the staff, and the deaconess institute at Kaiserswerth became famous. (Florence Nightingale obtained her only "formal" training in nursing there.) Four of the deaconesses and Pastor Fliedner journeyed to Pittsburgh, Pennsylvania, in 1849, to help establish a hospital under the leadership of Pastor William Passavant. Similar assistance was given to the founders of institutions on the Kaiserswerth plan in London, Constantinople, Beirut, Alexandria, Athens, and other localities.

Pastor Fliedner's work began with discharged prisoners (rather than the sick poor), in whom he became greatly interested through the reforms affected in England under Elizabeth Fry. Aided by both his first and second wives, he also established an orphanage and a normal school.

The *Protestant Sisters of Charity* was founded by Elizabeth Fry (1780 to 1845) of England, whose work among prisoners and the physically and mentally ill was based on reforms that had been instituted by John Howard (1726 to 1790) a quarter of a century before. Mrs. Fry became interested in the deaconesses at Kaiserswerth and visited the hospital to observe how they functioned. She then organized a small group of "nurses" in London to do similar work among the sick poor. She first called the group the Protestant Sisters of Charity, later changing it to the Institute of Nursing Sisters. (Unofficially they often were called the Fry Sisters or Fry Nurses.) The sisters were not affiliated with any church. Their training for nursing was extremely elementary. This group was in no way connected with the Sisters of Charity established earlier by Saint Vincent de Paul.

The *Sisters of Mercy* was a Roman Catholic society formed by Catherine McAuley (1787 to 1841) in Dublin, which later became an order and adopted a rule. The sisters visited Dublin hospitals and nursed victims of a cholera epidemic in 1832; their work grew rapidly and spread throughout the world, including the establishment of several Mercy hospitals in the United States.

The *Irish Sisters of Charity,* also a Roman Catholic group, was started by Mary Aikenhead (1787 to 1858). The sisters visited the sick in their homes and did volunteer nursing in the community during emergencies. They had limited nurses' training and, in 1892, founded a training school for laypersons in St. Vincent's Hospital in Dublin, in which they previously had assumed all nursing duties. They opened additional St. Vincent's hospitals in other areas of the world, including the United States, where they had gone in 1855 to nurse victims of a cholera epidemic in San Francisco.

Also during this period, several nursing sisterhoods were established under the auspices of the Church of England. One of these, the *Sisters of Mercy in the Church of England*, was organized in about 1850. The sisters had little if any formal preparation, but through practical experience acquired in district "nursing" and work in a cholera epidemic, they became quite proficient.

In 1854, a doctor founded another Anglican sisterhood, *St. Margaret's of East Grinstead*. The sisters worked entirely among the sick in the community; they were not associated with the hospitals in any way.

The Anglican order that did the most to improve hospital nursing during this period was *St. John's House*, founded in 1848 by the Church of England. Named for the parish in which it was located—St. John the Evangelist in St. Pancras, London—its purpose was to instruct and train members of the Church of England to act as nurses and visitors to the sick and poor. The original plan also stipulated that the order should be connected with "some hospital or hospitals, in which the women under training, or those who had already been educated, might find the opportunity of exercising their calling or of acquiring experience."[5] The first training program was successful, as were the 25 subsequent ones developed by St. John's House to meet changing needs, and the graduates were always in great demand.

Progress in medicine and science during these centuries was accompanied by accelerated interest in better nursing service and nurses' training. Neither was achieved to a significant degree, despite the fine work of dedicated men and women who belonged to the several nursing orders of the time. Limited in numbers and inadequately prepared for their nursing functions, the members of these orders could not begin to meet the need for their services. Such care as patients received in the majority of institutions was grossly inadequate.

In the mid-nineteenth century, therefore, the time was right—perhaps overdue—for the revolution in nursing education that originated under the leadership of Florence Nightingale and that influenced so greatly and so quickly (from a historical point of view) the nursing care of patients and, indeed, the health of the world.

KEY POINTS

1. A certain amount of the ritual, mysticism, and belief in spirits or gods pervaded the care of the sick in early civilizations.

2. Records of early civilizations emphasize treatment given by those designated as physicians or healers; there appears to have been men and women fulfilling nursing roles of some sort.

3. In early Egypt, India, China, Greece, and Rome, as well as in the lands of the Hebrews, setting rules of hygiene and sanitation, using herbs, and performing surgery were part of the care of the sick.

4. The Romans are generally credited with building the first hospitals, but in the Christian period, "houses for the sick" were available for the sick poor, often tended by men or women in religious and secular orders.

5. The art of medicine and nursing grew very slowly and was subject to the social climate of the times.

6. Noble women played a significant role in the care of the sick, but did so as a volunteer effort.

7. Military and religious orders of nurses grew strong during the Middle Ages and particularly during the Crusades.

8. The Dark Ages on the European Continent halted the progress of medicine; however, development continued in the Eastern Roman and Moslem Empires.

9. A startling effect of the Reformation was the almost total disappearance of male nurses.

10. By the nineteenth century, secular nursing was performed by "uncommon women"—prisoners and prostitutes—unkempt, unsavory, and disinterested. Except for members of a religious order, nursing had no acceptance, much less prestige.

11. Progress in medicine and science during the mid-nineteenth century was accompanied by interest in better nursing service. The time was right for the revolution in nursing originating under Florence Nightingale.

REFERENCES

1. Abrahamsen V. The goddess and healing. *J Holistic Nurs* 15:9–24, March 1997.

2. Dolan JA. *Nursing in Society*, 14th ed. Philadelphia: Saunders, 1978, p 98.

3. Bullough B, Bullough V. *The Care of the Sick: The Emergence of Modern Nursing.* New York: Prodist, 1978, p 57.

4. Ibid, p 6.

5. Moore J. *A Zeal for Responsibility: The Struggle for Professional Nursing in Victorian England*, 1868–1883. Athens, GA: University of Georgia Press, 1983, p 3.

Updates can be found at **www.kellysnursing.com**

The Influence of Florence Nightingale

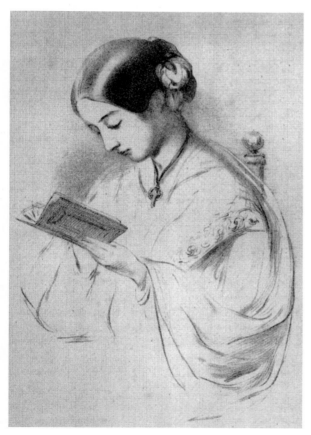

The young Florence Nightingale.
(Courtesy of Lucie Young Kelly, private collection)

It has been said that Florence Nightingale, an extraordinary woman in any century, is the most written-about woman in history. Through her own numerous publications, her letters, the writings of her contemporaries (including newspaper reports), and the numerous biographies and studies of her life, there emerges the picture of a sometimes contradictory, frequently controversial, but undeniably powerful woman who probably had a greater influence on the care of the sick than any other single individual.

Called the *founder of modern nursing*, Nightingale was a strong-willed woman of quick intelligence who used her considerable knowledge of statistics, sanitation, logistics, administration, nutrition, and public health not only to develop a new system of nursing education and health care, but also to improve the social welfare systems of the time. The gentle, caring lady of the lamp, full of compassion for the soldiers of the Crimea, is an accurate image, but no more so than that of the hardheaded administrator and planner who forced changes in the intolerable social conditions of the time, including the care of the sick poor. Nightingale knew very well that a tender touch alone would not bring health to the sick or prevent illness, so she set her intelligence, administrative skills, political acumen, and incredible drive to achieve her self-defined missions. In the Victorian age when women were almost totally dominated by men—fathers, husbands, brothers—and it was undesirable for them to show intelligence or profess interest in anything but household arts, this indomitable woman accomplished the following:

1. Improved and reformed laws affecting health, morals, and the poor

2. Reformed hospitals and improved workhouses and infirmaries

3. Improved medicine by instituting an army medical school and reorganizing the army medical department

4. Improved the health of natives and British citizens in India and other colonies

5. Established nursing as a profession with two missions— sick nursing and health nursing[1]

The new nurse and the new image of the nurse that she created, in part through the nursing schools she founded, in part through her writings, and in part through her international influence, became the model that persisted for almost 100 years. Today, some of her tenets about the "good" nurse seem terribly restrictive, but it should be remembered that in those times not only the image but also the reality of much of secular nursing was based on the untutored, uncouth workhouse inmates for whom drunkenness and thievery were a way of life. It was no small wonder that each Nightingale student had to exemplify a new image.

> The Nightingale nurse had to establish her character in a profession proverbial for immorality. Neat, ladylike, vestal, above suspicion, she had to be the incarnate denial that a hospital nurse had to be drunken, ignorant, and promiscuous.[2]

These historical idiosyncrasies should not, and do not, detract from the many Nightingale precepts that not only are pertinent today, but also are remarkably farsighted.

■ EARLY LIFE

Florence Nightingale was born on May 12, 1820, in Florence, Italy, during her English parents' travels there. She was named for the city in which she was born, as was her older sister, Parthenope, who was born in 1819 in Naples (known in ancient times by the Greek name *Parthenope*).

The family was wealthy and well educated with a high social standing and influential friends, all of which would be useful to Nightingale later. Primarily under her father's tutelage, she learned Greek, Latin, French, German, and Italian, and studied history, philosophy, science, music, art, and classical literature. She traveled widely with her family and friends. The breadth of her education, almost unheard of for women of the times, was also considerably more extensive than that of most men, including physicians. Scholars, as indicated in her correspondence with them, recognized her intelligence and education.

Nightingale was not only bright, but, according to early portraits and descriptions, slender, attractive, and fun loving, enjoying the social life of her class. She differed from other young women in her determination to do something "toward lifting the load of suffering from the helpless and miserable."[3] Later, she said that she had been called by God into His service on four separate occasions, beginning when she was 16.[4] This strong religious commitment remained with her, although she had increasingly little patience with organized religion or with traditional biblical exhortations. At one point she stated, "God's scheme for us was not that he should give us what we asked for, but that mankind should obtain it for mankind."[5] Apparently, the encouragement of Dr. Samuel Gridley Howe and his wife, Julia Ward Howe (who wrote "The Battle Hymn of the Republic"), during a visit to the Nightingale family home in 1844 helped to crystallize Florence's interest in hospitals and nursing. Nevertheless, her intent to train in a hospital was strongly opposed by her family, and she limited herself to nursing family members. There is some indication that this was the genesis of her firm belief that nursing required more than kindness and cold compresses.

Later, in *Notes on Nursing*, she wrote, "It has been said and written scores of times that every woman makes a good nurse. I believe, on the contrary, that the very elements of nursing are all but unknown."[6] At the same time, she added a few tart remarks about the need for education.

> It seems a commonly received idea among men and even some women themselves that it requires nothing but a disappointment in love, the want of an object, a general disgust, or incapacity for other things to turn a woman into a good nurse. This reminds one of the parish where a stupid old man was set to be schoolmaster because he was "past keeping the pigs." . . . The everyday management of a large ward, let alone of a hospital—the knowing what are the laws of life and death for men, and what the laws of health for wards (and wards are healthy or unhealthy, mainly according to the knowledge or ignorance of the nurse)—are not these matters of sufficient importance and difficulty to require learning by experience and careful inquiry, just as much as any other art? They do not come by inspiration to the lady disappointed in love, nor to the poor workhouse drudge hard up for a livelihood.[7]

Although remaining the obedient daughter, Nightingale found her own way to expand her knowledge of sick care. She studied hospital and sanitary reports and books on public health. Having received information on Kaiserswerth in Germany, she determined to receive training there—which was more acceptable because of its religious auspices. On one of her trips to the Continent, she made a brief visit and was impressed enough to spend 3 months in training and observation there in 1851 while her mother and sister went to Carlsbad to "take the cure." (The Nightingales were considered appropriately delicate Victorian ladies, although all lived past 80.) At the time she wrote positively about Pastor Fliedner's program, but she later described the nursing as "nil" and the hygiene as "horrible."[8] Her later effort to study with the Sisters of Charity in Paris was frustrated, although she got permission to inspect the hospitals there, as she had in other cities during her tours. She examined the general layout of the hospital, as well as ward construction, sanitation, general administration, and the work of the surgeons and physicians.

Apparently, these observational techniques and her analytical abilities then and later were the basis of her unrivaled knowledge of hospitals in the next decade. Few of her contemporaries ever had such knowledge.

In 1853, Nightingale assumed the position of superintendent of a charity hospital (probably more of a nursing home) for ill governesses run by titled ladies. Although she had difficulties with her intolerant governing board, she did make changes considered revolutionary for the day and, even with the lack of trained nurses, improved the patients' care. And she continued to visit hospitals. Just as Nightingale was negotiating for a superintendency in the newly reorganized and rebuilt King's College Hospital in London, England and France, in support of Turkey, declared war on Russia in March 1854.

■ CRIMEA—THE TURNING POINT

The Crimean War was a low point for England. Ill prepared and disorganized in general, the army and the bureaucracy were even less prepared to care for the thousands of soldiers both wounded in battle and prostrated by the cholera epidemics brought on by the primitive conditions. Not even the most basic equipment or drugs were available, and, as casualties mounted, Turkey turned over the enormous but bare and filthy barracks at Scutari across from Constantinople to be used as a hospital. The conditions remained abominable. The soldiers lay on the floor in filth, untended, frequently without food or water, because there was no equipment to prepare or distribute either. Rats and other vermin came from the sewers underneath the building. There were no beds, furniture, basins, soap, towels, or eating utensils, and few provisions. There were only orderlies, and none of these at night. The death rate was said to be 60 percent.

In previous wars, the situation had not been much different, and there was little interest on the battle sites; ordinary soldiers were accorded no decencies. But, for the first time, civilian war correspondents were present and sent back the news and photographs of these horrors to an England with a newly aroused social conscience. The reformers were in an uproar; newspapers demanded to know why England did not have nurses like the French Sisters of Charity to care for its soldiers, and Parliament trembled. In October 1854, Sidney Herbert, Secretary of War and an old friend of Florence Nightingale, wrote begging her to lead a group of nurses to the Crimea under government authority and expense. "There is but one person in England that I know of who would be capable of organizing such a scheme . . . your own personal qualities, your knowledge, and your power of administration, and, among greater things, your rank and position in society give you advantages in such work which no other person possesses."[9]

Nightingale had already decided to offer her services, and the two letters crossed. (She had also persuaded Mrs. Herbert that she should be selected.) In less than a week, she had assembled 38 nurses, the most she could find that met her standards—Roman Catholic and Anglican sisters and lay nurses from various hospitals—and departed for Scutari.

Even under the miserable circumstances found there, the army doctors and surgeons did not welcome Nightingale and her contingent. Dr. John Hall, chief of the medical staff, and his staff, although privately acknowledging the horrors of the situation, resented outside interference and refused the nurses' services. Hall and Nightingale soon developed a mutual hatred for each other. When Dr. Hall was honored with the KCB—Knight Commander of the Order of the Bath—she referred to him as "Knight of the Crimean Burial Grounds."[10]

Nightingale chose to wait to be asked to help. To the anger of her nurses, she allowed none of them to give care until 1 week later, when scurvy, starvation, dysentery, exposure, and more fighting almost brought about the collapse of the British army. Then the doctors, desperate for any kind of assistance, turned to the eager nurses.

Modern criticisms of Florence Nightingale frequently refer to her insistence on the physician's overall authority and her own authoritarian approach to nursing. The first criticism may have originated with her situation in the Crimean War. In mid-century England her appointment created a furor; she was the first woman ever to be given such authority. Yet, despite the high-sounding title that

Herbert insisted she have—General Superintendent of the Female Nursing Establishment of the Military Hospitals of the Army—her orders required that she have the approval of the Principal Medical Officer "in her exercise of the responsibilities thus vested in her. The Principal Medical Officer will communicate with Miss Nightingale upon all subjects connected with the Female Nursing Establishment, and will give his directions through that lady."[11] Although no "lady, sister, or nurse" could be transferred from one hospital to another without her approval, she had no authority over anyone else, even orderlies and cooks. What she accomplished had to be done through sheer force of will or persuasion. Her overt deference to physicians was probably the beginning of the doctor-nurse game.

Whatever the limitations of her power, Florence Nightingale literally accomplished miracles at Scutari. Even in the "waiting" week, she moved into the kitchen area and began to cook extras from her own supplies to create a diet kitchen, which for 5 months was the only source of food for the sick. Later, a famous chef came to the Crimea at his own expense and totally reorganized and improved military cooking. Nightingale managed to equip the kitchen and the wards by various means. One report is that when a physician refused to unlock a supply storehouse, she replied, "Well, I would like to have the door opened, or I shall send men to break it down."[12] It was opened, and he was recalled to London.

Miss Nightingale had powerful friends and control over a large amount of contributed funds—a situation that gained her some cooperation from most physicians after a while. Through persuasion and the use of good managerial techniques, she cleaned up the hospital; the orderlies scrubbed and emptied slops regularly; soldiers' wives and camp followers washed clothes; and the vermin were brought under some control. (Wrote Nightingale to Sidney Herbert, "the vermin might, if they had but unity of purpose, carry off the four miles of beds on their backs and march them into the War Office.")[13] Before the end of the war, the mortality rate at Scutari declined to 1 percent. When hospital care improved, Nightingale began a program of social welfare among the soldiers—among other things, seeing to it that they got sick pay. The patients adored her. She cared about them, and the doctors and officers reproached her for "spoiling the brutes." The soldiers wrote home, "What a comfort it was to see her pass even; she would speak to one and nod and smile to as many more, but she could not do it all, you know. We lay there by hundreds,

but we could kiss her shadow as it fell, and lay our heads on the pillow again content." And, "Before she came, there was cussin' and swearin', but after that it was holy as a church." And, "She was all full of life and fun when she talked to us, especially if a man was a bit down-hearted."[14] News correspondents wrote reports about the "ministering angel" and "lady with the lamp" making late rounds after the medical officers had retired—which inspired Longfellow later to write his famous poem "Santa Filomena." England and America were enthralled, and Queen Victoria and the Sultan of Turkey awarded her decorations.

But all did not go well. The military doctors continued in their resentment and tried to undermine her. There were problems in her ranks, dissension among the religious and secular nurses, and problems of incompetence and immorality. Later, she wrote:

> Rebellion among some ladies and some nuns, and drunkenness among some nurses unhappily disgraced our body; minor faults justified *pro tanto* the common opinion that the vanity, the gossip, and the insubordination (which none more despise than those who trade upon them) of women make them unfit for, and mischievous in the Service, however materially useful they may be in it.[15]

Her problems increased with the unsolicited arrival of another group of nurses under another woman's leadership, although the problem was eventually resolved. No doubt Nightingale was high-handed at times, and despite praise of her leadership, she was also called "quick, violent-tempered, positive, obstinate, and stubborn."[16]

Her personality continues to intrigue scholars, who have come to some interesting conclusions.[17] Certainly she drove herself in all she did. When the situation at Scutari was improved, she crossed the Black Sea to the battle sites and worked on the reorganization of the few hospitals there—with no better support from physicians and superior officers. There she contracted Crimean fever (probably brucellosis) and nearly died. However, she refused a leave of absence to recuperate and stayed in Scutari to work until the end of the war. She had supervised 125 nurses and forced the military to recognize the place of nurses. One that she did not supervise, but did respect, was Mary Seacole, a mulatto Jamaican woman, who set up her own "British Hotel" to serve food to soldiers. Seacole also gave care to casualties and was renowned for her skills. She was often on the battlefields.[18]

From her experiences, and to support her recommendations for reform, Nightingale wrote a massive report entitled *Notes on Matters Affecting the Health, Efficiency, and Hospital Administration of the British Army,* crammed with facts, figures, and statistical comparisons. On the basis of this and her later well-researched and well-documented papers, she is often credited with being the first nurse researcher.[19] Reforms were slow in coming but extended even to the United States when the Union consulted her about organizing hospitals. In 1859, she wrote a small book, *Notes on Nursing: What It Is and What It Is Not,* intended for the average housewife and printed cheaply so that it would be affordable. These and other Nightingale papers are still amazingly readable today—brisk, down-to-earth, and laced with many pithy comments. For instance, in *Notes on Hospitals,* written in the same year, she compared the administration of the various types of hospitals and characterized the management of secular hospitals under the sole command of the male hospital authorities as "all but crazy." And her words were prophetic: "If we were perfect, no doubt an absolute hierarchy would be the best kind of government for all institutions. But, in our imperfect state of conscience and enlightenment, publicity, and the collision resulting from publicity are the best guardians of the interests of the sick."[20]

Her knowledge was certainly respected, and many consulted her, including the Royal Sanitary Commission on the Health of the Army in India. When asked by the members of the commission what hospitals she had visited, she listed those in England, Turkey, France, Germany, Belgium, Italy, and Egypt, including all hospitals in some cities, and even Russian military hospitals. Her reforms in India extended beyond the medical and nursing facilities to raising the sanitary level of India.[21] Again, her insights were uncanny. In describing the proper method of analyzing the problem of sanitation and disease, she also suggested checking on "unwholesome trades fouling the water."

What is particularly astonishing is that all of this was done from her quarters. On her return from the Crimea, she took to her bed or at least to her rooms and emerged only on rare occasions. There is much speculation on this illness—whether it was a result of the Crimea fever, neurasthenia, or a bit of both, or whether she simply found it useful to avoid wasting time with people she did not want to see. She was famous now and had been given discretion over the so-called Nightingale Fund, to which almost everyone in England had subscribed, including many of the troops. However, newer studies seem to indicate that the brucellosis she contracted in the Crimea

became a serious chronic disease because it had been untreated and probably undiagnosed. She had debilitating, almost deadly symptoms over 32 years, yet amazingly she accomplished wonders.[22]

■ THE NIGHTINGALE NURSE

In 1860, Nightingale utilized some of the 45,000 pounds of the Nightingale Fund to establish a training school for nurses. She selected St. Thomas's Hospital because of her respect for its matron, Mrs. S. E. Wardroper. The two converted the resident medical officers to their plan, although apparently most other physicians objected to the school. The students were chosen, and the first class in the desired age range of 25 to 35 years and with impeccable character references numbered only 15. It was to be a 1-year training program, and the students were presented with what could be called terminal behavioral objectives that they had to reach satisfactorily. Students could be dismissed by the matron for misconduct, inefficiency, or negligence. However, if they passed the courses of instruction and training satisfactorily, they were entered in the "Register" as certified nurses. The Committee of the Nightingale Fund then recommended them for employment; in the early years, they were obligated to work as hospital nurses for at least 5 years (for which they were paid).

Students' time was carefully structured, beginning at 6 AM and ending with a 9 o'clock bedtime, which included a semimandatory 2-hour exercise period (walking abroad must be done in twos and threes, not alone). Within that time there was actually about a 9-hour work and training day (a vast difference from future American schools). This included bedside teaching by a teaching sister or the Resident Medical Officer and elementary instruction in "Chemistry, with reference to air, water, food, etc.; physiology, with reference to a knowledge of the leading functions of the body; and general instruction on medical and surgical topics," by professors of the medical school attached to St. Thomas's, given voluntarily and without remuneration.[23] The Nightingale school was not under the control of the hospital and education was its purpose. The Nightingale Fund paid the medical officers, head nurses, and matron for teaching students, beyond whatever they earned from the hospital in their other duties. Both the head nurses and matron kept records on each student, evaluating how she met the stated objectives of the program. The students were expected to keep notes from the lectures and records of patient observation and care, all of which were checked by the nurse teachers. At King's College Hospital, run by the Society of St. John's House, an Anglican religious community, midwifery was taught in similar style and with similar regulations, again under the auspices of the Nightingale Fund Committee. And, at the Royal Liverpool Infirmary, nurses were trained for home nursing of the sick poor under a Nightingale protocol, but were personally funded by a Liverpool merchant-philanthropist. As Nightingale said in 1863, "We have had to introduce an entirely new system to which the older systems of nursing bear but slight resemblance.... It exists neither in Scotland nor in Ireland at the present time."[24]

The demand for the Nightingale nurses was overwhelming. In the next few years, requests also came for them to improve the workhouse (poorhouse) infirmaries and to reform both civilian and military nursing in India. In response to these demands, Nightingale wrote many reports, detailing to the last item the system for educating these nurses and for improving patient care, including such points as general hygiene and sanitation, nutrition, equipment, supplies, and the nurses' housing conditions, holidays, salaries, and retirement benefits. (For India, she suggested that they had better pay good salaries and provide satisfactory working and living conditions, or the nurses might opt for marriage, because the opportunities there were even greater than in England.) She constantly reiterated that she could not possibly supply enough nurses but, when possible, she would send a matron and some other nurses, who would train new Nightingale nurses. She warned that one or two could not change the old patterns. "Good nursing does not grow of itself; it is the result of study, teaching, training, practice, ending in sound tradition which can be transferred elsewhere."[25]

Although Nightingale never headed a school herself, she selected the students and observed their progress carefully; with some she carried on correspondence for years. One of her favorites, Agnes Jones, was recommended to reform nursing at the Liverpool Workhouse Infirmary, which, with 12 other nurses, she did admirably, proving to the economy-minded governor that this kind of nursing also saved money. Nightingale often said that conditions there were as bad as those at Scutari, and indeed her young protégé died of typhus there. Nevertheless, reform of this pesthole showed England an example of what nursing care could be.

Despite her reputation and her personal acquaintance with Queen Victoria, her cabinet, and every prime minister during this time, Nightingale and her ideas ran into opposition. Although some doctors who understood what this new nurse could do were supporters, the idea of the nurse as a professional was not commonly accepted. Said one physician, "A nurse is a confidential servant, but still only a servant. . . . She should be middle-aged when she begins nursing, and if somewhat tamed by marriage and the troubles of a family, so much the better."[26] Maintaining standards was a constant struggle; even St. Thomas's Hospital slipped, and Nightingale, who had been immersed in the Indian reforms, had to take time to reorganize the program. What evolved over the years, from the first program, was one of preparation for two kinds of nursing practitioners: the educated middle- and upperclass ladies who paid their own tuition, and the still carefully selected poor women who were subsidized by the Nightingale Fund (Exhibit 2–1). The first were given an extra year or two of education to prepare them to become teachers or superintendents; a third choice was district nursing. "This nurse must be of a yet higher class and of a yet fuller training than a hospital nurse, because she has not the doctor always at hand and because she has no hospital appliances at hand."[27] The special probationers were expected to enter the profession permanently. The second group was prepared to be the hospital ward nurses.

In Nightingale's later years, she came into conflict with the very nurses who had been trained for leadership. In 1886, some of these nurses, now superintendents of other training schools, wanted to establish an organization that would provide a central examination and registration center, the forerunner of licensure. Nightingale opposed this movement for several reasons: nursing was still too young and disorganized; national criteria would not be as high as those of individual schools; and the all-important aspects of character could not be tested. She fought the concept with every weapon at her disposal, including her powerful contacts, and succeeded in limiting the fledgling Royal British Nurses' Association to maintaining a "list" instead of a "register."[28] (Nurse licensure came to South Africa before it came to England.) Nevertheless, it was a beginning and, although she was probably right about the standards, recognition of nurses was facilitated with the setting of national standards, however minimal.

Nightingale's prolific writings on nursing have survived, and some of them are still surprisingly apt. Often they reflect her concern about the character of nurses and her own determination that their main focus is on nursing (Exhibit 2–2). For instance, in her early writings on hospitals (before the Nightingale schools), she

■ **EXHIBIT 2–1.** Duties of Probationer under the "Nightingale Fund." St. Thomas's Hospital, 1860

You are required to be
- Sober
- Punctual
- Honest
- Quiet and orderly
- Truthful
- Cleanly and neat
- Trustworthy
- Patient, cheerful, and kindly

You are expected to become skillful
1. In the dressing of blisters, burns, sores, wounds and in applying fomentations, poultices, and minor dressings.
2. In the application of leeches, externally and internally.
3. In the administration of enemas for men and women.
4. In the management of trusses and appliances in uterine complaints.
5. In the best method of friction to the body and extremities.
6. In the management of helpless patients, i.e., moving, changing, personal cleanliness of, feeding, keeping warm (or cool), preventing and dressing bed sores, managing position of.
7. In bandaging, making bandages, and rollers, lining of splints, etc.
8. In making the beds of the patients, and removal of sheets whilst patient is in bed.
9. You are required to attend at operations.
10. To be competent to cook gruel, arrowroot, egg flip, puddings, drinks, for the sick.
11. To understand ventilation, or keeping the ward fresh by night as well as by day; you are to be careful that great cleanliness is observed in all the utensils; those used for secretions as well as those required for cooking.
12. To make strict observation of the sick in the following particulars: The state of secretions, expectoration, pulse, skin, appetite, intelligence, as delirium or stupor; breathing, sleep, state of wounds, eruptions, formation of matter, effect of diet, or of stimulants, and of medicines.
13. And to learn the management of convalescents.

Source: Kelly, L. *Dimensions of Professional Nursing.* New York: Macmillan, 1981, p 31.

reluctantly conceded that the nurse would have to be permitted visitors on her time off, distracting though that might be, and that spying on the nurse when she went out in her limited free time, although it had some advantages, was "no blessing in the long run and degrading to all concerned." Yet, nurses were to be held strictly to rules that limited their outside excursions to their exercise period, and it was preferred that they live adjacent to the patient wards. Nightingale's views moderated over the years, but her emphasis on morality and other personal qualities never wavered.

It was a time when salaries were low and petty thievery was common, and an accepted, desirable fringe benefit of a job (also recommended by Nightingale for nurses) was a daily allowance of beer, or even wine and brandy. But a Nightingale nurse who was found to be dishonest and drunken was dismissed instantly and permanently.

One principle from which Nightingale did not swerve was that nurses were to nurse, not to do heavy cleaning ("if you want a charwoman, hire one"); not to do laundry ("it makes their hands coarse and hard and less able to attend to the delicate manipulation which they may be called on to execute"); and not to fetch ("to save the time of nurses, all diets and ward requisites should be brought into the wards"). Then, as in many places now, status and promotion came through assumption of administrative roles, but Nightingale recognized that "many are valuable as nurses, who are yet unfit for promotion to head

---

■ **EXHIBIT 2–2. What a Nurse Is to Be**

A really good nurse must need be of the highest class of character. It need hardly be said that she must be—(1) Chaste, in the sense of the Sermon on the Mount; a good nurse should be the Sermon on the Mount in herself. It should naturally seem impossible to the most unchaste to utter even an immodest jest in her presence. Remember this great and dangerous peculiarity of nursing, and especially of hospital nursing, namely, that it is the only case, queens not excepted, where a woman is really in charge of men. And a really good trained ward "sister" can keep order in a men's ward better than a military ward-master or sergeant. (2) Sober, in spirit as well as in drink and temperate in all things. (3) Honest, not accepting the most trifling fee or bribe from patients or friends. (4) Truthful—and to be able to tell the truth includes attention and observation, to observe truly—memory, to remember truly—power of expression, to tell truly what one has observed truly—as well as intention to speak the truth, the whole truth, and nothing but the truth. (5) Trustworthy, to carry out directions intelligently and perfectly, unseen as well as seen, "to the Lord" as well as unto men—no mere eye-service. (6) Punctual to a second and orderly to a hair—having everything ready and in order before she begins her dressings or her work about the patient; nothing forgotten. (7) Quiet, yet quick, quick without hurry; gentle without slowness; discreet without self-importance; no gossip. (8) Cheerful, hopeful; not allowing herself to be discouraged by unfavorable symptoms; not given to depress the patient by anticipations of an unfavorable result. (9) Cleanly to the point of exquisiteness, both for the patient's sake and her own; neat and ready. (10) Thinking of her patient and not of herself, "tender over his occasions" or wants, cheerful and kindly, patient, ingenious and feat.

Source: From a Nightingale article on "Nurses, Training of, and Nursing the Sick," in *A Dictionary of Medicine*, edited by Sir Robert Quain, Bart, M.D., 1882.

---

nurses." Her alternative, however, would not be greeted favorably today—a raise after 10 years of good service!

Nightingale also commented on other issues considered pertinent today. Continuing education was a must, for she saw nursing as a progressive art, in which to stand still was to go back. "A woman who thinks of herself, 'Now I am a full nurse, a skilled nurse. I have learnt all there is to be learned,' take my word for it, she does not know what a nurse is, and she will never know: she has gone back already."[29] Although there is no evidence that she took any action to help end discrimination against women, she did support women's suffrage; she just didn't give it priority.[30] Nightingale believed that women should be accepted into all the professions, but she warned them, "qualify yourselves for it as a man does for his work." She believed that women should be paid as highly as men, but that equal pay meant equal responsibility. In a profession with as much responsibility as nursing, it was particularly important to have adequate compensation, or intelligent, independent women would not be attracted to it. Until the end, she was firm on the need for nurses to obey physicians in medical matters; however, she stressed the importance of nurse observation and reporting because the physician was not constantly at the patient's bedside as the nurse was. She was adamant that a nurse (and woman) be in charge of nursing, with no other administrative figure having authority over nurses, including physicians. She knew the importance of a work setting that gave job satisfaction. In words that are a far-off echo of nurses' complaints today, she wrote:

Besides, a thing very little understood, a good nurse has her professional pride in results of her nursing quite as much as a medical officer in the results of his treatment. There are defective buildings, defective administrations, defective appliances, which make all good nursing impossible. A good nurse does not like to waste herself, and the better the nurse, the stronger this feeling in her. Humanity may overrule this feeling in a great emergency like a cholera outbreak; but I don't believe that it is in human nature for a good nurse to bear up, with an ever-recurring, ever-useless expenditure of activity, against the circumstances that make her nursing activity useless, or all but useless. Her work becomes slovenly like the rest, and it is a far greater pity to have a nurse wasting herself in this way that it would be to have a steam engine running up and down the line all day without a train, wasting coals.

Perhaps I need scarcely add that nurses must be paid the market price for their labor, like any other workers; and that this is yearly rising.[31]

Obviously, Nightingale is eminently quotable in matters of health care and nursing today, in part because she was so far ahead of her time, and in part, unfortunately, because the errors of omission and commission in the field have a tendency to reappear or remain uncorrected.

Planner, administrator, educator, researcher, reformer, Florence Nightingale never lost her interest in nursing. As nearly as can be determined, her actual clinical nursing was limited to her early care of sick families, the short period at Kaiserswerth, a briefer interim of caring for victims of a cholera epidemic before the war, and then, of course, her experience in Crimea. Yet, her perception of patients' needs was uncanny for the time and frequently is still applicable today. In her *Notes on Nursing*, not only is there careful consideration of "Observation of the Sick" and crisp comments on "Minding Baby," but also pertinent directions on hygiene, nutrition, environment, and the mental state of the patient. At age 74, in her last major work on nursing, she differentiated between sick nursing and health nursing, and emphasized the primary need for prevention of illness, for which a lay "Health Missioner" (today's health educator?) would be trained.

When Nightingale died on August 13, 1910, she was to be honored by burial in Westminster Abbey. However, she had chosen instead to be buried in the family plot in Hampshire, with a simple inscription: "F.N. Born 1820, Died 1910."

KEY POINTS

1. Florence Nightingale was born to privilege and drawn to a host of philanthropic endeavors that would improve the human condition.
2. She cultivated friends in high places, and used their influence strategically.
3. The Crimean War provided an opportunity for Nightingale to transform the military hospital at Scutari into an efficiently managed institution. Through compassion, sanitary improvements, and good nursing care, the death rate was reduced from 60 percent to a fraction over 1 percent.
4. Civilian correspondents, who for the first time were present to give vivid pictures of the conditions of warfare to the public, reported these unprecedented gains to the home front.
5. A grateful public contributed generously to the Nightingale Fund. These monies were eventually used to establish the Nightingale Training School for Nurses at St. Thomas's Hospital.
6. In 1860, Florence Nightingale founded modern nursing at St. Thomas's Hospital in London with organized training programs that included both theory and practice, careful selection of students, and freedom from hospital control.
7. Nightingale felt strongly that nursing involved a separate body of knowledge and role function from medicine. She believed that physicians saved lives, but nurses helped people to live.
8. Nightingale resisted anything inflexible. For this reason she opposed graduation or registration, defining nursing as a progressive art in which to stand still is to regress.
9. In her careful observations and recording and her use of statistics in matters affecting health care and administration in the British army, in hospitals throughout Europe, and in the community, Nightingale is often credited with being the first nurse researcher.
10. Nightingale made many pertinent observations and recommendations on nurses and nursing practice, such as the need for nurses to be free from other duties so that they could concentrate on nursing, for holistic care, for home care, for continuing education, for adequate compensation, and for a satisfactory working environment.

REFERENCES

1. Barritt ER. Florence Nightingale's values and modern nursing education. *Nurs Forum* 12(4):10, 1973.
2. Ibid, p 34.
3. Bullough V, Bullough B. *The Care of the Sick: The Emergence of Modern Nursing.* New York: Prodist, 1978, p 69.
4. Dossey B. Florence Nightingale: A 19th century mystic. *J Holistic Nurs* 16:111–164, June 1998.
5. Barritt, op cit, p 10.
6. Seymer LR. *Selected Writings of Florence Nightingale.* New York: Macmillan, 1954, p 124.

7. Ibid, pp 214–215.

8. Bullough and Bullough, op cit, p 86.

9. Dolan JA. *Nursing in Society: A Historical Perspective*, 14th ed. Philadelphia: Saunders, 1978, p 159.

10. Kalisch P, Kalisch B. *The Advance of American Nursing*, 3rd ed. Philadelphia: Lippincott, 1995, p 32.

11. Seymer, op cit, p 28.

12. Dolan, op cit, p 161.

13. Kalisch and Kalisch, op cit, p 33.

14. Ibid, p 47.

15. Seymer, op cit, p 28.

16. Barritt, op cit, p 8.

17. Harris M. Remembering Florence Nightingale. *Home Healthcare Nurse* 20:291–293, May 2002.

18. Griffon P. "A somewhat duskier skin": Mary Seacole in the Crimea. *Nurs Hist Rev* 6:115–127, June 1998.

19. Dossey B. *Florence Nightingale: Mystic, Visionary, Healer.* Springhouse, PA: Springhouse, 1999.

20. Seymer, op cit, pp 222–223.

21. Hays J. Florence Nightingale and the India sanitary reforms. *Public Health Nurs* 6:152–154, September 1989.

22. Dossey B. Nightingale's Crimean fever. *J Holistic Nurs* 16:165–201, June 1998.

23. Seymer, op cit, p 244.

24. Ibid, p 234.

25. Ibid, p 229.

26. Dolan, op cit, p 169.

27. Monteiro L. Florence Nightingale on public health nursing. *Am J Public Health* 75:181–186, February 1985.

28. Helmstadter C. Florence Nightingale's opposition to state registration of nurses. *Nurs Hist Rev* 15:155–165, 167–168, 2007.

29. Pavey AE. *The Story of the Growth of Nursing.* London: Farber & Farber, 1938, p 296.

30. Selanders L. Florence Nightingale: The evolution and social impact of feminist values in nursing. *J Holistic Nurs* 16:227–243, June 1998.

31. Seymer, op cit, p 276.

Updates can be found at **www.kellysnursing.com**

Nursing in the United States

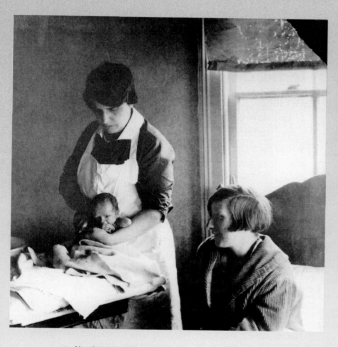

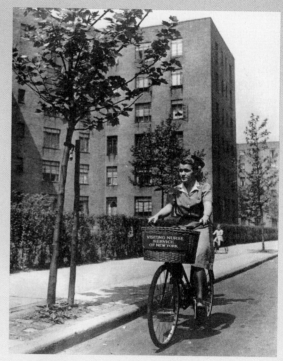

Nursing traces its roots to community practice. (*Left*, courtesy of the Visiting Nurse Association of Central Jersey; *right*, courtesy of the Visiting Nurse Service of New York)

The Evolution of the Trained Nurse, 1873 to 1903

Nursing in the United States between the American Revolution and the Civil War was probably no better or worse than that in Europe. As noted in Chapter 1, nurses from both Catholic and Protestant nursing orders came to America, and their nursing care, although semitrained, was the best offered. But there were not enough of them. Even given the occasional compassionate lady who might have ventured into hospitals to help with care in an epidemic or other emergency, the quality of lay nurses was about the same as that in England.

Early hospitals, privately managed and funded by endowments or public subscription, were modeled after those in Europe, with no improvement in quality; the mentally ill were confined in insane asylums, poorhouses, and prisons. Yet, by the time of the Civil War, social reforms had also reached America. One of the key figures was *Dorothea Lynde Dix* (1802 to 1887), a gentle New England schoolteacher, who became interested in the conditions under which the mentally ill existed when she went to teach a Sunday school lesson in a jail. She began to survey the needs of those forgotten people, and her descriptive reports and careful documentation eventually resulted in the construction of state psychiatric institutions (the first in Trenton, New Jersey). There was some lessening of inhumane care, even if there was no improvement in the understanding of the illnesses. Her crusade continued until her death, at which time some thirty psychiatric hospitals had been established in the United States and internationally.

■ THE CIVIL WAR

When the Civil War began in April 1861, there was no organized system to care for the sick and wounded. There never had been. For instance, camp followers, a few wives, women in the neighborhood, and "surgeons' mates" gave such basic care as existed during the American Revolution. It is possible that some of these women were employed by the army, because there are female names on the payroll lists as "nursing the sick."[1]

American women, considered by American men to be just as delicate and proper and unsuited for unpleasant service as their European counterparts, nevertheless rushed to volunteer. Within a few weeks, 100 women were given a short training course by physicians and surgeons in New York City, and Dorothea Dix, well known by then, was appointed by the Secretary of War to superintend these new "nurses." Meanwhile, members of religious orders also volunteered, and nursing in some of the larger government hospitals was eventually assigned to them because of the inexperience of the lay volunteers.[2,3]

Except for that group, almost none of the several thousand women who served as nurses during the war had any kind of training or hospital experience. They can be categorized as follows:

1. The nurses appointed by Miss Dix or other officials as legal employees of the army for 40 cents and one ration a day
2. The sisters or nuns of the various orders

3. Those employed for short periods of time for menial chores

4. Black women employed under general orders of the War Department for $10 a month

5. Uncompensated volunteers

6. Women camp followers

7. Women employed by the various relief organizations[4]

It is estimated that some 6000 women performed nursing duties for the Northern armies. The South used only about 1000 because of the attitude that prevailed for some time that caring for men was unfit for Southern ladies. (Nevertheless, a number of these ladies, such as *Kate Cummings*, who recorded her experiences, gave distinguished service under severe conditions in Southern hospitals.)[5]

US Army medical officers were no more pleased with the presence of females in their domain than were the British in Crimea. It was not that Miss Dix did not try for the serious minded; her recruiting specified only plain-looking women over 35 who wore gray, brown, or black dresses with no bows, curls, jewelry, or hoop skirts, and who were moral and had common sense. Presumably, those who did not qualify were among the many unofficial and unpaid volunteers. Some of the information on what the Civil War nurses did comes from the writings of Louisa May Alcott and Walt Whitman, both volunteers. In her journal, Alcott described her working day, which began at 6 AM. After opening the windows, because of the bad air in the makeshift base hospital, she was "giving out rations, cutting up food for helpless boys, washing faces, teaching my attendants how beds are made or floors are swept, dressing wounds, dusting tables, sewing bandages, keeping my tray tidy, rushing up and down after pillows, bed linens, sponges, and directions. . . ."[6] Volunteers also read to the patients, wrote letters, and comforted them. Apparently, even the hired nurses did little more except, perhaps, give medicines. But so did the volunteers, sometimes giving the medicine and food of their choice to the patient, instead of what the doctor ordered.

By 1862, enormous military hospitals, some with as many as 3000 beds, were being built, although there were still some makeshift hospitals: former hotels, churches, factories, and almost anything else available. There was even a hospital ship, the *Red Rover*, a former Mississippi steamer captured from the Confederates and staffed by nuns. Other floating hospitals were inaugurated and served as transport units, with nurses attending the wounded.[7] Discipline in the hospitals was rigid for nurses and patients alike, with the latter given strict orders to be respectful to the nurses. According to one Army hospital edict, the nurses, under the supervision of the "Stewards and Chief Wardmaster," were responsible for the administration of the wards, but many of their duties appeared to be related more to keeping the nonmedical records of patients and reporting their misbehavior than to nursing care. If the patient needed medical or surgical attendance, the doctor was to be called.[8]

Georgeanna Woolsey wrote that the surgeons treated the nurses without even common courtesy because they did not want them and tried to make their lives so unbearable that they would leave. The surgeons were often incompetent. As a temporary expedient, contract surgeons were employed with no position, little pay, and only minimal rank. Jane, another Woolsey sister who was also a volunteer nurse, wrote that although some were highly skilled, "faithful, sagacious, [and] tenderhearted," others were drunks, refused to attend the wounded, or injured the wounded more because of their incompetence.[9]

It was surgeons and officers of the latter type that the formidable nurse Mary Ann (Mother) Bickerdyke attacked. She managed to have a number of them dismissed (in part because of her friendship with General Grant and General Sherman). About this tough "Soldier's Friend," one physician stated, "Woe to the surgeon, the commissary, or quartermaster whose neglect of his men and selfish disregard for their interests and needs come under her cognizance."[10]

Another fighter was Clara Barton, who early in the war cared for the wounded of the Sixth Massachusetts Regiment. One story told about her is that while supervising the delivery of a wagonload of supplies for soldiers, she neatly extricated an ox from a herd meant for the Army so the wounded would have food.[11] (There are many other interesting aspects to her Civil War service.)[12]

Only in recent years has attention been given to the black nurses of the Civil War. Harriet Tubman, the "Moses of her people," not only led many black slaves to freedom in her underground-railroad activities before the war, but also nursed the wounded when she joined the Union Army. Similarly, Sojourner Truth, abolitionist speaker and activist in the women's movement, also cared for the sick and wounded. Susie King Taylor, born to slavery and secretly taught to read and write, met and married a Union soldier and served as a battlefront nurse for more than 4 years, although she received no salary or pension from the Union Army.[13]

There were other heroines, untrained women from the North and South, caring for the sick and wounded with a modicum of skills but much kindness, and, as in Crimea, the soldiers were sentimentally appreciative, if not discriminating. Even when paid, Civil War nurses had little status and no rank. One exception was Sally Tomkins, a civic-minded Southern woman, who efficiently took charge of a makeshift hospital and was made a captain of the cavalry by Confederate President Jefferson Davis so that she could continue her work. An investigative report by the US Sanitary Commission noted that nurses had not been well treated or wisely used.

> They have not been placed, as they expected and were fitted to be, in the position of head nurses. On the contrary, with a very inefficient force of male nurses, they have been called on to do every form of service, have been overtaxed and worn down with menial and purely mechanical duties, additional to the more responsible offices and duties of nursing.[14]

Nevertheless, the Civil War opened hospitals to massive numbers of women, well-bred "ladies," who would otherwise probably not even have thought of nursing. Some of these, such as Abby, Jane, and Georgeanna Woolsey, later helped lead the movement to establish training schools for nurses.

■ THE EARLY TRAINING SCHOOLS

The nursing role of women in the Civil War, however unsophisticated, and probably the fame of Florence Nightingale brought to the attention of the American public the need for nurses and the desirability of some organized programs of training. There had been previous elementary efforts in this direction: an organized school of nursing, founded in 1839 by the Nurse Society of Philadelphia under Dr. Joseph Warrington, awarded a certificate after a stated period of lectures, demonstrations, and experience at a hospital; a school of nursing for a "better type" of woman connected with the Women's Hospital in Philadelphia in 1861 gave a diploma after 6 months of lectures.

More physicians became interested in the training of nurses and, at a meeting of the American Medical Association in 1869, a committee to study the matter stated that it was "just as necessary to have well-trained, well-instructed nurses as to have intelligent and skillful physicians." The committee recommended that nursing schools be placed under the guardianship of county medical societies, although under the immediate supervision of lady superintendents; that every lay hospital should have a school; and that nurses be trained not only for the hospital but for private duty in the home.[15]

In 1871, the editor of *Godey's Lady's Book*, the most popular women's magazine of the time, wrote an editorial on "Lady Nurses" that was remarkably farsighted.

> Much has been lately said of the benefits that would follow if the calling of sick nurse were elevated to a profession which an educated lady might adopt without a sense of degradation, either on her own part or in the estimation of others. . . .
> There can be no doubt that the duties of sick nurse, to be properly performed, require an education and training little, if at all, inferior to those possessed by members of the medical profession. . . . The manner in which a reform may be effected is easily pointed out. Every medical college should have a course of study and training especially adapted for ladies who desire to qualify themselves for the profession of nurse; and those who had gone through the course, and passed the requisite examination, should receive a degree and diploma, which would at once establish their position in society. The graduate nurse would in general estimation be as much above the ordinary nurse of the present day as the professional surgeon of our times is above the barber-surgeon of the last century.[16]

Unfortunately, this idea of an educated nurse with professional status was a long time in coming. Nevertheless, in 1872, the New England Hospital for Women and Children, staffed by women physicians who were interested in the development of a school, acted on a statement in its bylaws of 1863 "to train nurses for the care of the sick." It was a 1-year program in which the students provided round-the-clock service for patients; there was no class work (although a few lectures were given during the winter months), and the duty extended from 5:30 AM to 9 PM, with a free afternoon every second week from 2 to 5 PM. At the end of the year, one student graduated—Melinda Ann (Linda) Richards, thereafter called America's first trained nurse. Of all the nurses who graduated from this primitive early program, she moved on to be a key figure in the development of nursing education. Richards, like some of the other students in the schools that evolved, had been a nurse in a hospital, although some schools would not accept them because they wanted to set a new image. This indicates that despite the frequent descriptions of criminal and thieving women who nursed, some nurses, although untrained in the later sense, must have been at least respectable, intelligent women.

Another outstanding graduate of the New England Hospital for Women and Children (1879) was Mary Mahoney, the first trained black nurse. A tiny, dynamic, and charming woman, she worked primarily in private duty in the Boston area, but was apparently always present at national nurses' meetings. In her honor, the Mary Mahoney Medal was initiated by the National Association of Colored Graduate Nurses, and the award was later continued by the American Nurses Association (ANA).

In 1873, three schools supposedly based on the Nightingale model were established.[17] The Bellevue Training School in New York City was founded through the influence of several society ladies who had been involved in Civil War nursing, including Abby Woolsey. Appalled by the conditions—900 patients, with three to five patients occupying strapped-together beds, tended by ex-convict nurses and night watchmen who stole their food and left them in filth—these women sent a young physician to England to confer with Nightingale. Then they raised funds to set up a nurses' training class for which they were given six wards. The hospital agreed to place these students under the direction of a female superintendent, provided that they also did the scouring and cleaning that had been done by the other "nurses"; they would not hire anyone to clean. Although the school attempted to follow Nightingale principles and reported that it was attracting educated women, its overall purpose was to improve conditions in a great charity hospital, and much of the learning was on a trial-and-error basis. Nevertheless, Bellevue had a lot of interesting firsts: interdisciplinary rounds where nurses reported on the nursing plan of care; patient record-keeping and writing of orders, initiated by Linda Richards, who became night superintendent; and the first uniform, by stylish and aristocratic Euphemia Van Rensselaer, which started a trend. And, of course, two of nursing's greatest leaders were Bellevue graduates—Lavinia Dock and Isabel Hampton Robb.

The Connecticut Training School in New Haven was started through the influence of another Woolsey, Georgeanna, and her husband, Dr. Francis Bacon. Through negotiation with the hospital, the superintendent of nurses was designated as separate from, and not responsible to, the steward (administrator) of the hospital, and teaching outside the wards was permitted. The threatened steward managed to make life so miserable for a series of superintendents that each resigned, but control remained with nursing. Meanwhile, all good intentions notwithstanding, the students soon were sent to give care in the homes of sick families, with the money going to the School Fund—and the school could boast that for 33 years it was not financed or directed by the hospital.

The Boston Training School was the last of that first famous triumvirate. Again, a group of women associated with other educational and philanthropic endeavors spearheaded its organization, but this time to offer a desirable occupation for self-supporting women and to provide good private nurses for the community. After prolonged negotiations that allowed the director of the school, instead of the hospital, to maintain control, the Massachusetts General Hospital assigned "The Brick" building to the school because it (The Brick) "stands by itself; represents both medical and surgical departments; and offers the hard labor desirable for the training of nurses."[18] Apparently, there was rather poor leadership and nurses continued to do dishwashing and other menial tasks, with little attention to training. When Linda Richards became the third director, she reorganized the work, started classes, and set out to prove that trained nurses were better than untrained ones. As an example, she cared for some of the sickest patients herself. By the end of 1876, she had charge of all the nursing in the hospital.

Other major training schools that were to endure into the next century were founded in the next few years, somewhat patterned after Nightingale's precepts. Their success and the popularity of their graduates resulted in a massive proliferation of training schools. In 1880, there were 15; by 1900, there were 432; and by 1909, there were 1105 hospital-based diploma schools. Hospitals with as few as 20 beds opened schools, and the students provided almost totally free labor. Usually the only graduate nurses were the superintendent and perhaps the operating room supervisor and night supervisor. Students earned money for the hospital; after a short period they were frequently sent to do private nursing in the home, with the money reverting to the hospital, not the school. Except for the few outstanding schools, all Nightingale principles were forgotten: the students were under the control of the hospital and worked from 12 to 15 hours a day—24 if they were on a private case in a home—and lessons, if any, were scheduled for an hour late in the evening, when someone was available to teach. (It was not necessary for all students to be available.) Moreover, if the "pupils" lost time because of sickness, which was almost always contracted from patients or caused by sheer overwork, the time had to be totally made up before they could graduate. Why then did training schools draw so many applicants? Because the occupational opportunities for untrained women were limited to domestic service, factory work, retail clerking, or prostitution. Even with the strict discipline, hard work, long hours, and almost no time off, after a year or two of training (the second year unabashedly free labor to the hospitals), the trained nurse could do private duty at a salary ranging from $10 a week to the vague possibility of $20 (if she could collect it), a far cry from the $4 to $6 average of other women workers. Of course, on these cases she was a 24-hour servant to the family and patient, lucky to have time off for a walk, and because there were necessarily months with no employment, even an excellent nurse was lucky to gross $600 a year.[19] Higher education for women was limited to typewriting or teaching, but these were seldom taught in universities. Those colleges and universities that did admit women rarely prepared them for professions. So the more famous hospital schools, particularly, had hundreds and even thousands of applicants in a year. On the other hand, there were a multitude of hospitals and sanitoriums of all kinds that were looking for students to meet their staffing needs, and for these, high-quality applicants were frequently lacking. Consequently, application standards were lowered rapidly. Apparently, most schools admitted a class of 30 to 35 (in some cases determined by their staffing and financial needs). Attrition, caused in part by the tremendously high rate of student illness and the unpleasant working and living conditions, was often 75 percent.

Student admission requirements varied, but all nurse applicants were female. Some hospitals accepted men in programs, but gave them only a short course and frequently called them attendants.[20] In 1888, at Bellevue Hospital, the Mills School was established with a 2-year course, but for a long time its graduates were also called attendants. Other early schools admitting men were at Grace Hospital, Detroit; Battle Creek Sanitorium, Battle Creek, Michigan; Boston City Hospital, Carney, and St. Margaret's, Boston; Pennsylvania Hospital in Philadelphia; and the Alexian Brothers hospitals in Chicago and St. Louis.[21] At first, the minimum age for all students was about 25, but later was lowered to 21 to prevent losing young women to other fields. Eight or fewer years of school were common, but usually good health and good character were absolute prerequisites. Obedience in training was essential, and a student could be dismissed as a troublemaker if the overworked girl grumbled, talked too much, was too familiar with men, criticized head nurses or doctors, or could not get along "sweetly" wherever placed. Married women and those over 30 were frequently excluded because they could not "fall in with the life successfully." And, of course, if they were divorced, they were naturally eliminated—"too self-centered with interests elsewhere." Blacks were also generally silently excluded. Over the years, training schools for black nurses were founded, the first being organized in 1891 at the Provident Hospital in Chicago.

In the 1890s, only 2 percent of nurse training was theory, containing some anatomy and physiology, materia medica, perhaps some chemistry, bacteriology, hygiene, and lectures on certain diseases. The leading schools developed their own institutional manuals, such as the simply written *Hand-Book of Nursing for Family and General Use*, written by a committee of nurses and physicians at the Connecticut Training School and published in 1878. The other great pioneering texts were *A Textbook of Nursing for the Use of Training Schools, Families, and Private Students*, by Clara Weeks Shaw (1885); *Nursing: Its Principles and Practice for Hospital and Private Use*, by Isabel Hampton (1893); *The Textbook on Materia Medica for Nurses*, by Lavinia Dock (1890); and the first scientific book written by a nurse, a textbook on anatomy, by Diana Kimber (1893).[22] Almost from the beginning, there were physicians who objected to so much education for nurses and devoted considerable medical journal space to their fulminations about the "overtrained nurse."

> Training, as we understand it, is drilling, and a person who is to carry out the instructions of another cannot be too thoroughly drilled. Pedagogy is another matter. We have never been able to understand what great good was expected from imparting to nurses a smattering of medicine and surgery. . . . To feed their vanity with the notion that they are competent to take any considerable part in ordering the management of the sick is certainly a most erroneous step.
>
> The work of a nurse is an honorable "calling" or vocation, and nothing further. It implies the exercise of acquired proficiency in certain more or less mechanical duties, and is not primarily designed to contribute to the sum of human knowledge or the advancement of science. . . .[23]

One physician even suggested a correspondence course for training nurses to care for the "poor folks," and a New York newspaper editorial proclaimed, "What we want in nurses is less theory and more practice."[24] But then, this was at a time when a leading Harvard physician held that serious mental exercise would damage a woman's brain or cause other severe trauma, such as the narrowing of the pelvic area, which would make her unable to deliver children.[25]

However, there were also farsighted physicians who supported not "teaching a trade, but preparing for a profession," as Dr. Richard Cabot noted in 1901. He listed reforms that included the following: (1) nurses should pay for their training and be taught by paid instructors; (2) nursing should be taught by nurses, medicine by physicians; and (3) the nurse's training should not be entirely technical. He added, "Subjects like French literature and history, which tend to give us a deeper and truer sympathy with human nature, are surely as much needed in the education of the nurse, who is to deal exclusively with human beings, as in the curriculum of the chemist or engineer, who deals primarily with things and not persons."[26] Meanwhile, students continued to live a slavelike existence, without outward complaint, poorly housed, overworked, underfed ("rations of a kind and quality only a remove better than what we might place before a beggar," said a popular journal), and unprotected from life-threatening illness (80 percent of the students in the average hospital graduated with positive tuberculin tests).[27] If they survived all this, no wonder they were expected to graduate as "respectful, obedient, cheerful, submissive, hard-working, loyal, pacific, and religious."[28] It was not professional education; it was not even a respectably run apprenticeship, because learning was not derived from skilled masters, but rather from their own peers, who were but a step ahead of them. These principles of sacrifice, service, obedience to the physician, and ethical orientation are embodied in the Nightingale Pledge, written in 1893 by Lystra E. Gretter, superintendent of the school at Harper Hospital in Detroit, a pledge still sometimes recited by students today.

I solemnly pledge myself before God and in the presence of this assembly;

To pass my life in purity and to practice my profession faithfully;

I will abstain from whatever is deleterious and mischievous and will not take or knowingly administer any harmful drug; I will do all in my power to maintain and elevate the standard of my profession, and will hold in confidence all personal matters committed to my keeping and all

family affairs coming to my knowledge in the practice of my calling;

With loyalty will I endeavor to aid the physician in his work, and devote myself to the welfare of those committed to my care.[29]

■ THE NURSE IN PRACTICE

In the late eighteenth and early nineteenth centuries, the graduate-trained nurse had two major career options: she could do private duty in home or, if she was exceptional (or particularly favored), gain one of the rare positions as head nurse, operating room supervisor, night supervisor, or even superintendent. The latter positions were, of course, much more available before the flood of nurses reached the market. Even so, in private duty, trained nurses often competed with untrained nurses who were not restrained from practicing in many states until the middle of the twentieth century. And, given the long hours and taxing physical work in home nursing, most private nurses found themselves unwanted at 40, with younger, stronger nurses being hired instead. Some of the more ambitious and perhaps braver nurses chose to go West to pioneer in new and sometimes primitive hospitals.

The practice of nursing was scarcely limited to clinical care of the patient. Job descriptions of the time appear to have given major priority to scrubbing floors, dusting, keeping the stove stoked and the kerosene lamps trimmed and filled, controlling insects, washing clothes, making and rolling bandages, and other unskilled housekeeping tasks, as well as edicts for personal behavior. Nursing care responsibilities included "making beds, giving baths, preventing and dressing bedsores, applying friction to the body and extremities, giving enemas, inserting catheters, bandaging, dressing blisters, burns, sores, and wounds, and observing secretions, expectorations, pulse, skin, appetite, body temperature, consciousness, respiration, sleep, condition of wounds, skin eruptions, elimination, and the effect of diet, stimulants, and medications," and carrying out any orders of the physician.[30] One of the more interesting treatments to modern nurses might be the vivid description of leeching, which included placing leeches, removing them from human orifices where they may have disappeared, and emptying them of excess blood.

At the end of the nineteenth century, the growth of large cities was marked in the United States. Although the cities had their beautiful public buildings, parks, and mansions, they also had their seamy sides—the festering slums where the tremendous flow of immigrants huddled. Between 1820 and 1910, nearly 30 million immigrants entered the United States, with a shift in numbers from Northern European to Southern European by the early 1900s. Health and social problems multiplied in the slum areas. In New York, for instance, it was not unusual to house 36 families in a six-story walk-up on a narrow 25 × 90-foot lot. Vermin, lack of sanitation, and the fact that many immigrants converted their crowded rooms into sweatshops made it easy for epidemics to rage through neighborhoods. Death from tuberculosis was common.

Somehow, Americans did not seem to feel a great need to serve the sick poor in their homes; after all, there were public dispensaries and charity hospitals. Nevertheless, in 1877, the Women's Board of the New York City Mission sent nurses, who received their training at Bellevue, into the homes of the poor to give care. In 1886, the Visiting Nurse Society of Philadelphia sent nurses not only to the poor but also to those of moderate means who could pay. In the same year, the nurses of the Boston Instructive District Nursing Association formally included patient teaching in their visits—principles of hygiene, sanitation, and aspects of illness. Other such agencies followed, but by 1900 it was estimated that only 200 nurses were engaged in public health nursing.

One of the key figures in community health nursing was Lillian Wald.[31] After graduating from New York Hospital School of Nursing and working a short time, she decided to enter the Women's Medical College. When she and another nurse, Mary Brewster, were sent to the Lower East Side to lecture to immigrant mothers on the care of the sick, they were shocked at what they saw; neither had known such abject poverty could exist. Wald left medical school, moved with Mary Brewster to a top-floor tenement on Jefferson Street, and began to offer nursing care to the poor. After a short while, the calls came by the hundreds from families, hospitals, and physicians. People were cared for, whether or not they could afford to pay. The concern of these nurses was not just giving nursing care but seeing what other services could be made available to meet the many social needs of the poor. Challenging the entire community to assume responsibility for these conditions of "poverty and misery" was an attitude strongly advocated by Lavinia Dock, who wrote in 1937:

> As I recollect it, this point of view turned rather toward exploration and discovery than simply toward good works alone, when Lillian D. Wald and Mary Brewster went in 1893, free from every form of control, "without benefit of"

managers, committees, medical encouragement, or police approval, into Jefferson Street (at first, then later into Henry Street), there to do what they could do; to see what they could see; and to publicize all that was wrong and remediable by making their findings known as widely as possible. . . .

> If I am not mistaken, it was Lillian Wald who first used the term public health nursing—adding the one word public to Florence Nightingale's phrase health nursing—in order to picture her inner vision of the possibilities of nursing services as widely and as effectively organized as were state and federal health services, and acting in harmonious cooperation with them, if not a part of them.[32]

After 2 years of such success, larger facilities, more nurses, and social workers were needed. In 1895, Wald, Brewster, Lavinia Dock, and other nurses moved to what was eventually called the Henry Street Settlement, a house bought by philanthropist Jacob H. Schiff. By 1909, the Henry Street staff had 37 nurses, all but 5 providing direct nursing service. Each nurse was carefully oriented and was able to demonstrate the value of understanding the family and the environment in giving good nursing care. Each nurse kept two sets of records, one for the physician and another recording the major points of the nurse's work.

The establishment of school nursing was also started by Lillian Wald, who suggested that placing nurses in schools might help to solve the problem of the schools having to send home so many ill children. (Health conditions in New York schools were so bad that in 1902, 10,567 children were sent home from school; local physicians did little in these settings.) Wald sent a Henry Street nurse, Lina L. Rogers, to a school on a 1-month demonstration project, which proved so successful that by 1903 the school board began to appoint nurses to the schools. It was not an easy job, and on occasion the schools were the sites of riots because mothers misunderstood the preventive measures that needed to be taken by the nurses. One amusing tale is found in the Children's Bureau records. On being notified that her child needed a bath, a mother wrote, "teacher, Johnny ain't no rose. Learn him, don't smell him."[33]

Industrial nursing also began to provide job opportunities for trained nurses. One of the earliest is generally credited to the president of the Vermont Marble Company in Proctor, Vermont, who in 1895 employed a trained nurse, Ada M. Stewart, to give "district nursing" service to the employees of the company. No public health nursing service was available at that time.

Miss Stewart often traveled about the town on a bicycle, wearing her nurse's uniform and a plain coat and hat, teaching company employees and sometimes other members of the community "habits for healthy living," caring for minor injuries, calling the doctor when indicated, and, at the schoolteacher's request, talking to school-children about hygiene and first aid. Miss Stewart's service was so helpful that in 1895 the marble company employed her sister, Harriet, to give similar service in other Vermont communities in which the company had mills and quarries.

The century ended with another war, in which nurses again proved their worth. The Spanish-American War lasted less than a year, but there was considerable loss of life. The Army was completely unprepared for it, and the hospital corpsmen were even less ready to cope with the sick and wounded. The National Society of the Daughters of the American Revolution offered to serve as an examining board for military nurses. The task of separating the fit from the unfit and the trained from the untrained among the 5000 applicants was overwhelming. Significant questions asked the volunteers were, "Are you strong and healthy?" and "Have you ever had yellow fever?" Although only a small percentage of the soldiers ever left the camps in the South to fight in Cuba, at one point fully 30 percent became ill from malaria, dysentery, and typhoid. Once more, some Army surgeons, particularly the Surgeon General, objected to the presence of trained women nurses, but their efforts to recruit male nurses were unsuccessful because glory, rank, and decent salary were lacking. Consequently, nursing was done by the dregs of the infantry squads. Finally, with serious outbreaks of typhoid killing the enlistees, women nurses from many training schools took over. Wearing their own distinctive school uniforms and caps, they included superintendents of nursing on leave from their noted schools, as well as new, young graduates. Their letters and journals relate the horrible conditions under which they worked. Some literally worked themselves to death in the Army hospitals in the South.

Meanwhile, a hospital ship, the *U.S.S. Relief*, sailed to Cuba with supplies, medicines, and equipment—along with Esther Hasson of New London, Connecticut, who would later become the first superintendent of the Navy Nurse Corps. They were just in time to receive the wounded of a naval battle, but again, the greatest problem was disease, including yellow fever, about which little was known. In testing the theory that the disease was caused by a certain type of mosquito, nursing gained its first martyr. Twenty-five-year-old Clara Maas of East Orange, New Jersey, volunteered to be bitten by a carrier mosquito. After being bitten several times, she died of yellow fever and is still considered a heroine in helping to prove the source of the disease.

The conditions under which soldiers and sailors were cared for continued to be horrendous. An investigation after the war indicated that the only redeeming aspect was the quality of the services of the women nurses, even though they were insufficient in number and were forced to work inefficiently. A recommendation was made for "a corps of selected trained women nurses ready to serve when necessity [to] arise, but, under ordinary circumstances, owing no duty to the War Department, except to report residence at determined intervals."[34] Still, the attitude of military authorities was hostile. One hospital commander surgeon objected to retaining women nurses, citing their "coddling" of patients, and the difficulty in preserving "good military discipline with this mixed personnel." So, although the number of women Army nurses had reached 1158 in September 1898, by the following July there were only 202. Despite this setback, a group of influential women, including some prominent nurses, eventually lobbied through a bill, and the Army Nurse Corps was established on February 2, 1901. Dita H. Kinney, Head Nurse of the US Army Hospital at Fort Bayard, New Mexico, became the first nurse superintendent. It took longer for the Congress to act on a Navy Nurse Corps, although it had the support of the Navy's Surgeon General; it finally became a reality in 1908.[35]

■ THE IMPACT OF NURSING'S EARLY LEADERS

Perhaps it was said best by Isabel Hampton Robb as she spoke to other early nursing leaders: "We are the history makers of trained nurses. Let us see to it that we work so as to leave a fair record as the inheritance of those who come after us, one which may be to them an inspiration to even better efforts."[36]

It was an amazing period of coordinated female leadership in what was barely becoming an accepted, respectable occupation in the last quarter of the nineteenth century. Yet, before the new century was far along, this intrepid coterie of nurses was responsible for setting nursing standards, improving curricula, writing textbooks, starting two enduring professional organizations and a nursing journal, inaugurating a teacher training program in a university, and initiating nursing licensure. They were a mixed group, but with certain commonalities: usually unmarried but, except for Lavinia Dock, not feminist; graduates of the better training schools; later functioning in some teaching and/or administrative capacity, most often as superintendent of a school; and involved in the early nursing organizations. Fortunately, many were also great letter writers and letter savers as well as authors, so that there are many fascinating insights into their lives. (See particularly the Christy series in *Nursing Outlook*, listed in the references.)

Nursing's first trained nurse, Linda Richards, had a continuing impact on the training schools because she spent much of her career moving from hospital to hospital in what seems to have been an improvement campaign. In those earliest days, almost any graduate was considered a prime candidate for starting another program, and some undoubtedly lacked the intellectual and leadership qualities needed, so that the new schools, if not actual disasters, were frequently of poor quality. Linda Richards apparently had the skill and authority to upgrade both the school and the nursing service, which were, after all, almost inseparable. However, she seemed willing to accept school management that tied the economics of the hospital to student education, usually to the detriment of the latter.

One of the most noted nursing figures is Isabel Hampton, who left teaching to enter the Bellevue Training School in 1881. Not only was she attractive and charming, but she was "in every sense of the word a leader, by nature, by capacity, by personal attributes and qualities, by choice, and probably to some extent by inheritance and training; a follower she never was."[37] In her two major superintendencies, she made a number of then-radical changes—cutting down students' workday to 10 hours and eliminating their free private-duty services. At Johns Hopkins, which she founded, she recruited fractious Lavinia Dock, who was still at Bellevue, to be her assistant. They must have made an interesting pair, for Lavinia, also a "lady," was outspoken and frequently tactless, particularly with physicians. Later, she was to say,

> A quite determined movement on the part of our masculine brothers to seize and guide the helm of the new teaching is . . . most undeniably in progress. Several . . . have lately openly asserted themselves in printed articles as the founders and leaders of the nursing education, which so far as it has gone, we all know to have been worked out by the brains, bodies and souls of women . . . who have often had to win their points in clinched opposition to the will of these same brothers and solely by dint of their own personal prestige as women. . . .[38]

M. Adelaide Nutting graduated in that first Hopkins class, and the three became friends.[39] Nutting followed Hampton as principal of the school when in 1894 Isabel was married to one of her admirers, Dr. Hunter Robb, and, as was the custom, retired from active nursing. (Letters of the time reveal the anger, dismay, and even sadness of her colleagues at her marriage. They were sure Dr. Robb was not nearly good enough for her, and besides, she was betraying nursing by robbing the profession of her talents.) Nevertheless, Isabel Hampton Robb maintained her interest in nursing and continued to be active in the development of the profession. In 1893, she was appointed chairwoman of a committee to arrange a congress of nurses under the auspices of the International Congress of Charities, Correction, and Philanthropy at the Chicago World's Fair. There, before an international audience of nurses, she voiced her concern about poor nursing education and stated that the term *trained nurse* meant "anything, everything, or next to nothing" in the absence of educational standards. At the same time, Dock pointed out that the teaching, training, and discipline of nurses should not be provided at the discretion of medicine. Similar themes were reiterated in other papers, as well as the notion that there ought to be an organization of nurses. Shortly after the congress, 18 superintendents organized the American Society of Superintendents of Training Schools for Nursing (later to become the National League of Nursing Education) to promote the fellowship of members, establish and maintain a universal standard of training, and further the best interests of the nursing profession. The first convention of the society elected Linda Richards president.

Another attendee at those early meetings was Sophia Palmer, a descendant of John and Priscilla Alden and a graduate of the Boston Training School, who, after a variety of experiences, organized a training school in Washington, DC, over the concerted opposition of local physicians who wanted to control nursing education. She approved the steps that were taken but was impatient with what seemed to be blind acceptance of hospital control of schools. "She had a very intense nature and, like all those who are born crusaders, had little patience with the slower methods of persuasion. . . . She was like a spirited racehorse held by the reins of tradition."[40] Within a short time, she and some of the others in the Society, including Dock and the new Mrs. Robb, recognized the need for another organization for all nurses. Although some of the training schools had alumnae associations, they were restrictive; in some cases, their own graduates could not be members, and any "outsider" could not participate. Therefore, if a nurse left the immediate vicinity of her own school, there was no way in which she had any organized contact with other nurses. In a paper given in 1895, Palmer stressed that the power of the nursing profession was dependent on its ability to organize individuals who could influence public opinion. Dock also made recommendations for a national organization. In 1896, delegates representing the oldest training school alumnae associations and members of an organizing committee of the Society selected a name for the proposed organization—Nurses' Associated Alumnae of the United States and Canada (to become the ANA in 1911)—set a time and place for the first meeting (February of 1897 in Baltimore), and drafted a constitution. At the end of that February meeting, held in conjunction with the fourth annual Society convention, the constitution and bylaws were adopted and Isabel Hampton Robb was elected president. Among the problems discussed at those early meetings were nursing licensure and the creation of an official nursing publication.

There were a number of nursing journals: the *British Journal of Nursing*, established by one of England's nursing leaders, Ethel Gordon Fenwick; and in the United States, the short-lived *The Nightingale*, started by a Bellevue graduate; *The Nursing Record* and *The Nursing World*, also short-lived; and *The Trained Nurse and Hospital Review*, which Palmer edited for a time, and which continued for 70 years. But the leaders of the new organizations wanted a magazine that would promote nursing and that was owned and controlled by nursing.

For several years there was discussion but no action, until another committee on the ways and means of producing a magazine was formed. In January 1900, they organized a stock company and sold $100 shares only to nurses and nurses' alumnae associations. By May, they had a promise of $2400 in shares, and almost 500 nurses had promised to subscribe. Admittedly, they had overstepped their mandate, which they reported to the third annual convention of the Nurses' Associated Alumnae, but they were given approval to establish the magazine along the lines formulated. The J. B. Lippincott Company was selected as publisher, and Sophia Palmer became editor, which she did on an unpaid basis for the first 9 months. (She had become director of the Rochester City Hospital in New York.) As the first issue went for mailing in October, it was discovered that the post office rules prevented its being mailed because the journal's stockholders were not incorporated. M. E. P. Davis and Sophia Palmer assumed

personal responsibilities for all liabilities of the new *American Journal of Nursing*, and it went out. The *Journal* was considered the official organ of the nursing profession, but the stock was still held by alumnae associations and individual nurses. It was Lavinia Dock who donated the first share of stock to the association, and by 1912 the renamed ANA had gained ownership of all the stock of the American Journal of Nursing Company, which it retained until 1996, when it was sold to Lippincott by the ANA.

One other major organization, the American Red Cross, was established by a nurse, Clara Barton, the schoolteacher who had volunteered as a nurse and directed relief operations during the Civil War. She also served with the German Red Cross during the Franco-Prussian War in 1870. (The establishment of the International Red Cross as a permanent international relief agency that could take immediate action in time of war had occurred in Geneva in 1864 with the signing of the Geneva Convention guidelines.) After her return to the United States, Barton organized the American Red Cross and persuaded Congress in 1882 to ratify the Treaty of Geneva so that the Red Cross could carry on its humanitarian efforts in peacetime. She also founded a Missing Soldiers Office to search for soldiers missing in the Civil War. (Twenty boxes of artifacts from that office were recently found.) Clara Barton, however, was not an active part of the nursing leadership that was molding the profession.

That group had another immediate goal. The Society recognized that nurses were at a disadvantage because they had no postgraduate training in administration or teaching, so a committee consisting of Robb, Nutting, Richards, Mary Agnes Snively, and Lucy Drown was formed to investigate the possibilities. At the sixth Society convention, they reported their success. James Russell, the farsighted dean of Teachers College at Columbia University in New York, had agreed to start a course for nurses if they could guarantee the enrollment of 12 nurses, or $1000 a year. The Society agreed. Members of the Society screened the candidates, contributed $1000 a year, and taught the course—hospital economics. Later, the students were also allowed to enroll in psychology, science, household economics, and biology. Anna Alline, one of the two graduates of the first class, then took over the total administration of the course.

There was one more major goal to be reached— licensure of nurses. Not only did the 432 hospital-based schools vary greatly in quality, but the market was also flooded with "nurses" who had been dismissed from schools without graduating, "nurses" from 6-week private and correspondence courses, and a vast number of those who simply called themselves nurses. It was inevitable that people became confused, for when they hired nurses for private duty in the homes, the "nurse" could present one of the elaborate diplomas from a $13 correspondence course that guaranteed that anyone could become a nurse, a real or forged reference, or a genuine diploma from a top-quality school. How could they judge? Consequently, because of the abysmal care given by individuals representing themselves as nurses, the public was once more disenchanted with the "nurse." Therefore, nursing's leaders were determined that there must be legal regulation, both to protect the public from unscrupulous and incompetent nurses and to protect the young profession by establishing a minimum level of competence, limiting all or some of the professional functions to those who qualified. The idea was not new; medicine already had licensing in some states, and many aspiring professions were also moving in that direction.

In September 1901, at the first meeting of the newly formed International Council of Nurses, which was held in Buffalo, a resolution was passed, stating that "it is the duty of the nursing profession of every country to work for suitable legislative enactment regulating the education of nurses and protecting the interests of the public, by securing State examinations and public registration, with the proper penalties for enforcing the same."[41]

In the United States, such licensing was a state function, so to gain the necessary legislative lobbying power, it was recommended that state or local nurses' associations be formed. In many ways the disagreements that arose in their formation were the forerunners of those that would center on the licensure process. Who should be eligible? In New York, for instance, Sylveen Nye, who became the state association's first president, thought that all nurses should be included and that standards could be raised later. Sophia Palmer, another key figure in its formation, believed that only "qualified" nurses should be permitted to belong—those who graduate from certain types of schools. Later, the question was, "Who should be eligible for licensure?"

As it was, New York had become the early leader in the licensure drive, for it had in place a Board of Regents that regulated education and licensure. In 1897, Palmer, in a smart political move, had already presented nursing's case to another emerging group of women who were gaining power and prestige—the New York Federation of Women's Clubs. They passed a resolution supporting her licensure concept, which included two major points—the need for a diploma from a school meeting certain standards, and insistence that the examining board consist only of nurses, as in other professions. Immediately Palmer organized a meeting with the secretary of the Board of Regents, who, then and later, was helpful and supportive, suggesting guidelines for action. (For instance, the licensed nurse

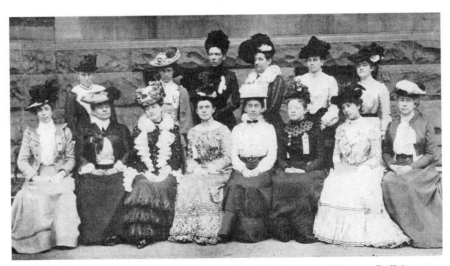

Foreign delegates and officers of the International Conference of Nurses, Buffalo, New York, 1901. (Courtesy of Lucie Young Kelly, private collection)

needed to be called something. Among the titles suggested by nurses were graduate nurse, trained nurse, certified nurse, registered nurse, and registered graduate nurse.) The Regents also suggested the formation of a state nurses' association. Once formed, the New York State Nurses' Association developed a licensure bill and embarked on a campaign to gain support for the proposed legislation. Opposition was foreordained. In a circular addressed to the women's clubs, Palmer accurately pinpointed the sources.

> The New York State Nurses' Association is preparing to apply for legislative enactments which will place training schools for nurses under the supervision of the Regents of the University of the State, with a view to securing by the authority of the law a minimum basis of education for the nurse, beyond which the safety of the sick and the protection of the public cannot be assured.
>
> While such a law cannot prevent the public from employing untaught women as nurses, if it so desires, it will prevent such women from imposing themselves upon the public as fully trained nurses.
>
> In this movement the Nurses' Association will meet with opposition: First, from the trained nurses of the State who are afraid to make an independent stand for their own and the public protection. Second, from all of the managers and proprietors of institutions which are not equipped for giving this minimum education, and which now conduct so-called training schools, for commercial advantages, and third, from all the vast army of so-called nurses who, without adequate nursing experience and education, undertake the grave responsibility of a nurse's work.[42]

And there was just that kind of opposition and more, for there were 15,000 untrained nurses in New York at the time, opposed to 2500 who were trained. In addition, some physicians objected to their lack of representation on the proposed nursing board, as did some nurses, including Nye. Moreover, some physicians did not see the necessity for any fancy standards and worried about over-education of nurses. Said one, "Nursing is not, strictly speaking, a profession. Any intelligent, not necessarily educated, woman can in a short time acquire the skill to carry out with explicit obedience the physician's directions."

Nevertheless, the bill became law on April 24, 1903. It was pitifully weak by today's standards, but daring for the times. Educational standards were set. A training school for nurses had to give at least a 2-year program and be registered by the regents. The board of five nurses was to be chosen by the regents from a list submitted by the New York State Nurses' Association. The regents, on the advice of the board, were to make rules for the examination of nurses and to revoke licensure for cause. The New York State Nurses' Association was given the right to institute proceedings and prosecute those violating the law, a responsibility that was not changed for some years. It should be remembered, though, that this, like all nurse licensure laws in those times, was permissive, not mandatory. That is, only the registered nurse (RN) title was protected. Untrained nurses could continue to work as nurses as long as they did not call themselves RNs.

New York was not the first state to register nurses. On March 3, 1903, North Carolina, and on April 1, 1903, New Jersey had passed laws. It was said that both were inspired by New York's initiative. (Virginia followed New York on May 14.) However, New York's law was the strongest. For instance, New Jersey's law omitted a board of any kind; North Carolina had a mixed board of nurses and doctors and allowed a nurse to be licensed without attending a training school if vouched for by a doctor. Partially because New York had the greatest number of trained nurses and because of the experience in regulation of the Board of Regents, the state's nurses were looked to as leaders in the further developments. The prestige, power, and authority of the Board of Regents was such that later, many training schools in other states and countries sought and received approval under New York's law—an action that also upgraded schools in those states. In fact, by 1906, more schools were registered outside the state than within it.

The enactment of the first nursing licensure laws was soon followed by like actions in other states; in a sense, it was the end of one era and the beginning of another. Nursing's leaders had shown themselves to be, as a whole, dedicated, strong, and remarkably bold. They set standards for nursing at a time when standards in long-established medicine were still quite weak. Despite internal dissension and the opposition of some powerful hospital administrators and physicians, they had had a licensing law passed—at a time when women had no vote. They literally created a young profession out of a woman's occupation. But the struggle to achieve full professionalism was far from over.

KEY POINTS

1. The work and ongoing interest of the volunteers who acted as nurses in the Civil War were influential in the establishment of the first training schools for nurses.

2. Students in the early training schools worked long hours, did many menial non-nursing tasks, and gave almost all the nursing care in hospitals.

3. War brought public attention to the need for nurses and the desirability of schools of nursing with an organized course of instruction.

4. In 1873, three schools established nursing education programs based to some degree on the Nightingale model.

5. The Nightingale school was known for its autonomy and financial independence; was staffed by nurse-faculty and controlled by nurses; and delivered care that was client oriented and based on the nurse's role in primary prevention. The earliest schools in the United States held few of these characteristics.

6. The major job market for the graduate trained nurse was home care or leadership positions in hospitals where students were the major workforce.

7. The large immigration waves of the late nineteenth century created poverty, festering slums, and the need for community health nursing services.

8. About 30 years after trained nursing began, nursing leaders in the United States were responsible for setting nursing standards, improving curricula, writing textbooks, starting two enduring nursing organizations and a nursing journal, inaugurating a teacher training program in a university, and initiating nursing licensure.

9. The original nursing practice acts did little more than protect the title "registered nurse," but it was a beginning.

REFERENCES

1. Selavan IC. Nurses in American history: The revolution. *Am J Nurs* 75:592–594, April 1975.

2. Wall B. Called to a mission of charity: The Sisters of St. Joseph in the Civil War. *Nurs Hist Review* 6:85–113, 1998.

3. Kalisch P, Kalisch B. *The Advance of American Nursing,* 3rd ed. Philadelphia: JB Lippincott, 1995, p 79.

4. Kalisch P, Kalisch B. Untrained but undaunted: The women nurses of the blue and gray. *Nurs Forum* 15(1):25–26, 1976.

5. Parsons M. Mothers and matrons. *Nurs Outlook* 31:274–278, 1983.

6. Kalisch and Kalisch (1995), op cit, p 59.

7. Leonard A. Catholic sisters and nursing in the Civil War. *Linc Her* 102(2):65–81, February 2000.

8. Lesniak RG. Expanding the role of women as nurses during the American Civil War. *Adv Nurs Sci* 32(1):33–42, January–March 2009.

9. Bullough V, Bullough B. *The Care of the Sick: The Emergence of Modern Nursing.* New York: Prodist, 1978, p 113.

10. Sartin JS. "Commissioned by God": Mother Bickerdyke during the Civil War. *Military Medicine* 168(10):773–777, October 2003.

11. Holder VL. From hand maiden to right hand—The Civil War. *AORN J* 78(3):448–450, 453–458, September 2003.

12. Oates S. *A Woman of Valor: Clara Barton and the Civil War.* New York: The Free Press, 1994.

13. Carnegie M. *The Path We Tread: Blacks in Nursing 1854–1984.* Philadelphia: Lippincott, 1986, pp 6–11.

14. Kalisch and Kalisch (1995), op cit, p 27.

15. Dolan JA. *Nursing in Society: A Historical Perspective,* 15th ed. Philadelphia: Saunders, 1983, p 194.

16. Ibid.

17. Kalisch and Kalisch (1995), op cit, p 88.

18. Dolan, op cit, p 206.

19. Kalisch and Kalisch (1995), op cit, pp 167–170.

20. Ibid, pp 135–136.

21. Dolan, op cit, pp 308–309.

22. Flaumenhaft E, Flaumenhaft C. American nursing's first text books. *Nurs Outlook* 37:185–188, July–August 1989.

23. Ingles T. The physician's view of the evolving nursing profession—1873–1913. *Nurs Forum* 15(2):123–164, 1976.

24. Ibid, p 148.

25. Bullough B, Bullough V. Sex discrimination in health care. *Nurs Outlook* 23:44, January 1975.

26. Ingles, op cit, pp 139–140.

27. Kalisch B, Kalisch P. Slaves, servants, or saints: An analysis of the system of nurse training in the United States, 1873–1948. *Nurs Forum* 14(3):230–231, 1975.

28. Ibid.

29. Kalisch and Kalisch (1995), op cit, p 171.

30. Ibid, p 174.

31. Buhler-Wilkerson K. Bringing care to the people: Lillian Wald's legacy to public health nursing. *Am J Public Health* 83:1778–1786, December 1993.

32. Our first public health nurse—Lillian D. Wald. *Nurs Outlook* 19:660, 1971.

33. Kalisch and Kalisch (1995), op cit, pp 271–274.

34. Ibid, p 216.

35. Ibid, pp 217–220.

36. Flanagan L. *One Strong Voice: The Story of the American Nurses Association.* Kansas City, MO: American Nurses Association, 1976, p 292.

37. Nutting MA. Isabel Hampton Robb—Her work in organization and education. *Am J Nurs* 10:19, 1910.

38. Ashley JA. Nurses in American history: Nursing and early feminism. *Am J Nurs* 75:1466, September 1975.

39. Poslusny S. Feminist friendship: Isabel Hampton Robb, Lavinia Lloyd Dock and May Adelaide Nutting. *Image* 21:64–68, Summer 1989.

40. Christy T. Portrait of a leader: Sophia F. Palmer. *Nurs Outlook* 23:746–747, December 1975.

41. Kalisch and Kalisch (1995), op cit, p 292.

42. Shannon ML. *The origin and development of professional licensure examination in nursing.* Unpublished Ed. D. dissertation. Teachers College, Columbia University, 1972, pp 57–58.

Note: Teresa Christy wrote a number of articles on the early nursing leaders in *Nursing Outlook* in January, March, May, June, and October 1969.

Updates can be found at **www.kellysnursing.com**

The Emergence of the Modern Nurse, After 1904

The period between 1904 and 1965 in particular was a time of multiple changes for nursing, many again precipitated by external forces, including the Depression, two world wars, and various social movements. But nurses created the changes within nursing. They included major shifts in education—type, location, curriculum, and student body—and alterations in practice, responsibility, economic status, and degree of autonomy. In 1903, the passage of the first nursing licensure laws set standards for nursing education and practice; in 1965, the development of new nursing roles and the American Nurses Association (ANA) position paper on nursing education opened the door for major revisions of those licensure laws and the emergence of the modern nurse.

■ NURSING BEFORE WORLD WAR I

After the licensure breakthrough, the leaders of nursing continued to look toward improvement of nurse training programs and, consequently, the improved practice of graduates of those programs. Most training schools remained under the control of hospitals, and the needs of the hospital superseded those of the school. For instance, it was not until 1912 that an occasional nurse received release time from hospital responsibilities to organize her thoughts and teach basic nursing, and superintendents were warned not to "neglect" patient care in favor of the school or they would face punishment. There was little support for improvement from physicians.

Before the Flexner Report of 1910, the education of the physician, although different, was sometimes less organized than that of the nurse. In the 1870s, few of the medical schools required high school diplomas and courses were completed in 2 years, whereas the nurses' program was being lengthened to 3 years. For the next 100-plus years, physicians complained of "overtrained nurses." Moreover, nursing was dominated by and primarily made up of women; it was not considered a profession, in part because it was not situated in an academic, collegiate setting. But to get into that setting as women, much less nurses, was a battle in itself. In essence, then, there were no major changes in the quality of education in the years that followed licensure, once those very limited standards were met. The hours were still long, and the students continued to give free service, with "book learning" as an afterthought.

The public, beginning to be aroused by poor conditions in factory sweatshops, showed surprisingly little interest in the exploitation of nursing students. Only in California, where an 8-Hour Law for Women was passed in 1911, was there any movement to include student nurses (not even graduate nurses). Yet, when the bill was introduced in 1913, it was fought bitterly not only by hospitals, as might be expected, but also by physicians and nurses. No doubt, some were influenced by a sentiment voiced by physicians who were saying that nursing would be debased by being included in a law enforced by the State Bureau of Labor. Stated one physician to nurses, "The element of sacrifice is always present in true service. The service that costs no pains, no sacrifice, is without virtue, and usually without value." Retorted Lavinia Dock, "I think nurses should stand together solidly and resist the dictation of the medical profession in this as in all other things. Many MD's have a purely commercial spirit toward nurses . . . and would readily overwork them. . . . If necessary, do not hesitate to make alliances with the labor vote, for organized labor has quite as much of an 'ideal' as the MD's have, if not more."[1] Although the bill finally passed, thanks to the persistence of Senator Anthony Caminetti, delegations of hospital representatives and physicians went to the governor to ask him to withhold his signature. When he asked where the people were who favored the law, a woman reporter told him that they were in the hospitals caring for the sick and unable to plead their own cause; he signed the bill.[2] But for years superintendents of nursing complained about the expense of hiring nurses who were now needed to do the work students had once done.

Although the Flexner Report brought about reform in medical schools, eliminating the correspondence courses and the weaker and poorer schools, Adelaide Nutting and other leaders were agitating for reform in nursing education. In 1911, the American Society of Superintendents of Training Schools for Nurses presented a proposal for a similar survey of nursing schools to the Carnegie Foundation. Then President Pritchitt, stating that the foundation's energies were centered elsewhere and ignoring nursing, directed a considerable amount of the foundation funds in such studies for dental, legal, and teacher education.

Although women were having a little more success in being accepted in colleges and universities, there was only limited movement to make basic nursing programs an option in academic settings. Apparently, before 1900 there was a short-lived program at Howard University, but it was almost immediately taken over by Freedman's Hospital Nursing School. There is also some evidence that the School of Medicine at the University of Texas in 1896 "adopted" a hospital school of nursing to prevent its closing for lack of funds. However, the University of Minnesota program, founded in 1909 by Dr. Richard Olding Beard, a physician dedicated to the concept of higher education for nurses, became the first enduring baccalaureate program in nursing. Even this was more similar to good diploma programs than other university programs. Although eventually the students had to meet university admission standards and took some specialized courses, they also worked a 56-hour week in the hospital and were awarded a diploma instead of a degree after 3 years. Other universities that took over hospital schools or started new ones, in part to obtain student services for their hospitals, started similar programs. Just prior to World War I, several hospitals and universities, such as Presbyterian Hospital of New York and Teachers College, offered degree options. These developed into 5-year programs with 2 years of college work and 3 years in a diploma school. This became a common pattern that lasted through the 1940s, but in 1916, when Annie Goodrich reported that 16 colleges and universities maintained schools, departments, or courses in nursing education, they were an assortment of educational hybrids.

Nursing practice had also not developed to any extent, with most graduate nurses still doing private duty in homes. A nurse, unless she became the favorite of one or more doctors who liked her work, found her cases through registries established by alumnae associations, hospitals, medical societies, or commercial agencies. The first two frequently limited the better jobs to their graduates; commercial agencies not only charged the nurse a fee but also did not distinguish between trained and untrained nurses. Finally, a county nurses' association gained control of a registry in Minnesota in 1904, and others followed. Nevertheless, private duty was an individual enterprise, with long hours, no benefits, and limited pay. (In 1926, some nurses were still working a 24-hour day at what averaged out to 49 cents an hour, less than what cleaning women made.)

However, in 1915, it is estimated that no more than 10 percent of the sick received care in the hospitals, and the majority of people could not afford private-duty nurses. From this need, a public health movement emerged that increased the demand for nurses. At first most of these nurses concentrated on bedside care, but others, like those coming from the settlement houses, took on broader responsibilities. Nevertheless, there were no recognized standards or requirements for visiting nurses. Therefore, in June 1912, a small group of visiting nurses, unofficially representing some 900 agencies and almost four times that many colleagues, founded the National Organization for Public Health Nursing (NOPHN) with Lillian Wald as the first president. It was an organization of nurses and lay people engaged in public health nursing and in the organization, management, and support of such work. The leaders of the group selected the term *public health nursing*, a term that Wald previously introduced, as more inclusive than *visiting nursing*; it was also reminiscent of Nightingale's *health nursing*, which had focused on prevention. One of the NOPHN's first goals was to extend the services to working- and middle-class people as well as to the poor.

Changes had also occurred in the first two nursing organizations. In 1911, the Associated Alumnae changed its name to the American Nurses Association (ANA), and in 1912, the Society of Superintendents adopted the name National League of Nursing Education (NLNE).

The Visiting Nurse Quarterly, the first American publication dealing exclusively with public health nursing, was offered to the NOPHN by its founder, the Cleveland Visiting Nurse Association. It became *Public Health Nursing*, the official journal of the NOPHN until 1952–1953, when *Nursing Outlook* absorbed it. Also in 1912, the Red Cross established the Rural Nursing Service. Wald, at a major meeting on infant mortality, had cited the horrible health conditions of rural America, the high infant and maternal mortality rates, the prevalence of tuberculosis, and other serious health problems, and suggested that the Red Cross operate a national service, similar to that found in Great Britain. Later, the name was changed to Town and Country Nursing Service to include small towns that had no visiting nurse service, and it was headquartered in Washington, DC. Although the Service provided nurses to care for the sick, conduct health teaching, and otherwise improve health conditions, it was not wholly successful.

Many communities did not choose to call in a national organization for assistance or could not afford the salaries of the nurses. (For a while, a wealthy woman contributed financial support to salaries, but withdrew funds because the rural nurses were not "ladies.") Nevertheless, the rural nurses carried on and proved to be a remarkably resourceful group, coping with an almost total lack of ordinary supplies and equipment. The Service survived primarily because the Metropolitan Life Insurance Company decided to use rural nurses for services to their policyholders, for many local Red Cross chapters had no interest in or understanding of the Service. (Red Cross involvement gradually decreased until, with increased government involvement in public health, it discontinued the program altogether in 1947.)

By 1916, public health nurses were being called on to be welfare workers, sanitarians, housing inspectors, and health teachers as well. A number of universities began offering courses to help prepare nurses to fulfill this multifaceted role, and Mary Gardner, one of the founders of the NOPHN and an interim director of the Rural Nursing Service, authored the first book in the field, *Public Health Nursing*.[3] One of the observations she made was that although broad-minded physicians recognized that public health nurses helped them produce results that would not have been possible alone, the more conservative feared interference by nurses and resented them. She noted that a service had a better chance of success if it was started with the cooperation of the medical profession, and pointed out ways nurses could avoid friction with physicians and still be protected from the incompetents.

Another outstanding public health nurse of that period was Margaret Higgins Sanger. She became interested in the plight of the poorly paid industrial workers, particularly women. Married with three children herself when she decided to return to work in public health, she was assigned to maternity cases on the Lower East Side of New York, where she found that pregnancy, often unwanted, was a chronic condition among the women. One of her patients died from a repeated self-abortion, after begging doctors and nurses for information on how to avoid pregnancy. That was apparently a turning point for Sanger. After she learned everything she could about contraception, she and her sister, also a nurse, opened the first birth control clinic in America in Brooklyn. She was arrested and spent 30 days in the workhouse, but continued her crusade.[4] She fought the battle for free dissemination of birth control information for decades, all over the world, against all types of opposition. As a result of her efforts, birth control education is generally accepted as the right of women and one nursing role. (Sanger herself was a most unusual person, and her life sometimes reads like a novel.)[5]

A new specialty for nurses that endured was anesthesia. In 1893, Isabel Robb mentioned this in her textbook, and apparently religious sisters gave anesthesia as early as 1877 in Catholic hospitals. However, the Mayo brothers trained two sisters who were nurses to take over these duties at Mayo Clinic. (Their friend, Alice Magaw, who succeeded them, was recognized for her brilliant work and is considered the "Mother of Anesthesia.")[6] The Mayos found a nurse more useful in anesthesia than an intern, who was also trying to learn surgery. In 1909, a course for nurse anesthetists was established in Oregon, as were others, and promptly these nurses were as exploited by hospitals. It was not until 1917 that the question was officially raised whether nurse anesthetists were practicing medicine, and it was ruled then that they were not, if paid and supervised by a physician. However, the legal answer was murky for more than 60 years, and the education of nurse anesthetists remained under the control of hospitals and doctors.

■ NURSES AT WAR

World War I was different from other wars fought by the United States because of both its international proportions and the kinds of weapons that were used. Immediately, the demand for nurses was increased. The Army Nurse Corps expanded greatly, as did the Navy Nurse Corps (although to a lesser extent). As the war continued, recruitment standards dropped, and applicants were accepted from nursing schools attached to hospitals with fewer than 100 beds. All nurses needed were certification of moral character and professional qualifications by their superintendent of nurses—and, of course, they had to be unmarried. Once more, untrained society girls were clamoring to be Red Cross volunteer nurses, without knowing what training was required or being willing to accept it. Afraid that Army nursing would fall into untrained hands as it had in Europe, Nutting, Goodrich, Wald, and others formed a Committee on Nursing to devise "the wisest methods of meeting the present problems connected with the care of the sick and injured in hospitals and homes; the educational problems of nursing; and the extraordinary emergencies as they arise."[7] Some weeks later, the committee was given governmental status and limited financial backing; most funds were contributions from nursing. The committee was able to estimate the number of available nurses and those in training, but, obviously, these were insufficient for both military and civilian needs.

The American Red Cross served as the unofficial reserve corps of the Army Nurse Corps. When these nurses, as well as those who were part of total multidisciplinary base units originating in hospitals, went to Europe, the home situation became desperate. Recruiting efforts were stepped up, first to attract educated women into nursing and then to encourage schools of nursing to somehow increase their capacity, even if it meant the unheard of—having local students live at home for part of their training. Interestingly enough, even though there were male nurses and they did volunteer, they were usually put in regular fighting units and their nursing skills went unused. Neither, apparently, did the Army choose to use black nurses. Only in mid-1917 would the Red Cross accept them, and then only if the Army Surgeon General agreed. Their eventual acceptance is credited to the efforts of Adah Thom, a black nurse.

Even with the patriotic fervor generated by the war, it was not easy to entice young women into nursing. High school students queried about their interest in nursing objected to the life of drudgery, strenuous physical work, poor education, severe discipline, lack of freedom and recreation as a student, and what they saw as limited satisfactory options for employment. However, schools did increase their capacity some 25 percent, and the pressures of the war brought about some educational changes. One of the more daring experiments of the times was the Vassar

Training Camp. The idea came from a Vassar alumna and member of the board of trustees to establish at Vassar in the summer of 1918 a preparatory course in nursing for college educated women. In the spirit of patriotism, more than 400 students aged 19 to 40, schooled in many professional fields, and representing more than 115 of the nation's colleges were recruited. More than half of the women had been teachers before selecting nursing. Each chose from 33 cooperating hospitals a school of nursing where the balance of their training would be completed in 2 years and 3 months. They were to be known as Vassar's Rainbow Division because the students wore various colored student uniforms representing the schools they had selected to complete their nursing studies. Of 439 students, 419 completed the summer camp, and 399 of these entered the affiliated schools.[8] Many of nursing's leaders arose from this group. Soon, five other universities opened similar prenursing courses and also admitted high school students. Because these programs were generally of considerably higher quality than those of the training schools, the movement of nursing education toward an academic setting received another nudge.

Meanwhile, nursing conditions in American military camps were reported as atrocious, and the Committee on Nursing convinced the Surgeon General to appoint Annie Goodrich to evaluate the quality of nursing service. Miss Goodrich, then an assistant professor at Teachers College, had experience inspecting training schools for New York State. She minced no words in her report—conditions were much worse than in civilian hospitals because there were not enough nurses to care for the patients and they found it impossible to deal with a constantly changing group of disinterested corpsmen. Goodrich recommended that nurse training schools be set up in each military hospital, where the students, under careful supervision, would give better care than aides or corpsmen. The suggested Army School of Nursing was to be centralized in the Surgeon General's Office under the supervision of a dean. After some dispute, but with the support of the nursing organizations and the influential Frances Payne Bolton of Cleveland, the Army School was approved in May 1918, with Annie Goodrich appointed dean. The 3-year course was based on the new *Standard Curriculum for Schools of Nursing*, published by the NLNE. Unlike civilian hospitals, duty hours did not exceed 6 to 8 hours. The military hospitals provided all medical and surgical experience, and gynecology, obstetrics, treatment of diseases of children, and public health were provided through affiliations in the second and third years. The response to the school was overwhelming, and it attracted many more students than it could accommodate.

The service of the nurse in the nightmarish battle conditions of World War I, coping with the mass casualties, dealing with injuries caused by the previously unknown shrapnel and gas, and then battling influenza at home and abroad, is a fascinating and proud piece of nursing history.[9]

■ BETWEEN THE WARS

In the 23 years between World Wars I and II, the Great Depression and adoption of the Nineteenth Constitutional Amendment in August 1920, which granted women the right to vote, affected nursing. Of the two, the latter had less immediate impact. Nurses showed relatively little interest in fighting for women's rights, and only one, Lavinia Dock, can be called an active feminist. "Dockie" was a maverick of the times. A tiny woman who loved music and was an accomplished pianist and organist, she also seemed to take on the whole world in her battle for the underdog. Early on, she decided that nurses could have no power unless they had the vote. Her speeches and writings were brilliant, but she did not move her colleagues. Nevertheless, she devoted a good part of her life to working for women's rights. In England, she joined the Pankhursts and landed in jail. Back in the United States, she picketed the White House, seizing the nearest, if not most appropriate, banner, "Youth to the Colors" (she was almost 60 then). Wrote her colleague, Isabel Stewart, "They all went into the cooler for the night. I think it just pleased her no end."[10]

For all her devotion to women's rights, Dock remained committed to nursing. She was editor of the *Journal*'s Foreign Department from 1900 to 1923, during which period she quarreled regularly with Editor Sophia Palmer and managed to ignore World War I because she was a pacifist. She was also involved with the International Council of Nurses and was the author of a number of books, including *Health and Morality* in 1910, in which she discussed venereal disease.[11] She was outspoken on the forbidden subject in open meetings, but had very moralistic opinions about treatment.[12] A number of nurses had become infected because physicians frequently refused to tell nurses when patients had the disease. Dock also regularly castigated her profession for withholding its interest, sympathy, and moral support from "the great, urgent throbbing, pressing social claims of our day and generation."[13]

But nursing had problems of its own. Immediately after World War I, there was a shortage of nurses because many who had switched careers "for the duration" returned to their own fields, and others appeared not to be attracted. In part, it was an image problem, one that was to continue to haunt nursing (see Chapter 11), but another quite real aspect was that nursing education was in trouble. As Isabel Stewart said, "The plain facts are that nursing schools are being starved and always have been starved for lack of funds to build up any kind of substantial educational structure."[14] Later, this problem was clearly pinpointed by a prestigious committee. In 1918, Nutting had approached the Rockefeller Foundation to seek endowment for The Johns Hopkins School of Nursing, stressing the need for improvement in the education of public health nurses. The meeting resulted in a committee to investigate the "proper training" of public health nurses, an investigation that quickly concluded that the problem was nursing education in general. The findings of the Goldmark Report (presented in more detail in Chapter 5) concluded that schools of nursing needed to be recognized and supported as separate educational components with not just training in nursing, but also a liberal education. Although the report had little immediate impact, it did result in Rockefeller Foundation support for the founding of the Yale School of Nursing (1924), the first in the world to be established as a separate university department with its own dean, Annie Goodrich. Although a few other such programs followed, progress lagged, for many powerful physicians reached the public media with their notions that nurses needed only technical skills, manual dexterity, and quick obedience to the physician. Charles Mayo, for instance, deciding that city-trained nurses were too difficult to handle, too expensive, and spent too much time getting educated, wanted to recruit 100,000 country girls.[15] But even popular journals recognized that student nurses were being exploited by hospitals and that the kind of student being encouraged into nursing by school principals was seen as not too bright, not attractive enough to marry, and too poor to be supported at home.

A study following close on the heels of the Goldmark Report soon reaffirmed the inadequacy of nursing schools and practicing nurses. *Nurses, Patients, and Pocketbooks* (see Chapter 5) pointed out that the hasty postwar nurse recruiting efforts had not improved the lot of the patient or nurse; in 1928, problems included an oversupply of nurses, geographic maldistribution, low educational standards, poor working conditions, and some critically unsatisfactory levels of care.

How could education be so poor with licensure in effect? Ten years after the passage of the first acts, 38 states had also passed such laws, but all were permissive, and although the title of "registered nurse" (RN) was protected, others could designate themselves as "nurses" and work. The first mandatory law was passed in New York in 1938 and implemented in 1944. At one point, Annie Goodrich cited a correspondence school that had turned out 12,000 "graduates" in 10 years. In addition, hospital schools of all sizes felt no need to meet standards that might deprive them of free student labor. Even those schools that chose to follow state board standards found them not too difficult, and follow-up was almost totally absent; most were approved on the basis of paper credentials. The states that did employ nurse "inspectors" ran into problems in withholding approval; members of the boards of nurse examiners were frequently as poorly qualified as the heads of schools, and the political pressures to avoid embarrassing the hospitals were overwhelming.

Even in New York State, where the state board was considered a model, the pressures on board members who also held jobs were unbelievable. They not only wrote all licensing examination questions, but also corrected all the papers and traveled throughout the state to give the practical exams. Writing about grading the lengthy open-ended questions, one board member complained: "The monotony is horrible; it stultifies the brain and one finds it impossible to work long at a sitting. So tiresome is it that one welcomes the diversion of a stupid answer."[16] By 1940, New York board members were each forced to grade 1994 tests as well as the practicals. Not until 1943 were exams scored by machine. Aside from grading fatigue, neither the test-writing skills of the authors nor the state of the art of testing gave any assurance that state boards guaranteed minimum levels of safe and effective practice for the newly licensed practitioner. Many nursing leaders called for grading of training schools as a starting point, but the Depression aborted any such action, although there were continued efforts to strengthen the licensing laws.

Unemployment after the stock market crash of 1929 also affected nursing. People who had no jobs could not afford private-duty nurses. It was estimated that 8000 to 10,000 graduate nurses were out of work, and notices warning nurses not to come to find work in specific areas became frequent in the *Journal*. A 1932 campaign by the ANA to promote an 8-hour day for nurses, hiring of nurses by hospitals, and discontinuance of some nursing schools met a cold reception. Even though they complained of the cost of training students, hospital administrators clung to the schools, perhaps because, despite financial figures to the contrary, students were obviously an economic asset. If one compared what the American Hospital Association said the students gave to hospitals in service ($1000) with an average of 7000 hours that students cared for patients—the hospital seemed to be crediting the contribution of student nurses at about 14 cents an hour. This was of questionable accuracy at best. However, even directors of nursing showed a reluctance to hire graduate nurses, and 73 percent of hospitals employed no graduates at all on floor duty in 1932.[17] By 1933, the desperate straits of unemployed nurses finally forced many to work in hospitals for room and board. Although some administrators believed this was taking advantage of unfortunate nurses, others thought that they were not worth food and lodging.

Some help finally came with the Roosevelt Administration, when relief funds were allocated for bedside care of the indigent, and nurses were employed as visiting nurses under the Federal Relief Administration (FERA). Under the Civil Work Administration (CWA), 10,000 unemployed nurses were put to work in public hospitals, clinics, public health agencies, and other health services. The follow-up Works Progress Administration (WPA) then continued to provide funds for nurses in community health activities. A few nurses also entered a new field that opened—airline stewardess.

By 1936, the number of diploma nursing schools had decreased from more than 2200 in 1929 to a little less than 1500 state-approved programs. There were about 70 "collegiate" programs, most merely of the liberal arts plus hospital school pattern. At this point, the NLNE presented its third revision of the *Curriculum Guide for Schools of Nursing*, with input from thousands of nurses around the country. A guide that was to endure (probably beyond its optimum usefulness), its major assumptions were that the primary function of the school was to educate the nurse and that the community to be served extended beyond the hospital. Numbers of academic and clinical hours as well as content were suggested.

An obvious problem was the lack of qualified teachers; even in so-called university programs, nurses did not meet the usual requirements for teaching. One outcome was that baccalaureate programs for diploma nurses began to offer specialized degrees in education, administration, or public health nursing. The other was a very slow movement to graduate education. For years, most of the graduate degrees held by nurses were in education, in part

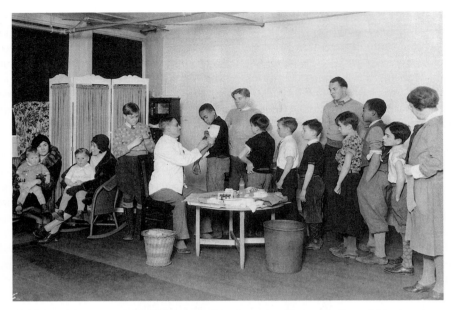

A child health center of the 1930s brought primary health care to the neighborhoods. (Courtesy of the Visiting Nurse Association of Central Jersey, Red Bank, New Jersey)

because Teachers College and other universities began to accept baccalaureate graduates for graduate preparation in education. In fact, some of the greatest leaders in nursing education either graduated from Teachers College or held teaching positions there. One such was Isabel Stewart, who arrived in 1908 for one semester and stayed for 39 years.[18] She succeeded M. Adelaide Nutting, who was the first nurse ever to receive a professorship in a university (1910) and who remained until 1925.[19] As early as 1932, Catholic University offered graduate courses in nursing, but that was uncommon. Apparently, the first, or nearly the first, nurse to earn a doctoral degree was Edith S. Bryan; it was in psychology and counseling from The Johns Hopkins University.

Another slow starter in American nursing was nurse-midwifery. In the 1920s, legislation such as the Sheppard-Tanner Act paid for nurses to give maternity and infant care, but nurse-midwives were not included. Still, lay midwives—some competent, some dangerously incompetent—provided a considerable amount of maternity care, particularly deliveries. When, in 1925, Mary Breckenridge founded the Frontier Nursing Service (FNS) in rural Kentucky, its staff was a mix of British

nurse-midwives and American nurses trained in midwifery in Britain. The outstanding services of the nurses on horseback (later in jeeps), who gradually increased their services to include other aspects of primary care, is an ongoing success story.[20] The FNS also founded one of the early nurse-midwifery schools (1936); the first was at the Maternity Center of New York City in 1932.

Of all the entrants into nursing, two groups got particularly short shrift—men and blacks. As the distorted image of the female nurse evolved, men did not seem to fit the concepts held by powerful figures in and out of nursing. Therefore, although men graduated from acceptable nursing schools, usually totally male, and attempted to become active members of the ANA, even forming a men's section, their numbers and influence remained small until the post–World War II era.

Black nurses, on the other hand, were caught in the overall common prejudice against their race. Individual black nurses, as noted earlier, broke down barriers in various nursing fields. As early as 1908, they organized the National Association of Colored Graduate Nurses (NACGN), both to fight against discriminatory practices and to foster leadership among black nurses. Although the

ANA had a nondiscrimination policy, some state organizations did not, and a rule that the nurse must have graduated from a state-approved school to be an ANA member eliminated even more black nurses. Finally, in 1951, the NACGN was absorbed into the ANA, which required nondiscrimination for all state associations as a prerequisite for ANA affiliation.[21] In 1924, it was reported that only 58 state-accredited schools admitted blacks, and most of these were located in black hospitals or in departments caring for black patients in municipal hospitals. Of these schools, 77 percent were located in the South; 28 states offered no opportunities in nursing education for black women. Most of the schools that trained black nurses were totally unacceptable, and many of those approved barely met standards. Moreover, there were some 23,000 untrained black midwives in the South, but no one made the effort to combine training in nursing and midwifery, which would have been a distinct service.

In 1930, there were fewer than 6000 graduate black nurses, most of whom worked in black hospitals or public health agencies that served black patients. Middle-class black women were usually not attracted to nursing because teaching and other available fields offered more prestige and better opportunities. It was not until a 1941 Executive Order, and the corresponding follow-through, that the federal government made any effort to investigate grievances and redress complaints of blacks.

The subsidized Cadet Nurse Corps of World War II also proved to be a boon for black nurses. Of the schools participating, 20 were all black and enrolled 600 black students; another 400 students were distributed among 22 integrated schools. It became clear that approved black schools were being held to a lower standard for a variety of reasons, some political. There were also overt and covert methods in the North and South to prevent more able black nurses from assuming leadership positions—some as simple as advancing the least aggressive. And for all the desperate need for nurses, the armed forces balked at accepting and integrating black nurses. Not until the end of the war and after some aggressive action by the NACGN and the National Nursing Council for War Service did this change.[22]

■ THE EFFECTS OF WORLD WAR II

Not just black nurses but nurses in general found that the exigencies of World War II created new opportunities, freedom, and also problems for nurses that proved to be long-lasting. As usual in wartime, nurses were in demand in the armed services. There were not enough nurses for both the home front and the battlefield, even with stepped-up efforts to encourage women to enter nursing programs. Finally, legislation sponsored by Congresswoman Frances Payne Bolton of Ohio was passed in 1943 establishing the Cadet Nurse Corps. The *Bolton Act*, the first federal program to subsidize nursing schools and nursing students, was a forerunner of future federal aid to nursing. For payment of their tuition and a stipend, students committed themselves to engage in essential military or civilian nursing for the duration of the war. The students had to be between 17 and 35 years old, in good health, and with a good academic record in an accredited high school. This new law brought about several changes in nursing. For instance, it forbade discrimination on the basis of race and marital status and set minimum educational standards. The antidiscrimination standard was not always implemented in good faith. The minimum educational standards, combined with the requirement that nursing programs be reduced from the traditional 36 months to 30, forced nursing schools to reassess and revise their curricula.[23]

Two other major efforts to relieve the nursing shortage had long-range effects in the practice setting. One was the recruitment of inactive nurses back into the field. For the first time, married women and others who could work only on a part-time basis became acceptable to employers and later became a part of the labor pool. The other change was the training of volunteer nurse's aides. Although the Red Cross initiated such training in 1919, nurses discouraged it later, particularly during the Depression.

During World War II, both the Red Cross and the Office of Civilian Defense trained more than 20,000 aides. At first, they were used only for non-nursing tasks, but the increasing nurse shortage forced them to take on basic nursing functions. After the war, with a continued shortage, trained aides were hired as a necessary part of the nursing service department. Their perceived cost-effectiveness stimulated the growth of both aide and practical nurse training programs, and eventually increased federal funding for both.

Finally, major changes occurred within the armed forces. Nurses had held only relative rank, meaning that they carried officers' titles but had less power and received less pay than their male counterparts. In 1947, full commissioned status was granted, giving them the same pay and prerogatives as other officers. At the same time, discrimination against black nurses ended, but, oddly

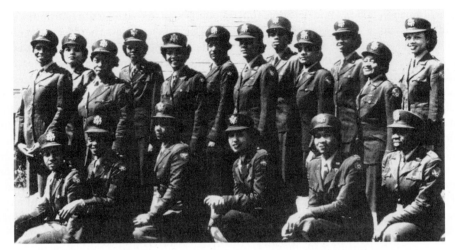

Black nurses' Army unit, World War II. (Courtesy of the Museum of Nursing History, Inc., Philadelphia)

enough, in the male-controlled armed services, it was not until 1954 that male nurses were admitted to full rank as officers.

As in all previous wars, nurses proved themselves able and brave in military situations. Many were in battle zones, and some became Japanese prisoners of war. Their stories have been told in films, books, plays, and historical nursing research, and are well worth reading.[24]

■ TOWARD A NEW ERA

The usual postwar nurse shortage occurred after World War II, but this time for different reasons. Only one in six army nurses planned to return to her civilian job, finding more satisfaction in the service. Poor pay and unpleasant working conditions discouraged civilian nurses as well. In 1946, the salary for a staff nurse was about $36 for a 48-hour work week, less than that for typists or seamstresses (much less men). Salaries were supposed to be kept secret, and hospitals, particularly, held them at a minimum. Split shifts were common, with nurses scheduled to work from 7 to 11 AM and from 3 to 7 PM, with time off between the two shifts. The work was especially difficult because staffing was short and nurses worked under rigid discipline. It was no small wonder that in one survey only about 12 percent of the nurses queried planned to make nursing a career; more than 75 percent saw it as a pin-money

job after marriage, or planned to retire altogether as soon as possible. Unions were beginning to organize nurses, and in 1949 the ANA approved state associations as collective bargaining agents for nurses. However, because the Taft-Hartley Act excluded nonprofit institutions from collective bargaining, most hospitals and home health agencies did not need to deal with nurses. In addition, the ANA non-strike policy took away another powerful weapon.

As noted, one answer that administrators saw was the hiring of nurse's aides. The use of volunteers and auxiliary help, such as practical nurses, aides, and orderlies—that is, anyone other than licensed or trained nurses—increased tremendously.

One group of workers that proliferated in the postwar era was practical nurses, defined by the ANA, NLNE, and NOPHN as those trained to care for subacute, convalescent, and chronic patients under the direction of a physician or nurse. Thousands who designated themselves as practical nurses had no such skills, and their training was simply in caring for their own families or, at most, aide work. Although the first school for training practical nurses appeared in 1897, by 1930 there were only 11 schools, and in 1947, still only 36. With the new demand for nurse substitutes, 260 more practical nurse schools opened by 1954, mostly in hospitals or long-term care institutions, and a few in vocational schools. Aiding the movement was funding from federal vocational education acts. There were, unfortunately, also a number of correspondence courses and other commercialized programs that did little more than expose the students to some books and manuals and present them with a diploma. By 1950, there were 144,000 practical nurses, 95 percent of them women, and although their educational programs varied, their on-the-job activities expanded greatly—to doing whatever nurses had no time to do. By 1952, some 56 percent of the nursing personnel were nonprofessionals, and some nurses began to fear that less expensive, minimally trained workers were replacing them.[25]

Nevertheless, with working and financial conditions not improving, the nursing shortage persisted. Soon a team plan was developed with a nurse as a team leader, who was primarily responsible for planning patient care, with less prepared workers carrying it out. Although the plan persisted for years, it did little to improve patient care; rather, it kept the nurse mired in paper work, away from the patient or required to make constant medication rounds. Practical nurses often carried the primary responsibilities for patient units on the evening and night shifts, with the few nurses available stretched thin, "supervising" these workers.

There were more nurses than ever at mid-century, but there were also tremendously expanded health services, a greater population to be served, growth of various insurance plans that paid for hospital care, a postwar baby boom with in-hospital deliveries, new medical discoveries that kept patients alive longer, and a proliferation of nurses into other areas of health care. Hospitals still were not the most desirable places to work, and economic benefits were slow in coming. Moreover, there were now more married nurses who chose to stay home to raise families. Studies done in 1941, 1944, and 1948 (see Chapter 5), all of which pointed out some of the economic and status problems of nurses, particularly in hospitals, went largely ignored.

When the Korean War broke out in 1950, the Army again drew nurses from civilian hospitals, this time from their reserve corps. War nursing on the battlefront was centered to an extent on the Mobile Army Surgical Hospitals (MASH), located as close to the front lines as possible. Flight nurses, who helped to evacuate the wounded from the battlefront to military hospitals, also achieved recognition. When that war was over and nurse reservists returned to their civilian jobs, it is possible that their experiences increased their discontent with working situations at home.

This was also a period of great medical and scientific discoveries, and physicians became increasingly dependent on hospitals for supportive services. As physicians cured patients or prolonged their lives, the corollary care required of nurses became more complex. It was not just a matter of patient comfort, but crucial life-and-death judgment. In the 1950s, Frances Reiter began to write about the nurse clinician, a nurse who gave skilled nursing care on an advanced level. This concept developed into the clinical specialist (see Chapter 15), a nurse with a graduate degree and specialized knowledge of nursing care who worked as a colleague of physicians. At the same time, the development of coronary and other intensive care units called for nurses with equally specialized technical knowledge, formerly the sole province of medical practice. In Colorado in 1965, a physician, in collaboration with a school of nursing, was pioneering another new role for nurses in ambulatory care. As nurses easily assumed responsibility for well-child care and minor illnesses, they combined their nursing knowledge with skills of medical management. What emerged was the "nurse practitioner" (NP) (see Chapter 15).

Nursing education was also going through a transition period in those decades. In the years immediately after World War II, the quality of nursing education came under severe criticism. There was no question that in the diploma schools, where most nurses were educated, there were frequently poor levels of teaching, inadequately prepared teachers, and a major dependence on students for services; often two-thirds of the hours of care were given by students.

The Brown Report in 1948 and a follow-up study in 1950 (see Chapter 5) that attempted to implement that report made it clear that nursing education was anything but professional. It was on the basis of these findings that national accreditation for nursing education by nurses was strengthened. With the reorganization of the nursing organizations, the National League for Nursing (NLN) assumed the responsibility for all accrediting functions in nursing. Dr. Helen Nahm, director of the accrediting service for the first 7 years, saw it as a culmination of all previous efforts to raise education standards—and as a last chance. Those schools that chose to go through the voluntary process and met the standards were placed on a published list, which for the first time gave the public, guidance counselors, and potential students some notion of the quality of one school compared with another. Eventually, accreditation proved a significant force in improving good schools and closing poor ones.

An impetus for collegiate nursing education was an advisory service funded by the Russell Sage Foundation for institutions of higher learning that were interested in enriching and improving their programs. The 1953 report by Dr. Margaret Bridgman, "Collegiate Education for Nursing," helped stimulate baccalaureate nursing programs to improve academically. In many cases, they were still quite similar to diploma programs, whose quality had improved considerably in the 1950s. The slow rate of growth of collegiate programs resulted in part from the uncertainty of nursing about what these programs should be and how they should differ from diploma education, and in part from the anti-collegiate faction in nursing that saw no point in higher education—a faction that was cheered and nurtured by a large number of physicians and hospital administrators. At times, it seemed to be a moot question whether any nurses were necessary. A postwar survey of the American College of Surgeons indicated that the vast majority believed, with few exceptions, that the needs of the sick could be met by nurse's aides or, at most, by practical nurses, and administrators were not averse to the "cheap is best" concept.

The establishment of associate degree (AD) nurse programs in community colleges was the most dramatic change in nursing education since its beginning. Based on a study by Dr. Mildred Montag at Teachers College, and funded by the W. K. Kellogg Foundation, pilot programs were established in a number of sites around the country in 1952. It was an idea whose time had come, for not only were community colleges the most rapidly expanding educational market of the time, but the late bloomer, the mature man and woman, and the less affluent student found this opportunity for a career in nursing and a college degree after 2 years of study highly attractive. Follow-up studies showed that these nurses performed well in what they were prepared to do—provide care at the intermediate level in the continuum of nursing functions as defined by Montag.[26] It was probably partially the influence of the AD programs, which were nondiscriminatory and generally nonpaternalistic in their relations with students, that helped loosen the restrictions on nursing students' personal lives in both diploma and some baccalaureate programs. Still, even into the late 1960s, some diploma schools excluded married students and men. The growth of AD programs ultimately outran all others in nursing except practical nurse programs.

Graduate education for nurses progressed slowly. Most degrees continued to be in education, in part because of the great shortage of teachers of nursing with graduate degrees, and in part because graduate schools of education

had part-time programs. In 1953, only 36 percent of nursing faculty had earned master's degrees, and some had no degree at all. In 1954, it was estimated that 20 percent of the positions held by nurses should require master's degrees and at least 30 percent baccalaureate degrees. However, only 1 percent of all nurses held master's and about 7 percent baccalaureate degrees, many not in nursing.

Part of the problem, of course, was financial, and, although private foundations such as the Commonwealth Fund provided some support for graduate education, federal funding made the crucial difference. It also controlled the direction of nursing education. Federal funding for the study of public health nursing from 1936 on created more baccalaureate-prepared nurses in public health than in any other field; support of psychiatric nursing increased the volume of nurses educated in that field. In 1956, the passage of the Federal Nurse Traineeship Act, which authorized funds for financial aid to registered nurses for full-time study to prepare for teaching, supervision, and administration in all fields, opened the door for advanced education for nurses at both the baccalaureate and graduate levels. Short-term traineeships also provided for continuing education programs. Another boost was the 1963 Surgeon General's Report (see Chapter 5), which specifically pointed out differences in the quality and quantity of nurses and their education and recommended both recruitment and advanced education. Following this, there was a new surge of federal aid to nursing. Nurse Traineeship programs continued to be enacted, although the struggle for funds, depending on the administration, was sometimes most difficult (see Chapters 12 and 19).

Master's programs for nurses still tended to focus on administration or education, even in schools of nursing. It was not until the 1960s that clinical programs developed. Clinical doctoral programs in nursing were almost nonexistent until the 1960s.

Nursing research also tended to take a slow path. Although there were studies of nursing service, nursing education, and nursing personality, most were done with or by social scientists. When nurses assisted physicians and others in medical research, it was just that—assisting. Nursing leaders realized that nursing could not develop as a profession unless clinical research focusing on nursing evolved. One of the first major steps in that direction was the 1952 publication of *Nursing Research*, a scholarly journal that reported and encouraged nursing research. The other was the ANA's establishment of the American Nurses' Foundation in 1955 for charitable, educational, and scientific purposes. The Foundation conducts studies, surveys, and research; funds nurse researchers and others; and publishes scientific reports. In 1956, the federal government also began to fund nursing research. Federal support in the 1960s provided research training through doctoral programs, including the nurse scientist program, and funding for individual and collaborative research efforts.

In all these changes, it can be seen that nursing's professional organizations had varied influence. At the same time, as organizations, they too were examining their roles and relationships. A study to consider restructuring, reorganizing, and unifying the various organizations was initiated shortly after World War II. In 1951, the NACGN was dissolved to merge with the ANA. In 1952, the National League for Nursing (NLN) was formed by the fusion of the NLNE, NOPHN, and the Association of Collegiate Schools of Nursing (ACSN). The ANA consisted of only nurse members, while the renamed NLN was composed of nurses, non-nurses, and agency members. The American Association of Industrial Nurses (AAIN) decided to continue, and the National Student Nurses' Association was formed. Practical nurses had their own organization. (See Chapters 24, 25, 26, 27, and 28 for details of the organizations.) Although there was an apparent realignment of responsibilities, the relationships between the ANA and NLN ebbed and flowed; sometimes they were in agreement, and sometimes they were not; sometimes they worked together, and at other times each appeared to make isolated, unilateral pronouncements. Some nurses longed for one organization, but there seemed to be mutual organizational reluctance to go in that direction. Still, it must be said that in those changing times each had some remarkable achievements—the NLN in educational accreditation, and the ANA in its lobbying activities, development of a model licensure law in the mid-1950s, and increased action in nurses' economic security.

Then, in 1965, the ANA precipitated (or inflamed) an ongoing controversy. After years of increasingly firm statements on the place of nursing education in the mainstream of American education, the ANA issued its first *Position Paper on Education for Nursing*. It stated, basically, that education for those who work in nursing should be in institutions of higher learning and that minimum education for professional nursing should be at least at the baccalaureate level; for technical nursing, at the associate degree level; and for assistants, in vocational education settings.

Although there had been increased complaints by third-party payers about diploma education being hidden in the costs for patient care and diploma schools had declined as associate and baccalaureate degree programs increased, there was an outpouring of anger by diploma and practical nurses and those involved in their education. It was a battle that persisted and became another divisive force in nursing (see Chapter 12). But, then, so was the beginning of the NP movement. There were nurses who feared it or saw it as pseudomedicine, detracting from nursing as a career. These issues remained unresolved for years.

Therefore, whether or not 1965 can be considered the gateway to a new era of nursing, it was the beginning of dramatic and inevitable changes in the education and practice of nursing and in the struggle for nursing autonomy.

■ EPILOGUE

Nursing history, of course, did not end in 1965; history is always just our yesterday. Therefore, it may be helpful to briefly review the 35-plus years that followed, even though they will be discussed in more depth in subsequent chapters.

The pattern of a nursing shortage followed by a presumed nursing oversupply continued during these years. By the early 1980s, the shortage was seen as acute, but it was followed in 1986 by layoffs and fears of layoffs as the prospective payment system required by the government for Medicare reimbursement resulted in shorter hospital stays for patients. Many hospitals found that they had more empty beds than they could afford and cut back on nursing personnel. The hospital was still the place where most nurses worked. Administrators, however, had not anticipated that because patients admitted were much sicker during their short stay, more nurses would be required to care for them. Moreover, nurses were being lured from hospitals by other health care opportunities, and soon a crisis in the nurse supply was declared. In an attempt to attract and keep nurses, considerable attention was given to their economic and general welfare, with funding for higher education made available, flexible scheduling, and salaries dramatically increased. On the other hand, by 1994, as health care facilities became concerned about what a national health care plan might mean to their survival, administrators attempted to cut back on the now well-paid RNs, hiring a variety of assisting personnel to provide the less complex care. In some communities, new graduates who had been recruited with a high-profile advertising campaign found that they could not necessarily get the jobs they wanted where they preferred to work. This was particularly true for some associate degree and diploma nurses. Nevertheless, predictions continued that in overall terms, a shortage particularly of nurses with advanced degrees was present and would continue into the new century. In short, the surplus/shortage cycle goes on, most definitely driven by economic forces and the whims of the health care industry as opposed to need.

In nursing education, the trends continued until nearly the end of the century: more RNs and licensed practical nurses (LPNs) continuing their education toward a baccalaureate degree; more second career individuals entering nursing; a moderate increase in baccalaureate programs; a spurt in programs that enabled those with a bachelor's degree in another field to move into a shortened master's program that led to licensure; a major increase in associate degree programs; and a decrease of diploma programs. Most dramatic was the emphasis on preparing clinical nurse specialists (CNSs) and nurse practitioners (NPs), with or without a master's degree. By the 1990s, there was general agreement that a master's degree was necessary for this level of practice, although many were still practicing without one; since in the 1970s, when NPs were gaining a foothold in health care, their background varied from RNs with NP training on a continuing education basis to graduate education. An increased need for NPs to provide primary health care was seen as part of the Clinton administration's national health care plan, and because enough would not be available, nursing education programs were emphasizing their preparation. Many were developing graduate programs that more or less blended the CNS and NP roles to create an advanced practice nurse (APN). (On the baccalaureate level, there was also a move to focus on preparation for primary health care, because the evolving trend toward care in the community as opposed to an institution called for these skills.)

The disagreement about the need for a graduate degree for NPs was as heated during the past quarter century as the still ongoing quarrel about the requirement of a baccalaureate-level degree for entry into professional practice. Over those years, a few states moved toward requiring the baccalaureate for basic nursing licensure, but almost all still granted RN licensure on the basis of the same test for all graduates. All states now require a separate license for the APN, usually granted after the individual's certification by a voluntary credentialing group, such as the American Nurses Credentialing Center (ANCC) and/or the various nursing specialty organizations' credentialing arms. The APN has some variety of prescriptive authority in every state and can be awarded staff privileges at the discretion of a facility. Direct reimbursement to APNs is available through most federal health entitlement programs, but state reimbursement differs from place to place. However, the American Medical Association (AMA) continued to object to such expansion of nursing practice without physician control, despite the fact that numerous studies showed how effective APNs were in providing care, and many individual physicians have accepted APNs as colleagues and partners in joint practice.

Nurses also continued to serve their country with distinction in the years after 1965. Their contributions were acknowledged in the Vietnam War[27] and the Persian Gulf War. A memorial to these nurses was erected in 1994, near the Vietnam memorial in Washington, DC—largely through the efforts and fund raising of nurses. Nurses also attained top ranks in the various armed services and were influential in bringing about significant changes.

Equally influential were those nurses who were elected to local, state, and national office or held key positions on the staffs of powerful legislators. Other nurses were appointed by US presidents to important offices, such as the heads of the Health Care Financing Administration (HCFA), Social Security Administration, and as the National AIDS Policy Coordinator. Nurses, overall, also became more active politically, and their input did affect legislation. One stunning result of nursing leadership and political influence as well as acceptance of the validity of nursing research was the establishment of the National Institute of Nursing Research as part of the National Institutes of Health.

As nurses became better educated and assumed more responsibility, they were able to positively affect patient care. In the best hospitals, nurse executives with appropriate graduate degrees were more commonly a part of the top decision-making team. Other nurses headed departments in infection control, managed care, quality assurance, staff education, and nursing research. Clinical nurse specialists were resources to nurses and others on the health care team. Nurses also participated in major institution-wide committees. They were particularly valuable on ethics committees, because serious ethical problems became more visible as a result of new technology, the problem of access to care, and the inclination of patients and families to demand participation in health-care decision making. Nursing also developed new patterns of patient care, in part to be more cost-effective. Nevertheless, it cannot be said that these patterns of nurse involvement and influence were present everywhere. In some situations nurses and physicians did not function as colleagues, and the administration did not support nurses as professional practitioners.

Alert professionals could have predicted most of the changes that emerged in these years, because their roots were in the past. Overall, there is every reason to be optimistic about nursing's role in health care, although progress is likely to be slowed if internal quarrels about education, practice, and research are not resolved. For success, it might be useful to return to the words of a nineteenth-century nursing leader: "To advance, we must unite."

KEY POINTS

1. The Flexner Report brought about reform in medical education, eliminating weak schools. A similar approach to improve the quality of nursing education was not well received.

2. Studies about nursing that pointed out deficiencies in nursing education and practice were often ignored because of the students' economic benefit to the hospital, but they seem to have had a cumulative effect that eventually brought about change.

3. By 1913, 38 states had licensing laws, but the absence of any provisions for a Board of Nursing or funding for its work often made the law useless.

4. The financial pressures of the Depression caused limited employment in home care and forced many nurses into hospital or community health practice.

5. Before the Depression, most graduate nurses worked in private duty, but public health nursing, school nursing, industrial nursing, midwifery, and other specialties gradually emerged under the leadership of nursing pioneers.

6. Major effects of World War II were the establishment of the Cadet Nurse Corps, legal elimination of discrimination on the basis of race or marital status, the introduction of flexibility in scheduling to bring inactive nurses back to the field, and the training of nurse's aides.

7. World War II sparked a growth in medical and scientific discovery that gave birth to advanced practice nursing delivered by the clinical nurse specialist and later by the nurse practitioner.

8. The Cadet Nurse Corps served as the prototype for associate degree nursing as community colleges grew and flourished in the postwar era.

9. Black nurses and male nurses were often discriminated against in nursing, but slowly gained status in the last half of the twentieth century.

10. Accreditation was established as the vehicle to distinguish between acceptable and good schools.

11. In 1952, nursing's organizations were restructured: the ANA had only nurse members; the NLN had nurse, non-nurse, and organizational membership.

12. War and the economics of health care have always exerted a significant effect on nursing.

13. The absence of agreement among nurses on education and practice issues has limited nursing's growth as a profession; the nurse practitioner movement and debate over education for "entry into practice" are good examples.

14. Much change in the education and practice of nursing has come about through external forces, rather than internal decisions.

REFERENCES

1. Kalisch P, Kalisch B. *The Advance of American Nursing*, 3rd ed. Philadelphia: Lippincott, 1995, p 208.

2. Ibid.

3. Gardner, MS. *Public Health Nursing.* New York: Arno Press, 1977.

4. Ruffing-Rahal MA. Margaret Sanger: Nurse and feminist. *Nurs Outlook* 34:246–249, September–October 1986.

5. Chesler E. *Woman of Valor: Margaret Sanger and the Birth Control Movement in America.* New York: Simon & Schuster, 1992.

6. American Association of Nurse Anesthetists (AANA). *Advancing the Art and Science of Anesthesia for 75 Years.* Park Ridge, IL: AANA, 2006.

7. Kalisch P, Kalisch B. *The Advance of American Nursing*, 2nd ed. Boston: Little, Brown, 1986, p 330.

8. Dreves K. Vassar training camp for nurses. *Am J Nurs* 75:2000–2002, November 1975.

9. Bledsoe H. American nurses for American men: A World War I diary. *Nurs Health Care* 18:11–18, January–February 1997.

10. Christy TE. Portrait of a leader: Lavinia Lloyd Dock. *Nurs Outlook* 17:74, June 1969.

11. Thoemmes Press. History of Nursing. http://www.thoemmes.com/social/nursing_intro.htm. Retrieved November 1, 2002.

12. Temkin E. Turn of the century nursing perspectives on venereal disease. *Image* 26:207–211, Fall 1994.

13. Ibid.

14. Kalisch and Kalisch (1995), op cit, p 243.

15. Bullough V, Bullough B. *The Care of the Sick: The Emergence of Modern Nursing*. New York: Prodist, 1978, p 113.

16. Shannon ML. *The origin and development of professional licensure examinations in nursing*. Unpublished Ed. D. dissertation. Teachers College, Columbia University, 1972, p 127.

17. Kalisch B, Kalisch P. Slaves, servants, or saints: An analysis of the system of nurse training in the United States, 1873–1948. *Nurs Forum* 14(3):222–263, 1975.

18. Christy T. Portrait of a leader: Isabel Maitland Stewart. *Nurs Outlook* 17:44–48, October 1969.

19. Christy T. Portrait of a leader: M. Adelaide Nutting. *Nurs Outlook* 17:20–24, January 1969.

20. January AM. Friday at Frontier Nursing Service. *Public Health Nurs* 26(2):202–203, March–April 2009.

21. Mosley M. Beginning at the beginning: A history of the professionalization of Black nurses in America, 1908–1951. *J Cultural Diversity* 2:101–102, 109, Fall 1995.

22. Carnegie ME. *The Path We Tread: Blacks in Nursing, 1954–1984*. Philadelphia: Lippincott, 1986.

23. Kalisch B, Kalisch P. The Cadet Nurse Corps in World War II. *Am J Nurs* 76:240–242, February 1976.

24. Sheehy S. US military nurses in wartime: Reluctant heroes, always there. *J Emerg Nurs* 33(6):555–563, December 2007.

25. Fairman J. Context and contingency in the history of post World War II nursing scholarship in the United States. *J Nurs Scholarsh* 40(1):4–11, January 2008.

26. Rines A. Associate degree education: History, development, and rationale. *Nurs Outlook* 25:496–501, August 1977.

27. Norman E. *Women at War: The Story of Fifty Military Nurses Who Served in Vietnam*. Philadelphia: University of Pennsylvania Press, 1990.

Updates can be found at **www.kellysnursing.com**

Major Studies of the Nursing Profession

Described here are the reports of research and studies that have guided nursing in the past and will always be considered milestones in the development of the field. The extent to which any of these studies has had a marked effect on the progress of nursing remains questionable. Nonetheless, the studies are noteworthy because they represent the efforts on behalf of nurses and other national health care experts to improve our knowledge of the nursing profession and contribute to its advancement. Detailed descriptions of many of these studies are found in previous editions of this text.

■ THE EDUCATIONAL STATUS OF NURSING (1912)

Conducted under the leadership of M. Adelaide Nutting, chairperson of the education committee of the American Society of Superintendents of Training Schools for Nurses, and published by the US Bureau of Education, this report resulted from a questionnaire study of what schools of nursing throughout the country were actually teaching their students at that time and the techniques employed. It also covered the students' working and living conditions. Although this study revealed many appalling practices, it did not create the stir in nursing or in the public that it should have. However, it did begin to establish nursing as a profession and to set a precedent for later studies. It also highlighted the need for continued investigation of educational practices in nursing, and—even as early as 1912—the need for schools of nursing to be independent from hospitals.

■ NURSING AND NURSING EDUCATION IN THE UNITED STATES: THE GOLDMARK REPORT (1923)

Also stimulated by Nutting, the Rockefeller Foundation funded a Committee for the Study of Nursing Education to investigate "the proper training of the public health nurse." It was chaired by Dr. C. E. A. Winslow, a professor of public health at Yale University, and included 10 physicians (two of whom were hospital superintendents), six nurses (Nutting, Goodrich, Wald, Clayton, Beard, and Ward), and two lay representatives. The secretary and chief investigator was Josephine Goldmark, who had already done a recognized field study. It soon became apparent that the scope of the study needed to be expanded to encompass nursing education in general. Goldmark gathered and synthesized the opinions of leading nurse educators and also surveyed and studied 23 schools of nursing and 49 public health agencies, seeking answers to questions about the preparation of teachers, administrators, and public health nurses; clinical and laboratory experience for students; financing of schools of nursing; licensure for nurses; and the development of university schools.

As the study pointed out, the education of nurses was still on an apprenticeship basis, a method abandoned by other professionals. Moreover, the quality of the teachers was poor; formal instruction was erratic, uncoordinated, and frequently sacrificed to the needs of the hospital; and students were often poorly selected. In essence, there was little training and almost no education. The conclusions of this landmark study did not result solely from the survey, but also from the firm opinions of its prestigious committee members and nursing leaders interviewed. Because some have still not been implemented, they have a remarkably contemporary ring.[1]

The major recommendations noted that public health nursing requires additional education to the basic hospital-oriented training; additional effort should be made to attract young women to a nursing career; state legislation should be enacted to define and license a subsidiary grade of nurses; lowering nursing education standards endangers public safety; neither the facilities nor education in the average hospital training school conforms to standards in other educational fields; and development, strengthening, and endowment of university schools of nursing are essential for adequate nursing services.

Although the recommendations related to education are usually given the most attention, the Goldmark Report did not neglect its original focus on public health nursing. Among other things, it was concluded that both bedside nursing care and health teaching for preventive care could be combined in one generalized service, as opposed to the separate services and agencies that were more common at the time, and were common in the Nightingale schools.

Although the 500-page report was published, it did not have the wide dissemination, interest, or impact of the Flexner Report. Only a few of the recommendations were given serious consideration on a wide scale. In part, this was owing to organized nursing's relatively early stage of development and nursing education being controlled by hospital administrators and physicians at the time of the Goldmark Report. On the other hand, positive results of the study were the Rockefeller Foundation's endowment of two university schools of nursing—Yale and Vanderbilt— and Frances Payne Bolton's endowment of Western Reserve. These represented significant forward steps in nursing education.[2]

■ NURSES, PATIENTS, AND POCKETBOOKS (1928)

This study was conducted by the Committee on the Grading of Nursing Schools, composed of 21 members representing the American Nurses Association (ANA), National League of Nursing Education (NLNE), National Organization for Public Health Nursing (NOPHN), American Medical Association (AMA) (which later withdrew), American College of Surgeons (ACS), American Hospital Association (AHA), American Public Health Association (APHA), and representatives of general education. Nurses contributed

about one-half of the $300,000 needed to finance the study; the remainder came from foundations and friends of nursing, such as Frances Payne Bolton, who also served on the committee. May Ayres Burgess, a statistician, directed the students.

The committee focused on three separate studies: supply of and demand for graduate nurses; job analysis of nurses; and grading of nursing schools. The first report, *Nurses, Patients, and Pocketbooks*, showed that there was an oversupply of nurses, with serious unemployment problems; that there was a geographic maldistribution, with most nurses remaining in large cities; that salaries and working conditions were poor; and that although in general both patients and physicians were satisfied with nurses' services (which were, of course, primarily in the private-duty sector), there was evidence of some serious incompetence.

■ A STUDY ON THE USE OF THE GRADUATE NURSE FOR BEDSIDE NURSING IN THE HOSPITAL (1933)

This was the first study done by the NLNE Department of Studies, which was established in 1932, with Blanche Pfefferkorn as its director. Prompted by previous findings of the Grading Committee, Miss Pfefferkorn and her coworkers made a comparative study of the bedside activities of the graduate and student nurse in the hospital to lend support to the gradually emerging belief (somewhat reluctantly accepted by hospital administrators) that nursing care should be given principally by graduate staff nurses, not by nursing students. The study helped to clarify the issues and laid a foundation for further reduction in the number of noneducational assignments given to students of nursing.

■ AN ACTIVITY ANALYSIS OF NURSING (1934)

This was a report of the second study sponsored by the Committee on the Grading of Nursing Schools. The principal purpose of this study, conducted by Ethel Johns and Blanche Pfefferkorn at the committee's request, was to gather facts about nurses' activities that could be used as a basis for improving the curricula in schools of nursing. It represents the first large-scale attempt to find out what nurses were actually doing on the job—in hospitals, in public health agencies, and on private duty—and this focused attention on nursing service as well as on nursing education encouraged a closer correlation of theory and practice.

NURSING SCHOOLS TODAY AND TOMORROW (1934)

This was the final report of the 8-year study conducted under the auspices of the Committee on the Grading of Nursing Schools. It provided statistics on the number of "trained and untrained" nurses and answered such questions as, what should a professional nurse know and be able to do, and how can hospitals provide nursing service? It described the nursing schools of the period and recommended essentials for a basic professional school of nursing.

A number of startling facts were brought to light. For instance, 42 percent of teachers in schools of nursing had not even graduated from high school; only 16 percent had a year or more of college. Again, it was pointed out that nursing was the only profession in which the student essentially provided all the service for her "learning" institution.

STUDY OF INCOMES, SALARIES, AND EMPLOYMENT CONDITIONS AFFECTING NURSES (EXCLUSIVE OF THOSE ENGAGED IN PUBLIC HEALTH NURSING) (1938)

The ANA initiated this questionnaire survey, which was launched in 1936 and was conducted through 23 state nurses' associations (SNAs) that agreed to participate. The data obtained from more than 11,000 private-duty, institutional, and office nurses were presented in the published report. This study undoubtedly had considerable bearing on the development of the ANA's economic security program.

ADMINISTRATIVE COST ANALYSIS FOR NURSING SERVICE AND NURSING EDUCATION (1940)

Blanche Pfefferkorn directed this study, which was sponsored jointly by the NLNE and AHA in cooperation with the ANA. This study, which focused on the purely business side of nursing service and education, produced some interesting and potentially useable data on the cost to the hospital of conducting a school of nursing and the economic value of the service rendered by nursing students.

THE GENERAL STAFF NURSE (1941)

As it became more and more common for hospitals to employ graduate professional nurses to provide bedside nursing care, which was formerly given almost entirely by students, the organizations most concerned—ANA, NLNE, AHA, and the Catholic Hospital Association (CHA)—felt the need to determine the status of general staff nurses as seen by directors of nursing, the nurses themselves, and others. A joint committee of these organizations was formed to undertake the study. The report indicates that general staff nurses had little status at the time. This was reflected in their hours of duty, their salaries, and personnel policies. This study gave impetus to a movement to try to upgrade the status of the general staff nurse.

NURSING FOR THE FUTURE (1948)

Esther Lucile Brown, a social anthropologist with the Russell Sage Foundation, conducted this study for the National Nursing Council, a large group of representatives of many health organizations and services that had functioned under other titles before and during World War II to recruit nursing students and coordinate military and civilian nursing needs.

The study, funded by the Carnegie Foundation for the Advancement of Teaching and the Sage Foundation (which published it), was to analyze the changing needs of the profession. Brown, who had already studied nursing as an emerging profession, gathered data by visiting nursing schools, attending workshops, and consulting with individual physicians and hospital administrators, as well as using both a nursing and a lay advisory committee.

The report of her findings was, ironically, not much different from those of earlier studies, indicating the slow progress of nursing education. At one point, Brown pondered "why young women in any large numbers would want to enter nursing as operated today."[3] Once more, the same inadequacies were pointed out, and once more, the closing of the several thousand small, weak schools was urged. In particular, Brown emphasized the necessity for the official examination of schools, publication and distribution of lists of accredited schools, and public pressure to eliminate the nonaccredited schools.[4]

In addition, she strongly recommended "that effort be directed to building basic schools of nursing in universities and colleges, comparable in number to existing medical schools, that are sound in organizational and financial structure, adequate in facilities and faculty, and well-distributed to serve the needs of the entire country."[5] Noting that many diploma schools still operated for the staffing benefit of the hospital, she found nursing education unprofessional.

The report was the first to make the point that nursing education, as a whole and not just an elite part, should be part of the mainstream of education, and that nurses could be divided into professional and practical groups.

■ NURSING SCHOOLS AT THE MID-CENTURY (1950)

Current national accreditation procedures for schools of professional nursing were influenced by the findings of this study of practices (in 1949) in more than 1000 schools of nursing. The study represented one attempt to implement the Brown Report. Conducted under the auspices of the National Committee for the Improvement of Nursing Services (a committee of the joint board of the six national nursing associations in existence at that time), the study covered such areas as organization of the schools, the cost of nursing education, curriculum content, clinical resources, student health, and others. The report contained statistics, tables, and graphs that schools used to evaluate their own performance as compared with that of others.

■ PATTERNS OF PATIENT CARE (1955)

This study was conducted under the direction of Frances L. George and Dean Ruth Perkins Kuehn of the University of Pittsburgh. Its main purposes were to determine how much nursing service was needed by a group of nonsegregated medical and surgical patients in a large general hospital, and how much of this service could safely be delegated to nursing aides and other nonprofessional personnel. The report, published by the Macmillan Publishing Company, New York, contained much practical information about staffing patterns and the allocation of duties, which was helpful to other nursing service administrators and of interest to all nurses. Variations of these suggested staffing patterns were used in many hospitals for years.

■ TWENTY THOUSAND NURSES TELL THEIR STORY (1958)

This is a report of a 5-year sequence of studies of nursing functions, initiated by the ANA and the American Nurses' Foundation (ANF), made possible by the financial support of individual nurses throughout the country, and made meaningful by the 20,000 nurses who were "guinea pigs" in one way or another for the study. The report of results, prepared under the direction of Everett C. Hughes, professor of sociology at the University of Chicago, who also helped with some of the 34 studies, was published by the J. B. Lippincott Company, Philadelphia.

These studies, intended to produce better care for patients, revealed what nurses actually were doing on the job, their attitude toward the nursing role as they saw it, and their satisfaction in their work.

The results formed the basis for the development of stated functions, standards, and qualifications of nurses prepared by each ANA section for its members. The studies also indicated that further research was needed in many rapidly developing areas of nursing practice, both clinical and nonclinical.

■ COMMUNITY COLLEGE EDUCATION FOR NURSING (1959)

Mildred Montag wrote Part I of this report of a 5-year Cooperative Research Project in Junior and Community College Education for Nursing. Lasser G. Gotkin wrote Part II. The project was sponsored by the Institute of Research and Service in Nursing Education at Teachers College, Columbia University, New York, and McGraw-Hill Book Company, New York, published the report.

This was an "action research" project, in that a program was developed with methods of evaluating its effectiveness built into the planning. Seven junior and community colleges cooperated in the study by establishing 2-year programs leading to an associate degree in nursing. Dr. Montag participated in the planning of all programs.

Part II of the report provides data obtained from 811 graduates of the junior and community colleges, presenting persuasive arguments for the establishment of more associate degree programs to prepare nurses for first-level positions in nursing. (See Chapter 13 for the effect of Montag's dissertation on nursing education.)

■ TOWARD QUALITY IN NURSING: NEEDS AND GOALS (1963)

The Consultant Group on Nursing, a 25-member panel of representatives from nursing, medicine, hospital administration, other areas of the health field, and the public, was appointed in 1961 by the Surgeon General of the US Public Health Service to advise him on nursing needs and to identify what role the federal government should take in ensuring adequate nursing services for the nation.

■ AN ABSTRACT FOR ACTION (1970)

This study was a direct result of a recommendation by the Surgeon General's Consultant Group on Nursing in its 1963 report, *Toward Quality in Nursing*. These experts recommended a national investigation of nursing education with special emphasis on the responsibilities and skills required for high-quality patient care. Although provision of funds for such a study was also recommended, no government funds were forthcoming.

Shortly thereafter, the ANA and National League for Nursing (NLN) established a joint committee to determine ways to conduct and finance such a study. The scope of the proposed study was enlarged to examine not only the changing practices and educational patterns of current nursing, but also probable future requirements. Confident that the problems of nursing ranged beyond the manpower problem, which the President's National Advisory Committee on Health Manpower was about to investigate, the ANF in the fall of 1966 voted to grant up to $50,000 to help launch a study. Impressed by this willingness of nursing to back its conviction that the study was needed, both the Avalon Foundation and the Kellogg Foundation granted $100,000 each to support the investigation. At the same time, an anonymous benefactor contributed $300,000.

In a meeting with the proposed head of the study, W. Allen Wallis, president of the University of Rochester and of the joint committee, it was decided that the study group to be set up would be an independent agency, functioning as a self-directing group with the power to plan and conduct its investigations as it saw fit. By January 1968, the new National Commission for the Study of Nursing and Nursing Education (NCSNNE) was fully established with 12 commissioners (three of whom were nurses); a project director, Jerome P. Lysaught; an associate director, Charles H. Russell; and a small staff. A timetable for the 3-year study was set, including the provision for a contingency operation (until January 1971) to initiate implementation of the recommendations.

The commission set as its major objective to "improve the delivery of health care to the American People, particularly through the analysis and improvement of nursing, and nursing education."[6] To meet this objective, two general approaches were used—the analysis of current practices and patterns and the assessment of future needs.

The project staff likened these methods to the work of Flexner in his study of American medicine, refined by the experience of professional studies conducted in the last quarter-century. A nursing advisory panel of 10 and a health professional panel were appointed to advise on plans for the study, suggest locations for site visits, and generally review and criticize each stage of the study.

Overall, there was an extensive search of the literature, questionnaires and surveys, 100 site visits, and a number of invitational conferences and meetings.[7]

The final report, entitled *An Abstract for Action*, was published in mid-1970 followed by a second volume of *Appendices* in 1971. A total of some 581 specific recommendations and subsumed recommendations emerged from the report.

The four key recommendations centered on the need for resources to study the impact of nursing practice on health care, the establishment of state master plans to ensure that nursing education is positioned in the mainstream of education, the formation of a National Joint Practice Commission (NJPC) and state counterparts between nursing and medicine, and the adoption of governmental measures to support nursing research.[8]

Eventually, all the major nursing organizations—the AMA, AHA, and other health groups—either published a statement of support for the report or endorsed it "in principle." The greatest concerns of the NLN were with the concept of "episodic" and "distributive" care and specific recommendations for nursing education.[9]

The determination of the commission and the project staff to begin implementation of the recommendations resulted in a commitment of funds for 1 year of implementation by the ANA and NLN. The Kellogg Foundation thereupon agreed to underwrite the project for 2 years and share with nursing the support for a third year. In 1973, the status of the implementation effort was reported in *From Abstract into Action*. The priority items of implementation were set as nursing roles and functions, nursing education, and nursing careers. By the summer of 1971, a newly organized NJPC had been established with 10 nurses and

10 physicians, each a practitioner engaged in direct patient care approximately 50 percent of the time.

Subsequently, NCSNNE attention was given to models of "episodic" and "distributive" care in education and practice, the study of new utilization patterns, and progress in nursing research. In terms of educational changes, much interest was focused on open curriculum, preparation of nurses in the expanded role, and some aspects of graduate education. In terms of careers, the commission looked at economic and social satisfactions, new approaches to extend the horizons of nursing, the impact of organizations, and the licensure dilemma.[10]

In summarizing the effect of the National Commission report on nursing and health care, it is necessary to recognize the difficulty in differentiating between changes that may have occurred through a normal process of evolving trends and those that could have been a direct result of NCSNNE recommendations. For instance, there was an upsurge of action in continuing education and open curriculum programs, and an increase in associate degree and baccalaureate programs. It is entirely possible that the report at least accelerated, if not initiated, action.

One specific action that occurred was the formation of the NJPC and its counterparts on the state, local, and institutional levels. Most states and some hospitals also formed such groups. The NJPC functioned well, and early on it made important statements.[11] However, in 1981, the AMA discontinued participation, and gradually the groups dissolved.

Overall, NCSNNE interests really did not have a very great impact. Most disappointing was the serious cutback of federal funds after a major increase in 1972. When Lysaught, in 1977, conducted a national survey to determine the progress made on the four major recommendations, he found it to be minimal, especially at the grassroots level. Perhaps remembering that the commission had repeated some of the recommendations of Brown's 1949 report, Lysaught suggested that the next years "should be characterized not by further search, but by accomplished fulfillment."[12]

■ EXTENDING THE SCOPE OF NURSING PRACTICE: A REPORT OF THE SECRETARY'S COMMITTEE TO STUDY EXTENDED ROLES FOR NURSES (1971)

At the request of the Secretary of Health, Education, and Welfare (HEW), a multidisciplinary committee was formed to study potential and actual new roles for nursing. The committee, which was chaired by Dr. Roger O. Egeberg, then Special Assistant for Health Policy at the Department of Health, Education, and Welfare (DHEW), consisted of 13 physicians and 13 nurses, as well as administrators and trustees of hospitals, administrators of schools of allied health, and knowledgeable DHEW staff. The purpose was to "examine the field of nursing practice, to offer some suggestions on how its scope might be extended, and to clarify the many ambiguous relationships between physicians and nurses."[13] The committee chose to view the subject from the perspective of the consumers of health services. The preface of the report ended with the statement:

> We believe that the future of nursing must encompass a substantially larger place within the community of the health professions. Moreover, we believe that extending the scope of nursing practice is essential if this nation is to achieve the goal of equal access to health services for all its citizens. . . .[14]

The report reviewed many current responsibilities of nurses, from simple tasks to expert, that were considered professional techniques necessary in acute life-threatening situations, and noted the nurse's role on the health team, as leader of the nursing team, and in counseling, teaching, planning, and assessing. Although recognizing that most nurses were not currently educationally prepared to assume extended roles, and that some were reluctant to accept these roles, the committee arrived at certain conclusions and recommendations it believed were significant in achieving extended roles for nursing. Legal considerations of the role were also reviewed (see Chapter 20).

The major recommendations related primarily to the need for collaborative efforts between nursing and medicine in providing health care services, curricular innovations, financial support, and appropriate legislation in developing expanded nursing roles, studies to assess the impact of extended nursing practice on the health care delivery system, and attitudinal surveys of health care providers and consumers to assess the acceptance of nurses in these roles. One outcome of this report was federal funding of, and increases in, nurse practitioner programs.

■ THE STUDY OF CREDENTIALING IN NURSING: A NEW APPROACH (1979)

There were two major considerations that precipitated a study of credentialing in nursing: an ongoing disagreement and confusion between the ANA and NLN on their respective roles in credentialing nurses, which was becoming somewhat acidulous by the mid-1970s, and increased activity by state and federal governments, presumably indicating public disaffection on the whole matter of health manpower credentialing (see Chapter 20). It was the action of the 1974 ANA House of Delegates "to examine the feasibility of accreditation of basic and graduate education" that stimulated two conferences on credentialing, under the sponsorship of the ANA Commission on Education. The outcome of these conferences, in which the NLN and the American Association of Colleges of Nursing (AACN) were also involved, was a recommendation that a feasibility study should encompass more than accreditation, that it should be broadened to include the assessment of credentialing mechanisms for organized nursing services, certification, and licensure, and "to formulate a proposal for studying the adequacy of these mechanisms, and to recommend future directions."[15]

In August 1975, the ANA contracted with the Center for Health Research, College of Nursing, Wayne State University, to (1) assess the adequacy of current credentialing mechanisms in nursing, including accreditation, certification, and licensure, for providing quality assurance to the public served; and (2) recommend future directions for credentialing in nursing.

When the NLN declined to cosponsor the study, the ANA proceeded to do so alone in August 1976. At that time, the Committee for the Study of Credentialing in Nursing (CSCN) was appointed—10 nurses and 5 others, with the later addition of Dr. Margretta Styles, a former dean of the Wayne State College of Nursing, as chairperson of the Committee. Inez G. Hinsvark, professor in the School of Nursing, University of Wisconsin, Milwaukee, was selected as project director.

The study was a complex task of some magnitude. It began with a comprehensive review of the literature and information, position papers, documents, and laws that were offered by various state agencies, nursing associations, and credentialing agencies.

The Committee's final recommendations included the following: principles to be applied to credentialing in nursing; position statements concerning definitions of nursing, entry into practice, control and cost of credentialing, accountability, and competence; credentialing definitions and their application to nursing (licensure, registration, certification, educational degrees, accreditation, charter, recognition, approval); and the establishment of a national nursing credentialing center.[16]

In 1979, the ANA Board of Directors established an independent taskforce for implementation of the report. The taskforce of 15 distinguished individuals (including 11 nurses) began its work with funding from the ANA, one SNA, some specialty nursing organizations, and a few other individuals and groups.

The Task Force on Credentialing in Nursing worked for 2 1/2 years, cooperating with 146 groups that were willing to be "resource groups." After considerable study of the original report, the major focus of the Task Force was the development of alternative structures and models of a credentialing center. Specific recommendations were also made on how the center could be implemented immediately through a coalition of nursing organizations.

This report was presented to representatives of national nursing organizations considered as potential coalition members and some of the nursing press on April 24, 1982. Although 73 resource groups had endorsed the principle of a national nursing credentialing center, it was immediately clear that if implementation meant giving up control of their own credentialing activities, the national organizations, including the ANA, were not interested. Although all groups expressed interest in continued dialogue, and some still endorsed the concept or principle of a center, a planned meeting of the credentialing organizations to be held later did not occur. The Task Force dissolved itself after the meeting; its final report was distributed through the ANF.[17]

◼ SELECTED STUDIES RELATED TO NURSING SUPPLY AND DEMAND (1975 to 1980)

In the late 1970s and early 1980s, the number of studies about, and important to, the nursing profession increased. Some were national studies that were federally funded and included such topics as the career patterns of nurses, trends in the registered nurse (RN) supply, job availability for new graduates, and the distribution, salaries, and job responsibilities of nurse practitioners. For instance, one major study of this kind, *Analysis and Planning for Improved Distribution of Nursing Personnel and Services*, which was contracted to the Western Interstate Commission for Higher Education (WICHE) by the then DHEW in 1975, was geared to strengthen nurses' abilities to analyze and plan for improved distribution of nursing personnel and services, explore ways to reduce uneven distribution, and involve nurses in health planning.[18]

For a number of reasons, the early 1980s produced especially significant nursing studies. Ironically, all began and may have been somewhat influenced by the nursing shortage then at its peak, and almost all the reports were released as the shortage appeared, at least, to be subsiding. However, by the mid-1980s, the nursing shortage had once again intensified, and new studies and commissions were called for.

A report released in late 1980, although not directly related to nursing, created a stir in the nursing community because of its implications for the profession. The Graduate Medical Education National Advisory Committee (GMENAC) had been charged by the Secretary of the Department of Health and Human Services (DHHS) to advise on physician supply and demand.[19] The committee consisted primarily of physicians. The overall conclusion was that there would be an oversupply of physicians by 2000, and many recommendations were related to this point. However, the recommendations repeatedly stated that the number of physician assistants (PAs), nurse practitioners (NPs), and certified nurse midwives (CNMs) being graduated from educational programs each year should not be increased until the need for them could be determined. Moreover, the "medical" services of NPs and PAs were to be under the supervision of a physician, and third-party reimbursement was to be made only to the employing institution or physician. Although not all the recommendations were so negative, many nurses saw the report as one more act of interference by medicine with nursing's professional development.

One study referred to frequently during this time was related to nurse employment in Texas.[20,21] Released in 1980, it was replicated in many other states and helped to stimulate national studies exploring the factors that affected nurses' employment satisfaction, particularly in hospitals. Spurred by the severe nursing shortage, the purpose of *Conditions Associated with Registered Nurse Employment in Texas* was to determine the reasons for nurses' working or not working in nursing and to decide how they might be attracted back into the workforce.

The findings of the study indicated that the chief component of job dissatisfaction was that hospital policies and administration attitudes kept nurses from providing patients with professional care.[22] Major dissatisfactions also included inadequate salaries and benefits, the amount of paperwork, and lack of both hospital and nursing administrative support. A number of innovative ideas generated by the nominal group were later adopted by a number of hospitals across the country, with some evidence of success.

■ EFFECTS OF FEDERAL SUPPORT FOR NURSING EDUCATION ON ADMISSIONS, GRADUATIONS, AND RETENTION RATES AT SCHOOLS OF NURSING (1982)

In some ways, this report was overshadowed by the congressionally mandated Institute of Medicine (IOM) report (1983, reported later). Prepared by Abt, a professional consultant company, for the Health Resources Administration, the study examined federal assistance to nursing education from only one perspective: its impact on the number of students entering, continuing in, and graduating from basic nurse training programs.

Although there were frequent references to lack of data and problems in the statistical analysis of the data, it was clearly stated that federal funds had important effects: increased admissions and graduations in the 10 years studied. It was also noted that, although it was unrealistic to expect federal support to produce massive changes in the size of the nursing workforce in a short time, the impact over the decade had been appreciable.

■ MAGNET HOSPITALS: ATTRACTION AND RETENTION OF PROFESSIONAL NURSES (1983)

In 1981, the Governing Council of the American Academy of Nursing (AAN) appointed a Task Force on Nursing Practice in Hospitals, charging it "to examine characteristics of systems impeding and/or facilitating professional nursing practice in hospitals." The prestigious nurse administrators who comprised the taskforce chose to focus on those hospitals across the country that seemed to have created nursing practice organizations that served as "magnets" for professional nurses; that is, they were able to attract and retain a staff of well-qualified nurses and consistently provided high-quality care.

Specific criteria were as follows: Nurses considered the hospital a good place to work and practice; the hospital had the ability to recruit and retain professional nurses; and it was in a geographic area in which it had competition for staff. The Center for Health Care Research and Evaluation (CHCRE) at the School of Nursing, the University of Texas at Austin, was selected as the site for data collection, tabulation, and analysis.

A total of 165 institutions were nominated; the final sample was 41. The magnet hospitals were primarily private, nonprofit institutions, with the majority in the 201- to 700-bed range. The occupancy rate was 72 to 98 percent. The educational preparation of the directors of nursing was primarily at the master's level, with about 12 percent holding doctorates and about 7 percent baccalaureates. Associates or clinical directors were also primarily prepared at the master's or doctorate level, although 19 percent held no degree. About one-half of the head nurses and about 43 percent of the area supervisors held no degree. The taskforce members conducted interviews of selected staff and the nurse executive. The staff nurses' responses revealed the importance of high standards, clearly enunciated, with adequate administrative support to ensure that standards can be met. Specifically, they expressed the importance of the visibility, accessibility, and support of the director of nursing; participatory management; decentralized responsibility; and low patient-to-RN ratios, with qualified staff, and consultation from clinical specialists. Personnel policies that reflect the hospitals' concern with employees' needs and interests were also stressed, as were opportunities for professional practice. These opportunities included involvement in community outreach, development and operation of a career ladder, and opportunities to teach patients and families.

The nurse administrators, although taking more of a conceptual view and being somewhat more abstract in answering the same questions, seemed to agree almost entirely with the staff nurses about what created the positive environment that made their nursing services a magnet for RNs.

The report concluded that change was possible, because some of these hospitals had enjoyed magnet status for some time, whereas others had changed rather dramatically in a relatively short time prior to the study. This positive change seemed to have followed a change in key leadership people such as the hospital administrator and the director of nursing.

Although the magnet hospitals had certain differences, there were also critical similarities. A key point was that there was a "fit" of vision and competence between the nurse administrator and the hospital's chief executive officer (and presumably the board of trustees). Without such a balanced power structure, change cannot occur.[23]

By the early 1990s, the magnet hospital study gave birth to the Magnet Recognition Program of the American Nurses Credentialing Center (ANCC). This program recognizes quality patient care, nursing excellence, and innovations in professional nursing practice. Magnet Recognition provides consumers with the ultimate benchmarks to recognize the quality of care that they have the right to expect from a health care organization. The original Magnet research study of 1983 identified 14 characteristics that differentiate organizations that were best able to recruit and retain nurses during the shortages of the time. These characteristics became the ANCC Forces of Magnetism and provide the conceptual framework for today's Magnet appraisal process.

■ NURSING AND NURSING EDUCATION: PUBLIC POLICIES AND PRIVATE ACTIONS (1983)

The findings of this significant study, mandated by Public Law 96-76, the Nurse Training Act Amendments of 1979 (NTA), and contracted to the IOM by the DHHS, were presented in 1983. A 6-month interim report in July 1981 had raised strong protests in the nursing community, and there were some adjustments in the final report.

The original purpose of this study was in some ways similar to that of the Abt study in that it was prompted by the question of whether further substantial outlays for nursing education were needed to ensure an adequate supply of nurses. However, it went further. As expressed in the legislative history, the intent of the mandate was to secure an objective assessment of the need for continued federal support, to make recommendations for improving the distribution of nurses in medically underserved areas, and to suggest actions to encourage nurses to remain active in their profession.

The study committee was composed of institute members and recognized experts in public policy and disciplines related to nursing. Out of the 26 members, only 9 were nurses. The study's findings were based primarily on the synthesis and interpretation of data secured from existing sources. This became a controversial point when the interim report was released, because much of the data, though garnered from open hearings, contained very different recommendations than when originally presented. Criticism by the nursing field focused primarily on the fact that, as compared to the GMENAC committee, controlled by physicians, here nurses were in the minority, which could suggest "a view of nursing as an occupation that is not clinically valued and that must have others assume leadership and major input in making recommendations regarding what is best for it."[24]

Moreover, although no actual recommendations were made, certain statements were interpreted to mean that the IOM committee tended to see nursing in relation to resource allocation and cost rather than quality. There was the implication that the minimum baccalaureate degree advocated by those in the nursing field might result in increased salaries, fewer nurses, and a lower quality of care. A major concern, of course, was that the IOM report, being mandated by Congress, would also greatly influence legislation affecting nursing when nursing education and research were both highly dependent on federal funds.

Whether or not these statements were only intended to raise questions for further exploration, or whether nursing's negative attitude toward the report or the follow-up of additional data from varied sources affected the attitude of some members of the committee, may never be known. Nevertheless, the final report presented some farsighted recommendations. Significantly, the addition of considerable new information received in the interim between the reports was noted.

The recommendations had a major impact on nursing. For instance, within 6 months, legislation was introduced to place a National Institute of Nursing within the National Institutes of Health. The 1985 legislation creating the National Center for Nursing Research and later legislation finally resulting in the National Institute of Nursing Research were the culmination of these initiatives. This unprecedented action can be directly traced to the IOM statement that lack of adequate funding for nursing research had inhibited the development of nursing investigations, and that the federal government should establish an organizational entity in the mainstream of scientific investigation.

The recommendations of the IOM panel focused on the following:

1. Alleviation of the shortages and maldistribution of nurses
2. An increase in financial aid for students and the development of recruitment strategies to attract a variety of nontraditional students
3. Improvement of employment conditions
4. Expansion of the federal government's support of graduate education for nurses and NP education
5. More emphasis on the education for, and practice of, geriatric nursing
6. Federal establishment of an organizational entity to place nursing research in the mainstream of scientific investigation
7. Further research on the knowledge and competencies of nurses with various levels of education and practice
8. Continued federal support for the collection and analysis of timely data on the national nursing supply, education, and practice.[25]

A surprisingly large number of these recommendations were acted on in the next decade, except that federal funding was not forthcoming to the extent recommended.

■ THE NATIONAL COMMISSION ON NURSING STUDY (1983)

The National Commission on Nursing was formed as an independent commission sponsored by the AHA, the Hospital Research and Educational Trust, and the American Hospital Supply Corporation. Composed of 30 leaders in the fields of nursing, hospital management, medicine, government, academia, and business, it was charged, during its 3-year charter, with developing and implementing action plans to provide practical solutions for institutions and organizations confronting nursing problems. One-half of the group were nurses. In part because of its sponsorship and because a hospital administrator (distinguished though he was) was chairman, organized nursing at first regarded the National Commission with some suspicion. Once more, there was concern about a non-nursing-sponsored group potentially making decisions about nursing. Yet the commission did, indeed, prove to be an independent entity. With a respected nurse as staff director, the commission began, like the IOM group, to study data about nursing, relying primarily on the literature, policy statements, surveys and studies, and hearings.

Those in the nursing field received the *Initial Report and Preliminary Recommendations*, published in September 1981, with considerable enthusiasm and perhaps some astonishment. The report was seen as much more positive than the IOM report of the same period.

In summary, the key recommendations focused on nurses and physicians participating in a collaborative relationship in which nurses are included in clinical decision making and have authority and responsibility for their own practice; administrators establishing a suitable practice environment, including involvement of the nurse administrator as part of the top management team; the establishment of salaries, benefits, and educational opportunities for nurses commensurate with their responsibilities as professionals; the need for diverse nursing constituencies to join together to formulate and support common policies in education, credentialing, and standards of practice; the promotion of accessibility and educational mobility in higher education through educational articulation for undergraduate nurses and RNs; the continuation of funding for nursing education; the appropriate utilization of nurses related to the competency obtained in the specific educational program; collaboration between educational institutions and practice agencies to provide good clinical experience for students, practice opportunities for faculty, and continuing education for RNs; and the implementation and maintenance of nationally accepted standards for licensure. On the controversial issue of baccalaureate education for professional nursing practice, it was seen as a "desirable goal," with consideration given to regional differences in the availability of programs, funds, faculty, and students. Specific goals for each set of recommendations were presented, with concomitant demonstration and research projects recommended.[26]

As noted, nursing generally responded favorably to the *Initial Report.* So did the AMA. The AHA, however, received negative reactions from a number of their constituent organizations and administrators. In the interim between the initial and final reports, the National Commission published the results of a survey of innovative nursing programs and projects, and sponsored an invitational conference to learn about evolving trends and innovative approaches to nursing in hospitals, to which chief executive officers, trustees, medical directors, and chief nurses from hospitals with successful models came as a team and discussed strategies and solutions to nursing problems.

When the final report was released, some disappointment by nurses was inevitable because certain recommendations were seen as less strong. For instance, in relation to nursing education, the recommendations were more muted than those in the initial report advocating the baccalaureate degree for professional nursing practice, instead also supporting all types of education programs and stressing educational mobility.[27]

Omitted was the statement urging appropriate utilization of nurses according to educational background. On the other hand, a new recommendation strongly urged that a high priority be given to nursing research and to the preparation of nurse researchers.[28]

Why the changes? New data, new analysis, and new discussion might be one answer. But another is pragmatic: Nurses alone cannot bring about recommended changes, however desirable they may be; they need the cooperation of physicians and hospital administrators—especially to support changes in the practice setting. The fine art of compromise is necessary to get most plans moving, and the National Commission was certainly concerned that its work not be filed away as simply another report never acted on, particularly because one of the primary motives for the study was the nursing shortage, which by 1983 was no longer considered serious (although a more severe nursing shortage reemerged a few years later).

The chairman summarized their conclusions:

> . . . if we are going to make any progress at all, the first priority would seem to be better educated, more highly qualified nurses; reformed relationships among health professionals; and new types of organizational structures. Action must be long-range. Short-term solutions alone are difficult and costly; they hamper nursing's ability to keep up with the present, let alone prepare for the future.[29]

By the mid-1980s, there was talk of another national nursing shortage. This time, it occurred against the backdrop of turbulent changes in the health care system such as prospective payment for Medicare and Medicaid, a rising number of patients needing high-tech care or treatment of chronic illness, spiraling health care costs, and a federal budget deficit that limited the availability of funds for all federal health care initiatives. As a result, health care providers faced severe financial and resource constraints, and nurses (along with other health care personnel) struggled to meet the demands of a caseload of patients with higher acuity levels than ever before. The supply of nurses seemed unable to meet the quality and quantity of the new types of demand. Some aspects of the nursing shortage stemmed from characteristics of the profession that had always made recruitment difficult, and some originated beyond nursing, within the context of the health care system and society in general.

Thus, in the mid-1980s, several public and private agencies launched studies to examine the extent of the nursing shortage, the characteristics of the nurse supply, and recommendations for the future. Many of the studies were based on and often made reference to the earlier landmark studies of the 1980s, especially the reports of the National Commission and the IOM. These studies from the late 1980s are reviewed in the following.

■ OFFICE OF TECHNOLOGY ASSESSMENT STUDY OF NURSE PRACTITIONERS, PHYSICIAN ASSISTANTS, AND CERTIFIED NURSE-MIDWIVES (1986)

In December 1986, the Office of Technology Assessment (OTA) issued Health Technology Case Study 37, *Nurse Practitioners, Physician Assistants, and Certified Nurse-Midwives: A Policy Analysis*. The study was prepared in response to a request by the Senate Committee on Appropriations to update a previous OTA case study, *The Cost and Effectiveness of Nurse Practitioners*. The advisory panel of 21 experts with backgrounds in health policy, medical economics, health insurance, medicine, nursing, and consumer advocacy based its final report on an extensive review of the literature and consultation with many individuals who were knowledgeable about NP, PA, and CNM practice. Basically, the panel found that

> . . . these practitioners have not been used to their fullest potential. Major obstacles to the greater employment and appropriate use of NPs, PAs, and CNMs are that most third-party payers do not cover . . . the provision by NPs, PAs, and CNMs of many services that are typically and characteristically provided by physicians, and, in those instances where third party payers do cover the services of NPs, PAs, and CNMs, the payments are most often indirect (i.e., to the employing physicians or institutions) rather than direct (i.e., to the NPs or CNMs).
>
> Moreover, NPs and CNMs are more adept than physicians at providing services that depend on communication with patients and preventive actions. . . . Patients are generally satisfied with the quality of care provided by NPs, PAs, and CNMs, particularly with the interpersonal aspects of care.[30]

Although nursing welcomed this report, the AMA was not enthusiastic.[31] However, in the interest of patient welfare, the need to negotiate nursing and medical roles in a rapidly changing health care environment was evident.[32]

■ SECRETARY'S COMMISSION ON NURSING (1988)

In 1987, in response to reports of widespread difficulties recruiting RNs, Health and Human Services Secretary Otis R. Bowen, MD, established the Secretary's Commission on Nursing (SCON). He directed this 25-member panel to advise him on problems related to the recruitment and retention of RNs, and to develop recommendations on how the public and private sectors could work together to implement immediate and long-range solutions for enhancing the adequacy of the supply of RNs.

The SCON report was important for several reasons. First, it documented the pervasiveness and seriousness of the nursing shortage. It also reinforced the themes of previous nursing studies in pushing for improvements in the working conditions and status of nurses. However, perhaps because of the seriousness of the nursing shortage at the time, its tone was more emphatic than that of previous studies with regard to the need to actively promote nursing's unique role in the health care delivery system and to ensure the participation of nurses in policy formation and clinical decision making.

Based on its Interim Report of July 1988, the commission concluded that the shortage of RNs was widespread, cutting across all health care delivery settings. Furthermore, the shortage was primarily a result of increased demand as opposed to a contraction of supply, with projections into the future indicating a continued imbalance between supply and demand. The commission's final report included 16 specific recommendations with 81 directed strategies designed to alleviate the shortage and ensure a healthy nurse labor market in the future.

With regard to the utilization of nursing resources, the recommendations called for the provision of adequate support services for nurses, utilization of the most appropriate mix of nursing personnel, and adoption of labor-saving technologies, such as automated information, to increase RN productivity and improve internal management of nurse resources.

In the area of nurse compensation, the commission members urged health care delivery organizations to increase RN compensation by providing a one-time adjustment to increase RN relative wages, implement innovative compensation options for nurses, and expand pay ranges based on experience, performance, education, and demonstrated leadership.

As for nurse decision making, the commission recommended that nurses have greater representation on policy-making, regulatory, and accreditation bodies. Such representation would facilitate nurses in making unique, critical, and effective contributions to the health care delivery system. Furthermore, the panel members urged employers, as well as the medical profession, to recognize the appropriate clinical decision-making authority of nurses in relationship to other health care professionals.

Noting the downturn in nursing school enrollments during the mid-1980s and its implications for the future supply of nurses, SCON also offered recommendations aimed at facilitating the education of nurses.[33]

COMMONWEALTH FUND: WHAT TO DO ABOUT THE NURSING SHORTAGE (1989)

Responding to the severe nursing shortage in the mid-1980s, when between 1984 and 1986 the average vacancy rate for nursing positions in hospitals increased from 11 to 20 percent, the Commonwealth Fund conducted a national nursing study. The Commonwealth Fund report explored why the shortage existed when the number of nurses per capita was at an "all-time high" and the number of hospital beds continued to decline.[34]

Although the study's conclusions and recommendations were similar to those of other national studies, the methodology was different. Basically assuming that nursing "labor markets were highly local and variable," the researchers collected in-depth data for six major metropolitan areas: Boston, Chicago, Houston, Los Angeles, New York, and Pittsburgh. The investigators urged hospitals to provide more-desirable compensation packages and encouraged organizations involved with education to develop programs that would "make nursing a more available and desirable career."[35]

NATIONAL COMMISSION ON NURSING IMPLEMENTATION PROJECT (1991)

The National Commission of Nursing Implementation Project (NCNIP) was launched by the Tri-Council (ANA, NLN, AACN, and American Organization of Nurse Executives) with Kellogg Foundation funding to implement select recommendations of the 1983 studies on nursing from the Institute of Medicine and the National Commission on Nursing. Vivien De-Back, PhD, RN, was project director. Representatives from other health care, consumer, and business groups joined the nursing organizations to form a 12-member governing body.[36]

The publication of *Nursing's Vital Signs* was intended as an "information collage" rather than an "end of project report," and included descriptions of "innovative approaches and experiences for nurses in practice, education, and research to help them stay in step with change."[37] One of the most significant outcomes was the development of the 3-year *multimedia advertising campaign* to improve the image of nursing. The Ad Council directed the campaign, which was expected to yield $20 million in donated media time and space. This successful National Nursing Image Campaign was seen as partially responsible for increasing nursing school enrollment. A number of conferences were also held on differentiated practice (nursing assignments according to competence, experience, and educational background), and nursing informatics.

COMMISSION ON THE NATIONAL NURSING SHORTAGE (1991)

In 1990, DHHS Secretary Louis Sullivan, MD, signed a 1-year charter for a new 15-member Commission on the National Nursing Shortage (CONNS). He appointed a nurse and health researcher, Caroline Bagley Burnett, MSN, ScD, as executive director, as well as 11 other members.

The CONNS charter extended from February 1990 to June 1991.[38] Over that time period CONNS analyzed ongoing public and private sector initiatives related to three focal areas.

The first initiative related to the focal areas of recruitment, educational pathways, retention, and career was a project to identify long-term care facilities that participate in career development or have such programs, examine their strategies, and document their effectiveness in recruiting and retaining personnel. The second was to identify the variables contributing to successful recruitment and retention, somewhat like the AAN's Magnet Hospital study, and the third involved data collection and analysis requirements. CONNS developed a number of recommendations for the three focal areas, somewhat reiterating recommendations made by previous groups studying the same shortage problems. They also recommended continued monitoring of activities emanating from their recommendations and projects.

Perhaps because the nursing shortage seemed to ease or because it takes time to flesh out such projects and receive government funding, the follow-through on recommendations was not what CONNS would have wanted. Momentum was indeed lost.

HEALTH PROFESSIONS EDUCATION FOR THE FUTURE: SCHOOLS IN SERVICE TO THE NATION (1993–Pew Health Professions Commission No. 1)

This report by the Pew Health Professions Commission, funded by the Pew Charitable Trusts, was a follow-up to its

1991 report that declared that the education and training in the health professions were not adequate to meet the health care needs of the American people. Two years later, the commission was even more convinced that professional education was out of sync with the health care system that was emerging. The commission considered the need for change in the allied health professions, dentistry, medicine, nursing, pharmacy, public health, health care administration, and veterinary medicine, and presented both general strategies and recommendations that related to all the health professions and others specific to each profession.

It was pointed out that during the 1980s and early 1990s, each of the major professional groups had been studied by a variety of influential bodies. Their recommendations concerning education included many of the themes advanced by the Pew Commission. Yet nothing much happened to implement these recommendations. Why? Among other things, professional identity and territoriality, a stagnant mindset, the lack of institutional rewards for changed behavior, and the tendency to preserve tradition rather than risk change were all seen as obstacles. "Change is not the natural vocation of most who have selected an academic career."[39]

In relation to nursing, a greater diversity in nursing— racial, ethnic, and gender—was seen as a plus, along with the trend toward higher education. The value of CNMs and NPs as important sources of primary care was noted, as was the important role of nurses in care of the aging population, health promotion and disease prevention, providing cost-effective care, and management of care. The multiple educational pathways into the professions were seen as an asset, as was nursing's community orientation in education and practice.

The commission proposed six strategies for nursing education, placing "great emphasis on nursing's proven ability to integrate care by working with a variety of social service providers in the community and linking together teams that effectively meet the health care needs of the public."[40]

■ REFORMING HEALTH CARE WORK-FORCE REGULATION: POLICY CONSIDERATIONS FOR THE TWENTY-FIRST CENTURY (1995–Pew Health Professions Commission No. 2)

The second phase of the work of the Pew Health Professions Commission resulted in a report by the Taskforce on Health Care Workforce Regulation. The Taskforce, a separate group selected to conduct this study, consisted of eight members involved with regulation, international health manpower, and consumer groups, as well as health policy analysts. No health professionals were involved.

The group began its work by discussing and articulating a set of principles for a health care workforce regulatory system and stated the belief that the regulation of the health care workforce would best serve the public interest by

- Promoting effective health outcomes and protecting the public from harm;
- Holding regulatory bodies accountable to the public;
- Respecting consumers' rights to choose their health care providers from a range of safe options;
- Encouraging a flexible, rational, and cost-effective health care system that allows effective working relationships among health care providers; and
- Facilitating professional and geographic mobility of competent providers.[41]

The interest in, and concern about, health care personnel credentialing seems to make periodic appearances. In the early 1970s, a number of blue-ribbon panels, committees, and taskforces were formed for the same purposes, with strong federal government involvement. These are described in considerable detail in the fifth edition of this book.[42] Although the recommendations of 1977 were an impetus for a number of changes in the credentialing process, for example, sunset laws for licensure boards, there were also strong objections by the various professions. Then, the federal government, with a new administration, seemed to lose interest in pursuing the issues. Periodically, some controversial issue, such as institutional licensure, again has reared its head, but this Pew Taskforce was the first in about 20 years to consider the topic so thoroughly. Nursing did create a taskforce to study credentialing in nursing in 1979 (discussed earlier in this chapter), but its primary recommendation for a multi-organizational credentialing center was not acceptable to most other nursing organizations.

The ANA and other nursing organizations had strong criticisms of the 1977 report, and again had some strong disagreements about the Pew recommendations. The ANA did agree that health care workforce regulation could benefit from a thorough examination of its current functioning and supported some of the proposals. The major objections raised were in relation to the vagueness of the goals and the lack of specific means to achieve them. The

National Council of State Boards of Nursing (NCSBN) took another tack. This group cited the advances nursing had made in relation to each recommendation.

The reader should be alerted that the Pew recommendations relate to health care workforce regulation in general. The entire Pew Report is too detailed to be discussed here, but should be studied because of the potential impact on credentialing. The eighth edition of *Dimensions of Professional Nursing* includes an overview of the ANA and NCSBN's critique and comments.

Just what long-term follow-up there will be to this report is not yet clear. However, Pew did fund three projects in regulatory reform: Maine, Southern Regional Education Board (SREB), and Citizen Advocacy Center (CAC). Earlier, Pew gave grants to several states for broad inquiry into workforce and health care reform. Indirectly this Pew study may have significantly influenced growth of the nurse licensure compact (NLC), which is operative in 23 states as of 2010 (see Chapter 20).

■ CRITICAL CHALLENGES: REVITALIZING THE HEALTH PROFESSIONS FOR THE TWENTY-FIRST CENTURY (1995–Pew Health Professions Commission No. 3)

In the continuing effort to "assist workforce policymakers and educational institutions to produce health care workers who meet the changing needs of the American health care system," the Pew Health Professions Commission presented this third report, which immediately followed the report on credentialing. It was noted that within another decade, 80 to 90 percent of the insured population in the United States will receive its care through integrated systems that combine primary, specialty, and hospital services.[43] These circumstances create some "realities" cited as affecting the nation's 10 million health care workers, such as the closure of possibly 60 percent of hospital beds; massive expansion in ambulatory and community settings; surpluses in the supply of physicians, nurses, and pharmacists; consolidation of the over 200 allied health professions into multi-skilled areas of practice; demands for public health professionals to meet the needs of the market-driven health care system; and fundamental alterations in the way health professions schools organize, structure, and frame their programs of education, research, and patient care.[44]

The commission made recommendations to all health professionals in general, and specifically to allied health, dentistry, medicine, nursing, pharmacy, and public health. For all health professions,

1. All health professional schools must *enlarge* the scientific bases of their educational programs to include the psychosocial-behavioral sciences and population and health management sciences in an evidence-based approach to clinical work.

2. Although legitimate areas of specialized study should remain the domain of individual professional training programs, key areas of preclinical and clinical training must be *integrated* as a whole, across professional communities, through increased sharing of clinical training resources, more cross-teaching, more exploration of the various roles played by professionals, and the active modeling of effective team integration in the delivery of efficient, high-quality care.

3. The next generation of professionals must *be prepared* to practice in more intensively managed and integrated systems. Specifically, the clinicians of the future will be required to use sophisticated information and communications technology to promote health and prevent disease, to sharpen their skills in areas ranging from clinical prevention to health education to the effective use of political reforms to change the burden of disease, to be more customer or consumer focused, and to be ready to move into new roles that ask them to strike an equitable balance between resources and needs.

4. There is a substantial body of literature that concludes that culturally sensitive care is good care. This means two things for all health professional schools. First, they must *continue* their commitment to ensuring that the students they train represent the rich ethnic diversity of our society. Important investments and many successes have been achieved, but this is an obligation that must be continued at each institution until it is no longer an issue. Second, *diversifying* the entering class is not sufficient to ensure understanding and appreciation of diversity. Cultural sensitivity must be a part of the educational experience that touches the life of every student.

5. Every professional school must be willing to *develop* partnerships and alliances that have not been a part of education in the past—partnerships with managed care for training, clinical research, and tertiary care referrals; with computer and software companies to develop information and communications systems; with integrated systems to support health services research; and

with state government to determine the best ways to meet the health needs of the public.

6. All health professions must *recognize* that the current health professions regulatory system needs to change. Health professionals must work with state legislators and regulators to ensure that regulation is standardized where appropriate, accountable to the public, flexible enough to support optimal access to a competent workforce, and effective and efficient in protecting and promoting the public's health, safety, and welfare.[44,45]

For nursing,

- *Recognize* the value of the multiple entry points to professional practice available to nurses through preparation in associate, baccalaureate, and master's programs; each is different, and each has important contributions to make in the changing health care system.

- *Consolidate* the professional nomenclature so that there is a single title for each level of nursing preparation and service.

- *Distinguish* between the practice responsibilities of these different levels of nursing, focusing associate preparation on the entry-level hospital setting and nursing home practice; baccalaureate on the hospital-based case management and community-based practice; and master's degree for specialty practice in the hospital and independent practice as a primary care provider.

- *Strengthen* existing career ladder programs to make movement through these levels of nursing as easy as possible.

- *Reduce* the size and number of nursing education programs (1470 basic nursing programs as of 1990) by 10 to 20 percent. These closings should come in associate and diploma degree programs. These closings should pay attention to the reality that many areas have a shortage of educational programs and many more have a surplus.

- *Encourage* the expansion of the number of master's level NP training programs by increasing the level of federal support for students.

- *Develop* new models of integration between education and the highly managed and integrated systems of care that can provide nurses with appropriate training and clinical practice opportunities, and can model flexible work rules that encourage continual improvement, innovation, and health care work redesign.

- *Recover* the clinical management role of nursing and recognize it as an increasingly important strength of training and professional practice at all levels.[46]

The ANA, although noting that many of the recommendations were "timely and laudable," considered some of those related to nursing "controversial." The major objections were to Recommendations 3 and 4. First, David Keepnews, a nurse attorney and director of the ANA Office of Policy, refuted the assumption that there was or would be a surplus of nurses. Although some nurses are having a more difficult time finding suitable positions in hospitals and others are being downsized, he said the reality is that there are not enough qualified nurses hired to give good nursing care to the increasingly sick patients requiring complex care. As health care systems place greater emphasis on profit, the growing need for nursing care is unmet. Moreover, the recommendation about placing AD nurses in entry-level positions to care for those patients ignores the continued need for baccalaureate nurses to be involved in direct clinical care, rather than just managing care. Of additional concern was that there was no proposal on making baccalaureate education more accessible and affordable for AD and diploma nurses, although career ladders were encouraged.

Despite these legitimate concerns voiced by the ANA, the Pew Report is well worth reading. There is a great deal of information about the changing nature of health care, interesting case studies, and useful backup information regarding the recommendations. Because the report includes all the health professions, it also enables nurses to understand better how the changing health care scene affects their colleagues and the issues facing them. A number of noted nurses as well as community and health professions leaders were members of the commission, and substantial resources were put into researching the problems and issues. Whether or not all nurses, or for that matter, other health professionals, agree with the recommendations, these could also have a definite impact on health policy.

■ NURSING STAFF IN HOSPITALS AND NURSING HOMES (1996)

In response to a legislative mandate from Congress, a 15-member IOM committee was charged to "determine whether and to what extent there is need for an increase in the number of nurses in hospitals and nursing homes in order to promote quality patient care and reduce the incidence among nurses of work related injuries and stress."[47] The committee consisted of prominent nurses in nursing education, service, health policy, and consulting, as well as physicians, health care administrators, governmental representatives, and a law professor. Carolyne Davis, a nurse consultant who had also headed the Health Care Financing Administration (HCFA) in a previous administration, was the co-chair. Hearings were held in Washington, DC, and Irvine, California, where representatives from the ANA, AACN, and the American Organization of Nurse Executives (AONE), as well as others, testified. There was also an advisory panel of health care and nursing organization representatives.

Although the committee members expressed "shock" at the lack of current data relating to the quality of care in hospitals, they presented a number of key conclusions and recommendations.

Key Conclusions

- The aggregate number of RNs is adequate to meet national needs, but their distribution and mix of educational preparation may not be adequate to meet either the current or future demands of a rapidly changing health care system.
- The roles of RNs in hospitals are changing, requiring increased professional judgment in the management of complex systems of care.
- Nurse assistants, under the direction of RNs, are assuming increased responsibility for direct patient care and often are not trained to do such work.
- A clear need exists to monitor and evaluate the impact of the rapidly changing care delivery systems on the quality of patient care and the well-being of nursing staff.
- Although RN-rich staffing ratios in hospitals are sometimes associated with improved outcomes, they are essentially proxy measures for organizational attributes that grant nurses greater status, autonomy, and control over their practice.
- Although it has improved somewhat in recent years, the quality of nursing home care still leaves much to be desired.
- The shortage of nursing staff at all levels in nursing homes hurts care delivery and leads to increased rates of complications.
- The presence of RNs on all shifts and an RN-rich nursing ratio are related to improved quality of nursing home care and potential long-term cost savings.
- Except for back injuries, especially among nursing assistants in nursing homes, evidence of the linkages between staffing levels and work-related injuries is inconclusive.

Recommendations on Staffing and Quality in Hospitals

Recommendation 1. The committee recommends that hospitals expand the use of RNs with advance practice preparation and skills to provide clinical leadership and cost-effective patient care, particularly for patients with complex management problems.

Recommendation 2. The committee recommends that hospitals have documented evidence that ancillary nursing personnel are competent and that such personnel are tested and certified by an appropriate entity for this competence. The committee further recommends that the training for ancillary nursing personnel working in hospitals be structured and enriched by including training of the following types: appropriate clinical care of the aged and disabled, occupational health and safety measures, culturally sensitive care of the aged and disabled, culturally sensitive care, and appropriate management of conflict.

Recommendation 3. The committee recommends that hospital leaders involve nursing personnel (RNs, LPNs, and nurse's aides [NAs]) who are directly affected by organization redesign and staffing reconfiguration in the process of planning and implementing such changes.

Recommendation 4. The committee recommends that hospital management monitor and evaluate the effects of changes in organizational redesign and reconfiguration of nursing personnel on patient outcomes, patient satisfaction, and nursing personnel themselves.

Recommendation 5. The committee recommends that the National Institute of Nursing Research (NINR) and other appropriate agencies fund scientifically sound research on the relationships between quality of care and nurse staffing levels and mix, taking into account organizational variables. The committee further recommends that the NINR, along with the Agency for Health Care Policy and Research (AHCPR) and private organizations develop a research agenda on quality of care.

Recommendation 6. The committee recommends that an interdisciplinary public-private partnership be organized to develop performance and outcome measures that are sensitive to nursing interventions and care, with uniform definitions that are measurable in a uniform manner across all hospitals.

Recommendations on Staffing and Quality in Nursing Homes

Recommendation 1. The committee recommends that Congress require by 2000 a 24-hour presence of RN coverage in nursing facilities as an enhancement of the current 8-hour requirement specified under the 1987 Omnibus Budget Reconciliation Act (OBRA 87). It further recommends that payment levels for Medicare and Medicaid be adjusted to enable such staffing to be achieved.

Recommendation 2. The committee recommends that nursing facilities use geriatric nurse specialists and geriatric NPs in both leadership and direct care positions.

Recommendation 3. The committee recommends that the training for nurse assistants in nursing homes be structured and enriched by including training in the following: appropriate clinical care of the aged and disabled, occupational health and safety measures, culturally sensitive care, and appropriate management of conflict.

Recommendation 4. The committee recommends that research efforts on staffing levels and skill mix specifically address the relationship of LPNs and nurse assistants to quality of care.

Recommendation 5. The committee recommends that, in view of the increasing case-mix acuity of residents and the consequent complexity of the care provided, nursing facilities place greater weight on educational preparation in the employment of new directors of nursing.

Recommendation 6. The committee recommends that the Secretary of Health and Human Services fund additional research and demonstration projects on the use of financial and other incentives to improve quality of care and outcomes in nursing homes.

Recommendations on Work-Related Injury and Stress

Recommendation 1. The committee recommends that hospitals and nursing homes develop effective programs to reduce work-related injuries by providing strong leadership, instituting effective training programs for new and continuing workers, and ensuring the appropriate use of existing and emerging technology, including lifting and moving devices and needleless medication delivery systems.

Recommendation 2. The committee recommends that all hospitals and nursing homes screen applicants for patient care positions filled by nurse assistants for past history of abuse of patients and residents, and criminal records.

Major nursing organizations generally endorsed the recommendations and commended the committee for its work. However, some complained that the recommendations lacked "a sense of urgency" in addressing the critical issues affecting quality of care. Although agreeing that more research on how staffing affects the quality of patient care was needed, the ANA maintained that there was enough anecdotal evidence of serious problems from both nurses and consumers. A press release cited reduced RN staffing as a "clear and present danger to all health care consumers," particularly with hospitals' increased reliance on unlicensed personnel to provide a growing range of patient care services. The ANA also called for public accountability of hospitals and other institutions concerning staffing mix, credentials, and patient outcomes.

The AONE noted that, as health care is increasingly being delivered outside the hospital, nurses and others are moving into these settings and must be functional to serve patients in new ways. Within institutions, more efficient ways must be found to provide care. One aspect cited was freeing nurses from tasks not requiring professional expertise, such as delivery of food trays.

■ STRENGTHENING HOSPITAL NURSING (1996)

The ongoing concern about the quality of patient care and nursing's role in improving that care triggered several projects funded by major foundations. *Strengthening Hospital Nursing* is a program to improve patient care that is jointly supported by the Robert Wood Johnson Foundation (RWJF) and the Pew Charitable Trusts and concluded in 1996.[48] Fifty-seven hospitals and 23 hospital consortia had been awarded planning grants by the two foundations in 1989. Two years later, 12 hospitals and 8 consortia were chosen from among the original planning grantee pool and were awarded 5-year implementation grants of $1 million each. The hospitals and consortia spanned the nation. Despite the tremendous changes in health care delivery since the end of the 1980s, the principles guiding the grantees as they pursued their projects and achieved related outcomes did not change. These were to

- Create a substantive, shared vision known to everyone at all levels of the organization.
- Commit to a patient-centeredness philosophy for patient care delivery—focusing on the needs of the patient as the common goal of services and interventions provided by caregivers and management.
- Endorse a continuity of care system that provides and integrates consistent, appropriate, and efficacious care across service settings.
- Ensure high-quality and responsive service experiences for patients and caregivers that are satisfying and efficient both for those providing care and those receiving care.

The grantees pursued their goals through various projects, and their activities and outcomes were reported in over 100 publications in nursing and other health care journals, books, and newsletters.[49] The health care organizations had been asked to "foster the development of innovative systems to strengthen patient care through collaborative efforts of all patient care providers."[50] A clear challenge was the ever-present demand in modern health care to "do it better with less." The summaries of the grantees' efforts, presented in the final report, as well as other publications, provide an excellent overview of what can be accomplished, problems notwithstanding.

■ THE QUALITY CHASM SERIES (2000 to 2006)

During the period of 2000 to 2006, a series of 11 research documents from the Institute of Medicine (IOM) proved to Americans that no individual has the assurance of high-quality health care. Health care is plagued with inappropriate utilization of services and errors in practice. The first two reports set aims to achieve quality in health care and propose a plan to redesign a failing system. The needed transformation is substantial given the chasm between what is and what should be. Other reports in this series and all of these works have significant implications for nurses and nursing.

In 2000, the IOM released its landmark report, *To Err Is Human: Building a Safer Health System*. This report revealed that thousands of people were injured by the very health system from which they sought help. Tens of thousands of Americans die each year and hundreds of thousands are injured due to medical errors and incidents and accidents sustained in the delivery system. This report and its companion, *Crossing the Quality Chasm*, "have had

a profound impact on how health care is viewed. The information and perspectives moved conversations regarding patient safety and quality care from inside health care institutions to the mainstream of media, corporate America, and public policy. The reports raised awareness of the depth and complexity of quality challenges and prompted the marked expansion of quality improvement efforts through research and other means."[51]

The most significant barrier to improving patient safety identified in *To Err Is Human* is a "lack of awareness of the extent to which errors occur daily in all health care settings and organizations. This lack of awareness exists because the vast majority of errors are not reported, and errors are not reported because personnel fear they will be punished."[52] While these statements describing the essence of the challenges facing health care are simple and straightforward, the level and complexity of effort needed to address them is not. Since the release of the two reports, broad-based efforts have begun to bring more sophistication and precision to measuring and improving the safety and quality of health care. Nevertheless, substantial work in both academic and practice settings remains to be done.

Since the release of *To Err Is Human* and *Crossing the Quality Chasm*, the IOM has produced nine additional related reports. The IOM Quality Chasm Series (see Table 5–1) includes reports "linking quality to a range of issues, from health professions education, to health care in rural America, to improving health care quality for mental health and substance-abuse systems. Threaded through this series are key concepts of the framework presented in the original two reports. In each report, facets of the framework are expanded or applied to specific populations or system characteristics. The language of most of the reports tends to group members of health care disciplines by the terms "providers" or "clinicians," with an occasional mention of specific professional groups such as medicine or nursing. Generally speaking, the content of the reports is directly or indirectly applicable to all health care professionals. Consequently, each of the 11 reports has implications for aspects of nursing practice, research, education, and public policy engagement."[53]

The series describes external drivers that can improve the safety and quality of health care, including nursing care. External drivers that influence the quality of nursing care include regulation and legislation, accrediting organizations, efforts to link payment with performance, the need for interdisciplinary collaboration, the commitment of professional organizations, and public engagement.

■ **TABLE 5–1. The IOM Quality Chasm Series**

To Err Is Human: Building a Safer Health System, 2000[54]

Crossing the Quality Chasm, 2001[55]

Leadership by Example: Coordinating Government Roles in Improving Health Care Quality, 2002[56]

Fostering Rapid Advances in Health Care: Learning From Systems Demonstrations, 2002[57]

Priority Areas for National Action: Transforming Health Care Quality, 2003[58]

Health Professions Education: A Bridge to Quality, 2003[59]

Patient Safety: Achieving a New Standard for Care, 2003[60]

Keeping Patients Safe: Transforming the Work Environment of Nurses, 2004[61]

Quality Through Collaboration: The Future of Rural Health Care, 2004[62]

Preventing Medication Errors: Quality Chasm Series, 2006[63]

Improving the Quality of Health Care for Mental and Substance-Use Conditions: Quality Chasm, Series, 2006[64]

■ COLLEAGUES IN CARING (2002)

Colleagues in Caring, a national program funded by the RWJF, was initiated in 1996. The intent of this program was to control the market-driven changes in health care that create periodic shortages—surpluses in the nurse workforce. The key is seen as regional/local collaboration among all levels of nursing practice and education. The program is based on the assumption that most of the factors underlying nursing care requirements are local in nature, such as the employment market, demand-need patterns, and population demographics.[65]

Regional recipients of the grant awards were responsible for carrying out five major tasks.

1. Assessing current and projected nursing care needs throughout the area
2. Developing a system for estimating future nursing workforce needs
3. Analyzing the capacity of the region's nursing workforce to meet these needs and of the area's educational infrastructure to produce the numbers and types of nursing professionals required
4. Developing a regional nursing workforce consortium
5. Establishing a formal mechanism to keep the consortium in place over the long term

Within these consortia, there is formal collaboration among all levels of nursing schools to

- Enable individual nurses to pursue a continuum of education throughout their professional careers, from LPN to the doctorate.
- Prepare RNs to meet the regional nursing care needs at all levels.
- Develop a regional cadre of RNs for leadership roles as clinicians, educators, and service managers.
- Develop or refine workplace settings that differentiate the practice of nurses based on the education and experience of its nurses.

Grantees were to receive up to $200,000 over a 3-year period, in addition to providing matching and in-kind support for the project. Grantees were located in Alaska, Arizona, Hawaii, California, Colorado, Connecticut, District of Columbia, Maryland, Minnesota, Mississippi, Missouri, New Jersey, New Mexico, Ohio, South Carolina, South Dakota, Tennessee, Texas, and West Virginia and were joined by a growing number of independently funded program sites that are moving their collaboratives toward implementing permanent systems of nursing workforce planning. The grantees chose various means of achieving their objectives, with some reporting their approach, progress, and results in the literature. Most of these studies were initiated and brought to completion by talented individuals who recognized the importance of acquiring pertinent and timely nursing data.

This dedication and interest in studying the profession will take on even more importance as we acquire new technologies and research capabilities and move forward into the twenty-first century.

■ THE FUTURE OF NURSING (2010)

This was a 2-year effort of the IOM and the RWJF to find solutions to the continuing challenges facing the nursing profession, and to build upon nursing-based solutions to improve quality and transform the way Americans receive health care.

Through its deliberations, this IOM/RWJF committee developed four key messages:

- Nurses should practice to the full extent of their education and training.
- Nurses should achieve higher levels of education and training through an improved education system that promotes seamless academic progression.
- Nurses should be full partners, with physicians and other health care professionals, in redesigning health care in the United States.
- Effective workforce planning and policy making require better data collection and information infrastructure.

This report is designed as a framework for change in the nursing profession and the health care delivery system. Its nurse-led solutions are directed to policy makers, national state and local government leaders, payers, health care researchers, executives and professionals, as well as to licensing bodies, educational institutions, and philanthropic and advocacy groups, especially those representing the consumer. These issues are not new, but deserve to be looked at through a fresh and creative lens of problem solving.[66]

KEY POINTS

1. Studies of the nursing profession provide a rich resource for understanding the evolution of the discipline over time.
2. These studies attest to public and private sector interest in nursing's professional advancement.
3. Despite the rather decisive findings of many of these studies, there has been relatively little ability to influence public policy.
4. The ability of a study to move the profession forward is often very subtle, but real.
5. The cyclical shortages and surpluses in the nursing workforce have generated much government and philanthropic interest.
6. Change is slow, but philanthropy and the profession itself are moving it along more incisively than government.

REFERENCES

1. Goldmark J. *Nursing and Nurse Education in the United States.* New York: Macmillan, 1923.
2. Garling J. Flexner and Goldmark: Why the difference in impact? *Nurs Outlook* 33:26–31, January–February, 1985.
3. Brown EL. *Nursing for the Future.* New York: Russell Sage Foundation, 1948, p 45.
4. Ibid, pp 132–170.
5. Ibid, pp 48, 178.
6. National Commission for the Study of Nursing and Nursing Education. *An Abstract for Action.* New York: McGraw-Hill, 1970, p 75.
7. Lysaught J. *An Abstract for Action.* New York: McGraw-Hill, 1970.
8. Ibid, pp 156–161.
9. Report of the Task Force. *Nurs Outlook* 21:111–118, February 1973.
10. Lysaught J. *From Abstract into Action.* New York: McGraw-Hill, 1973.
11. Nurse and medical practice act must permit flexibility, NJPC says. *Am J Nurs* 74:602, April 1974.
12. Lysaught J, Christ MA, Hagopian G. Progress in professional service: Nurse leaders queried. *Hospitals* 52:120, August 16, 1978.
13. US Department of Health, Education, and Welfare. *Extending the Scope of Nursing Practice.* Washington, DC: US Department of Health, Education, and Welfare, 1971, p 2.
14. Ibid, p 4.
15. *The study of credentialing in nursing: A new approach.* A report of the committee (mimeographed). Milwaukee, WI: University of Wisconsin, January 1979, p 3.
16. Ibid, pp 82–92.
17. de Tornyay R. *Report of the meeting convened by the task force on credentials in nursing.* Kansas City, MO: American Nurses Foundation, 1983.
18. Lum J. WICHE panel of expert consultants report: Implications for nursing leaders. *J Nurs Admin* 9:11–19, July 1979.
19. *Report of the Graduate Medical Education National Advisory Committee to the Secretary, Department of Health and Human Services, volume 7.* Washington, DC: US Department of Health and Human Services, 1981.
20. Wandelt M, Pierce PM, Widdowson RR. *Conditions Associated With Registered Nurse Employment in Texas.* University of Texas at Austin: Center for Research, School of Nursing, 1980.

21. Wandelt M, Pierce PM, Widdowson RR. Why nurses leave nursing and what can be done about it. *Am J Nurs* 81: 72–77, January 1981.

22. Ibid.

23. Task Force on Nursing Practice in Hospitals. *Magnet Hospitals: Attraction and Retention of Professional Nurses.* Kansas City, MO: American Academy of Nursing, 1983.

24. Jacox A. Significant questions about IOM's study of nursing. *Nurs Outlook* 31:28–33, January–February 1983.

25. Nursing and Nursing Education. *Public Policies and Private Actions.* Washington, DC: National Academy Press, 1983, pp 1–23.

26. National Commission on Nursing. *Initial report and preliminary recommendation.* Chicago: National Commission on Nursing, 1981, p 5.

27. National Commission on Nursing. *Summary report and recommendations.* Chicago: National Commission on Nursing, 1983, p 15.

28. Ibid, p 11.

29. Ibid, p xi.

30. *Nurse Practitioners, Physician Assistants, and Certified Nurse Midwives: A Policy Analysis.* Washington, DC: Office of Technology Assessment, 1986, pp 5–7.

31. Ibid, p 6.

32. Jacox A. The OTA report: A policy analysis. *Nurs Outlook* 35:262–267, November–December 1987.

33. *Secretary's Commission on Nursing, final report, volume I.* Washington, DC: US Department of Health and Human Services, 1988.

34. Minnick A, Roberts MJ, Curran CR, et al. What do nurses want? Priorities for action. *Nurs Outlook* 37:214–218, September–October 1989.

35. *What to Do about the Nursing Shortage.* New York: The Commonwealth Fund, 1989, p 20.

36. *Nursing's Vital Signs, Shaping the Profession for the 1990s.* Battle Creek, MI: W. K. Kellogg Foundation, 1989, pp 9–13.

37. Ibid, p 9.

38. *Secretary's Commission on the National Nursing Shortage, final report.* Washington, DC: US Department of Health and Human Services, 1992.

39. O'Neil E. *Health Professions Education for the Future: Schools in Service to the Nation.* San Francisco: Pew Health Professions Commission, 1993, p 9.

40. Ibid, p 87.

41. *Reforming Health Care Workforce Regulation.* San Francisco: Pew Health Professions Commission, 1995, p vii.

42. Kelly L. *Dimensions of Professional Nursing.* New York: Macmillan, 1985, pp 440–451.

43. *Critical Challenges: Revitalizing the Health Professions for the Twenty-First Century.* San Francisco: Pew Health Professions Commission, 1995, p v.

44. Ibid.

45. Ibid, p vi.

46. Ibid, pp vi, vii.

47. Wunderlich G, Sloan F, David C. *Nursing Staff in Hospitals and Nursing Homes: Is It Adequate?* Washington, DC: Institute of Medicine, 1996.

48. Donaho B. *Celebrating the Journey: A Final Report.* St. Petersburg, FL: Strengthening Hospital Nursing: A Project to Improve Patient Care, 1996.

49. Ibid, pp 14–15.

50. Ibid, pp 109–114.

51. Kohn LT, Corrigan JM, Donaldson MS, Eds. *To err is human: Building a safer health system.* A report of the Committee on Quality of Health Care in America, Institute of Medicine. Washington, DC: National Academy Press, 2000, p 150.

52. Ibid, p 155.

53. Wakefield M. Chapter 4: The Quality Chasm Series: Implications for Nursing. Washington, DC: National Academy Press. http://www.ahrq.gov/QUAL/nurseshdbk/docs/WakefieldM. Retrieved March 17, 2010.

54. Kohn, loc cit.

55. Institute of Medicine. *Crossing the quality chasm: A new health system for the 21st century.* Washington, DC: National Academies Press, 2001.

56. Institute of Medicine. *Leadership by example: Coordinating government roles in improving health care quality.* Washington, DC: National Academies Press, 2002.

57. Institute of Medicine. *Fostering rapid advances in health care: Learning from systems demonstrations.* Washington, DC: National Academies Press, 2002.

58. Institute of Medicine. *Priority areas for national action: Transforming health care quality.* Washington, DC: National Academies Press, 2003.

59. Institute of Medicine. *Health professions education: A bridge to quality.* Washington, DC: National Academies Press, 2003.

60. Institute of Medicine. *Patient safety: Achieving a new standard for care.* Washington, DC: National Academies Press, 2003.

61. Institute of Medicine. *Keeping patients safe: Transforming the work environment of nurses.* Washington, DC: National Academies Press, 2004.

62. Institute of Medicine. *Quality through collaboration: The future of rural health.* Washington, DC: National Academies Press, 2005.

63. Institute of Medicine. *Preventing medication errors: Quality chasm series.* Washington, DC: National Academies Press, 2006.

64. Institute of Medicine. *Improving the quality of health care for mental and substance-use conditions: Quality chasm series.* Washington, DC: National Academies Press, 2005.

65. Colleagues in Caring Project. http://www.aacn.nche.edu/CaringProject/about.htm/. Accessed June 17, 2002.

66. Robert Wood Johnson Foundation. Initiative on the Future of Nursing. http://www.rwjf.org/humancapital. Retrieved October 12, 2010.

HELPFUL WEBSITES FOR PART I

Agency for Health Research and Quality (AHRQ): http://www.ahrq.gov

American Association for the History of Medicine (AAHM): http://www.histmed.org

American Association for the History of Nursing, Nursing History Review: http://www.aahn.org/nhr.html

American Historical Association: http://www.theaha.org

American Nurses Association Centennial Exhibit: Voices from the Past, Visions of the Future: http://www.ana.org/centenn/index.htm

American Nurses Association Hall of Fame: http://www.ana.org/hof/index.htm

Archives of Nursing Leadership: http://www.nursing.uconn.edu/archive.html

Army Nurse Corps: http://www.army.mil/cmh-pg/anc/anchhome.html

Black Nurses in History: http://www.umdnj.edu/camlbweb/blacknurses.html

Boston University, The History of Nursing Archives: http://www.bu.edu/speccol/nursing.htm

Carnegie Foundation for the Advancement of Teaching: http://www.carnegiefoundation.org

Clendening History of Medicine Library—Florence Nightingale Resources: http://clendening.kumc.edu/florence

The Commonwealth Fund: http://www.commonwealthfund.org

Florence Nightingale Museum, London: http://www.florence-nightingale.co.uk/

Frontier Nursing Service: http://www.achiever.com/freehmpg/kynurses/fns.html

Images from the History of Medicine: http://www.ihm.nlm.nih.gov/

Institute of Medicine of the National Academies: http://www.iom.edu

The Lycos Network: http://www.members.tripod.com/~DianneBrownson/history.html

Medical History on the Internet: http://www.anes.uab.edu/medhist.htm

Men in American Nursing History: http://www.geocities.com/Athens/Forum/6011/

Nurses in the U.S. Navy—Historical bibliography: http://www.history.navy.mil/faqs/faq50-1.htm

Robert Wood Johnson Foundation: http://www.rwjf.org

The Rockefeller Foundation: http://www.rockefellerfoundation.org

Royal College of Nursing Archives: http://www.rcnscotland.org/Archivuk.htm

University of Connecticut School of Nursing: www.nursing.uconn.edu/nurhis

University of Pennsylvania, School of Nursing, Center for the Study of the History of Nursing: http://www.nursing.upenn.edu/history

University of Virginia, School of Nursing, Center for Nursing Historical Inquiry: http://www.nursing.virginia.edu/centers/history.html

W. K. Kellogg Foundation: http://www.wkkf.org

PART II

Contemporary Professional Nursing

The Health Care Setting

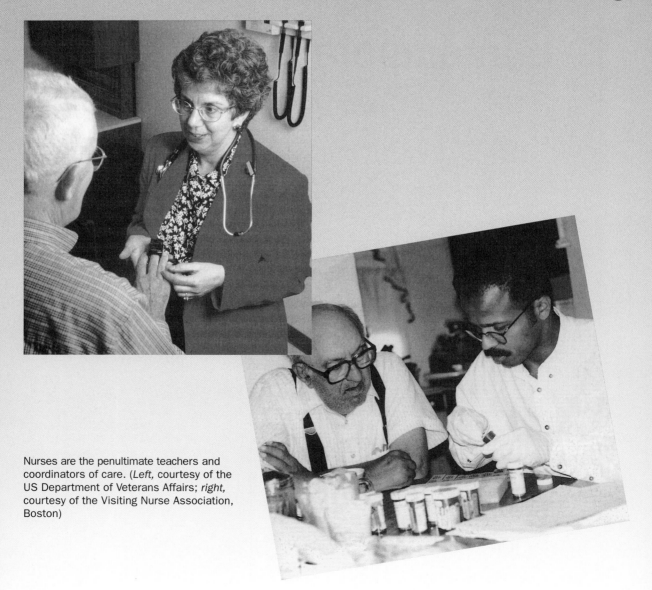

Nurses are the penultimate teachers and coordinators of care. (*Left,* courtesy of the US Department of Veterans Affairs; *right,* courtesy of the Visiting Nurse Association, Boston)

The Impact of Social and Scientific Changes

As a vital social service, and as one of the health professions, the changes, problems, and issues of society affect nursing in general, in addition to those that are specific to health care. Change has become a defining characteristic of our lives as we approach the twenty-first century. In contrast to other times, the direction and nature of today's change is unpredictable, turbulent, and often disarming. Our reliance on trends is inadequate, but the astute observer can identify patterns. This sensitivity to the underlying dynamics of change can determine whether you are in control or being controlled by the times.[1]

Surrounded by constant change, nurses (and others, for that matter) are tempted to ignore its potential effects on the profession or at best to cope with problems only when they become inescapable. Professions that ignore the nature of social change find themselves scrambling to catch up, rather than planning to advance—reacting, rather than acting. When the public justifiably accuses the professions of being unresponsive to their needs, it is, in part, because those professions have not been astute enough to observe emergent patterns of change, or have been too insular to see the necessity of becoming a part of them. It is a luxury that no profession, least of all nursing with its intimate person-to-person contact, can afford. The purpose of this chapter is to review some of the major changes in the last few decades to determine their impact on nursing.

■ A GLOBAL PERSPECTIVE

For a 50-year period that ended with the 1990s, global military and ideological preoccupation caused the diversion of financial, human, and material resources to essentially unproductive purposes. With the collapse of the former Soviet Union and movement to a more cooperative world order, we could no longer hide from the severest consequences of those years of social neglect. Furthermore, where democracy was the choice, there were many hard lessons to be learned before a better life materialized for the majority. Neither could more affluent, industrialized countries dismiss the problems of less-developed countries (LDCs) as belonging to someone else. Modern communications has opened territorial boundaries, challenged old ways, and forced us to realize that as people of this earth, we have some common responsibility for the worldwide human condition. There is a moral imperative to strive for some equitable distribution of the finite and often deteriorating resources at our disposal. There is still much anguish in the world, but also reason to anticipate a much kinder and more equitable future.

In 2000, the United Nations Millennium Development Goals (MDGs) were ratified by the 191 member states of the general assembly (Exhibit 6–1). There will be concerted action to achieve these eight goals by 2015. This declaration commits world leaders to combat poverty, hunger, disease, illiteracy, environmental degradation, and discrimination against women. The MDGs are derived from this declaration, and all have specific targets and indicators.

Health is at the heart of the MDGs. All of the goals either directly or indirectly hold implications for health. Achieving these goals is not possible without progress on food security, gender equality, the empowerment of women, wider access to education, and better stewardship of the environment. At the midpoint between 2000 and 2015, the analysis shows encouraging signs of progress, particularly in child health; it points to areas where current gains need to be sustained (particularly in relation to AIDS, tuberculosis [TB], and malaria) and areas where there has been little or no movement. Data reported for 2009 show major differences in progress between and within countries and regions.

In all, we are left with evidence of a changing world, much for the better . . .[2]

The proportion of undernourished children under 5 years of age declined from 27 percent in 1990 to 20 percent in 2005.

Some 27 percent fewer children died before their fifth birthday in 2007 than in 1990.

Even better gains were documented in infant mortality, from 148 deaths per 1000 live births in 1955 to 59 in 1995, and a projected 29 in 2025.

On average over 80 percent of the world's children are immunized against diphtheria, tetanus, whooping cough, polio, measles, and TB as compared with 5 percent in the 1970s. Some countries boast rates of 90 percent and higher.

Fifty-one million of the world's children are unregistered at birth.

One hundred fifty million children 5 to 14 years old are engaged in child labor.[3]

The proportion of pregnant women in the developing world who had at least one antenatal care visit increased from slightly more than half at the beginning of the 1990s to almost three-quarters a decade later.

The global maternal mortality ratio has barely changed since 1990. Every year an estimated 536,000 women die in pregnancy or childbirth. Most of these deaths occur in sub-Saharan Africa.

Seventy million girls and women in 29 countries have experienced female genital mutilation (FGM). More than 18 percent have had this procedure performed on them by health care providers. This is referred to as the "medicalization of FGM."[4]

One-third of 9.7 million people in developing countries who need treatment for HIV/AIDS were receiving it in 2007.

The MDG target for reducing the incidence of TB was met globally in 2004.

Twenty-seven countries reported a reduction of up to 50 percent in the number of malaria cases between 1990 and 2006.

For developing countries, the good news is that by 2025, infectious diseases such as poliomyelitis, leprosy, guinea worm disease, filariasis, and hepatitis B, which together afflict and disable hundreds of millions of people, will have been eliminated or reduced to very low prevalence levels.[5]

Gaps between the richest and poorest countries remain huge, but are gradually closing, at least in terms of premature deaths. For example, in 1995, 76 percent of people who died in the World Health Organization's (WHO's) African region were under 50. By 2025, the proportion will fall to 57 percent.

The number of people with access to safe drinking water rose from 4.1 billion in 1990 to 5.7 billion in 2006. About 1.1 billion people in developing regions gained access to improved sanitation in the same period.

In 2005, an estimated 1.1 million people died from diabetes.

Almost 80 percent of diabetes deaths occur in low- and middle-income countries.

Almost half of diabetes deaths occur in people under the age of 70 years; 55 percent of those who die from diabetes are women.

WHO projects that diabetes deaths will double between 2005 and 2030.

Clearly, the problem of population growth, a major societal concern for a number of years, is no less urgent now. Between 1955 and 1998, the estimated world population grew from 2.8 to 5.8 billion, or more than doubled, increasing to almost 7 billion in 2010.[6] Annual births have leveled at about 134 million per year since their peak at 163 million in the late 1990s and are expected to remain constant. However, deaths are only around 57 million per year. Because births outnumber deaths, the world's population is expected to reach 9 billion in 2040. The greatest rate of growth continues to be in the LDCs. The People's Republic of China and India represent approximately 37 percent of the world's population, with the nearest challenger being the United States with 309 million or 4.54 percent of the total in April 2010. This is despite the slow but growing success of birth control. WHO reports that although there were only three countries below the population replacement level in 1955, 102 will achieve that status by 2025.[7]

The health of infants and children largely depends on the status of women in a society, and the person who is the most compromised and least empowered on her own behalf is the girl-child. The United Nations' (UN's) Fourth World Conference on Women in Beijing in l995 brought girls into a new position of prominence. This represented the culmination of a long struggle to recognize women's rights throughout their lifespan. The problems of women and the girl-child are reflections of one another and perpetuate a vicious cycle that compromises the advancement of a total society. Seeking to document progress since Beijing, nongovernmental organizations were surveyed during 1998 about progress in the key areas of education, health, negative traditional practices, protection against violence, and economic exploitation. The greatest gains were seen in the girl-child's access to primary education, but they may be transient given the current level of philanthropic and government interest in this area. Progress in secondary education was virtually nonexistent. There is great frustration in trying to improve school retention rates because adolescent girls drop out to marry, bear and raise children, or work, or because they do not see the relevance of what they are learning. The shortage or absence of female teachers to act as role models is a major obstacle.[8] The literate woman has fewer pregnancies and better spacing of children, provides better nutrition for her children, and is more inclined to seek primary care services when they are needed and where they are available.[9]

Good progress is documented in health and nutrition and few gender biases are noted. This seems consistent with reported decreases in mortality and morbidity. Although there have been claims of gender discrepancy in food allocations, there is no significant distinction in nutritional status to support this statement.

The areas of negative traditional practices, violence, and economic exploitation loom as the most threatening to the girl-child, and ironically beg the most for the intervention of government. The life situations that these words signify are varied: FGM, infanticide, commercial sexual exploitation, incest, and more. Even where legislation is in place, enforcement may be weak. It is difficult to determine whether the trend toward urbanization will exacerbate problems of exploitation and violence for the girl-child and women.

Of equal concern is the older woman, who is a product of her life and times. Although women generally live longer than men, it does not mean that these years will be lived free from disability or hold any quality. Many women face old age before their time, given the role that inequality and discrimination have played in their earlier years. Women Watch, the UN Internet gateway on the advancement and empowerment of women, provides good information on the global agenda for women:

www.un.org/womenwatch

With gains in the health of infants and children, the working-age population (aged 20 to 64) is growing and currently represents half of the world's population. There are, however, 15 million deaths yearly from among this group, many of which are preventable. AIDS claims 1.8 million adult lives; TB, 2 to 3 million; and multi-drug resistant HIV-related co-infections and mutant strains of infectious diseases present new threats to health and well-being.[10] This information, combined with the earlier observation that our greatest success in stemming mortality is among the aging and the very young, reaffirms the potential for an ominous dependency ratio.

Further focusing on the issue of family planning, women have been brought to the center of the debate and empowered themselves. The discussion has turned to family planning as a personal right as never before, and nongovernmental organizations that work with women at the local level have proven to be major allies. Critics caution that statements on women's rights and family planning establish battle lines between women and the family. They cautioned that in some cultures the woman literally belongs to the family, and decisions about family are made in that forum. In contrast, because America is a land of immigrants, many Americans have fewer family ties. In many developing countries, the extended family is the only vehicle for survival, and personal choices are subordinated to tradition or common practice. Taking an opposing position or exercising independent choice may cause the woman to be ostracized from the protection of the family. This example is offered to demonstrate the complexity of the issue and the degree to which it strikes at the heart of culture.

> As we begin the 21st century, members of the global community are becoming more alike despite the persistence of pockets of extreme need, and the problems of women are assuming more prominence. The gains that we have experienced can probably trace their origins to the Declaration of Alma-Ata, the culminating statement of a 1978 international conference jointly sponsored by WHO and UNICEF. This pronouncement set the stage for worldwide support of primary care as the vehicle through which to achieve *Health For All.* This was a statement on social justice and had very modest expectations. WHO has recently rekindled its commitment to primary care, seeking to shift a vast proportion of resources invested in cure to a prevention and health promotion agenda, which it anticipates could cut 70% of the world-wide disease burden.[11]

International programs have frequently been the recipients of philanthropic dollars. Usual patterns of giving are seriously challenged by the observation that for change to be successful it must begin at the local level. Furthermore, there is a growing preference for nongovernmental organizations to invest their dollars in places where there is strength on which to build. This is a radical departure from the ethic that has prevailed in international giving over the years.

■ UNITED STATES POPULATION

As of July 2010, the US population was estimated at about 309 million people, 22 million more than in 2002.[12] The 2010 census marks the 220th anniversary of the first census, taken in 1790 when the United States had just under 4 million residents. The 2010 census is barely under way, and promises some interesting comparisons.

The demographic profile of the nation is clearly the result of declining fertility and mortality rates. Baby boomers have moved solidly into their 60s. The median age for the population increased from 32.8 in July 1990 to over 35 in the 2000 census. There were 6.4 million more women than men in 1990, and 5.1 million more in 2000. Women outnumber and outlive men to the extent that 70 percent of women are without the support of a spouse in their declining years, compared with men, only 40 percent of whom find themselves in this predicament. The

greatest future population growth will be among the old-old—those over 85—who numbered 3 million in l994 and are expected to increase to 19 million by 2050.[13] This graying of America is a critical factor when we anticipate the country's future needs for health care.

Ten percent of those over 65 are poor or near poor; women, blacks, and Hispanics have a higher poverty rate. Social security is the major source of support for many. Still, the economic level of the elderly varies widely, with some having income and assets from a variety of sources. More than 22 percent of Americans over 85 live in nursing and convalescent homes. On a given day such facilities are caring for one out of every 20 Americans over 65.[14] Of those who live in these arrangements, a disproportionate number are women, generally unmarried or widowed.

The elderly, better educated than ever, have had a significant influence on legislation. With organizations such as the American Association of Retired Persons (AARP) as their lobbyists, and with politicians' appreciation of their voting power, the elderly are clearly a political force. Given their growing numbers, factors that affect the elderly must be considered in the context of social and political events that affect all Americans.

Each generation is a product of its times. The aged of the turn of the century faced the Great Depression as children, were the patriots of World War II, and knew economic deprivation in a time without social welfare programs. Their natural allies may be today's 30-something young adults. They are alternately called generation X, because at first they defied classification, or the 13ers, being the 13th generation in American history. Their relationship with their parents, the boomers, sets the stage for an intergenerational crisis. They are a generation who inherited the repercussions of the excesses of their elders: a toxic environment, national debt, unemployment, economic recession, AIDS, and recurrent TB. The fact that the Cold War is over hardly seems an even exchange. Many were raised by grandparents of the silent generation or wartime America (the aged in our developing plot), whereas their parents, the boomers, were caught up in divorce or the supermom phenomenon. Most will suffer a loss in living standards when compared with their parents, a hard blow to Americans who were always expected to better their lot with each ensuing generation. Determined to regain what they have lost, the 13ers have focused on strengthening the family, asking for very little governmental assistance throughout their lifetime, pursuing conservative politics and investments, and favoring the needs of the very young over the very old (mostly the boomers as they continue to age). Where the boomers were caught up in quick change and episodic relationships, generation X will look to reestablish traditional institutions and invest in traditional social systems.[15] This portends a whole new brand of volunteerism, a movement from adhocracy to a more long-term commitment, but with a no-nonsense attitude about what should be accomplished. We can see their influence as they demand a tough attitude toward crime and violence, prefer "workfare" to "welfare," and look to balance the national budget, even if there is some jeopardy to entitlement programs.

The rising millennial generation, called generation Y, is another factor in the intergenerational equation, bringing with it values and attitudes more aligned with the baby boomers than with generation X. Where the genexers were disillusioned and pessimistic, generation Y seems to embody the optimism and idealism that baby boomers themselves held dear. There has been a drop in alcohol consumption, drug usage, out-of-wedlock pregnancy, and homicides among generation Y, and a renewed emphasis on family and religious values. Although it is still too early to characterize them properly, generation Y seems to look to their parents and admire their accomplishments. Each generation has characteristics that will affect its employer/employee and client/provider relationships. The "boomer" bosses and the "generation X and Y" workers do not necessarily agree on the meaning of work in their life. Much of the dispute over staffing and mandatory overtime can be traced to generational differences. Generation Y is of particular interest: by 2020 this group will comprise 32 percent of the population. Generation Y is ethnically diverse, with minorities constituting 34 percent of its total. It is intensely computer driven and skeptical of government and the media, although it is well aware of societal issues and problems.[16] Any further "read" on their qualities may be premature.

There have also been a number of other notable changes. The South and West have accounted for the greatest percentage of population growth; over 35 percent of the population lives in the South. However, the West is currently growing at a slightly faster rate. Almost half the national population lives in 41 metropolitan areas that have populations of over 1 million. The newest census figures show some stabilization in the loss of population from rural areas and an upturn in rural land values.

The influx of immigrants to the United States has added to the diversity of America and is responsible for most of the recent population growth. One international migrant enters the United States every 35 seconds. Despite much publicity about illegal aliens, most immigrants enter legally; however, if both groups were counted, the numbers in the last decade would surpass even the record 8.8 million admitted in the first decade of the twentieth century. Unlike the great European migrations, the new immigrants are primarily from Latin America and Asia (particularly Korea and the Philippines). The Hispanic or Latino population, which can be of any race, grew from about 9 percent of the country's population in 1990 to 13 percent in 2000, and nearly 67 million people of Hispanic origin (who may be of any race) will be added to the nation's population between 2000 and 2050. Their numbers are projected to grow from 35.6 million to 102.6 million, an increase of 188 percent. Their share of the nation's population would nearly double, from 13 percent to 24.4 percent. The Asian population is projected to grow 213 percent, from 11.9 million in 2000 to 33.4 million in 2050. Their share of the nation's population would double, from 3.8 percent to 8 percent—a 58 percent increase. The black population is projected to rise from 35.8 million to 61.4 million in 2050, an increase of about 26 million or 71 percent. The black population would then account for 14.6 percent in 2050, as opposed to a current 12.7 percent of the population. Hispanics are the youngest population group, showing a median age of 26.9 years as compared with 38 for white non-Hispanics.[17]

People who identified themselves as black comprised 12 percent of the US population in 2000. The non-Hispanic white population represented roughly 69 percent of the total population in 2000, as opposed to 76 percent in 1990, and is projected to be 50.1 percent of the total population in 2050. The country's minority population grew by 43 percent between 1990 and 2000 to account for 31 percent of the nation's people. This growth was largely fueled by immigration.[18]

Acceptance of the new immigrants has varied. One concern is their assimilation into the community. It has been noted that for the first time in our history the majority of immigrants speak just one language (Spanish) and tend to live in ethnic enclaves served by media communicating in Spanish. Some Asians have also tended to cluster in ethnic neighborhoods and work in ethnic groups. The fact that foreign-born black and Hispanic people are sometimes more likely to have jobs than those native born has caused resentment (although there is also resentment if the newcomers are receiving public assistance).

The same is true of Asians, many of whom have the entire family working long hours to support a small shop or business and often pressure their children to perform well in school.

It is impossible to adequately profile a population without considering the family, which has been a support system in health and illness, and the traditional context for childbearing and child rearing. The new millennium has represented a period of restabilization for the American family that shrunk to its smallest ever, 2.62 people, in 1992 and rebounded to 3.2 people in the 2000 census. According to 2000 census figures, the American family is changing in dramatic ways. Some things to consider include the following[19]:

- Of 70.8 million children under 18, 69 percent live in households with two parents, 27 percent live with one parent, and 4 percent live with neither parent.
- In families where children live with one parent, 38 percent of those parents are divorced, 35 percent were never married, 19 percent are separated, and 4 percent are widowed.
- In two-parent families, it continues to be common for both parents to work outside the home, and the single-parent family is usually headed by a working woman.
- The number of families headed by single mothers has increased 25 percent since 1990 to more than 7.5 million households.
- For most of the past decade, about one-third of all babies were born to unmarried women, compared with 3.8 percent in 1940.
- The number of single fathers has also increased; single fathers now head more than 2 million families.

The need for child care arrangements, the growing popularity of flexible working hours, and the choice of working from home are some of society's responses to family needs. Four million American children live with grandparents. Nearly 22 million adult children are living with one or both parents. These patterns may be owed, in part, to the return to traditionalism of the X and Y generations.

Births to unmarried and teen mothers deserve reinterpretation. Although there is concern over a recent increase in births to older teenagers after years of decline, this does not correctly define the overall trend. Instead, much of the rise is due to significant increases in births among unmarried women in their 20s and 30s. Between 2002 and 2006, the rate at which unmarried women in that age group were having babies increased from 13 to 34 percent. The percentage of babies born to unmarried women in the United States is starting to look more like Europe's. Data show the proportion of babies born to unmarried women is about 66 percent in Iceland, 55 percent in Sweden, 50 percent in France, and 44 percent in the United Kingdom. In many of those countries, couples are living together instead of getting married. This is also the situation in the United States where about 40 percent of births to unmarried women occur in households where couples are cohabitating.[20]

The number of abortions, which peaked in 1990 with 1.6 million, dropped to an estimated 1.2 million in 2005. That is 8 percent fewer than in 2000.[21] The typical woman selecting abortion is likely to be young, white, and unmarried with no previous live births, and having the procedure for the first time. Having additional children no longer qualifies families on public assistance for access to more resources under many current welfare policies. However, public dollars are not readily available for abortion services, making it more of an option for women with money or insurance. Further, given the controversy around the procedure, fewer physicians are willing to risk the personal danger to those who continue to offer abortion services. In 2008, the number of abortion providers in the United States dropped to 1787, representing a 2 percent decline from 2000.[22] In the midst of these circumstances, abortion continues to be a legal option, but is becoming de facto unavailable to many women.

The last 50 years have been an economic roller coaster in the United States. There have been several periods of unparalleled prosperity interspersed with periodic recession. Since 1995, there have been fewer poor people, and median family income has been higher. About one-half of the nation's poor continue to be either under 18 or over 65. In 2008, according to the Organization for Economic Cooperation and Development (OECD), child poverty in the United States was about 20 percent and poverty among the elderly was as high as 23 percent.[23] Government data show that 3.5 million children under the age of 5 are at risk of hunger in the United States. The situation is most critical in 11 states, Louisiana having the highest rate, followed closely by North Carolina, Ohio, Kentucky, Texas, New Mexico, Kansas, South Carolina, Tennessee, Idaho, and Arkansas, where more than 20 percent of children under 5 are allegedly at risk of going hungry. Children are

■ **EXHIBIT 6–2.** The 2008–2009 Poverty Threshold Measured According to the Department of Health and Human Services Poverty Guidelines

Persons in Family Unit	48 Contiguous States and District of Columbia	Alaska	Hawaii
1	$10,830	$13,530	$12,460
2	$14,570	$18,210	$16,760
3	$18,310	$22,890	$21,060
4	$22,050	$27,570	$25,360
5	$25,790	$32,250	$29,660
6	$29,530	$36,930	$33,960
7	$33,270	$41,610	$38,260
8	$37,010	$46,290	$42,560
For each additional person, add	$3,740	$4,680	$4,300

Source: *Federal Register* 74(14):4199–4201, January 23, 2009.

at the greatest risk in rural areas.[24] Poor children are twice as likely as non-poor children to suffer stunted growth or lead poisoning, and to be kept back in school. They also score significantly lower on reading, math, and vocabulary tests when compared with other children.[25]

There is currently work under way by the Department of Health and Human Services (DHHS) to redo the federal poverty thresholds, making them more realistic to today's economy. These thresholds are used to determine eligibility for federal programs (see Exhibit 6–2). State eligibility is another issue, and those thresholds vary from state to state.

In March 2010, the Patient Protection and Affordable Care Act was signed into law. This legislation promises to reduce the number of insured in the United States by 32 million people. (See Chapter 19 for more detail on this legislation.) In fact, there are 47 to 50 million uninsured Americans and 14 million of them are individuals 30 or younger who can afford insurance but typically choose not to have it.[26] Currently, only 30.2 percent of the poor have no health insurance of any kind, but poor people or those with incomes below the poverty level comprise 27.1 percent of the uninsured. Additionally, the foreign-born population was without health insurance 32.5 percent of the time, as compared with the native-born population at 13.6 percent.[27] Furthermore, there is a special population more correctly called the medically indigent. These people are either uninsured or have inadequate insurance once confronted with medical necessity. The medically indigent are

neither poor enough for Medicaid nor old enough for Medicare. They are middle-class people with little savings who are commonly employed in part-time or episodic jobs that provide inadequate or no benefits. The new legislation promises to directly confront many of these problems, but only time and experience will determine how well it performs.

Poverty is also associated with homelessness. Six hundred thousand people are homeless in this country at any point in time, and 7 million people will be homeless at some point during their lifetime. Over two-thirds of the homeless are unattached men in their late 30s, and one-fifth are families with a woman in her early 30s as head of household. Homelessness has become a way of life for some and is a transient incident for others. The circumstances that accompany homelessness are psychiatric disability, substance abuse, or just plain poverty. The homeless are at high risk for HIV/AIDS and TB. Thirty to forty percent of the male homeless are veterans. About 39 percent of the homeless have come from institutional living of some sort or were in foster care as children.[28]

The homeless have been caught in a vicious cycle—no home, no address, unsafe public shelters, no place to leave children while looking for a job, and much more. Recent public policy initiatives have begun to chip away at these problems. The homeless have been very successful in securing advocates who are vocal and influential. The homeless have gained a voice, and this is to our advantage.

But they have also experienced significant backlash. They have lost the sympathy of middle America. Generational changes, problems with health care, and crime on the streets have all tested our patience and brought us back to basics. We seem to want more order in our lives, and we expect government to take charge. Citizens want their streets and public buildings back, and they want them clean and uncluttered. They want to move freely about their cities without fear of personal harm. The declining crime rates in many of our major cities are applauded. The homeless are a reminder of our shortcomings as a society, and we would prefer not to be reminded.

■ THE NATION'S HEALTH

The health status of the US population as a whole is, according to statistics, better than ever. Health status is determined in several ways: using mortality statistics (life expectancy and death rates), which are easily obtained, and morbidity statistics (the incidence and prevalence of illness). The latter are much more difficult to obtain and are less accurate because most diseases are not reportable, and reports, surveys, and research can be interpreted in a number of ways.

The past years have seen an increase in life expectancy for all Americans. The most significant increase was among black women, whose average life expectancy increased by 12.3 years between 1950 and 2000. Across racial groups, women live longer than men. National Vital Statistics data show that, in 2008, women of every race lived 5 years longer than men of the same race. These trends have been consistent over time. Newborn baby boys can expect to live to be 75 on average and girls can expect to be 80. For the first time, life expectancy for black males reached 70 years.[29]

Maternal/child health statistics provide many stories about the health and social expectations of a people. Despite a 21-percent decline in the infant mortality rate between 1990 and 1999, the United States continues to have a higher rate than many other industrialized countries. The overall infant mortality was 6.7 deaths per 1000 live births. Further, infant mortality rates varied widely according to the race of the mother, with the highest rate (13.8) for infants of black mothers, which is more than four times higher than the groups with the lowest rates: 2.9 for infants born to Chinese mothers and 3.4 for Japanese mothers. Infant mortality rates were higher for mothers who began prenatal care late or had none at all, were

teenagers, did not complete high school, were unmarried, or smoked during pregnancy. Infant mortality rates were also higher for male infants, multiple births, and infants born preterm or at low birth weight.[30]

There is substantial proof of the social inequity in health among the people of the United States. Blacks are particularly compromised, even though years of progress have moved them closer to the mainstream in this country. Although the statistics are confusing, some general statements can be made. All Americans have shared in life expectancy gains, but a gap persists between blacks and others in the incidence of asthma, diabetes, HIV/AIDS, and some forms of cancer. Death from heart disease, stroke, and diabetes were 20 to 60 percent more prevalent in minority populations.[31] The largest discrepancies in health outcomes for minorities came in the areas of cardiovascular disease, HIV/AIDS, cancer, and diabetes. They were less likely to receive sophisticated treatments such as angioplasty, bypass surgery, kidney transplantation, or combination drug therapy for HIV/AIDS.[32]

AIDS continues to be the leading cause of death for 25- to 44-year-old blacks. And in 2000, more than 8000 Hispanics in the United States were infected. Although the daily headlines about HIV/AIDS have disappeared, the disease has not, particularly among minority groups in the United States. Whereas the black and Hispanic communities each constitute an estimated 12 percent of the nation's population, they account for more than half of all people diagnosed with HIV/AIDS each year.[33]

Blacks, Hispanics, and Native Americans have experienced a particularly sharp rise in the prevalence of type 2 diabetes in recent years. Diabetes is the epidemic of our times, but for certain minority populations it is especially devastating. The prevalence of diabetes among blacks aged 40 to 74 has doubled in just 12 years, from 8.9 percent to 18.2 percent. More than 10 percent of all Mexican Americans aged 20 or older have diabetes, and the incidence jumps to almost 24 percent among those aged 45 to 74. Among the Pima Indians of Arizona, about 50 percent of those between the ages of 30 and 64 have diabetes.[34] These distinctions should not be oversimplified, nor can they be satisfactorily explained.

Statistics are sometimes deceiving. There has been a significant decline in chronic disease in general, but when race is added as a variable, almost all of the gain has been among whites. Other minority groups seem more vulnerable to specific health problems: Asians have the greatest incidence of TB, Hispanics suffer more fatal and disabling strokes, Puerto Rican children more asthma, and blacks have the most consistently compromised health status. Simple answers are impossible. Pointing fingers at the availability of health insurance may also be naive. Hispanics are relatively poor as a group and are unlikely to have insurance, yet they stay healthy longer than any other group, including whites and blacks.[35]

Because cancer is still a major cause of death, 2010 data from the American Cancer Society are pertinent[36]:

- About 555,500 deaths are expected from cancer in the United States, more than 1500 a day; cancer is the second leading cause of death.
- Approximately 9 million Americans alive today have a personal history of cancer.
- Seventy-seven percent of cancers are diagnosed in individuals 55 years of age or older.
- One of every two men and one of every three women will develop cancer over the course of their lifetime.
- Five to ten percent of cancers are attributable to heredity.
- Cancer of the lung and bronchus is the leading cause of cancer deaths for both sexes, accounting for 31 percent of all deaths in men and 25 percent in women.
- The next most common cause of cancer death in men is the prostate (11 percent) and in women the breast (15 percent).
- Scientific evidence suggests that one-third of cancer deaths are related to nutrition, physical inactivity, obesity, and other lifestyle factors and could have been prevented.
- Certain cancers related to infectious exposures, such as hepatitis B virus (HBV), HIV, helicobacter, and others, could have been prevented through behavioral change, vaccines, or antibiotic use.
- Many of the more than 1 million skin cancers diagnosed in 2010 could have been prevented by protection from the sun's rays.
- The 5-year survival rate is 82 percent for those cancers detected by screening or self-examination, such as prostate, cervical, oral, breast, colon, skin, rectal, testis, and skin cancers.
- Black Americans are more likely to develop cancer and die from it than persons of any other racial or ethnic group.

The leading causes of death in the United States are heart disease, cancer, stroke, chronic obstructive pulmonary disease, accidents/unintentional injuries, diabetes, Alzheimer's disease, influenza/pneumonia, kidney disease, septicemia/blood poisoning, suicide, chronic liver disease/cirrhosis, hypertension, Parkinson's disease, and homicide, in that order. Perhaps the most discouraging news is, as has been true for decades, many of these causes of death are premature, often owing to lifestyle, and are preventable. In 1979, the DHHS launched the first of three *Healthy People* initiatives in an attempt to improve the well-being of Americans. Each includes a set of objectives and measurable indicators to move the country toward very precise goals. The first program was *Healthy People: The Surgeon General's Report on Health Promotion and Disease Prevention.*[37] The goal was to decrease mortality for every age group in the population, and additionally to increase the independence of America's oldest citizens. The 1990 targets for the first of the *Healthy People* programs were achieved with the exception of those for adolescents and seniors. It is disputable whether there was actually a lack of progress or the monitoring and surveillance systems were faulty.

Healthy People 2000 benefited from this earlier experience and was built on an expanded science base, allowing more sophisticated disease prevention and health promotion goals[38]:

- Increase the years of healthy life for all Americans.
- Reduce the disparities in health that exist among different populations in this country.
- Provide all Americans with access to disease prevention and health promotion services.

These broad goals were further developed into objectives and then organized into 22 priority areas (Exhibit 6–3). After the mid-course review of 1995, objectives and some priority areas were revised. Progress was mixed and precise measurement was hampered by the absence of baseline information in many areas and deficient surveillance systems. The process of *Healthy People 2000* has been as important as the content. This has been a true initiative of the American people. States and local communities have networked under this program, becoming aware of their deficiencies and investing in programming for health and wellness. Government and the private sector have partnered to make *Healthy People 2000* work, sharing the credit where there has been success and frustration where the absence of information or resistant patterns of living thwart progress. The latest phase of *Healthy People* began in January 2000. With *Healthy People 2010,* the emphasis is on health status and the nature of life—quality years, not just longevity. A broadened perspective has come from the development of the science of prevention, improved data systems and surveillance activities, consumer demand for promotion of health, and a renewed appreciation of the public health. *Healthy People 2000* put a participatory and decentralized process into operation; *Healthy People 2010* will capitalize on those dynamics. The agenda continues to be a variation on the following theme: to increase quality and years of healthy life, and to eliminate health disparities between America's people. *Healthy People 2010* consists of 28 focus areas (see Exhibit 6–3), each further defined by health indicators and targeted goals that were chosen because of their ability to motivate, their relevance as broad public health issues, and the availability of data to measure progress. Individuals from all segments of American life have been personally involved in designing the goals, objectives, and indicators, and in data collection and monitoring.[39] The information that comes from these programs is a rich source for understanding America's problems, strengths, and changing character. The student is encouraged to go to websites associated with *Healthy People* for more detail. A good place to start is

---

■ EXHIBIT 6–3. Focus/Priority Areas—US Department of Health and Human Services, Healthy People Programs

Healthy People 2000

1. Physical Activity and Fitness
2. Nutrition
3. Tobacco
4. Substance Abuse: Alcohol and Other Drugs
5. Family Planning
6. Mental Health and Mental Disorders
7. Violent and Abusive Behavior
8. Educational and Community-Based Programs
9. Unintentional Injuries
10. Occupational Safety and Health
11. Environmental Health
12. Food and Drug Safety
13. Oral Health
14. Maternal and Infant Health
15. Heart Disease and Stroke
16. Cancer
17. Diabetes and Chronic Disabling Conditions
18. HIV Infection
19. Sexually Transmitted Diseases
20. Immunization and Infectious Diseases
21. Clinical Preventive Systems
22. Surveillance and Data Systems

Healthy People 2010

1. Access to Quality Health Services
2. Arthritis, Osteoporosis, and Chronic Back Conditions
3. Cancer
4. Chronic Kidney Disease
5. Diabetes
6. Disability and Secondary Conditions
7. Educational and Community-Based Programs
8. Environmental Health
9. Family Planning and Sexual Health
10. Food Safety
11. Health Communication
12. Heart Disease and Stroke
13. HIV
14. Immunizations and Infectious Diseases
15. Injury and Violence Prevention
16. Maternal, Infant, and Child Health
17. Medical Product Safety
18. Mental Health and Mental Disorders
19. Nutrition
20. Occupational Safety and Health
21. Oral Health
22. Physical Activity and Fitness
23. Public Health Infrastructure
24. Respiratory Diseases
25. Sexually Transmitted Diseases
26. Substance Abuse
27. Tobacco Use
28. Vision and Hearing

Source: US Public Health Service. http://web.health.gov/healthypeople/.

http://www.cdc.gov/nchs/healthy_people.htm. Explore indicators, baseline data, targeted goals, and current progress.

The program is a tall order, but the evidence already presented in this chapter builds a good case for claiming progress. There is some drop in drug use by teens, except for alcohol. The smoking rate of the general population has fallen, but for teenagers of both sexes, both black and white, it has risen. Government action, however, has banned smoking in many public places and on public transportation. There has also been governmental intervention in the use of alcohol; all states are in compliance with the National Uniform Drinking Age Law after raising the drinking age to 21. The death rates for coronary artery disease and stroke have declined significantly; the latter by 16 percent and the former by 12 percent.

There has been a notable improvement in the major risk factors for cardiovascular disease. Adults claim they exercise more, although it is not clear what and how much is meant, and at any rate, this is primarily a phenomenon of the middle and upper-middle classes, particularly among young and middle-aged adults. Nevertheless, one-fourth of the population admits that they engage in no physical activity, and there is general concern that children are getting very little exercise.

Although Americans, again probably mostly middle class, eat fewer fatty foods, they still eat too much. More Americans of all ages are overweight than ever before: 14 percent of children between 6 and 11, 12 percent of youth between 12 and 17, and 35 percent of people over 20. Positively, more people than ever before know their blood pressure reading and cholesterol levels, and the mean serum cholesterol level for the population has dropped. The outcomes are compelling, but the evidence is often contradictory and deserving of continued scientific investigation.

Yet there are other concerns. TB has emerged as a serious public health threat, particularly in inner cities. TB has become closely associated with AIDS, where resistance to infection is very low and the extensive use and sometimes abuse of antibiotics has helped to create a multi-drug-resistant strain of TB.

In addition, data show that one in five adults suffers from at least one mental disorder, about the same for men as for women except that more women suffer from depression. More disturbing, the figures are similar for children and young adults. Anxiety disorders, substance abuse, and antisocial personality problems are more common in this young group. It is not known if mental illness, however mild, might also have a part in the escalating rate of suicide, particularly among young men. Suicide is also significant among the elderly. Certainly, violence is a major factor in death rates. The Centers for Disease Control and Prevention (CDC) reported suicide and homicide as leading causes of premature death for Americans. Although declining among the general population, they remain as major causes of death among those 15 to 24.

The most resistant areas seem to be those associated with chronic disease. And the number of those who experience limitation in activities of daily living owing to chronic conditions continues to mount. Again, the evidence is inconsistent; other studies report a decline in chronic disability for those over 65. However, even here the major gains are among whites if the data are more carefully analyzed.

Healthy People 2010 is looking more toward communities to strengthen their own capabilities to promote and protect health and ensure access to services. Perhaps the greatest achievement of *Healthy People 2000* is the capacity it has built for surveillance and monitoring patterns in health and living, thereby making us aware of our own needs.

The work of *Healthy People* has taken on a life of its own and moved into the work of *Healthy People 2020*. Each decade the DHHS has released a comprehensive set of national public health objectives, and each has been known as *Healthy People*. The initiative has been grounded in the notion that setting objectives and providing benchmarks to track and monitor progress can motivate, guide, and focus action. Building on the work of *Healthy People 2010*, the objectives from that report are retained, modified, or archived. New objectives and priority areas have been added at the discretion of the study committee. *Healthy People 2020* is still in the formative stage. The reader is referred to http://healthypeople.gov/hp2020/.

Any discussion of today's health issues would be incomplete if environmental factors were not considered. Americans feel imperiled by a variety of factors that accompany modern life. These include food additives, contamination of food products, transportation dangers, and inadequately tested medications. However, the fact that, by broad statistical measures, Americans have never been safer should not be a cause to underestimate the real hazards. The effect on health may not be seen for decades, and there may not be a clear indication of which of the many interacting factors is clearly responsible for an illness or death.

Some occupational illnesses have been identified, and to varying degrees, safety standards have been set and enforced by the Occupational Safety and Health Administration (OSHA) and the Environmental Protection Agency (EPA). Consumer groups and unions have claimed that such protection is generally insufficient, whereas industry complains that it is so overregulated that expenses for compliance are unreasonable. Some conditions, such as byssinosis (brown lung disease), caused by cotton dust in the textile industries, and silicosis (black lung disease), caused by silica, particularly in mining, are clearly recognized as job-related diseases. It is generally accepted that other occupation-related disabilities are caused by benzine, formaldehyde, waste anesthesia gases, asbestos, ethylene oxide (a sterilizing agent in hospitals and medical products industries), diisocyanate (a chemical used to produce plastic products), vinyl chloride, lead, and radiation, to name a few. Clearly, some of these are particular hazards for nurses, along with the danger of AIDS, hepatitis B and C, airborne pathogens, and accidents (see Chapter 30). The Nurses' Environmental Health Watch publishes information on hazards for nurses and how to avoid or minimize them.

Public health experts and environmentalists cite other environmental hazards. The depletion of the stratospheric ozone layer caused by chlorofluorocarbons (CFCs) used in sprays, refrigeration and air conditioning systems, industrial blowing agents, insulating foams, metal cleaning and drying, garment cleaning, sterilization of medical supplies, and liquid fast freezing cause skin cancer and potential changes in the world's climate. The Clean Air Act has set limitations for sulfur oxides, suspected particulate matter, nitrogen oxides, carbon monoxides, hydrocarbons, lead, and other pollutants emitted by various industries and automobiles, but there is a constant battle to determine what the limit should be.

Acid rain, resulting from emissions from coal-burning plants and factories—chiefly sulfur dioxide and nitrogen oxides that are chemically changed in the atmosphere—is suspected of destroying freshwater life, damaging forests and crops, and possibly threatening human health. Cited by the EPA as probably the most serious environmental problem in the United States is hazardous wastes. These are by-products of the manufacturing process of many products, but the large-scale generators are chemical manufacturers, petroleum refiners, and metal production companies. Careless dumping of these wastes, for instance, in areas where they leak into a water supply or cause an

explosion, has resulted in serious danger to whole communities. Scientists contend that it is possible to contain wastes safely if certain caveats are observed, and some manufacturers are making an effort to clean up sites. Meanwhile, dangerous old waste dumps are continually being discovered.

The deadly chemical dioxin, an unwanted by-product of herbicides, pesticides, and other industrial products, has been given considerable attention, particularly since the question was raised as to its effect on soldiers and civilians in Vietnam, where it was a chemical contaminant of the defoliant Agent Orange. There is some belief that others, such as inhabitants of the Love Canal area and those exposed to dioxin in train wrecks or factory explosions, suffer from a variety of conditions, including kidney and liver ailments, birth defects, and cancer. In other environmental situations, contamination by polybrominated biphenyls (PPBs) and polychlorinated biphenyls (PCBs), now banned, has resulted in the required destruction of food products because of danger to human beings.

Almost daily, there is some report in the media about product or environmental dangers, whether noise, food additives, safety failure of equipment, toys, autos, clothing, hazardous wastes, acid rain, radioactive leaks, unsafe drinking water, or even human destruction from nuclear weapons, germ warfare, or anthrax. Some feel that this is a hysterical reaction to unproven claims. Others ignore the entire issue. Still others feel that with or without more definitive data, a stronger effort must be made to improve the environment. Certainly, the clearly visible smog in so many urban areas is evidence that there is room for improvement.

■ TECHNOLOGICAL, SCIENTIFIC, AND MEDICAL ADVANCES

There is little question that the technological advances of recent years have been amazing and, combined with scientific advances in medicine, the health care delivery system in the United States has experienced a major transformation.

Some of the most significant technological and scientific changes affecting patient care can be categorized as follows:

• *Developments in diagnosis and treatment*, such as automated clinical laboratory equipment, artificial human organs, improved surgical techniques (such as microsurgery, bloodless surgery, and an endless variety of nonintrusive techniques that reduce the need for surgery) and equipment (such as lasers and the use of computers to both diagnose and provide treatment options).

- *Information management,* such as electronic systems for rate calculation, billing, accounting, transfer of information and funds, maintenance of databases, and record keeping and transmission of clinical documentation. These databases enable not only management, but also clinical decisions. The criteria for systems development have been speed, accuracy, and equity—ensuring that providers make their decisions based on information that is dependable and reflects the state-of-the-art of the science, that the least amount of effort possible is needed for coordination, and that all parties are paid promptly for what they do.

- Developments *affecting health care supplies and services,* such as widespread adoption of plastic, other inexpensive and improved materials, and equipment such as specialized carts, conveyers, and pneumatic tubes.

- Improvement in the *management processes and structural design* of health facilities, aimed at more efficient utilization of personnel, equipment, and space, and increased consumer satisfaction. This involves sensitivity to the needs and preferences of both the internal (employee) and external consumer (recipient of service).

- *Mass communication,* which not only increases the opportunity to educate the consumer, but can be a powerful influence in molding public opinion. Consumers can be empowered on their own behalf and make more knowledgeable decisions about their choice of providers.

Clearly, technology plays an important role in health care. Scientific and medical advances have gone beyond the imagination of science fiction. Almost all have raised many ethical issues and sometimes legal complications in relation to access, quality of life, and right to life. (Some of these issues are discussed in Chapters 10 and 22.) The rapidity of technological development has caught almost everyone unprepared. For instance, the progress of genomic medicine and the process of cloning are no longer a hypothetical and distant frontier, but today's reality. Further, there is the issue of cost. Progress is expensive, and with new treatments and new equipment there is the constant need to update. This is frequently criticized as adding to the cost of health care, but these new medical and nonmedical technologies are believed to improve human services and the quality of our lives.

Futurists have labeled the first 100 years of the new millennium as the century of biotechnology. The year 2003 held the announcement that the human genome had been sequenced, although much work remains to understand how this "instruction book for human biology" carries out its multitude of functions.[40] Equipped with this genetic road map, and once we know how each gene functions, we can learn how to fix what needs fixing. This opens the floodgates for genetic engineering to conquer cancer, eliminate cystic fibrosis and muscular dystrophy, create new body parts from stem cells, reset our biological clock, and much more. It also presents ethical dilemmas of monumental proportion. Who is to have access to your genetic information? It seems noble to use genetic fingerprinting on criminals, but will the rest of us be far behind? How easily we will be tempted to tamper with the personal characteristics that make someone an individual: IQ, physical appearance, athletic ability, and gender, to name a few.

We would be remiss to move from this section without offering comments about the use of computer technology. Although the initial use was often for operations purposes, clinical information was quickly integrated into these systems as the level of reimbursement became driven by observations about the patient's condition and the services provided. Nurses have always been positioned in the midst of clinical information, given their continual presence and comprehensive role.

Nursing information systems (NISs) are an integral part of the information system existing in every health care organization. There are also hospital information systems (HISs), systems for long-term care facilities, systems for home care agencies, and so on. These systems are designed to be easily adapted to computerization, but can also operate with paper and pencil. Information systems exist to promote efficiency, effectiveness, and accountability, and those qualities can be enhanced through the proper use of computers. But quite to the contrary, often information requirements and their entry into computer systems may prove to be very disruptive and painful to employees. If the information is not relevant and both computer software and hardware are not friendly and useful, communication can be less effective than before.

Over the last several years, there has been a great deal in the nursing literature about the use of computers in education and practice. The variety of uses continually increases, and more nurses are becoming experts. Nurses, like others, must find fast, effective ways to turn raw data into useful, organized information. Information systems can assist in patient assessment, designing care, monitoring progress, documentation and charting, discharge coordination, staffing and scheduling, and tracking acuity, cost, and quality. Computers can also enrich clinical decisions and offer prompts to alternate solutions for relatively common problems. Computer terminals at the patient's bedside, in the examining room, or even in the patient's home can ease the burden of record keeping, improve accuracy, and eliminate duplication of information. If used properly, computers can also improve the exchange of information between nurses and other health care professionals and staff. Critical paths are one example of a clinical information system that is exceptionally suited to computerization, although they may operate with paper alone. Ideally, *critical paths* (also known as *caremaps*) are the product of interdisciplinary consensus on the preferred course of treatment for a specific condition, the anticipated response of the patient, and the manner in which organizational systems should respond in support of the patient and provider. The path serves as a prompter to clinical decision making and alerts the provider to situations in which the patient is not responding as anticipated. The path is uniquely suited to evidence-based practice. The existence of the path documents the plan of care and allows the nurse to limit charting to exceptions to the path, thus reducing paperwork.

Computer technology is used widely in nursing education and research. Computer-assisted instruction (CAI) is used in such areas as drill and practice, simulations, and tutorials. Internet courses allow independent learning and self-pacing. Interactive television (ITV) broadcasting brings educational programming to many who would otherwise be absent opportunities. Nursing informatics is a component in every basic curriculum, and there is the expectation that students bring some computer skills. Nursing research depends on computer technology for data collection and analysis, retrieval of information, and communication between researchers with similar scientific interests. This increased use of electronic media is demonstrated in the Sigma Theta Tau Center for Nursing Scholarship International Library, where just about all its holdings are in electronic format; it is a library without paper.

The ideal electronic system would be fully interactive and link the point at which care is given with every department and service from accounting to materials management, computer-assisted clinical prescribing and monitoring drug interactions, ancillary services, clinical decision-making support, and computerized patient records, including bedside information systems. Such a system would allow multiple record correction from a single point of data entry. More descriptively, the nurse enters an order for a diagnostic procedure that requires a preparatory regimen including medication and special diet. As the order is placed, the procedure is scheduled for the time of day that is most comfortable for the patient as identified in the nursing history, the pharmacy receives the order for medication, transport is notified when to pick up the patient, diet is changed, inventories are updated where supplies were used, the episode enters the quality assurance loop, and the nurse is alerted to any possible adverse reactions. Given the amount of nursing effort invested in coordination of services, the value of information technology is limitless. For nurses this means learning to use the new technology for the benefit of the patient, but continually maintaining the emphasis on individuality and human contact, which no machine can provide, as well as protecting the patient's privacy and advocating on the patient's behalf.

■ EDUCATION

Trends in education affect nursing in a number of ways: (1) the kind, number, and quality of students entering the nursing programs and the background they bring with them; (2) the introduction of new technology to better respond to the needs of the learner; and (3) the impact of social demands on education, which are eventually extended to education in the professions, including nursing. Usually it is not just one social or economic condition that brings about change in education, nor is there only one kind of change. For instance, overexpansion by most institutions of higher education when baby boomer admissions were at their height created a large pool of unemployed college graduates in the early 1970s. Some of these, as well as college students with a worried eye to the future, looked for educational programs that seemed to promise jobs immediately on graduation, among them nursing. Thus, what had once been a trickle of mature, second-degree students into nursing became a steady stream. As the baby boom group diminished, overextended institutions of higher education and their nursing programs found it necessary to use marketing strategies of all kinds to attract enough students. They discovered the working adults in the community, who were a relatively untapped pool.

To attract and retain these nontraditional students, higher education had to make the college experience more flexible and individualized. Successful schools became innovative without sacrificing their integrity. This standard was applied to every aspect of the academic experience: fulfilling requirements for graduation, course scheduling, and more.

The more mature student brought a lot of life experience to college with them, and it became necessary to find approaches to award academic credit for what a person knows regardless of when, where, or how that knowledge was acquired. The concepts of independent study and credit by examination have been explored by an increasing number of colleges, and a variety of mechanisms that have wide acceptance are being used to grant credit in all areas of study, including nursing. These chiefly include teacher-made examinations, standardized tests, and portfolio development. One example of standardized testing is the College Level Examination Program (CLEP), which was developed some time ago by the College Board through funding by the Carnegie Foundation. CLEP is the most widely accepted credit-by-examination program in the United States today, helping students of all ages earn college degrees faster by getting credit for what they already know. It provides testing in a variety of general and specialized courses for which most colleges and universities award credit.

Over time, the higher education community has responded to public pressure for nontraditional routes to educational credentials. One model has been the external degree route as an option to traditional college attendance. Some external degree programs are marginally legitimate operations that have given the whole concept a bad name with meaningless mail-order degrees. But increasingly, respected, accredited educational institutions have established creative but rigorous processes to ensure the quality of their graduates. The true external degree university does not give any courses itself, but functions as a clearinghouse to verify the competence of the degree recipient through testing and/or studies completed in a variety of acceptable settings. A particularly successful example of the external degree exists at Excelsior College, previously Regents College, which includes associate, baccalaureate, and master's degree programs in nursing.

Other flexible educational options are programs that concentrate coursework in weekends, evenings, summers, or a combination of these. We see more outreach programs for isolated geographic areas or even workplaces with enough employees interested in coursework. These satellite or outreach programs have thrived on the technology associated with distance education. Distance education is discussed at greater length in Chapter 12.

Equally significant are other happenings in higher education. Cost, to student and institution, is an ongoing controversy. As government aid declines, the cost to the student for higher education increases. Because there are not as many tax benefits to encourage charitable giving, colleges and universities have a major problem in balancing costs, quality, and service to students. Two-year colleges are under particular pressure because of their very low tuition. On the other hand, despite the cry for higher quality, there is less state interest. This translates to a lack of funding to improve public community colleges or public higher education in general. The public only seems ready to put its dollars where quality already exists and has become critical of providing remedial instruction in basic skills to students who come ill prepared for college, but somehow were admitted. Although what may be needed is a reassessment of the mission of publicly funded colleges and universities, the response has been to raise tuition and vigorously market to attract new and different students. Nursing continues to be a very popular program for community colleges, offering occupational preparation in 2 years. Financial problems of private colleges are just as serious, and many smaller colleges have been forced to close their doors, as have some nursing programs.

The public also identifies college tuition cost as a major concern, followed closely by student attitude, drug problems, and the poor quality of academic programs, including a demonstrated lack of faculty interest in teaching. The cost of a college education is outpacing inflation. Nontraditional students have found the cost of college of particular concern because they are often ineligible for financial aid, which is historically reserved for full-time students. The influence of organized nursing in Washington, DC, made government traineeship dollars available to nurses for part-time study as early as 1989. However, all students who rely on government funding may have problems, because the standard has moved away from grants to loans that have to be repaid. Experts say that this may have a negative effect on students from low-income backgrounds, who are often reticent to go into debt for education. And further, colleges and universities whose students have a poor record of repayment will be penalized.

Completing a baccalaureate degree in 4 years is no longer guaranteed. Graduate study is also more drawn out and frequently earned in a part-time program. Retention rates in higher education are also of concern, but the information is guarded. Many people believe that an institutional emphasis on research as opposed to teaching is part of the problem; faculty, especially in universities, tend to be rewarded and promoted largely on the basis of their research productivity.[41] Loudly voiced public discontent has forced such institutions to work on ways to reestablish teaching as a priority.

In 2001, undergraduate students consisted of an almost equal number of men and women; Asians made up the vast majority of foreign students. Almost 83 percent of freshmen were white, 12.7 percent were black, 3.7 percent were Asian American, and 11 percent were Hispanic. Where these students were not emancipated and parental income was an issue, families earned less than $50,000 a year. Lack of financial aide kept 170,000 students from college. Half of full-time students work 25 hours a week, which affected their academic performance. Almost 14 percent of students spoke a language other than English at home. Almost 40 percent expected to eventually complete a graduate degree and described themselves politically most often as middle of the road. The motivation for higher education was closely associated with a future work life, and the financial security it represented, but there was also the inquisitiveness to learn more about things "that interest me." A college is often selected because of its academic reputation and the observation that graduates get good jobs. Freshmen believed that the government should do more to preserve the environment, that we should be less concerned about protecting the rights of criminals, that employers should be allowed to require drug testing, that handguns should be controlled, that a national health care plan is necessary, that wealthy people should pay more taxes, and that racist and sexist speech should be prohibited on campus. Only slightly more than half thought that abortion should be legal (56 percent) and that undocumented immigrants should be denied access to public education (55 percent). For more than 70 percent, a major objective in their life was to raise a family and be well-off financially.[42] Whether or not students' attitudes change during their college years has never been measured accurately, but it can be assumed that at least some changes occurred. Meanwhile, the data are, at the least, interesting to consider and very much representative of generation Y, which is coming of age to provide leadership in the society. One basic difference between nursing and non-nursing students is often their age. Many individuals select nursing for a midlife or later-life career change. Consequently, the average age of associate degree students is almost 40; baccalaureate enrollees are generally in their mid- and late 20s.

■ THE WOMEN'S MOVEMENT

Nursing, from its beginnings in America, was primarily made up of women, and some nurses have always been involved in the women's movement. For example, Lavinia Dock was active and prominent in the early struggles for suffrage, and Margaret Sanger fought courageously to bring birth control to the poor. However, feminist women and nurses have historically had an uneasy alliance. A group of nurse activists describe this relationship as follows:

> Much of the energy in the women's movement has been directed toward opening up nontraditional fields of study and work for women. Nursing has been seen as one of the ultimate female ghettos from which women should be encouraged to escape. . . . Feminists have sometimes failed to look beyond the inaccurate sexist stereotypes of nurses and to acknowledge the multiple dimensions of professional nursing.[43]

Being a suffragette was not easy in the late nineteenth and early twentieth centuries, and often women did not support the movement. That reaction may have been caused, in part, by the negative, even vindictive portrait newspapers painted of those in the movement, as illustrated by a few typical quotes: "organized by divorced wives, childless women, and sour old maids," "unsexed women," "entirely devoid of personal attractions," "laboring on the heels of strong hatred towards men." Whether the opposition resulted from the fear of overthrowing "the most sacred of our institutions (marriage)"[44] or any other threat to the status quo is a moot point. Despite the success of the women's movement, most notably the passage of women's suffrage in 1921, discrimination against women has not ended. Women still face many formidable economic, social, and political barriers.

Women in all occupations, professions, and walks of life have encountered these barriers, and the success of the women's movement attests to the fervor and commitment with which they have fought to improve women's status. It is no surprise that the women's movement has been considered one of the major phenomena of the twentieth century.

Over the years, there has been a proliferation of women's organizations concerned with women's rights.

Among the most active groups is the National Organization for Women (NOW), founded in 1966 and made up of women and men who support full equality for women in truly equal partnership with men and ask for an end to discrimination and prejudice against women in every field of importance in American society.

The founding of NOW offered one of the most politically radical agendas of the twentieth century: Men and women would share equally in public and private responsibilities—in paid work and in the rearing of children.

NOW activities are directed toward legislative action to end discrimination, and it attempts to promote its views through demonstrations, research, litigation, and political pressure. It is interesting that the first president of NOW, Wilma Scott Heide, was a nurse and feminist, demonstrating that nursing and feminism can find common ground.

Another prominent women's organization is the National Women's Political Caucus (NWPC). The NWPC was founded in 1971 as the first national political organization to promote women's entry into politics at leadership levels. The main thrust of the NWPC is to ensure that women's issues are given more attention by facilitating the election of women to political office.

Although many of the issues that women have confronted are slow to be resolved, the women's movement has been the major catalyst in raising awareness and instigating action on sex discrimination and women's rights. The impact of the movement can be observed in both legal and social changes occurring, slowly but surely, in women's roles. However, children are still being socialized into stereotyped male and female roles by books, toys, and the influence of parents, teachers, and others—a problem that feminists and others continue to address. According to NOW, "a feminist is a person who believes women (even as men) are primarily people; that human rights are indivisible by any category of sex, race, class or other designation irrelevant to our common humanity; a feminist is committed to creating the equality (not sameness) of the sexes legally, socially, educationally, psychologically, politically, religiously, economically in all the rights and responsibilities of life."[45]

In 1975, the International Women's Year culminated in a UN-sponsored conference in Mexico City, intended to develop a 10-year plan to improve the status of women, particularly stressing education and health care. More than 1000 UN delegates and 5000 feminists and interested spectators attended; however, despite a document of official recommendations, the highly politicized meeting was not as successful as had been hoped. Most serious was the division of interests of the women. The caucus of third-world women, for instance, showed little interest in the concerns of Western women.

Equal pay and day-care centers are not issues in countries where most women have no voting or property rights. The recommendations that emerged were a mixture and focused on encouraging governments to ensure equality in terms of educational opportunities, training, and employment; to ameliorate the "hard work loads" falling on women in certain economic groups and in certain countries; and to ensure that women have equal rights with men in voting and participating in political life.

In 1979, the UN General Assembly adopted "... what is essentially an international bill of rights for women." However, the treaty, known as the United Nations Convention on Elimination of All Forms of Discrimination Against Women, has yet to gain worldwide recognition or acceptance. In 1994, 128 countries had ratified the treaty, and few had made any significant efforts to eliminate discrimination against women. Notably, although the United States was part of the General Assembly consensus in adopting the convention, the Senate has yet to ratify it.

In 1985, a UN Third World Conference on Women was held in Nairobi, Kenya. It pulled together the disparate views that had kept women apart in Mexico a decade earlier and focused them into a document called *Nairobi Forward-Looking Strategies for Advancement of Women to the Year 2000.* The strategies evolved from three basic objectives: equality, economic and social development, and peace.

The focus of the meeting in Kenya on development was unable to ignite the spark to unify women and drive them on to some very challenging positions, which were certain to create personal jeopardy. Also, however eloquent the rhetoric in 1985, the resources to fund the platform were nonexistent at international or national levels. The 10 years between Kenya and Beijing, which was the site for the UN Fourth World Conference on Women, were unique and changed the dynamics of the international women's movement.

Telecommunications came into its own, and although not penetrating every corner of the world, networks began to be built, and women began to realize that there was a common agenda. The barriers that had existed between women of the developing and industrialized worlds were realized for what they were: self-imposed limitations on their ability to join together and become a unified force.

Digging beneath the surface, there was a common cause. The other variable that happened on the scene at the same time as telecommunications, and perhaps was strengthened because of it, was the growing presence and power of nongovernmental organizations (NGOs). It is the NGOs that can speak out boldly, rise above government in many instances, and often find the dollars to do what has to be done. It is the NGOs that penetrate down to the grass roots, cement the marriage of public and private sector resources, and know the capacity for success in most ventures. The magic of women's networks fashioned and strengthened by NGOs and the ability to sustain communications brought 50,000 participants to Beijing. The agenda was also "right" for the times. The legal and legislative focus of 1985 gave way to discussions of personal security. The Platform for Action included issues on the empowerment of women, reproductive health, valuing women's unpaid work, the equal right of women to inherit, women's rights as human rights, and violence against women.[46] Particular attention was given to the girl-child and her right to nurturing and protection.[47] Not surprisingly, the United Nations has lagged in follow-through. However, pieces of the platform are already being mobilized through the growing global web that has begun to connect women's groups.

In the United States, resistance to the women's movement was epitomized by the death of the proposed Equal Rights Amendment (ERA) to the Constitution, three states short of the 38 needed for ratification (see Chapter 17). Ten years after it was passed by Congress, and despite an extension of the deadline for ratification from 1979 to 1982, Indiana in 1977 was the last state to ratify. More than 450 national organizations endorsed the amendment, and polls showed that more than two-thirds of US citizens supported it, but to no avail. The conservative opposition, including fundamentalist Christian churches, the so-called Moral Majority, the John Birch Society, the Mormon Church, and the American Farm Bureau, led a well-financed, smoothly organized, and politically astute campaign. Antiamendment forces assured state legislators that the Fourteenth Amendment offered sufficient protection to women, and claimed that the ERA would cause the death of the family by removing a man's obligation to support his wife and children; would legalize homosexual marriages; would lead to unisex toilets; and most damaging, would lead to the drafting of women for combat duty. Advocates of the ERA were later criticized as lacking political finesse and alienating women who were potential supporters—blacks, pink-collar (office) workers, and housewives. Amendment supporters lay heavy blame on men, particularly in legislature and business.

In the 1980s and early 1990s, feminists were determined to concentrate women's new consciousness and resources in building legislative strength to eventually pass the ERA and to mount a campaign for reproductive freedom, including abortion and recognition of all human rights, including gay and lesbian rights; democratization of families; more respect for work done in the home; and comparable pay for the work done outside it. Since 1973, when the US Supreme Court decided *Roe v. Wade*, women have had the right to seek an abortion, at least in the first trimester. The basis for this decision was a woman's right to privacy. Efforts to overturn *Roe* have not been successful, but antiabortion forces have succeeded in eliminating Medicaid funding of abortion for poor women (Hyde amendment), and in requiring a waiting period prior to abortion and parental consent for minors who seek an abortion.

Three decades after Betty Friedan published *The Feminine Mystique* (called by the futurist Alvin Toffler, "the book that pulled the trigger of history"), changes can be clearly identified, even though some of the results have varied.

In terms of the ERA, Congress voted down another ERA bill in 1983. The bill was defeated by six votes. Yet both friends and foes of equal rights note that the campaign for the amendment, along with other social forces, made a definite impact on American life.

The glass ceiling is still intact and full-time employed women are being paid only 78 cents for every dollar earned by men. Women of color continue to fare even worse, with an African American woman receiving, on average, only 69 cents for every dollar earned by a white man, and a Hispanic woman receiving only 59 cents to the same dollar. Women have to work more than 3 extra months in a year to achieve the same pay that men received. A report, *A New Look Through the Glass Ceiling: Where Are the Women?*, commissioned by Congress and based on data compiled by the General Accounting Office (GAO) from the *Current Population Survey*, shows that 71 percent of all employed women and 73 percent of female managers work in 10 industries. The results confirm what most women already know from experience: women who are full-time managers are paid less and advance less often than male managers. The data also revealed an alarming setback: the wage gap between female managers and their male counterparts widened between 1995 and 2000 in 7 of the 10 industries. The higher women advance, the larger the wage gap between men and women grows. In addition to adverse consequences in the present, the wage gap threatens women's retirement security because lower pay leads to a pension gap and reduced Social Security benefits.[48]

A growing number of lawsuits and union negotiations have challenged the male/female pay ratio based on the comparable worth theory. This theory, going beyond equal pay for equal work, calls for equal pay for different jobs of comparable worth. The intent is to revalue all jobs on the basis of the skills and responsibility they require. Neither the Equal Pay Act nor the Civil Rights Act brought about reform at any level of the workforce. A landmark case resulted in the state of Washington being ordered in 1984 to pay female workers up to $1 billion in back wages and increases because of such pay inequity. However, shortly thereafter, the decision was reversed on appeal. Generally, federal and state governments, as well as the courts, were not supportive of comparable worth. For example, in 1985, the US Civil Rights Commission rejected the comparable worth concept. That same year, a court of appeals ruling written by Judge Anthony M. Kennedy, who was later appointed to the Supreme Court, approved a state's relying on market rates in setting salaries even if it knowingly pays less to women as a result.

The need to give equal attention to home, family, and career along with a variety of other personal interests, once attributed to women, is becoming increasingly important to both sexes. Modern times call for the emergence of a new leadership style, which focuses on quick responses to change and the ability to bring out the best in people. This is not only a response to the values that women have brought to the workplace, but is totally consistent with what today's employees want for themselves.

The issue of women's rights is closely related to the problems, activities, and goals of women working in the health service industry. Between 75 and 85 percent of all health service workers are women, and the largest health occupation, nursing, is almost totally female. These female-dominated occupations are also expanding rapidly, but men continue to dominate the positions of authority within the health care system.

The reasons so many women are in health care are that, first, they are an inexpensive source of labor; second, they are available; and third, they have been safe and not a threat to physicians. The rise of nurses as autonomous practitioners certainly is a threat to that traditional power base.

More than any other factor, the absence of professional autonomy for nurses is considered a direct result of sex discrimination in nursing, with the end result that the patient and client ultimately suffer. The movement of nurses toward autonomy is seen partially as the result of the women's movement, and the struggles in achieving autonomy have certainly enhanced interest in the movement. The fight against sexual discrimination has gained new impetus in nursing, as well as in other segments of society, and has spilled over to include the consumer movement of women's health.

■ LABOR AND INDUSTRY

Because nursing is part of the health care industry and unions are making new efforts to organize nurses and others in health care, the status of labor unions is an important socioeconomic factor. Unions represented 12.4 percent of the workforce in 2010, which is significantly reduced from its high of 20.1 percent in 1983, the first year for which comparable data are available.[49]

Beginning with President Reagan's breaking of the air controllers' illegal strike in August 1981 by firing and subsequently replacing the air controllers, the unions have had special difficulties. Some employers simply threaten to file for bankruptcy, and the courts have supported their right to abrogate any existing union contract under those circumstances. Others find that they can withstand long strikes because they are legally permitted to make permanent job replacements, and the unemployed and workers in lesser-paid fields are willing to take the strikers' jobs. (Note that President Clinton signed an executive order making it illegal for employers who participate in federal government contracts to permanently replace strikers.) Given the compromised position of most employees, employers are demanding (and getting) paybacks of benefits and pay in new contracts, citing competition as the reason. Union leadership has been blamed by many for not seeing the economic problems of being greedy in earlier years. What has also made it easier for management is the growing tendency of people to prefer to work part time, a trend that is predicted to increase. Although this is particularly true of women, including nurses, who have young families or simply need to contribute to the family income, there are also a surprising number of men who make this choice. Both women and men may be attending school, beginning their own business, testing out a different field, working at a second job, or simply looking for more flexibility and independence. Some like the variety and the fact that they need not get involved in the politics and problems of the workplace. On the other hand, wages may be lower (not necessarily true for nurses), there is little opportunity for career advancement, and some temporary workers complain of being dumped on by regular employees. Industry has found these contingency workers economically advantageous. Employers do not usually pay for any benefits, which can be a considerable savings, and they can bring in these workers at busy times, while maintaining a minimum workforce. It sometimes provides a way around union work rules and, at times, a way to confront striking unions. The negative side is that part-time or short-term workers may not have the same commitment to the company, and unless they return to the same place frequently, they need orientation and perhaps even training. Yet, it is quite possible that the availability of these workers and full-time replacements has made strikes a less popular union tool.

Despite these problems, by the beginning of 1990 there was some optimism in the ranks of labor. For the first time in over a decade, younger, more sophisticated labor leaders had replaced nearly all the old guard. Also, both labor and industry were stressing the need for harmony. In 1989, union membership grew, although with a greater overall growth in the workforce, the percentage continued to diminish. There was considerable growth in governmental unions, but the service industries, accounting for most of the growth in the labor force, had only 6 percent union participation. All seemed to be good candidates for organization. Because women are a large part of the latter group (they are also considered easier to organize), the unions are beginning to tackle "women's issues" such as abortion and the safety of women on the job. However, their interest has not extended to placing women in the top echelon of the labor federation's hierarchy.

Management, criticized for its authoritarian approach, is trying new techniques to increase worker satisfaction. Although far from widespread, there does seem to be growing interest in involving workers in decision making. Most American companies have reform programs in which workers and supervisors discuss operations. In industry these may be called quality circles; in health care they may be called shared governance. Some labor experts say that these reforms (also known by such names as *job redesign*, *work humanization*, *employee participation*, *workplace democracy*, and *quality of work life*) are more cosmetic than real because few workers participate in the companies'

most important decisions, and that in a difficult situation most managers revert to an authoritarian stance. Others say that this new management style is necessary now that the nation is engaged in vigorous international competition. Similar techniques have been used in Europe and Japan for some time, and production success, particularly in Japan, was envied by American industry. Whether there will be backsliding when economic times are worse is the question.

In summary, American unions had been in decline for some years, with the presence of a federal administration that favored big business and created incentives for the country's financial recovery to occur through the development of small business and industry. This antilabor sentiment was acted out through management-friendly appointments to the Supreme Court and the National Labor Relations Board (NLRB), the governmental unit critical to facilitating efforts at organizing and unionization. At the same time, more basic employee guarantees were being provided through legislation and regulations, decreasing the need for union protection. A final observation is that the American union tradition had been built on an adversarial relationship between labor and management. This has proved to be inconsistent with the employee-employer relationships that have produced quality outcomes in other countries. Conversely, recent presidential appointments to the NLRB have been pro-union. The only sure prediction is that American labor is in a state of transition, but the direction of change is currently uncertain. This transition will be further discussed in Chapter 30.

■ THE CONSUMER REVOLUTION

The consumer revolution, said to have begun when Theodore Roosevelt signed the first Pure Food and Drug Act in 1906, has been an accelerating phenomenon since the 1950s. Although the term is often interpreted differently, it might be broadly defined as the concerted action of the public in response to a lack of satisfaction with the products or services they receive. The publics are, of course, different, but often overlapping. A woman unhappy about the cost and quality of auto repairs might be just as displeased by the services of her gynecologist, the cost of hospital care, or the use of dangerous food additives.

There have probably always been dissatisfied consumers, but the major difference now is that many are organized in ad hoc or permanent organizations and have the power, through money, numbers, and influence, to force providers to be responsive to at least some of their demands. The methods vary but include lobbying for legislation, legal suits, boycotts, and media campaigns. One of the most noted, albeit highly criticized, consumer activists is Ralph Nader, whose Center for Study of Responsive Law produced a blitz of study group reports in the early 1970s that exposed abuses in a wide range of fields. His Health Research Group has been one of the most influential in health consumerism. There is an increasingly strong force moving in that direction, especially with the better-educated and more aggressive generations and the elderly. Consumers, who first concentrated their efforts against the shoddy quality of work and indifferent services offered on material goods, have now turned to the quality, quantity, and cost of other services, particularly in health care. Fewer patients and clients are accepting without protest the "I know best" attitudes of health care providers, whether physician, nurse, or any of the many others involved in health care. The self-help phenomenon in which people learn about health care and help each other ("stroke clubs" and Alcoholics Anonymous, for instance) has extended to self-examination. Interest in health promotion and illness prevention has also been manifested by the involvement of consumers in environmental concerns.

The dehumanization of patient care, which is contrary to all the stated beliefs of the professions involved, is repeatedly castigated in studies of health care. Although complaints often are directed at the care of the poor, too often it is a universal deficiency. The concerted action of organized minority groups led to the development of the American Hospital Association's Patient Bill of Rights (see Chapter 22), which received widespread attention in 1973, followed by a rash of similar rights statements specifically directed to children, the mentally ill, the elderly, pregnant women, the dying, the handicapped, patients of various religions, and others. The whole area of the rights of people in health care, which focuses to a great extent on patients' rights to full and accurate information so that they can make decisions about their care and the accountability of health care plans, has major implications for nurses.

The creation of the Agency for Healthcare Research and Quality (originally the Agency for Healthcare Policy and Research) is another example of the growth of consumerism in the health care industry. The agency was charged by Congress to work with the medical community to reach consensus on the preferred treatment of a select group of common conditions that the Institute of Medicine (IOM) identified. This was a direct response to the frustration that government and the public experienced over inconsistencies in the medical management of these conditions, and that the absence of adequate explanations usually resulted in the patient deferring to the provider. These consensus statements were translated into consumer-friendly language and provided as public information.

The growth of managed care has created a consumer revolution of another type. With the current competition between hospitals and even nursing homes to fill their beds, consumer satisfaction has emerged as a significant outcome indicator. Institutions are placing a priority on the courtesy that employees show to consumers and conduct frequent surveys to identify where indignities and impatience may continue to exist. It is right and proper that the "customer" be treated with courtesy and respect, but the consumer cannot always be "right" where decisions often require knowledge and skill accrued over a lifetime of professional service. The goal is commendable, but caution must be exercised before we lose sight of the ultimate end of improving the human condition.

It has been hard for many Americans to adjust to the limited options provided by some managed care plans. Responding to the allegation that quality, and even safety, is often compromised, President Clinton established an Advisory Commission on Consumer Protection and Quality in the Health Care Industry, which authored a *Patient's Bill of Rights*. This bill of rights has had many of its aspects put into legislative form, but none has become law. The following consumer protections have been major concerns:

- Holding managed care plans liable for decisions on withholding care that cause harm to patients
- Ensuring that treatment decisions are made by the patient and the patient's chosen health care provider
- Ensuring that physicians and nurses can report quality problems with health plans or settings for care without retaliation (whistle-blowing protection)
- Preventing health care professionals from being rewarded for limiting a patient's care
- Requiring hospitals to publicly disclose information on nurse staffing and adverse clinical outcomes in patients
- Protecting nurses who voice concern about poor staffing from retribution

- Requiring health care institutions considering a merger or acquisition to report on the anticipated effect this would have on the community
- Ensuring patient access to clinical trials

This list is not all inclusive, but it provides an indication of the range of public concern over health care. These ideas about patient rights and protections were cast into legislation, which has lingered for many Congressional sessions with little progress. In fact, many states moved forward in the interim to guarantee these and many more consumer protections at the state level.

Other consumers are concerned with the power issue and are insisting, with some success, on increased representation on governing boards of hospitals and other health care institutions, accrediting boards, health planning groups, and licensing boards. What lies ahead in terms of more regulation, such as an overall federal consumer protection law and state laws that are actually enforced, is not yet known. However, the consumer movement continues to gain strength, and some further action is inevitable. The nursing community has a history of supporting public policy that builds the strength of consumerism. These sentiments are prominent in *Nursing's Agenda for Health Care Reform*, organized nursing's directive for public policy reform.[50]

KEY POINTS

1. Nursing and health care must exist within the socioeconomic and technological changes that have occurred and are occurring.
2. The shrinking world makes it impossible for any country to exist in a vacuum, monopolizing the use of resources and ignoring the pain of the rest of the planet.
3. As developing countries make progress, their problems will become more like those of the industrialized world.
4. The complexity of our human problems demands a social model for the delivery of health services, accepting the fact that health care, housing, education, workplace safety, and a host of other concerns interrelate in the search for quality of life and vie for the same resources.
5. Health care and its support systems exist within a cultural context, and it becomes dangerous to impose an alien value system.
6. We are entering a period of social stabilization in this country. Social structures may not look the same, but there is a recommitment to traditional values.
7. In the United States, demographics are our destiny; we are faced with an aging and chronically ill population.
8. Our most prominent health problems could be significantly reduced through healthier living—diet, weight control or reduction, exercise, stress reduction, and rest.
9. No cure has been found for HIV/AIDS, but massive strides in managing the disease make a long and productive life possible.
10. A nation's health is often judged in terms of its infants and children. Despite recent efforts, America's children are still significantly needy.
11. The declining presence of the traditional family in this culture demands the creation of new services, programs, and public policy.
12. A fragile environment requires that we take every precaution to prevent its further deterioration.
13. High-tech advances will not stop but must be counterbalanced by a conscious and generous dose of caring and humanism.
14. Nurses stand at the center of an information-rich environment, the most strategic position for the twenty-first century.
15. Our centralized structures have failed, and we are decentralizing to rebuild from the bottom up.
16. Americans are demanding personal expression in their work, hours that complement a private life, and participation in decisions that impact the quality of their workplace.
17. Suspicion of our most basic institutions has moved us to demand more accountability from professionals.
18. We are in a period of active consumerism that will only intensify as Internet information increases in quality.

KEY POINTS

19. Americans are returning to self-reliance after a crippling period of dependence on institutions and government to make our decisions and do our bidding.

20. There is a growing expectation that government should guarantee certain health care protections to its people.

21. The traditional hierarchical model has become flattened, and we are responding to needs with networks and ad hoc systems.

22. Americans will live with less, they will sacrifice, but they will never give up their right to choose.

REFERENCES

1. Begun J, White K. Altering nursing's dominant logic: Guidelines from complex adaptive systems theory. *Complex Chaos Nurs* 2:5–15, Summer 1995.

2. World Health Organization. The World Health Report 2008. http://www.who.int/whr/2008/en/index.html/. Retrieved March 20, 2010.

3. UNICEF. The State of the World's Children 2009 (Special Edition). http://www.unicef.org/rightsite/sowc/pdfs/SOWC_SpecEd_CRC_ExecutiveSummary_EN_091009.pdf/. Retrieved March 24, 2010.

4. Ibid.

5. Ibid.

6. US Census Bureau. US & World Population Clock. http://www.census.gov/main/www/popclock.html/. Retrieved April 2, 2010.

7. World Health Organization, loc cit.

8. UNICEF, loc cit.

9. Joel L. Teach a woman, educate the world. *Am J Nurs* 94:7, July 1994.

10. AVERTing. HIV and AIDS. http://www.avert.org/world-stats.htm/. Retrieved March 20, 2010.

11. The World Report 2008, Executive Summary, loc cit.

12. US & World Population Clock, loc cit.

13. Census 2000. http://www.usatoday.com/graphics/census2000/United States/state.htm/. Retrieved June14, 2001.

14. Centers for Disease Control (CDC). FastStats. http://www.cdc.gov/nchs/fastats/nursingh.htm/. Retrieved March 20, 2010.

15. Law Practice Today. http://www.abanet.org/lpm/lpt/articles/mgt08044.html. Retrieved March 24, 2010.

16. CBS News. The Millenials Are Coming. http://www.cbsnews.com/stories/2007/11/08/60minutes/main3475200.shtml/. Retrieved March 30, 2010.

17. US Census Bureau News. More Diversity, Slower Growth. http://www.census.gov/Press-Release/www/releases/archives/population/001720.html/. Retrieved April 4, 2010.

18. Diner H. Immigration and US History. http://www.america.gov/st/diversity-english/2008/February/20080307112004ebyessedo0.1716272.html/. Retrieved March 18, 2010.

19. US Census Bureau News. 50 Million Children Lived With Married Parents in 2007. http://www.census.gov/Press-Release/www/releases/archives/marital_status_living_arrangements/012437.html/. Retrieved April 10, 2010.

20. Washington Post. Number of Unwed Mothers Has Risen Sharply in the US. May 14, 2009. http://www.washingtonpost.com/wp-dyn/content/article/2009/05/13/. Retrieved March 10, 2010.

21. Jayson Sharon. Report: Overall Abortion Rates Continue to Drop. January 18, 2008. http://www.usatoday.com/news/health/ 2008-01-16-abortion-rates_N.htm/. 22. Idem. Retrieved March 16, 2010.

22. Ibid.

23. Organization for Economic Cooperation and Development (OECD). Country Note: USA. http://www.oecd.org/dataoecd/47/2/41528678.pdf. Retrieved April 8, 2010.

24. CBS News. 3.5 M Kids Under 5 on Verge of Going Hungry. http://www.cbsnews.com/stories/2009/05/07/health/main4998190.shtml. Retrieved April 2, 2010.

25. Children's Defense Fund. http://www.childrensdefense.org/. Retrieved June 17, 2002.

26. CNN Money. Young Invincibles Imperil Health Care Reform (April 9, 2010). http://money.cnn.com/2010/04/09/news/economy/health_reform_young_invincibles_threat/. Retrieved April 10, 2010.

27. US Census Bureau. Income and Poverty Status of Americans Improve, Health Insurance Coverage Stable, Census Bureau Reports. http://www.census.gov/. Retrieved April 10, 2002.

28. Homelessness: Programs and the People They Serve. http://www.huduser.org/publications/homeless/homelessness/content.html. Retrieved June 17, 2002.

29. Reuters. US Life Expectancy Reaches a New High. http://www.reuters.com/article/idUSTRE57I6BF20090820. Retrieved April 3, 2010.

30. Health Resources Service Administration (HRSA). Child Health USA: 2008–2009. http://mchb.hrsa.gov/chusa08/hstat/hsi/pages/206im.html. Retrieved April 2, 2010.

31. National Center for Health Statistics. Healthy People 2000. http://www.cdc.gov/nchs/about/otheract/hp2000/2000ind icators.htm. Retrieved August 15, 2000.

32. Connolly C. US minorities get lower quality health care: Moral implications of widespread pattern noted. *Washington Post*, March 21, 2002, A4.

33. American Red Cross. HIV/AIDS Facts. http://www. redcross.org/services/hss/Tips/February/answer00.html. Retrieved June 29, 2002.

34. National Report Says Minorities Hard Hit by Diabetes: National Diabetes Education Program Responds. http://www.niddk.nih.gov/welcome/releases/. Retrieved July 1, 2002.

35. National Center for Health Statistics. Retrieved August 15, 2000, ibid.

36. American Cancer Society. Cancer Facts and Figures 2010. http://www.cancer.org/docroot/home/index.asp/. Retrieved March 22, 2010.

37. US Public Health Service. *Promoting health/preventing disease: Objectives for the nation.* Washington, DC: US Department of Health and Human Services, 1980.

38. US Public Health Service. *Healthy People 2000.* Washington, DC: US Department of Health and Human Services, 1990.

39. US Public Health Service. *Laying the foundation for Healthy People 2010—The first year of consultation.* Washington, DC: US Department of Health and Human Services, 1999.

40. National Institutes of Health, National Human Genome Research Institute. The Human Genome Project Completion. http://www.genome.gov/11006943/. Retrieved April 9, 2010.

41. The Boyer Commission on Educating Undergraduates in the Research University. Reinventing Undergraduate Education. http://naples.cc.sunysb.edu/Pres/boyer.nsf/webform/overview/. Retrieved April 10, 2010.

42. The Chronicle of Higher Education. The Nation. http://chronicle.com/free/almanac/2001. Retrieved June 20, 2002.

43. Vance C, Talbot S, McBride A, et al. An uneasy alliance: Nursing and the women's movement. *Nurs Outlook* 33:281–285, November–December 1985.

44. Christy T. Liberation movement: Impact on nursing. *AORN* 15:67–68, April 1972.

45. National Organization for Women. Resolved: The Pursuit of Feminist Ideals Is Detrimental to the Achievement of Gender Equality. November 11, 1995. http://www.now.org/history/debate.html. Retrieved November 1, 2002.

46. Shepherd D. Beijing conference ignited profound hopes among world's women, but frustration sets in. *The Earth Times* August–September 1996.

47. NGO Working Group on Girls. *Clearing a path for girls.* New York/Geneva: UNICEF, 1998.

48. National Organization for Women. Women Deserve Equal Pay. http://www.now.org/issues/economic/factsheet.html/. Retrieved April 2, 2010.

49. US Department of Labor, Bureau of Labor Statistics. Union Members Summary. http://www.bls.gov/news.release/union2.nr0.htm. Retrieved March 22, 2010.

50. American Nurses Association. *Nursing's agenda for health care reform.* Washington, DC: American Nurses Publishing, 1991.

Updates can be found at **www.kellysnursing.com**

CHAPTER 7

Health Care Delivery: Where?

Health care today is provided in a variety of settings, such as hospitals, nursing homes, community health centers, clinics, and the homes of patients and clients. More than 12 million workers are involved in providing these services.[1] The size and complexity of the health care system alone create problems in the quality of service provided.

It is generally agreed that some of the essential ingredients of optimum health services, wherever they are given, include a cooperative interdisciplinary approach to care; a spectrum of services, including diagnosis, treatment, rehabilitation, education, and prevention; a system that coordinates these services and ensures continuity; and a program of evaluation and research concerning the adequacy of services in meeting patient and community needs. Put another way, organizations offer various types of services that could be categorized as primary care, and so on. For optimum benefit, they are further structured to allow fluid movement of patients through these services. Although it is not practical to proceed with our discussion using these definitions, because there is considerable overlap, they are necessary for you to understand and are presented in Exhibit 7–1.

This chapter and the next are intended to provide an overview of current health care delivery, its organization, and its workers. Specific details on how the nurse may function in these various settings are presented in Chapter 15.

■ THE HEALTH CARE ENVIRONMENT: ISSUES OF COST AND QUALITY

Before describing the settings in which health care is delivered, it is essential to understand some of the changes that have occurred in the last several decades—changes that relate directly to the public's concern about the cost and quality of health care. As often happens, the public's dissatisfaction with something translates itself into legislation by those they elected. In this case, because the cost of health care rose so rapidly, legislation, regulations, and executive orders proliferated at both the state and national levels. The strategy was to clamp down on the people (providers) and places delivering health care and force them to treat their patients with more economic prudence. (See Chapters 17 and 19 on how laws are made and how legislation affects health care.) Government impact is particularly great on health care because almost every sector of the industry receives a large portion of its revenues from government entitlement programs, grants, and contracts. The government's share of health care expenditures increased dramatically after the establishment of the Medicare and Medicaid programs. By 1995, the government's share was more than 45 percent of the total expenditures in this country. Moreover, others who pay for health care (payers) such as health insurance companies, including the well-known Blue Cross and Blue Shield, tend to follow the payment patterns set by the government.

National health expenditures in the United States surpassed $2.3 trillion in 2008, more than three times the $714 billion spent in 1990, and over eight times the $253 billion spent in 1980. In 2008, US health care spending was about $7,681 per resident and accounted for 16.2 percent of the nation's Gross Domestic Product (GDP); this is among the highest of all industrialized countries. The GDP is the total value of goods and services produced in the United States and is an indicator of total economic production,

■ EXHIBIT 7–1. Definitions

Primary care: "(a) a person's first contact in any given episode of illness with the health care system that leads to a decision of what must be done to help resolve his problems; and (b) the responsibility for the continuum of care, i.e., maintenance of health, evaluation and management of symptoms, and appropriate referrals."[a]

Secondary care: the point at which consulting specialty and subspecialty services are provided in either an ambulatory, residential, or community hospital inpatient setting.

Tertiary care: the point at which highly sophisticated diagnostic, treatment or rehabilitation services are provided, frequently in university medical centers or equivalent settings.

Quaternary care: advanced levels of medicine that are highly specialized and not widely used. Experimental medicine, service-oriented surgeries, and other less common approaches to treatment and diagnostics comprise the bulk of quaternary care. The term is an extension of tertiary care, which is more common and less specific.

Vertical integration of services: an arrangement between organizations that provide different services with the goal of creating a continuum of care.[b]

Horizontal integration: an arrangement between organizations that provide similar services, such as a chain or network of hospitals.[b]

Acute care: those services used in the treatment of illness or disability that have as their purpose the restoration of normal life processes and function.

Long-term care: "those services designed to provide symptomatic treatment (palliative), maintenance, and rehabilitative services for patients of all age groups . . ."[a]

[a]US Department of Health, Education, and Welfare. *Extending the Scope of Nursing Practice*. Washington, DC: US Department of Health, Education and Welfare, 1971, pp 3–11.
[b]Sullivan EJ, Decker PJ. *Effective Leadership and Management in Nursing*, 4th ed. Menlo Park, CA: Addison Wesley Longman, 1997, p 21.

or total economic output. Total health care expenditures grew at an annual rate of 4.4 percent by 2008, a slower rate than earlier years, yet still outpacing inflation and the growth in national income.[2] Over the years, government dollars as a percentage of total dollars spent on health care have also increased. In 1960, private funds, including private insurance and out-of-pocket dollars, paid for over three-quarters of health care in the United States. By 1998, the government's share was almost half. By 2002, the government was funding 60 percent of health care for the American public.[3]

As shown in Exhibit 7–2, hospital care and physician/clinical services combined account for half (51 percent) of the nation's health expenditures.

A variety of factors have been blamed for the high cost of health care in the United States. Until 1983, both Medicare and Medicaid and most health insurance plans traditionally paid for the full and reasonable cost of care on a retrospective basis, that is, whatever the provider said it cost, within certain limits. (Medicare/Medicaid law and its changes are described more fully in Chapter 19.) With the high cost of new technology used for both diagnosis and treatment as well as consumer demand for the newest and the best, costs soared. In 1983, federal regulations entitled Prospective Payment [System] (PPS) for Medicare Inpatient Hospital Services were developed because hospital costs were the most expensive component of the industry, and there was fear that Medicare funds would run out.

Under PPS, disorders of the human body were divided into major diagnostic categories with hundreds of subgroups called diagnostic related groups (DRGs). A patient is assigned to one of approximately 500 subgroups depending on age, principal diagnosis, and the presence or absence of surgery or other major procedures and complications or comorbidity (case mix). One all-inclusive reimbursement amount is identified for each patient, regardless of whether the patient's care requires fewer or more dollars than anticipated. The concept is one of shared risk, recognizing that within each DRG there will be a range of patients whose needs differ; they cross-subsidize one another, and, as a group, generate enough resources to compensate the hospital. Those who clamor for more

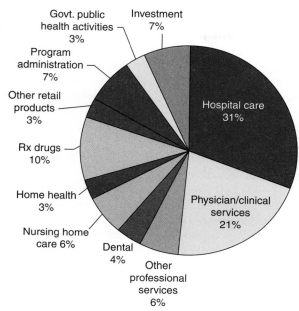

National Health Expenditures, 2008

- Govt. public health activities 3%
- Investment 7%
- Program administration 7%
- Other retail products 3%
- Rx drugs 10%
- Home health 3%
- Nursing home care 6%
- Dental 4%
- Other professional services 6%
- Hospital care 31%
- Physician/clinical services 21%

Total = $2.3 trillion

EXHIBIT 7–2. How is the US health care dollar spent? (*Source:* Centers for Medicare and Medicaid Services, Office of the Actuary, National Health Statistics Group)

case-specific calculations have missed the principle of shared risk.

If a patient is discharged without using all of the dollars reserved for his or her care, the hospital is allowed to keep all or part of the surplus. This has resulted in accusations that patients are being discharged sicker and quicker, with more complex and highly technological care being required in the home or nursing home. Some hospitals are exempt from the DRG model, and there are exceptions, but they are becoming rarer. The predetermined cost of an episode of illness based on select patient-centered assessments (case mix) that drive the payment system for services has been expanded past the hospital market. Case mix methodologies (mandated for Medicare) have been developed for nursing homes (the Minimum Data Set [MDS] and Resource Utilization Groups [RUGs]), for home care (the Outcome and Assessment Information Set [OASIS]), for hospital-based ambulatory care (Ambulatory Payment Classifications [APC]), and for provider professional

services (the Resource-Based Relative Value Scale [RBRVS] and Current Procedural Terminology [CPT]). Many states have seized on the case mix and PPS model to apply to other public welfare programs, such as Medicaid.

The whole process of admission, discharge, and the use of hospital resources during the length of stay is monitored for Medicare by government intermediaries (Peer Review Organizations), and payment for any service may be denied retrospectively, after the service is given. A similar system of oversight has been adopted on a state-by-state basis for other programs under state jurisdiction. There is much concern that patient acuity or intensity is not adequately considered, especially in relation to the nursing care needed. Shaped by these economic models, hospital utilization has been greatly reduced, and patients are considerably sicker because admission tests are now done on an outpatient basis, and there are no grace periods for postacute or postsurgical recovery before discharge.

The 1980s was a time of competition and aggressive business practices. Hospitals followed suit and looked to new strategies for financial survival. One strategy was aggressive marketing, aimed particularly at self-paying patients and those with private sector insurance. Although it is sometimes denied, administrators encouraged physicians to admit patients who were likely to be dischargeable early. Some hospitals closed units that were costly and unlikely to be fully reimbursed, such as burn and trauma units, and encouraged regionalization.

Patient dumping, transferring certain high-resource patients to government hospitals, was another cost-saving technique, although in 1989 a law was enacted penalizing hospitals that dump. Hospitals looked for other ways to fill beds with paying patients, such as those requiring long-term care. They developed subacute and skilled nursing units, emergicenters, surgicenters, and home care services. Hospitals established neighborhood primary care clinics, so that as the healthy and relatively healthy became ill, they would reach out to the parent hospital for their continuing care. They used helicopters to bring in emergency patients from distant areas and advertised their services and their physicians in media campaigns. Some created profit-making components that included equipment rental, health promotion and education classes, and even hotels and contracts with noted fast-food companies. They merged with other hospitals or agencies to share services and markets, sometimes even developing into national chains. Many of these tactics have become standard practice, even to creating health care malls that include doctors' offices; a hospital; ambulatory care; laboratory, pharmacy, optometry, physical therapy, and physical fitness services; as well as home care services, restaurants, gift shops, banking, and parking. Although copycat economics has been criticized, nonprofit hospitals maintained that these approaches were needed for survival. In fact, in the 1980s and 1990s, many small hospitals, especially in rural areas, simply went out of business, despite the needs of the population, and more closures are predicted as we move more deeper into the twenty-first century.

Care of the 46.3 million uninsured people in this country creates serious problems for hospitals.[4] These are the medically indigent—the working poor. They are neither old enough for Medicare nor poor enough for Medicaid. They may be unemployed, between jobs, or caught in episodic or part-time positions and unable to afford private health insurance. Then there are the homeless who come to emergency rooms, without Medicaid, even though they may be eligible. As a class these individuals and others create the bad debt burden for US hospitals.

Hospitals have always given free care, and usually the cost was absorbed by increasing the bills of paying patients. This historic technique, called cost shifting, has backfired. This strategy had the ultimate consequence of billing patients with private insurance at a higher rate and indirectly contributing to increased premium rates. Insurers and employers did not accept this situation quietly. The practice of cost shifting was tested in the courts and found to be illegal. Instead, in most states, the burden of uncompensated care is assumed by hospitals and the state jointly. One approach is for the state to provide dollars equal to all or part of the amount of uncompensated care, which is then distributed to those hospitals that carry a heavy burden of debt. It has become part of every hospital's legacy to assume some debt, because government entitlement programs (Medicare/Medicaid) do not pay the full cost of the care of their patients.

Even though creative and humane solutions have surfaced to spread the cost of caring for the medically indigent, the issue remains whether this is the health care industry's problem or a public health responsibility to be addressed by the society as a whole.

Many small employers are choosing not to provide health care benefits. Large corporations are opting to become self-insured, promote wellness and prudence among employees, and fund their own risk. Almost everyone is imposing some sort of benefits management. This may be as little as requiring that anticipated medical care

episodes be precertified or to move all employees into a managed care plan where their choices are to some degree limited. Still other employers may set up their own managed care networks.

Freedom of choice is declining, and many of us are being forced into healthy living. The economic crisis in health care has made many Americans reevaluate their lifestyle and become more self-sufficient in decisions about their health and economically prudent in their choices. Some companies reward employees who have healthy lifestyles or allow the buyback of unused portions of health benefits. In return, employees are paying larger copayments and deductibles.

The Medical Savings Account (MSA) is a program enabled through federal and in many cases state legislation, and also supports this philosophy of personal responsibility. Consumers are allowed to set aside pre-tax dollars to be used for medical expenses. The amount is capped at a preset amount, the gross salary is reduced by a like amount, and any dollars remaining in the account at the end of the year are forfeit. This money can be used for copayments, deductibles, and uncovered health care expenses. In some situations, a separate account may be set up to cover dependent care expenses. This account operates in the same manner as an MSA, but is reserved for child or elder care expenses. Success is contingent on an ability to accurately predict your expenses.

A combination of all these factors brought back interest in national health insurance, a concept that had not been popular since the Great Society years of the Johnson Administration. (See Chapter 19 for more details.) Aside from South Africa, the United States is the only country that does not guarantee its citizens a right to health care. Although there seems to be a trend in these other countries to privatize a portion of their health care, and certainly there are problems, including costs, several national polls indicated that Americans were ready for government to guarantee universal access to health care. Actually, both the American Nurses Association (ANA) and the National League for Nursing (NLN), as well as the American Public Health Association (APHA) have supported the concept of universal access to health care services for years, but the American Medical Association (AMA) and other powerful groups that influence health policy oppose it. Debate should be careful to divide the issues. The funding of health care and the provision of services are two different issues.

On March 23, 2010, President Obama signed into law the Health Care Bill, which promised to transform the US health care system. Though much resistance remains, the legislation aims to assure universal access through a myriad of public/private sector arrangements. The legislation includes prohibitions on exclusions for pre-existing conditions, expanded coverage for children, mandatory coverage with various subsidies for the poor and lower income individuals, eventual closure of the "donut hole" in the Medicare prescription plan, expanded Medicaid coverage, and more.[5] The reader should be alert that the passage of legislation is the first step in a long and tortuous course of action; the development of rules and regulations are the next stage before implementation. Additionally, universal access does not mean socialized medicine or that the government would move into the role of a provider.

Given the burden of caring for the uninsured, some solution is necessary, and this is an ethical dilemma as well as a public policy issue. The question of quality is no less unsettling. Beyond state licensing of health care facilities, which presumably ensures safety, the Joint Commission on Accreditation of Healthcare Organizations (JCAHO), described later, puts its stamp of approval on institutions and agencies that meet specific quality criteria. There is some cynicism as to whether this is simply a paper tiger, but the value of accreditation is certainly evident in some circumstances: Federal funding for certain kinds of services is exclusive to accredited facilities. A number of consumer groups—some formal, some loosely organized, some interested in specific kinds of care such as nursing homes, and some servicing a large group such as the American Association of Retired Persons (AARP), who see high-quality health care as one of their concerns—are also active in evaluating health care or lobbying for improvements. In addition, the federal government has released the names of hospitals with high mortality rates, which some have said is unfair because certain hospitals have more at-risk patients. There are predictions that quality of care will be the hottest issue of the millennium, and that the public expects health practitioners to take responsibility for ensuring high-quality care. Although both physicians and nurses have peer review systems in place, to one extent or another, the warning is that unless improvements are made, government oversight, such as the federally funded Peer Review Organizations (PROs), will increase. PROs monitor the services provided to Medicare recipients to ensure that admission, discharge, and use of resources during the hospital stay are appropriate. If there is any doubt, payment is jeopardized.

So, there has been movement, although it is incremental. Americans are making conscious decisions about the degree of personal health care risk they are willing to assume and about the degrees of freedom they are willing to sacrifice for cost saving. More than ever before, their voices are heard and they are in control of decisions about their health. The growing prominence of managed care supports the use of nontraditional settings for service and coordination, and continuity of services has been proven to be a wise choice and not a luxury. Women, children, and primary care have become our priorities. The enrollment of the poor into managed care plans that also serve the middle class has finally put teeth into the statement, "Health care is a right and not a privilege." We continue to fix the parts that do not work as we had wanted them to be, never seeing the need to undo as failure. Our health care system is, as ever, as diverse and pluralistic as our population.

■ MANAGED CARE

It is impossible to speak of health care without giving significant attention to managed care. What it is. What it is not. What it hopes to accomplish.

Managed care is not a place, but an organizational structure. Neither is it one type of organization, such as a health maintenance organization (HMO). It is based on specific principles that govern the relationship between insurers and providers, such as the observation that cost and utilization are linked. One nonnegotiable rule is to remove the temptation of using volume to increase profit. The common financial arrangement is prepayment of a periodic fee based on capitation. The technique of prepayment shifts the risk to the provider, although it is not used in every plan. Capitation means that the insured (or someone on the insured's behalf, perhaps an employer) agrees to periodically prepay a fixed amount that is established independently from the actual service utilization practices of the enrollees. With capitation, prudent utilization can create profit for the provider, whereas over-utilization can create a financial liability. In some models, risk is even shifted to the insured, for example, in the choice to go to a provider outside of the network available to enrollees for an additional fee. The goal of managed care is to require the decision makers—the consumers, payers, and providers—to carefully consider the merit of services, procedures, and treatments in view of the resources available. In many instances, a primary care provider is expected to assume the responsibility for oversight and become the gatekeeper, ensuring that care is timely and necessary. Particular vigilance is directed toward the major drivers of cost: hospitalization, specialists, and high technology.

Physicians, and perhaps advanced practice nurses (APNs), are seen as the dominant influence because they generate most of the cost through their clinical management. To offset this, the insurer moves to establish a level of control over them. This is done clinically by the use of clinical pathways/protocols that present preferred approaches to a situation. The ultimate goal is standardization, though appeals are possible and expected. Control is achieved financially by seeking a more or less exclusive relationship between the provider and the insurer, thereby creating financial dependency. The most controlled model is the staff HMO, where physicians and nurses are salaried and must usually agree to work exclusively for that HMO. Except for staff HMOs, most providers continue to see patients from a variety of plans. The need to ensure coordination and avoid duplication is truly respected and has created a very prominent role for nurses in case management.

Many of the decisions internal to the managed care organization (MCO) are based on observations of populations as opposed to individuals—what works best for most of the people most of the time. Although contrary to our usual mindset, this could reap much benefit as we struggle to reverse our eroding public health.

Managed care includes the HMO and an endless number of hybrids. The HMO is both an insurer and a provider. Two models are common: the staff model and the individual practice association (IPA). In the staff model, the HMO operates its own facilities and provider professionals are employees. In the IPA, service is delivered through a network of community-based physician or APN offices, and the providers are independent contractors. The HMO is a prepaid health plan, and the consumer pays a single monthly or annual fee. In addition, small copayments are customary for each visit or service. In HMOs, primary care providers (MDs, DOs, APNs) act as gatekeepers, managing common medical conditions and authorizing access to services and specialty care, and the consumer is usually expected to use the services of in-network providers. It has been verified through extensive data collection that APNs are especially suitable for this primary care role.

There are a variety of other managed care models. With the exception of the HMO, there is little clarity on these other models, except that they differ in regard to the following:

- The ability to secure services from providers who are outside the plan's panel (network)
- Direct access to specialists without going through a gatekeeper
- Payment on a fee-for-service or capitated basis
- The amount of copayment or deductible (if relevant)

As of 2010, managed care had captured 50.3 percent of the health care market or about 154 million individuals. Medicare funds 23.1 percent of these enrollees, Medicaid 67.7 percent, and commercial companies enroll 74.6 percent.[6]

Managed care has been promoted as a solution to the escalating costs and fragmentation for Medicare and Medicaid. Mandated managed care enrollment of Medicaid recipients creates a whole new set of problems. MCOs find it difficult to create plans to operate on the limited dollars available through Medicaid. The industry had similar objections to Medicare managed care enrollees, seeing fees as too low to cover the cost of care for the elderly, who are high users. Some researchers have said that one reason HMOs had a history of cost-effectiveness was that their self-selected enrollees were more conservative users of health services, who were attracted by the HMO philosophy of preventive care and health maintenance. This profile does not necessarily apply to Medicare and Medicaid recipients.

There are concerns about quality, disallowing providers to share full information about state-of-the-science treatment and treatment options that should be considered, limitations on choice even if you do know what options exist, incentives paid to providers to push the least expensive choice, and so on. Nearly all states have passed "patient protection" or consumer-oriented laws and/or regulations dealing with managed care. State legislation was an intense focus from 1992 through 2002, with dozens of measures enacted yearly, amid major media attention, anecdotal stories of patients denied treatment, and several major lawsuits. The US Congress has not enacted comparable managed care consumer legislation, although there has been some less strident policy. This activity has dropped off dramatically since 2002, in part because so many states already had laws in place. State legislatures and regulatory agencies, consumers, and managed care entities had reached a reasonable operational balance.[7]

MCOs will have hit their stride when they compete on the basis of quality as opposed to cost. Many now seek accreditation by the National Committee for Quality Assurance (NCQA). The NCQA was established in 1979 by the trade associations for HMOs and managed care. It has become independent and conducts a very rigorous, voluntary accreditation of these plans. Many employers and state agencies require NCQA accreditation as a condition of doing business. Others look to the health plan report card, which provides data from the NCQA's Health Plan Employer Data and Information Set (HEDIS), showing measures of plan performance. The quality assurance infrastructure for managed care is taking shape.

The battle over managed care liability is still raging in state capitals after reaching some degree of closure in Washington. The Employee Retirement Income Security Act (ERISA) was enacted to ensure that employees receive the pension and other benefits promised by their employers. Twenty-one years after the passage of ERISA, the Supreme Court held, in 1995, that ERISA was meant only to ensure uniform administration of employee benefit plans and was not intended to replace the role of the state in regulating the quality of the health care. Then, on June 20, 2002, the US Supreme Court held that states can challenge managed care coverage decisions and hold them responsible for their actions (over the objections of the industry).[8] This is clearly an affirmation of states' rights in health care. However, either managed care or the philosophy it preaches has played a significant role in stemming the increasing cost of health care, and there is promise in these approaches.

■ SELF-CARE

Obviously, most people spend the greater portion of their lives in relative health. The constitution of WHO defines health as a state of complete physical, mental, and social well-being, and not merely the absence of disease or infirmity, which, although it serves as a broad philosophical declaration, is more an optimum goal than a reality.

On a practical level, the Public Health Service's National Center for Health Statistics defines health implicitly in its use of disability days, when usual activities cannot be performed.

Self-care can be defined as the process whereby a layperson functions effectively on his or her own behalf in health promotion, disease prevention, disease detection, and treatment. It is not new and ranges from a simple matter of resting when tired to a more careful judgment of selecting or omitting certain foods or activities, or a semi-primary care activity of taking one or more medications self-prescribed or prescribed by a professional provider at some other point of care. Health care advice comes gratuitously from family, friends, neighbors, and the media (often with a product to sell). People also actively seek, although informally, information or advice from groups, a health professional acquaintance, or the Internet; however, self-care often becomes a matter of trial and error. Increasingly, a new consumer mentality has included the help of others with similar conditions or concerns, so that the individual has support and reinforcement as needed, but can also detect at what point he or she needs professional help.

In some cases, a person may have had some level of professional care previously, and may again, but a certain amount of informed self-diagnosis is not only less expensive for the public, but may also serve a useful purpose for the individual. For instance, a mother who has been taught to take her child's temperature can give much more accurate information to a doctor or nurse practitioner (NP), or avoid a call altogether if she also knows how temperature relates to a child's well-being. A blood pressure reading taken properly at home is more likely to identify hypertension quickly than is a yearly physical examination. The sale of do-it-yourself medical tests, stethoscopes, blood pressure devices, and other medical devices has become a rapidly growing business. Then, the Internet allows us to interpret our data and weigh our options.

In a keynote address to the American Hospital Association Convention in 1996, Newt Gingrich talked about Americans regaining control of health. He noted the range of over-the-counter diagnostics and the ability of people to eventually enter those indicators into a computer, either in their home or at a public kiosk conveniently located for that purpose. The response to this information will be the most common explanation for the symptoms; the best treatment at this point in time; cautions about when and if to seek professional help; who is most qualified to give that help if it becomes necessary; and their credentials, experience, and success rate. This scenario is not some invention of the imagination, but in many ways has become the here and now. Given adequate support systems, 85 percent of health care could be self-provided.

Areas of activity that well describe the self-care domain are as follows[9]:

1. Monitoring, assessing, and diagnosing—monitoring your own body and using diagnostic techniques to establish a database for decisions about personal health and illness. Examples: breast self-examination, pregnancy testing, cholesterol and blood sugar screening, urine testing, tracking weight and blood pressure, diagnosing minor illness, and so on.

2. Supporting life processes—teeth brushing, bathing, nutrition, and exercise.

3. Therapeutic and corrective self-care—care of minor acute and stabilized chronic illnesses, even serious conditions such as kidney disease requiring dialysis and brittle diabetes that are of such a long-term quality that they become part of the individual's self-image.

4. Prevention of disease and maladjustment states—taking into consideration risk factors for certain illnesses such as cardiac conditions, diabetes, hypertension, methods of maintaining psychological well-being (e.g., stress reduction techniques), guided imagery, and yoga.

5. Specifying health needs and care requirements—advocating on your own behalf, setting the parameters for your treatment, and rejecting anything less.

6. Auditing and controlling the treatment program—women and minorities demanding better care, holding provider professionals accountable to the client on the client's terms. Should that be unacceptable, finding another provider.

7. Grassroots or self-initiated health care—using peers as therapists: Weight Watchers, smoking cessation programs, and peer support for a variety of problems.

Besides consumerism, another factor that encourages self-care is cost and convenience. For instance, emergency rooms are frequently filled with patients who have minor conditions that could have been prevented or self-treated at home at an earlier stage.

Nursing incorporates a philosophy of holism and empowerment. It is empowering for an individual to be capable and self-sufficient in taking charge of his or her own health and the health of those for whom he or she is responsible, such as children, the elderly, and the disabled. To be encouraged to be dependent is to be crippled. Centers with this philosophy are often found in churches where the parish nurse teaches, counsels, supports, and makes recommendations.

The focus should be on wellness and prevention of illness in approaching self-care. The nurses' greatest contribution should be educating and reeducating to healthful lifestyles. Many of the major causes of illness are learned behaviors that can be unlearned. The strongest support for this approach appears to come from business, the insurance industry, and union leaders (perhaps because of the increasing cost and overuse of health insurance that is often a workplace benefit). Reimbursement for these services is becoming more common, and they are regularly included by HMOs.

The natural relationship between disease prevention and health promotion, education, and counseling has become obvious. These strategies have become linked to a popular interest in a healthy lifestyle. Workplace programs have become common, seeing a link between job productivity, satisfaction, and health. Some employers have provided exercise periods and facilities; choices of low-fat, low-salt, and low-cholesterol foods in employee cafeterias; and health education programs. Schools are reemphasizing good health habits and involving parents. Among the bestselling books are those on diet, exercise, and stress reduction; radio and television have also climbed onto this popular bandwagon.

■ ALTERNATIVE/COMPLEMENTARY MEDICINE

Although alternate or complementary medicine may not fit correctly in this chapter, it does fit with self-care. Which term is used to describe this movement can also evoke emotional responses. Alternative medicine is any healing practice that does not fall within the realm of conventional medicine taught in traditional Western medical schools. Complementary medicine is different from alternative medicine. Whereas complementary medicine is used together with conventional medicine, alternative medicine is used in place of conventional medicine. In Western culture, alternative medicine is often opposed to evidence-based medicine and commonly encompasses therapies with a historical or cultural, rather than a scientific, basis. Commonly cited examples include naturopathy, chiropractic, herbalism, traditional Chinese medicine, Unani, Ayurveda, meditation, Reiki, Tai Chi, aromatherapy, yoga, biofeedback, hypnosis, homeopathy, acupuncture, and nutritional-based therapies, in addition to a range of other practices. These techniques are commonly grouped under the umbrella term complementary and alternative medicine or CAM. Some practitioners in alternative medicine oppose this grouping, preferring to emphasize differences of approach, but nevertheless use the term CAM, which has become standard.

Are we speaking of a rejection of traditional Western medicine or new strategies to augment that tradition? According to a nationwide government survey released in December 2008, approximately 38 percent of US adults aged 18 years and over and approximately 12 percent of children used some form of CAM.[10] The first and landmark study on CAM spending was completed in 1997 and reported the cost to the consumer at about $27 billion.[11] American consumers spent an estimated $34 billion on CAM in 2007. CAM accounts for over 11 percent of out-of-pocket spending on health care in the United States. This information comes from the first national estimate of dollars spent on CAM in 10 years. Increasing numbers of medical colleges have also started offering courses in alternative medicine. For example, in three separate research surveys that surveyed 735 schools (125 medical schools offering an MD degree, 25 schools offering a doctor of osteopathic medicine degree, and 585 schools offering a nursing degree), 60 percent of the medical schools, 95 percent of the osteopathic medical schools, and 84.8 percent of the nursing schools teach some form of CAM.[12] Of special note is the fact that Americans make more visits to alternative care providers than to primary care physicians. In response to public pressure, many health plans are recognizing some of these optional treatments, and mainstream health facilities are establishing departments or clinics that specialize in CAM therapies. According to the American Hospital Association's *Annual Survey of Hospitals,* the number of hospitals offering CAM services has more than doubled, from 7.9 percent in 1998 to 19.8 percent in 2006. Most of these facilities are located in urban areas. Patient satisfaction (86 percent) seems to be the metric of choice in the evaluation of CAM services. The greatest challenges faced by hospitals in implementing programs are budgetary constraints (67 percent) and physician resistance (46 percent).[13]

By 1998, over 40 percent of adults used some form of alternate therapy. Their frequency, in rank order, were herbal therapy, chiropractic, massage, vitamin therapy, homeopathy, yoga, acupressure, acupuncture, biofeedback, hypnotherapy, and naturopathy. A common observation was that alternative care practitioners spend more time with their patients, about four times more than a physician, and are more holistic. The most common reasons for seeking alternative therapy are chronic pain, specifically back pain; arthritis; anxiety; depression; allergies; insomnia; and menopause. Evidence is mounting that complementary therapy has made a difference in these conditions.[14] How much can be attributed to the mind-body connection is yet to be determined.

In 1992, the National Institutes of Health (NIH) created an Office of Alternative Medicine (OAM) with a budget of $2 million to examine the efficacy of these methods. Interest was so strong that by 1998, the OAM became the National Center for Complementary and Alternative Medicine (NCCAM) with a $68.7 million budget in 2000.[12]

■ AMBULATORY CARE

It is not practical to discuss the institutions involved in the various types of health care delivery under the headings of primary care and so on, because there is considerable overlap of functions. For instance, hospitals and HMOs may deliver all levels and types of care, even encouraging or sponsoring self-care activities on the part of individuals and community groups. Therefore, institutions and agencies are presented as more traditional units of service, such as ambulatory care, hospitals, emergency services, and long-term and home care. Additionally, there are some venues for care that are better described as programs; they integrate and coordinate a wide variety of services on behalf of the patient. Such programs are considered separately and include long-term care (LTC), hospice, and managed care entities. An MCO is an insurer, but it can also be a provider and it is included here because of that potential.

Ambulatory care consists of those health care services that do not require an overnight stay in any health care facility and are consequently community based. The patient or client comes to the provider, as compared with home care where the provider goes to the recipient. The shared characteristic between ambulatory services and home care is that they are both community based. However, respecting their differences, home care is treated separately.

Ambulatory care is rapidly becoming the dominant mode of service delivery in this country. Once ambulatory care was almost exclusively provided in physicians' offices, hospital emergency rooms, and outpatient clinics. Today, there is a broad range of services, and many can trace their roots to hospitals.

Physician Office Practice

Except for home care and nurse-managed centers (NMCs), most ambulatory services currently involve physician-patient contact. Various sources indicate that the vast majority of care given by physicians is on an ambulatory basis; only about 10 percent of the people seen are ever admitted to a hospital. Most patient visits for health (or sick) care have been made to health care practitioners in solo, partnership, or private group practice. This is the major mode of organization for physicians and other health care providers who are acknowledged to be licensed to practice independently, such as dentists, chiropractors, podiatrists, and optometrists. Although there is a growing acceptance of nurses practicing independently or in partnership with a physician, most people must be educated to that concept.

Physicians in private practice provide a range of health services and operate on a contractual basis with the patient (usually unwritten) or the insurer (definitely written). Specific services may be provided for a fee, or patients may be serviced as part of a managed care plan with a small or no copay for each office visit, regardless of which services are provided. When patients require hospitalization, they pay (or their insurer pays) the hospital for services provided, except for the physician, who maintains an independent status and is paid directly and separately. If a referral is made to specialists (secondary care), those specialists receive their fees, and the primary care physician sees the patient again when specialist services are no longer warranted, or in many cases both continue to see the patient simultaneously, and bill concurrently. For various reasons, more physicians are salaried and employed by health care institutions or health care plans, in which case patients do not pay physicians separately, and the office itself may be run and staffed by institutional personnel. Anesthesiologists, pathologists, radiologists, and other specialists based in the hospital often bill patients separately, sometimes under contract to the hospital, which gets part of the fee.

Most patient visits to physicians are made in an office. If an emergency arises, the patient may be seen in a hospital emergency room where the physician has staff privileges. Few make house calls, although this is beginning to change as physicians want to increase their market. A small percentage of physicians (usually in urban areas) do not have hospital staff privileges, in which case the patient may be seen in the hospital by a referred colleague. From a business and tax viewpoint, private practice may be a corporation or partnership or may have some other designation.

Little is known about how physicians distribute their time in office practice among history taking and examinations, diagnosing, therapy, teaching or counseling, supervising or teaching staff, and paperwork; most appear reluctant to have outsiders look into their work. Nor is there much information on how doctors interact, or what the doctor-patient relationship consists of, how decisions are made, how quality is monitored, or how much traveling and meeting time is devoted to continuing education.

Patients who can choose their own point of entry into the health care system usually start with a visit to a physician's office, and there is increasing concern that, for all the importance of that choice, people do so on an unsophisticated and relatively uninformed basis—someone's recommendation, proximity to the home, or, at best, a blind choice from a list provided by the local medical society or the managed care plan. Frequently, people do a preliminary diagnosis of their own symptoms and choose a specialist on the basis of what they understand to be the problem. Because that physician may have no contact with the other specialists the individual has chosen at random, continuity and comprehensiveness of care are often lacking.

A physician's private practice setting often consists of only the physician (solo practice) and some full-time or part-time clerical help or a medical assistant, office nurse, or physician's assistant (PA). Group practices are increasingly popular, with one or more physicians in the same specialty or a multiple-physician specialty conglomerate with all the workers previously cited plus x-ray and laboratory facilities with the appropriate personnel, and other supportive health professionals and services such as health education and physical therapy. More and more of these practice modes also include APNs as employees or as partners (see Chapter 15).

To a great extent, physicians may choose whom they are willing to treat in their offices. Some patients are members of managed care plans associated with the physician; others pay personally or have traditional fee-for-service insurance. Many physicians refuse to treat Medicaid recipients because of the low-paying fee structure, and the totally uninsured may have no option but to seek care in hospital emergency rooms.

Nurse Private Practice

Nurses have been in private practice since formal nursing programs were started (see Chapters 3 and 4). In a manner of speaking, private-duty nursing was and is a private practice for which the individual nurse has professional and financial responsibility.

In a contemporary model of private practice, the nurse has an office where patients are seen, although he or she may also make house calls. In this form of independent practice, nurses have the same economic and managerial requirements as physicians, with the added concern that reimbursement by third-party payers is still limited or, even if legal, nurses often have to fight with intermediaries to start to establish their track record. In many states, the APN, who is the most common candidate for independent practice, is required to establish a collaborative relationship with a physician. Despite all this, there are many nurses in independent or group practices who are making it. Some may simultaneously hold other positions, such as teaching posts. There are also nursing faculty who carry a private practice to enhance their faculty role and do not depend on that income.

NPs or clinical nurse specialists (CNSs) who practice in an isolated area and are the sole source of health care for a population are in a somewhat hybrid situation. They may work under specified protocols, are in telephone contact with backup physicians, diagnose illnesses and prescribe medications, and have admitting privileges in local hospitals, or any combination of these. The nurses may be paid by the community or state, or by some other special arrangement. The primary care given is whatever is within the scope of that nurse's practice. These entrepreneurial practices are discussed in Chapter 15.

Community Health Centers

Out of the social unrest of the 1960s and early 1970s emerged the neighborhood health center (NHC), an ambulatory practice with mandated community involvement in both policy-making and facility operations. The NHC movement was stimulated by funding from the Office of Economic Opportunity (OEO) during the Johnson Administration. In many ways, NHCs were similar to the early charitable dispensaries, which were established because of the hospitals' lack of interest in ambulatory care and disappeared in the 1920s because of poor financing, poor staffing, and physician disapproval.

Now more commonly called community health centers (CHCs) and including migrant health centers, they serve some 6 million Americans, usually poor, in about 2000 locations nationwide. They may be freestanding, with a backup hospital for special services and inpatient care, or legally part of a hospital or health department, functioning under that institution's governing board and license, but with a community advisory board.

CHCs are primarily found in medically underserved urban areas, where the minority poor, the homeless, and various ethnic groups rely on hospital ambulatory services for primary care. In many cases, the hospital clinic service and the emergency service, often expensive, overcrowded, fragmented, and disease oriented, are inappropriately used. Their ineffectiveness is a major reason for the rise of the CHCs, called by some "one-stop health shopping" at acceptable, affordable prices, with interest in providing holistic health care. Often, they are at least partially staffed by the ethnic group served, so that communication is improved, and a real effort is made to provide services when and where patients and clients need them in a caring and understanding atmosphere. Use of nontraditional workers, such as family health workers, and an emphasis on using a health care team have been characteristic.

Although much of the health care given by CHCs is excellent, their problems have caused a drop in number from the peak development of the 1970s. Problems include tensions between community advisory boards and administrators of the center or the backup hospitals, and funding. Maintaining CHCs is extremely expensive, and most patients can pay only through Medicare or Medicaid, if at all. Few centers are self-supporting. CHCs qualify for funding through the Public Health Service as a Federally Qualified Health Center (FQHC).[15] When external funds are not available, severe program and personnel cuts are often necessary. The future of CHCs remains uncertain, in part because of a sociological question: Are they perpetuating a separate kind of care for the poor?

Nurse-Managed Centers

NMCs are a variation on the theme of the CHC. They are introduced separately because of some details that set them apart. The NMCs are managed and staffed by nurses and therefore offer the ultimate autonomous practice opportunity for nurses. NMCs may also be called nurse-run clinics or designated as community nursing organizations (CNOs). They guarantee direct client access to nursing services, offer services that are reimbursable, place the accountability for both the services provided and the management of the center with nurses, and allow nurses to practice to the fullest extent of their legal scope of practice. They are firmly rooted in classic nursing and public health.

NMCs are not new creations, but can trace their roots to the early 1900s and the tradition of the visiting nurse and public health nursing. Neither must all NMCs be community based. A modern-day example of an NMC can be observed in the Loeb Center established at Montefiore Hospital in New York by Lydia Hall in the early 1960s. Hall characterized the Loeb center as a nursing facility with the qualities of public health being offered in an institutional setting.

NMCs achieved prominence in the 1970s and 1980s owing to the troublesome gap between nursing service and nursing education, a scarcity of student clinical experiences with a wellness focus, and the continuing resistance to NPs in the medically dominated delivery system. The NMC movement was aided significantly by philanthropic support and government awards through the Division of Nursing. The Robert Wood Johnson Foundation funded 39 freestanding health clinics based on nurses as principal providers.[13] There are currently 300 NMCs. The merits of NMCs, especially with underserved populations, were a perfect vehicle to move the reimbursement agenda for nurses forward.

CNOs provide services to Medicare Part B beneficiaries for a single predetermined all-inclusive fee (capitation). A CNO is an NMC; it may also be characterized as a nursing HMO. The CNO is required to offer enrollees a package that includes home care, ambulatory services, prosthetics, durable medical equipment and supplies, speech and hearing services, social services, physical therapy, and optionally, medical day care and case management. Among the full range of community services only pharmacy, laboratory, and x-ray are excluded from the capitated rate. Although the CNOs were created by legislation in 1987, the difficulties in rate setting and disputes over the right of nurses to practice without physician oversight delayed final implementation. After years of dispute between the profession and the regulatory agencies, four demonstration sites were authorized to go forward in 1991. They were positively evaluated in 1996, and were authorized for a continued period of demonstration. Demonstration sites for CNOs were cautiously selected from among applicants with an existing history of success with the NMC concept. The capitated rates negotiated for the CNOs needed to be counterbalanced by patients who represent less at-risk clients. To further minimize their financial risk, many NMCs have been successfully designated as FQHCs, which facilitate Medicare and Medicaid reimbursement.

NMCs may be freestanding and entrepreneurial, or affiliated with a college of nursing or a health care institution. In any of these relationships, they may become part of a managed care network, fulfilling the functions of a primary care provider. The services offered by an NMC may be narrow in scope or diverse. They can offer all of the traditional primary care services, diagnosing and treating minor illness and managing chronic conditions.

Where physician collaboration is required by state law, those relationships are created. By their nature, NMCs can provide so much more:

- Services for life transitional and developmental changes related to birthing, parenting, puberty and adolescence, midlife, aging, divorce, and death.

- Services for organizations and businesses including expert consultation, clinical case management, education for management and employees, and employee wellness programs.

- Services for those experiencing life-altering crises and for informal caregivers, such as families of Alzheimer's patients.

- Services for longer term continuity of care, designed to enhance quality of life for individuals and families experiencing chronic illness, physical and developmental disabilities, and the challenges associated with aging.

A few exemplary NMCs are as follows:

- Genesis/Tampa General Health Center for Women and Children is affiliated with Tampa General Hospital.

- University of Rochester School of Nursing Community Nursing Center is a vehicle for faculty practice with both education and research goals accomplished through a diversified range of direct and subcontracted services.

- Alcorn State University Division of Nursing, Nursing Center in Natchez, provides care of adolescents and their families living in rural southwest Mississippi.

- The Block Nurse Program in Cleveland is a neighborhood-based home care service for older persons that integrates formal health care and informal support services.

- Community Health Clinic of Lafayette, Indiana, provides comprehensive family-focused care to women, children, and male adults up to age 65 and concentrates on the uninsured.

- Mercy Mobile Health Program of Atlanta brings primary care, HIV testing, substance abuse counseling, and other services to underserved populations in a fully equipped van.

- UCLA School of Nursing Health Center, Union Rescue Mission, is a large facility bringing primary care to the homeless. This is one of several NMCs run by the school.
- Community Health Services of Scottsdale, Arizona, provides family health care for individuals of all ages, and at least half are privately insured.
- In Lansing, the University of Michigan's NMC serves veterans through a capitated contract with the Department of Veteran's Affairs. This is one of nine NMCs operated by the University.
- The University of Texas—Houston Health Science Center School of Nursing's NMC offers some care to traditionally underserved populations, but focuses more on occupational health and primary care for the employees of local companies and organizations.

It should be noted that some of the most successful NMCs have been birthing centers established by certified nurse midwives (CNMs). Models for NMCs have also been developed by CNSs within such specialty areas as cardiovascular, oncology, low-birthweight babies, chronic obstructive pulmonary disease, diabetes, and so on. The chronically ill need primary care, too.

NMCs have a tradition of serving the most vulnerable populations. Further, registered nurses (RNs) employed with NMCs are significantly more educated than the nursing staff complement in other health care settings, with 31 percent holding a baccalaureate degree and 37 percent a master's degree.

The future of NMCs will depend on their success as participants in managed care and in making strategic decisions to diversify or focus their services. Further, our commitment to the underserved is consistent with our history, but to grow and flourish the vast middle class must also become our consumers.

Other Health Centers and Clinics

There are endless variations on CHCs, and nurses are responsible for knowing that they exist. **Rural health centers**, developed under federal financing such as regional health and the Appalachian projects or funded by communities or foundations, are the rural corollary to CHCs and also qualify for FQHC funding—existing to serve people, usually poor, in medically underserved areas. Because few physicians are available, care is often given by NPs and PAs linked to physicians at other sites.

Mental health centers or community mental health centers are intended to provide a wide range of mental health services to a particular geographic catchment area. They may be sponsored by state mental health departments, psychiatric hospitals or departments of hospitals, or the federal government. Staffed by teams of mental health personnel, they may consist of single physical entities or networks, but tend to focus on short-term care, including crisis intervention. The Community Mental Health Center Act (1963) and its later amendments facilitated the development of comprehensive services and stimulated the community mental health movement. It was intended, in part, to prevent the warehousing of mental patients and assist their reintroduction into the community.

Unfortunately, deinstitutionalization moved faster than the available community services, and even today there are mental patients living on the streets (estimated at one-fourth to two-fifths of the homeless population) or in deplorable, but less available, single-room occupancy hotels. Although there are good halfway houses, day care centers, and semisupervised living arrangements, the services have not caught up with the demand.

There is general agreement that what is needed is a spectrum of services ranging from providing suitable housing to managing serious psychiatric and physical illness, and adequate coordination of these multiple community services.

A particular concern is management of the chronically mentally ill, who need the services of mental health professionals as well as social workers, and have more than their share of physical problems. The noninstitutionalized mentally ill must be reached in many settings, including the streets, shelters, board-and-care facilities, and jails.

A large portion of the mentally ill qualifies for government entitlements. Seen as a group with special needs, their health care is frequently carved out or treated separately and differently than programs for the general population of the poor and disabled. In many instances, psychiatric NPs are designated as the primary care providers or case managers for these patients. These are nurses with a graduate degree and dual preparation as a psychiatric–mental health nursing clinical specialist and an NP.

Women's clinics are usually owned and operated by women concerned about women's health problems and dissatisfied with the quality of care for women and the attitudes of many male health care providers. Most emerged out of the women's movement, along with the consumer and self-care movements. Services may include routine gynecological and maternity care, and family planning, as well as some general health care. Emphasis is on self-help, mutual support, and noninstitutional personal care. Both CNMs and lay midwives are used, as are NPs and supportive physicians, although many staff are laypeople. In a number of cities and towns, conservative groups and medical societies have harassed the clinics, and some have had to become involved in lengthy and expensive legal suits. These should not be confused with women's health care centers developed and operated by hospitals to target this specific clientele.

Family planning clinics, of which the clinics of Planned Parenthood are most notable, provide a spectrum of birth control and women's health services and information.

Abortion clinics are sponsored by community and other groups, as well as proprietary organizations, or may be located in a physician's private practice. There may also be abortion services offered in conjunction with a women's health or family planning clinic. However, harassment by antiabortion activists, including picketing and sometimes violent actions, as well as cutbacks in funding by the government and other external funding sources have resulted in limitation of services and even closings in the last few years. A recent US Supreme Court decision considered the harassment of patients and professionals and came down in favor of the public's right to access these facilities.

Renal dialysis centers were spurred into massive growth by the inclusion of treatment for end-stage renal disease patients in the 1972 Medicare amendment. At one time, the treatment of those with chronic kidney disease by using expensive artificial kidneys was a sensitive matter of "who shall live?" When Congress decided that all should have that opportunity and funded it, the cost rose to unexpected millions of dollars. Many centers are freestanding, mostly physician owned or developed by proprietary organizations, but they also exist in hospitals. A whole new coterie of specialists at all levels has developed. The desired emphasis now is the less-expensive home dialysis.

Another group of burgeoning facilities are those for rehabilitation of drug abusers. Most common are the **methadone maintenance programs** (substituting methadone for heroin, along with certain rehabilitative measures), which have had varying success. Drug-free programs include self-help and **therapeutic resident programs, halfway houses, counseling centers,** and hotlines.

Adult day care centers are agencies that provide health, social, psychiatric, and nutritional services to infirm individuals who are sufficiently ambulatory to be transported between home and center. Psychogeriatric day care centers were first opened in 1947 under the direction of the Menninger Clinic. Studies ordered by Congress in 1976 showed day care centers to be cost-effective, but no national policy on reimbursement followed. Funding now comes from uncoordinated and disparate sources; therefore, some communities have set priorities as to who can use the services.

Still, day care has been shown to be superior to nursing homes for eligible individuals because of lower costs, improved health and functional outcomes, and a heightened quality of life. Unresolved issues are related to their use for young adults with debilitating diseases, the feasibility of rural centers, and the need for regulation and licensing. Currently, governmental distinctions exist between **medical and social day care.** The former requires some presence of health care personnel or some available health care services.

■ AMBULATORY CARE ALTERNATIVES TO INSTITUTIONS

The 1980s brought increased complaints about the expense of health care, particularly in hospitals, and ushered in the competitive model. The core of the model is that consumer choice and market forces rather than regulation should be used to control health care costs.

As a result, alternative health care delivery modes, particularly in ambulatory care, developed and expanded. Among these are the **surgicenters,** independent proprietary facilities for surgery that do not require overnight hospitalization. The first was established in 1970 in Phoenix, Arizona, and they have gained popularity. Some are specialized, such as the plastic surgery centers, but in general the centers can perform any surgery that does not require prolonged anesthesia. Surgicenters are said to be able to perform up to 40 percent of all surgical procedures, including face lifts, cataract surgery, vasectomy, breast biopsy, dilatation and curettage, knee arthroscopy, and tonsillectomy. Because of low overhead, surgicenters can charge as little as one-third of hospital costs for the same procedure, and patients like being able to return to home, or even work, the same day.

When it was evident that this new delivery mode was not only well accepted, but also reimbursable by insurance plans, many hospitals joined the movement and set up day surgery centers. Although payers greeted them enthusiastically at first because of the cost savings, within a few years the unregulated fees soared.

Emergicenters may be for-profit or nonprofit, public or private, freestanding or owned by another entity. The term freestanding refers to the fact that the facility may be sponsored or affiliated with a hospital, but is not owned by it. These centers are designed to treat episodic, nonurgent health problems. Since they first opened their doors in 1976, many more have sprung up around the country. When owned or sponsored by a hospital, the emergicenter can also be a strategic business move. As a hospital satellite, the more seriously ill will be referred to the sponsoring institution unless the patient exercises the right to choose another facility. Typically, emergicenters are in shopping centers or commercial and industrial areas, and have a high patient turnover, a short (15- to 20-minute) waiting period, and a cost that may be 30 to 40 percent lower than that of hospital emergency rooms.

Closely related are **wound care centers** that treat chronic nonhealing wounds, **pain clinics, incontinence clinics,** and so on. Staff may also coordinate access to other needed services. All these centers have the potential to be lucrative businesses and are natural markets for advanced practice nursing. Government regulation is still largely nonexistent.

Although some women are again turning to home births attended by midwives, a more popular and growing alternative to hospital births is the **childbearing center**, also called **birth center** or **childbirthing center**. These centers made their appearance in 1973, when the alienated and questioning middle class became disenchanted with hospital maternity care. The demonstration nurse midwifery model was the Maternity Center of New York. Now an increasing number of out-of-hospital centers are operating. Some are operated by or utilize CNMs; others are sponsored by physicians or lay midwives.

There are both freestanding (autonomous) childbirthing centers and a variation of the concept in hospitals. Both allow for more humane care in a high-quality, home-like setting with the father and other children present—all costing considerably less than hospital care. If only one in four pregnant women had access to and used birthing centers, millions and perhaps billions of health care dollars would be saved.

Another humanistically oriented as well as cost-saving mode of care is the **hospice**. The hospice movement was pioneered in Great Britain by Dr. Cicely Saunders at St. Christopher's Hospice in London. The first widely recognized hospice in the United States was Hospice, Inc., established in 1971 in New Haven, Connecticut. Modeled after St. Christopher's, its focus is on improving the quality of patients' last days or months of life so that they can live until they die.

The number of patients served by hospices increased from about 1 million in 2004 to nearly 1.5 million in 2008, and the number of hospices grew from 3600 to almost 5000. More than 90 percent of hospices in the United States are certified by Medicare. Most of this explosive growth has been driven by for-profit companies.[16] Medicare classifies hospices into four types: hospital based, home health agency based, skilled nursing facility (SNF) based, and independent. The first three are part of a larger institution; the independent, of which there are very few, are corporate entities. Hospices may offer inpatient care, home care, or a mix of the two. But whatever the setting, in reality it is a concept, an attitude, and a belief that involves support of the family as well as the dying patient. It can be carried out in an ordinary hospital setting, with extraordinary perception. The hospice functions on a 24-hour, 7-day-a-week basis; backup medical, nursing, and counseling services are always available. The typical hospice team consists of a physician and some combination of nurses; medical social workers; psychiatrists; nutritionists; pharmacists; speech, physical, and occupational therapists; and clergy or pastoral counselors. The staff meets regularly both to discuss treatment plans and to provide support to one another. Because they are close to both patient and family, team members may suffer from burnout and stress; therefore, counseling is available for them as well. Hospices frequently rely on well-trained volunteers, who provide respite care, companionship, transportation, patient teaching, and bereavement support. The family is also considered part of the team.

Most hospices serve cancer patients primarily, but many also care for patients with progressive neurologic diseases and now AIDS. Except for the latter two groups, the majority of hospice patients are elderly. Any patient whose physician certifies that he or she has a life expectancy of less than 6 months is eligible for hospice care. Patients must be aware of their diagnosis and prognosis. Most patients die at home, surrounded by their families, and free of technological, life-prolonging devices. Symptom control is a vital step, and pain-relieving medications are dispensed at a level that will ensure that the patient is virtually pain-free at all times. Psychological comfort is considered as important as physical comfort, and the counseling, support, and companionship of hospice staff help relieve the fear, depression, and anxiety of patients and their families alike.

A number of studies have shown that hospice care is less expensive than traditional care, and partial or full reimbursement is being offered by most commercial insurance carriers and MCOs. In 1986, hospice became a permanent Medicare benefit and an optional Medicaid benefit, but at least 80 percent of the care is supposed to be provided in the home, and patients relinquish the right to curative therapy. Difficulties are surfacing as modern drug therapy extends life beyond those 6 months, and it additionally becomes difficult to determine whether a procedure or course of treatment is curative or palliative in its intent.

■ HOSPITALS

In 1946, at the close of World War II, there were 6000 American hospitals. With the passage of the Hill-Burton Act to fund hospital expansion and the burgeoning of hi-tech, the system grew to a high of 7200 acute care hospitals. In the current climate that discourages hospital use for anything but major illness, the number of community-based hospitals has been reduced to approximately 5010.[17]

Hospitals are generally classified according to size (number of beds, exclusive of newborn bassinets); type (general, mental, tuberculosis, or other specialty, such as maternity, orthopedic, eye and ear, rehabilitation, chronic disease, alcoholism, or narcotic addiction); ownership (public or private, including the for-profit, investor-owned proprietary hospitals or nonprofit voluntary hospitals, which may be owned by religious, fraternity, or community groups); and length of stay (short or long term). Hospitals vary from fewer than 25 to more than 2000 beds. The most common type of hospital has been the voluntary, general, short-term hospital, followed by the local government, general, short-term hospitals. The two major groups in terms of size are short-term general hospitals, averaging 160 beds, and long-term hospitals, averaging 900 beds. Many hospitals have been forced to close. Causes cited by the American Hospital Association (AHA) include federal funding cutbacks, pressure by insurance companies and businesses to reduce health care expenditures, and changing health care practices (such as those described earlier). If not closed, the small hospitals are likely to become part of a multi-institutional system, a major trend in health care delivery. These may comprise two or more hospitals owned, leased, sponsored, or contract managed by a central

organization. They can be for-profit or nonprofit. Advantages can include improved access to capital markets, joint purchasing, technology, economics of scale, shared use of technical and management staff, richer referral networks, and the opportunity to specialize among the facilities.

The terms teaching and nonteaching are also used to describe hospitals. Teaching hospitals are associated with medical schools and maintain accredited residency programs in which medical students, residents, and specialty fellows are taught (house staff). Teaching hospitals have been awarded Graduate Medical Education (GME) funding from both state and federal governments and have traditionally been reimbursed at higher rates for patients they treat. This was out of respect for the fact that teaching hospitals often pursued diagnostic and treatment alternatives that were more costly, all for the sake of learning. The teaching designation does not derive from programs or experiences that the hospital may provide for other health professionals or allied health workers.

These hospitals (about 9 percent) usually have more than 400 beds and are in medical centers proximate to the associated medical school (in which case they are often quaternary care centers). The extra funding that once derived from the teaching hospital status is drying up quick, and one of the most confounding questions in health care is where the money for medical education will come from.

Because of all these variations, it is difficult to draw one picture of the hospital as an entity. Exhibit 7–3 shows a common organizational pattern of a general hospital, which illustrates both the lines of authority and the kinds of services available. Exhibit 7–4 shows the organizational structure for a multifacility corporation consisting of hospitals, clinics, home care, and an SNF. The day-to-day operations take place at the facility or program level. Strategic planning and decisions about mission, market share, and the broad policy making occur at the corporate level. It is also common to consolidate specific service areas at the corporate level where they serve all the facilities.

Examples of consolidated services may be personnel recruitment, nursing education, purchasing, and so on. Larger and more diverse systems will have more complex organizational structures. A hospital that has outreach facilities, home health services, or a long-term care facility differs greatly from a 50-bed community hospital. Smaller hospitals may have fewer diverse clinical services and few, if any, education programs, but there are almost always business and finance departments, physical

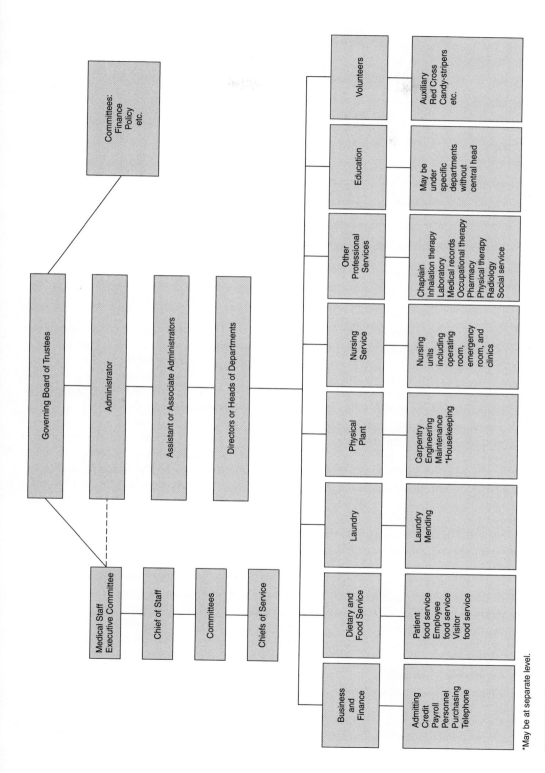

EXHIBIT 7–3. One common organizational pattern of a general hospital.

*May be at separate level.

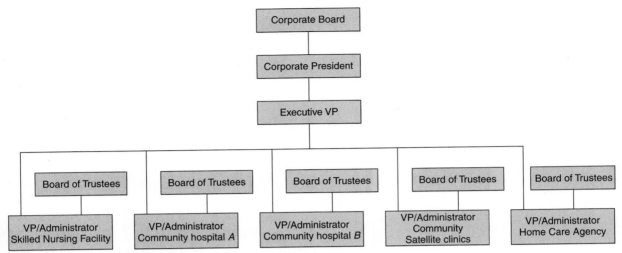

EXHIBIT 7–4. Organizational structure for a multifacility corporation.

plant (maintenance of all kinds), laundry, supplies and store-room, dietary and food services, clinical nursing units (inpatient and outpatient), and the other professional service units, such as laboratories, radiology, other diagnostic and treatment units, pharmacy, and perhaps social service. Some hospitals are now outsourcing laundry and dietary in the belief that this is less expensive than maintaining their own equipment and dealing with all of the human resource problems that inevitably come with the service area.

The physical layout of a hospital varies from single story to highrise, and may include large or small, general or specialized patient units; special intensive care units; operating rooms; recovery rooms; offices (sometimes including providers' private offices); space for diagnostic and treatment facilities; storage rooms; kitchens and dining rooms; maintenance equipment; work rooms; meeting rooms; classrooms; chapel; waiting rooms; and gift and snack shops. Most hospitals have some form of emergency services, such as an emergency room, but many no longer maintain their own ambulance services. A great many have outpatient or ambulatory services, and perhaps an extended care or cooperative care unit for patients who do not need major nursing service; some provide home care.

The nursing service department has the largest number of personnel in the hospital, in part because of around-the-clock, 7-day-a-week staffing. Other departments, such as radiology and clinic laboratories, may maintain some services on evenings and weekends and

may be on call at night. There is a trend to have other clinical services available on weekends and evenings. For instance, a patient who needs rehabilitation exercises or other treatments in the physical therapy department fails to receive this necessary care during the evenings and weekends when that department follows the usual 9 to 5, Monday through Friday staffing pattern.

Hospitals are licensed by the state and presumably are not permitted to function unless they maintain the minimum standards prescribed by the licensing authority. ("Presumably" because the process of closing a hospital owing to inadequate facilities or staff is long, difficult, and not always successful.) However, to be eligible for many federal grants, such as Medicare, and to be affiliated with educational programs, accreditation is necessary. The Joint Commission (formerly JCAHO) accreditation is voluntary and is a stamp of quality. In 1992, the Joint Commission put a new accreditation system in place. The Joint Commission began to reject the assumption that if good care was provided, the results would be positive. Proof of positive clinical and performance outcomes was required, and quality was measured on an ongoing basis rather than at one point in time. Visits are made by an inspection team (which may or may not have a multidisciplinary makeup) that reviews various records and minutes of meetings, interviews key people, and generally scrutinizes the hospital. Reports are made that include criticisms and recommendations for action. Accreditation may be postponed, withheld, revoked, granted, or renewed on the basis of the inspection and review of the hospital's report and self-evaluation. Nurses are included on the inspection team, and there is nursing input into the standards for nursing service. To be eligible for the Joint Commission accreditation survey, the hospital must be registered or listed by the AHA, have a current unconditional license to operate as required by the state, and have a governing body, organized medical staff, nursing service, and other supporting services. The Joint Commission's board of trustees consists of representatives from the AMA, the American College of Surgeons, the Academy of Medicine, and the American Dental Association. Additionally, since 1992 there have been several consumer representatives and a seat that is filled by a designated representative of organized nursing. This individual is identified by a coalition of the major nursing organizations. Additionally, a nurse selected by the ANA sits on the professional-technical advisory group for each of the Joint Commission's accreditation programs.

Joint Commission accreditation is particularly necessary, because it holds "deemed" status with the Centers for Medicare and Medicaid Services (CMS); that is, if a hospital is accredited by the Joint Commission, CMS accepts this credential as verification of quality and allows reimbursement for service to Medicare beneficiaries. The Joint Commission accreditation is not exclusive to hospitals, but is also available for ambulatory care, behavioral health care, home care, laboratory services, long-term care, and office-based surgery.

Voluntary hospitals are usually organized under a constitution and bylaws that invest the board of trustees with fiduciary responsibility. This governing board is generally made up of individuals representing various professional and business groups interested in the community. Although unsalaried and volunteer (except for proprietary hospitals, in which members are often stockholders), board members are usually extremely influential citizens and are often self-perpetuating on the board. This type of membership originated because at one time administrators of hospitals did not have a business background, and because of the need to raise money to support hospitals. (Most trustees still see recovery of operating costs as their most crucial hospital problem.) Some consumer groups have complained that most members are businessmen, bankers, brokers, lawyers, and accountants, with almost nonexistent representation of women, minorities, consumers in general, and labor. Physicians also complain of lack of medical representation, although they work closely with the board and are subordinate to it only in certain matters. Because of these pressures, boards are gradually acquiring broader representation.

Public hospitals usually do not have boards of trustees. Hospital administrators are directly responsible to their administrative supervisors in the governmental hierarchy, which may be a state board of health, a commissioner, a department such as the Veterans' Administration, or a public corporation with appointed officials. Presumably, all are ultimately responsible to the public.

Although administrator is still the generic term for the managerial head of a hospital, in recent years this title has included a variety of designations, such as president and chief executive officer (CEO). The hospital administrator, the direct agent of a governing board, implements its policies, advises on new policies, and is responsible for the day-to-day operations of the hospital. Hospital or health administration, like any other, encompasses planning, organizing, directing, controlling, and evaluating the resources of an organization. In large institutions, the administrator has a staff of assistants or associates, each responsible for a division or group of departments. Most hospitals have recognized that the nurse executive should hold one of these positions (most frequently designated as a vice president) in order to participate in the policy-making decisions that inevitably affect the largest hospital department. Department heads or supervisors are next in the line of authority; these individuals are also gradually becoming specialists by education and experience in their area of functional or clinical responsibility.

The medical or professional staff is an organized entity made up of provider professionals who are admitted to membership by the incumbents. Subsequently the Board of Trustees, who is ultimately responsible for the welfare of the patients, approves their appointment. Members of the staff are granted the privilege of using the hospital's facilities for their patients. A typical classification of medical staff includes honorary (not active), consulting (specialist), active (attending physicians), courtesy (those not wishing full status but occasionally wanting to attend private patients), and house staff (any salaried professionals including physicians and APNs). Through their committees, including the Credentials Committee, the professional staff is an impressive power in the hospital, for it is often in a position to control not only medical practice, but also all patient care.

In hospitals where the professional staff is more progressive, there are nurses and other nonphysician representatives on committees concerned with patient care, and decisions are made jointly. Although the professional staff is still overwhelmingly physician dominated, it is not unusual for other provider professionals to have practice privileges of some sort. The 1983 stand of the Federal Trade Commission that medical rules should permit hospitals to grant staff membership to CNMs, APNs, and other nonphysician health professionals, and 1984 Joint Commission guidelines giving hospitals the option of granting such privileges, were major breakthroughs.

There is some feeling among the nursing leadership, however, that such approval should not come from the medical staff but, if nurses are involved, from the nurses themselves. Although not widespread, in some hospitals nursing staff bylaws enable nurses to be self-directed and self-governed, and allow for this orderly change within nursing. With such a mechanism, adjunct nursing staff, including community-based NPs, could, after having been approved by the nurse credentialing committee, admit and provide care to hospitalized clients.

Since 1982, there have been dramatic changes in hospitals, and even more are expected. Much is owing to health care economics and the criticism hospitals have received for their part in causing costs to escalate. The government-mandated PPS for hospitals, utilizing DRGs to determine payment, was a landmark event. Among other things, the PPS is responsible for the drop in length of stay (LOS), which by 2006 was 4.8 days nationwide.[18] Additionally, a competitive model accelerated the growth of for-profit corporations that bought, built, and leased hospitals and other facilities and operated them under a corporate mantle. Although the type of governance varies, the motive is profit. One executive reported his company's strategy as acquiring hospitals in areas with favorable business factors, creating sophisticated facilities that provide a broad base of services, and involving physicians in profit sharing. Comprehensive long-term care facilities, rehabilitation, and psychiatric hospitals, as well as home care, were cited as increasingly profitable ventures. There has been some criticism that the investor-owned hospitals do not give as good a quality of care as the non-profits, but these claims have been challenged. In fact, clinical outcomes are comparable, but the nonprofits give more care to the medically indigent and poor.

This hybridization has led the hospitals down some varied paths. Besides their diversification into areas such as freestanding outpatient surgery programs (the most successful), outpatient diagnostic centers, cardiac rehabilitation services, substance abuse programs, inpatient rehabilitation units, outpatient surgery satellites, industrial

medicine clinics, sports medicine programs, home health services, and women's health programs (which have proved to be successful for the vast majority of hospitals developing them), some hospitals have also initiated health information telephone hotlines, medical equipment rentals, weight reduction programs and counseling, fitness programs, TV programs, wellness centers and babysitting services in shopping malls, advertising and public relations businesses, cleaning services, catering services, and even a graphics design business. Some states have threatened to not only tax these for-profit entities, but to cut the subsidies of hospitals so engaged. Oddly enough, among the reported financial losers are wellness and health promotion programs, even though the vast majority of hospitals are said to offer such programs.

Certainly, hospitals have had to adjust to many changes and face serious problems, aside from the ongoing issues of cost and quality. Because of heightened public awareness of the dangers of infectious waste, more attention must be given to its safe disposal, which is a costly operation. Inner-city hospitals are being drained by bad debt, created in caring for the medically indigent, including illegal aliens. Hospital emergency rooms are crowded to capacity, but are being used more for primary care than for true emergency care.

There is no doubt that hospitals have the opportunity to remain a pivotal component in health care, but the system and consumer preferences are changing around them. They will either move with the times or be discarded. The choice falls to each institution. Fewer inpatient beds will be needed. They must move into the community, rather than expect the community to come to them. Managed care plans will seek out those hospitals that actively manage their patients and curry favor with consumers.

Consumer satisfaction and cost are the primary concerns of managed care entities. This is not to cast aside quality; rather, there is an assumption that a given baseline standard of quality is ensured. Competition will prevail among hospitals. The most potent marketing tool available is bringing to the public assurances of the adequate presence of professional nurses.

■ GOVERNMENT FACILITIES

In the federal government, at least 25 agencies have some involvement in delivering health services. Those with the largest expenditures in direct federal hospital and medical services are the Veterans' Administration, which operates the largest centrally directed hospital and clinic system in the United States; the Department of Defense (members of the military and dependents); and the Health Resources and Services Administration (HRSA) of the Department of Health and Human Services (DHHS). The HRSA operates one Public Health Service (PHS) hospital devoted to Hansen's disease, and provides care for federal prisoners and Coast Guard personnel. The Indian Health Service (IHS) operates hospitals, health centers, and satellite health clinics for Native Americans and Alaska natives. A variety of DHHS agencies provide indirect funding or contracts for clinics, drug and alcohol rehabilitation centers, maternal-child and family planning centers, neighborhood health centers, and the National Health Service Corps.

State and local governments also have multiple functions and multiple services in health care delivery, directly through grants and funding to finance their own programs, and indirectly as third-party payers. Although most states have some version of a state health agency or department of public health, health services are often provided through other state agencies, a situation that creates territorial battles, duplication, and gaps. In most states, operation of psychiatric hospitals and the Medicaid program, two of the most important state health functions, is by departments other than an official state agency for health. In direct services, some states operate psychiatric, TB, or other hospitals and alcohol and drug rehabilitation programs; provide noninstitutional mental health services; fund public health nursing programs and laboratories; and provide services for maternal-child health, family planning, crippled children, immunization, TB, chronic respiratory disease control, and venereal disease control. All are considered traditional public health services, in addition to environmental health activities.

On a local level, services offered by a health department depend a great deal on the size, needs, and demands of the constituency. There appears to be little information about local health departments or health officers. Those with considerable visibility are in large urban centers, where health problems are complex and generally unresolved.

Some large municipalities operate hospitals that provide for the indigent or working poor who are not covered by Medicaid or private insurance.

Some health departments run school health services and screening programs. Some run duplicate services that are already offered by other state or local agencies. There are few data on how much state and local agencies coordinate their services to avoid duplication or omission, but lack of coordination or cooperation is not uncommon. Although there is a great deal of criticism of most local health services in relation to high cost, waste, corruption, and poor quality, attempts to terminate any of them, particularly hospitals in medically underserved areas, become political conflicts, with representatives of the poor complaining that no other services are available and that the loss of local jobs will create other hardships. With all the politically sensitive issues involved, most health care experts are pessimistic about reorganization or major improvement of the health systems at any government level.

One emergent trend that may somewhat dilute these politics is the talk about privatizing both Medicare and Medicaid. Several states have chosen to give their poor a voucher to buy into the managed health care plan of their choice. Others are requiring that Medicaid recipients enroll in managed care plans offered for their use. Plans that wish to compete for this market must attempt to have enrollees also include non-Medicaid recipients. This forces health care facilities that have primarily served the poor to rise to the cost-efficiency and attractiveness expectations of the private sector, and substantially reduces the infrastructure that is directly under government control. In the same spirit of seeking simplification, talk on Capitol Hill questions whether the existing federal systems (Veteran's Affairs, stateside military health care facilities) should continue to exist as separate entities or should continue to exist at all, the option being to award vouchers for use in the private sector to all individuals having a right to government entitlement programs.

■ EMERGENCY MEDICAL SERVICES

Ambulance services, originally a profit venture of funeral directors, are a vital link in transporting accident victims or those suffering acute overwhelming illnesses (such as myocardial infarctions) to a medical facility. In most cases, providing such services, either directly or through contracts, has now become the responsibility of a community—a responsibility that is not consistently assumed. The unnecessary deaths owing to delayed or inept care have received considerable attention, which was probably responsible for some important federal legislation.

With continued federal and state funding and regulation, the previously diverse ambulance and rescue services of volunteers, firefighters, police, and commercial companies are being coordinated with regional systems. Several hundred are now in place. Criteria include training of appropriate personnel; education of the public; appropriate communication systems, transportation vehicles, and facilities; adequate record keeping; and some participation by the public in policy making.

Under these laws, a variety of emergency medical technicians (EMTs) have been trained and staff many ambulance services, including mobile intensive care units, which have very sophisticated equipment.

■ HOME HEALTH CARE

Home health care is probably more of a nurse-oriented health service than any other, originating with Florence Nightingale's health nurses and the pioneer efforts of such American nurses as Lillian Wald. Nevertheless, what Wald worked for in the late nineteenth century—comprehensive services for the patient and family that extend beyond simple care of the sick—is even more pertinent today. Today the terms public health nurse, community health nurse, and home health nurse are often used interchangeably. But they are not the same. Home health care nursing is the delivery of personal care services to an individual in a site other than an institution. Community and public health nursing involve delivering services to a population, and through this action improving the quality of life for the larger society.

Home care includes a broad spectrum of services, from home birthing to hospice care. Medical services are primarily provided by the individual's private or clinic physician, although in some instances agencies will employ or contract for a physician's services. In addition, home-maker–home health aide services may be required in conjunction with (or sometimes following) nursing and therapy. These consist of bathing, personal grooming, assistance with self-help skills, meal planning and preparation, and general housekeeping services. Among the other home health services that may be available are medical supplies and equipment (expendable and durable), nutrition, occupational therapy, physical therapy, speech pathology services, and social work. Other services, which may be provided through coordinated efforts of the agency and the community, include audiological services, dental services, home-delivered meals (for example, Meals on Wheels), housekeeping services, information and referral services, laboratory services, ophthalmologic services, patient transportation and escort services, podiatry services, prescription drugs, prosthetic and orthotic services, respiratory therapy services, and x-ray services. The NLN, describing a model of home health services, also included

as highly desirable environmental and social support services such as barber/cosmetology services, handyman services, heavy cleaning services, legal and protective services, pastoral services, personal contact services, recreation services, and translation services. Some might be developed as volunteer efforts.

Certified home health operates under various auspices. The major types are visiting nurse associations (VNAs), public agencies, hospital-based agencies, and proprietary agencies. In 2007, there were a total of 9284 Medicare certified home health agencies: VNAs numbered 475, whereas there were 1132 public agencies in 2006. VNAs and public agencies have experienced significant decline in recent years. In 1975, they were 23 and 55 percent of the home care market, respectively. Freestanding proprietary agencies with 4919 agencies in 2006, and hospital-based agencies at 1503 in 2007 dominated the market.[19]

VNAs are freestanding, voluntary, nonprofit organizations governed by a volunteer board of directors and supported by contributions as well as revenues received for care and services delivered. VNAs are the oldest and have been the classic providers of home care services. Depending on the location and resources, the spectrum of services may vary greatly, but generally includes at least skilled nursing and other professional services. Many VNAs also operate adult day care centers, wellness clinics, hospices, and Meals on Wheels programs. The mission of VNAs has always been to provide quality care to all people, regardless of their ability to pay. Volunteers have played a large role in assisting VNAs to accomplish their mission through fundraising, friendly visiting, telephone reassurance, and assistance with clinic and office work.

Public agencies are government agencies operated by a state, county, city, or other unit of local government. In addition to providing home health care services, these agencies have a major responsibility for preventing disease and community health education.

Hospital-based agencies are operating units or departments of a hospital. The number of hospital-based agencies has grown substantially since the initiation of prospective payment for inpatient hospital services in 1983. The attraction of a hospital-based agency is particularly strong where consumers have had a positive inpatient experience. Although hospitals are required to give discharged patients several options to choose from, the myth or reality of continuity of care is a strong incentive.

Proprietary agencies are freestanding for-profit home health agencies. They have been characterized by aggressive development of new services, especially in the area of high-tech home care, and by brisk and sophisticated marketing activities. They have often provided the competitive impetus and organizational model for other home health agencies to rethink their service delivery patterns and structures.

Home care in the United States is in a state of crisis. Financial support from Medicare and Medicaid has been a major factor fueling the growth of the home care industry. Medicare is the largest single payer for services. In 2006, Medicare spending accounted for 37 percent of total home care revenue and Medicaid for 19 percent. Other major payor sources in 2006 were out of pocket (10 percent), private insurance (12 percent), and state and local government (19.9 percent).[20] Although home care represents a relatively small percentage of total Medicare and Medicaid expenditures, it has been the fastest-growing category of expenses for both of these programs. Governments' need to keep a tight rein on health care costs and the anticipated growth of home care created an uncomfortable situation. The response was the Balanced Budget Act of 1997, designed to demand efficiencies by reducing the number of federal dollars to the program, and moving home care onto a PPS by October 2000. FY 2000 witnessed a slight slowing in dollars from Medicare and Medicaid to home care, with a rebound in FY 2001, and continued decisive growth.[21]

Medicare-certified home health agencies meet standards set by the federal government for type of services, quality of care, and organizational structure and oversight, and are paid through the PPS. It is difficult to isolate any reason for the industry decline in 2000 with subsequent dramatic and continued recovery. Was this due, in part, to the changes in Medicare home health reimbursement enacted as part of the Balanced Budget Act of 1997, or how much of this change was due to the growth of subacute care as an institutional option to home care for individuals needing skilled services? Perhaps it is program diversification in home care, including telephonic monitoring and other creative programs enabled by today's technology, that has prompted restructuring. Or maybe it is just culling out weaker agencies as the going gets tough.

Both Medicaid and Medicare are already working to move their beneficiaries into managed care programs. Managed care companies are pressuring home health agencies to provide fewer visits at lower cost, without compromising quality, and at the same time demonstrating positive results (outcomes) of the care provided. Growth in managed care plans and their desire to bundle

payment for acute and postacute services has influenced a number of freestanding agencies, especially VNAs, to affiliate with or become part of larger integrated health systems. Within these relationships the home health agency often relinquishes at least some autonomy in return for a secure and often expanded referral base.

Some of the VNAs and other agencies that have survived best now plan on a more businesslike basis, and new organizational patterns have emerged. One includes the development of a holding company or corporate structure with both a nonprofit (traditional VNA) and a for-profit subsidiary. The for-profit branch may provide a variety of profitable services, such as home health aides, chore services for the frail elderly, presurgery counseling before hospital admission, vocational rehabilitation, and more recently, establishing a pharmacy for home infusion therapy solutions. The after-tax profits from this corporation are then donated to the nonprofit corporation to provide the free services that have sometimes kept VNAs on the point of bankruptcy.

If family or significant others are absent in a patient's life or are unwilling to take on the necessary responsibility, home care may not be the most desirable approach for dependent individuals. On the other hand, with the participation of health professionals who have a commitment to this aspect of health care, reasonable assurance of quality, and adequate financing, home health care has tremendous potential for filling a health care gap and has been demonstrated to increase effectiveness and reduce costs of health care for a number of diagnoses.

The focus on managed care and reducing health care costs presents many challenges and uncertainties to the home care industry. Conversely, it also offers a powerful role for home care and community health nurses in particular. Managed care plans are placing a growing emphasis on preventive care, education, and training as the most cost-effective forms of health care. It is exciting to anticipate a return to the roots of home care through provision of services that community health nurses have always been committed to and are uniquely qualified to render.

■ LONG-TERM CARE

LTC services for chronic diseases and conditions comprise one of the fastest-growing components of the industry. In part this is owing to the success of medical science in saving those who might have died at any earlier stage of life, and in part to the fact that the nuclear family has no place for the incapacitated who, years ago, were simply cared for at home with no public help. LTC signifies much more than the chronic disease hospital and the nursing home. A whole range of options has evolved with the intent of supporting consumer choice and avoiding institutionalization.

The concept of hospice as originally conceived—a cluster of seamless services that support the patient's movement back and forth, depending on comfort and ability—has found renewal in many **life care communities** for older Americans.

Assisted living offers the frail elderly and disabled a comprehensive package of nontraditional services, such as personal care, chore services, or companionship. Assisted living is a social, not a medical program. It rejects the concept of dependency and requires that the beneficiary retain control of his or her life. "Independence, individuality, choice, privacy and dignity are its mantra."[22] Assisted living assumes that care that requires a nursing home can be offered in the home and at lower cost. Given acceptance of that requirement, there is the opportunity to age in place.

There are those who do fine with **long-term home care, medical, or social day care**, and a variety of other stand-alone programs.

Even as we support a return to community and home care services, we know that for many it just is not enough. The multiple backup services, social and health related, that are needed are not easy to organize or to coordinate, and are even less likely to be reimbursed. Therefore, despite much rhetoric, institutional care, although considerably more expensive and often lessening the individual's quality of life, still appears to be necessary for part of the population.

There are two major categories of long-term care institutions: long-term stay or **chronic disease hospitals** (for example, psychiatric, rehabilitation, chronic disease, and TB) and **nursing homes.** Long-term stay hospitals are declining, given the trend toward deinstitutionalization and the development of special care units in nursing homes that are often geared to longer-term situations. Further, the title of chronic disease hospital is a euphemism when most nursing home residents also have limited prospects for community reentry given their frailty, and we are trying to normalize life as much as possible. That means deposing the medical model. The average nursing facility resident needs assistance with four or five activities of daily living (eating, transfer, toileting, dressing, and bathing); this is their prime concern.

In 2004, 16,100 licensed nursing facilities were reported with over 1.7 million beds and an occupancy rate of 86 percent.[23] Special care units have become common for Alzheimer's, AIDS, ventilators, special rehabilitation, and hospice. Most nursing homes have an average of 107 beds, and 53 percent of nursing homes are owned or operated by a chain. Forty-seven percent are independently operated, and 65.5 percent are run for profit. The overwhelmingly greatest numbers of nursing home residents are Medicaid recipients. The reader is reminded that Medicare is an episodic program assuming some return to health and improvement in functional ability; Medicaid is designed for continuing care.

Nursing homes can be classified according to the levels of care offered and whether they are certified for the Medicare or Medicaid programs. According to government regulations, an SNF that provides inpatient skilled nursing and restorative and rehabilitative services must provide 24-hour nursing services, have transfer agreements with a hospital, and fulfill other specific requirements. An intermediate care facility (ICF) provides inpatient health-related care and services to individuals not requiring SNF care. Nursing homes may be certified for either or both levels; about 25 percent are not certified at all. If certified, the Peer Review Organization (PRO) monitors them; some are also accredited by the Joint Commission. All Medicare-certified beds are skilled; Medicaid may be skilled or intermediate. Fourteen percent of SNFs are hospital based. The certificate of need process in most states has kept the hospital-based market from expanding, but it is a natural use for unoccupied hospital beds. The tendency is to eliminate the skilled and intermediate distinction, and instead calculate reimbursement on the specific resource needs of each resident.

The organizational structure of a nursing home is often much like that of a hospital, but there are usually fewer diagnostic and therapeutic departments. Generally, both short- and long-term care are offered. The nursing home may or may not be associated with a particular hospital. Some extended care facilities have expansive services providing a continuum of care from skilled nursing to home care. In recent years, nursing homes have become much more clinically sophisticated; giving intravenous (IV) fluids is common, as are tube feedings and the use of oxygen. Most extended care facilities are moving rapidly to establish subacute and special care units, as noted earlier in this section. These units require a greater presence of professional nurses.

Although about 12 percent of nursing home residents are under 65, the rapid growth of the over-85 population has made the care of the frail elderly and chronically ill a public concern. It has been noted that the population of those over age 85, who are most apt to need long-term care and financial assistance for such services, is increasing seven times as fast as the population as a whole, and elderly Americans who will need some sort of help, now over 6.5 million, will climb to 19 million by 2040. One expert has said that actuarially, the odds are nearly one in two that an individual would need LTC between the age of 65 and death, largely because of chronic disabilities.

The cost of nursing home care is quite high on a long-term basis, and often the patient and spouse must spend down their assets until the patient is eligible for Medicaid. Not too long ago this could have reduced the spouse to poverty, but now legislation allows the spouse to keep both assets and a monthly income at a more reasonable (but still not generous) level. Some elderly are still often upset that their hard-earned savings, which they had hoped to leave to their children, are almost wiped out when nursing home care is necessary. The attitude in this country has turned to financial creativity to avoid impoverishment, such as reverse mortgages and viatical settlements (a cash advance for a life insurance policy on yourself). Long-term care insurance is also becoming more common. The assumption that there is a right to leave assets in an estate by having government pay for your care is becoming very unpopular.

Nursing homes are considered good business opportunities for investors, many of whom believe that more elderly will have good investments in years to come and can pay the ever-increasing rates. And these are the kinds of clients they seek—not the Medicaid patients, with relatively low reimbursement and heavy government oversight.

The variability in the resources needed among LTC patients has caused the federal government to initiate a refinement of the current rate-setting system for nursing homes. As of July 1, 1998, Medicare adopted a PPS for nursing home reimbursement. The system is based on a case mix methodology that is driven by a resident-specific clinical assessment. Medicaid may well follow suit, and already has in many states. This clinical assessment, called the minimum data set (MDS), places a resident in one or another of 44 categories of a case mix. The case mix, Resource Utilization Groups (RUGs), has proven the sensitivity to explain over 50 percent of the variance in resource use among nursing home residents.[24] Put more simply, residents will have the opportunity to obtain the resources they need for quality care if the assessment is done in a timely, accurate, and complete fashion.

Aside from the cost, the quality of nursing homes is an even more difficult issue. The CMS releases periodic data on nursing homes that participate in the Medicare and Medicaid programs. The nursing home industry has been plagued with criticisms about failure to ensure personal cleanliness and grooming, the absence of a stimulating environment, and deficiencies in food handling and storage (the most common criticisms). The ANA commented that one problem in quality was insufficient staffing, especially numbers and availability of registered nurses—not a new issue. The ANA was unsuccessful in its attempt to have 24-hour RN coverage for nursing homes included in legislation for nursing home reform. Owners and managers said these regulations were too tough and expensive; health groups said that they were too weak. One key compromise was the requirement for 24-hour licensed nurse coverage, with an RN on duty on the day shift. Coupled with a generous waiver clause where it was difficult to recruit, it was still possible that nursing home patients could be staffed entirely without an RN.

One happier note is that advanced practice nurses (NPs/CNSs) can make some of the required visits to nursing home residents, and that nurse's aides must be certified (CNAs) after completing a minimum of 75 hours of training. Nurse's aides give up to 85 percent of the care and are often given little or no training. Among other improvements are requirements for a full-time social worker in facilities with more than 120 beds; rehabilitation and dental services; no admissions of mentally ill patients except those with Alzheimer's or related dementia; and residents' guarantee of freedom from abuse, excessive medication, and punitive physical or chemical restraints. Other rights have also been spelled out over the years.

There will probably still be complaints about the quality of life, if not the quality of physical care, in nursing homes. In some areas, ombudsmen for the institutionalized elderly regularly make checks to prevent or detect abuses. There are also a few adopt-a-grandparent or similar programs that give the residents caring social contacts outside the home. It has been noted that the factors generally regarded most highly by residents as important to quality of care were an adequate, competent, caring staff; a homelike environment; properly prepared and varied food; activities; the ability to make some of their own choices; and medical care. No doubt, if these were present in most nursing homes, people would not be as reluctant, even frightened, to be admitted to them.

KEY POINTS

1. There has been increasing concern over the cost of health care since we started down the road to universal coverage in 1965 with Medicare and Medicaid.

2. In search of cost-efficiency and quality, existing health care structures will have to adjust or get out of the way of progress.

3. The United States is slowly but decisively moving toward universal health care, but the process is sometimes circuitous and always incremental.

4. The confusion, fragmentation, and costs of health care have supported a return to self-care for many and created significant interest in alternate/complementary medicine.

5. Regulation of the health care industry will increase, despite our basic distaste for the presence of government in our lives. Alternative therapies and managed care are being targeted.

6. Health care will continue to move into the community and present with new models that allow choice and the normalization of life.

7. Managed care dominates the health care market, but there will always be other choices.

8. Within managed care plans, APNs will begin to dominate as primary care providers and case managers.

9. Ambulatory care will continue to consist of a range of creative programs and avoid standardization.

10. Primary care of the chronically ill will increase as a market.

11. Hospitals will either become one benchmark on a continuum of integrated services, or establish themselves as the hub for a cadre of community health services.

12. Home care must become integrated in systems of care; the freestanding agency is in jeopardy.

13. Nursing homes will serve only the frailest and most disabled.

14. New models will service intermediate levels of disability and acuity, such as subacute care and assisted living.

REFERENCES

1. National Institute for Occupational Safety and Health (NIOSH). Health Care Workers. http://www.cdc.gov/niosh/topics/healthcare. Retrieved April 10, 2010.

2. Kaiser Family Foundation. US Health Care Costs. http://www.kaiseredu.org/topics_im.asp?imID=1&parentID=61&id=358. Retrieved April 2, 2010.

3. Physicians for a National Health Program. Government Funds 60% of US Healthcare Cost. July 9, 2002. http://www.pnhp.org/news/2002/july/government_funds_60.php. Retrieved March 20, 2010.

4. *USA Today*. Five Faces of the Uninsured. September 25, 2009. http://www.usatoday.com/money/industries/health/2009-09-22-faces-uninsured_N.htm. Retrieved April 5, 2010.

5. CBSNews. The Health Care Bill. April 1, 2010. http://www.cbs.com. Retrieved 2, 2010.

6. Managed Care Fact Sheets. Positioning You for Change in Health Care. April 14, 2010. http://www.mcareol.com/factshts/factnati.htm. Retrieved April 14, 2010.

7. National Conference of State Legislatures. Managed Care Laws and Regulations, Including Consumer and Provider Protections. June 2009. http://www.ncsl.org/Default.aspx?TabId=14320. Retrieved April 14, 2010.

8. Lueck S, Greenberger R, Rundle R. Court backs patient appeals in battle over HMO coverage. *Wall Street Journal*, June 21, 2002. http://blogs.wsj.com/law. Retrieved March 22, 2010.

9. Sharp N. Community nursing centers coming of age. *Nurs Manage* 23:18–20, August 1992.

10. National Center for Complimentary and Alternative Medicine. CAM Use in the USA. November 19, 2009. http://nccam.nih.gov/news/camstats. Retrieved April 14, 2010.

11. Eisenberg DM, Davis RB, Ellner SL, et al. Trends in alternate medicine use in the United States, 1990–97. *JAMA* 280:1515–1567, 1998.

12. Medscape Today. Medical Schools Embrace CAM Uncritically. http://www.medscape.com/viewarticle/565472_3. Retrieved April 14, 2010.

13. Hospital and Health Networks. CAM: An Increasing Presence in US Hospitals. January 20, 2009. http://www.hhnmag.com/hhnmag_app/jsp/articledisplay.jsp?dcrpath=HHNMAG/Article/data/01JAN2009/090120HHN_Online_Ananth&domain=HHNMAG. Retrieved April 10, 2010.

14. Brody J. Alternate medicine makes inroads, but watch out for curves. *New York Times*, April 28, 1998, p A3.

15. Rural Assistance Center. Federally Qualified Health Centers. http://www.raconline.org/info_guides/clinics/fqhc.php. Retrieved April 4, 2010.

16. Kaiser Health News. Why Are Fewer Patients Enrolling in Hospice? February 18, 2010. http://www.kaiserhealth-news.org/Columns/2010/February/021810Gleckman. aspx. Retrieved April 14, 2010.

17. American Hospital Association. Fast Facts on U.S. Hospitals. November 11, 2009. http://www.aha.org/aha/resource-center/Statistics-and-Studies/fast-facts.html. Retrieved April 4, 2010.

18. Centers for Disease Control and Prevention (CDC). 2006 National Discharge Survey. http://www.cdc.gov/nchs/fastats/hospital.htm. Retrieved April 4, 2010.

19. The National Association for Home Care and Hospice. *Basic statistics about home care.* Washington, DC: The Association, 2008.

20. Ibid.

21. Ibid.

22. Joel L. Assisted living: Another frontier. *Am J Nurs* 98:7, January 1998.

23. CDC. 2004 National Nursing Home Survey. http://www.cdc.gov/nchs/fastats/nursingh.htm. Retrieved April 3, 2010.

24. Joel L. The economics of nursing home practice. *Am J Nurs* 97:7, December 1997.

Updates can be found at **www.kellysnursing.com**

8 CHAPTER

Health Care Delivery: Who?

A hundred years ago, the trained health workforce consisted of physicians, dentists, some pharmacists, and nurses. Now there are more than 200 acknowledged health occupations and professions, with more being developed every day. In 2008, the estimated number of health care industry employees was over 14.3 million, or about 10 percent of the workforce—one out of every 10 American workers. Health care will generate 3.2 million new wage and salary jobs between 2008 and 2018, more than any other industry, largely in response to rapid growth in the elderly population and longer life expectancies.[1] This does not include others who are self-employed or independent contractors. It does include a vast array of people both involved in health care as a business and indirectly supporting the work of direct caregivers. There are secretaries, clerks, accountants, receptionists, messengers, security force, maintenance, record room staff—the list is endless. As health care has entered the mainstream of business, we have seen the appearance of highly paid administrators, consultants, lawyers, strategic planners, and marketing professionals, and consumers have been critical. Not only has the health care workforce expanded, but also the jobs have changed. Medical records provide a good example. The rapid growth of people covered by government and private health insurance has required more paperwork—and more people to tend to the paperwork once it has been completed. Informatics and computers have become the backbone of operations. Bills are generated by computers and are electronically transmitted for payment. Information on the recipients of care and the services provided is essential for budget decisions, strategic planning, staffing, and more.

The overwhelming growth of personnel is in direct care positions. Many new occupations and suboccupations have emerged because of specialization; other jobs have flourished on the peculiar assumption that several less-prepared workers can accomplish more than a qualified professional. Most of these workers are not licensed; many are trained in on-the-job programs, and even more are trained in a variety of programs with no consistent standards. Others have standardized programs approved by the state or some private sector authority. Generally, this entire group of workers is categorized as allied health professionals or personnel (AHP).

The most recent figures on the employment in health care by segment of the industry and projected changes are displayed in Exhibit 8–1. There are two departments of government that are highly invested in collecting these data: the Bureau of Health Professions, Health Resources and Services Administration of the Department of Health and Human Services (DHHS), and the Bureau of Labor Statistics of the Department of Labor (DOL). It is their work that is considered official. It is difficult to draw conclusions but interesting to make comparisons between these data, because each department uses the indicators most appropriate to its mission. The DHHS focuses on the supply side of the equation, whereas the DOL is most concerned with the number of jobs that are held. The number of jobs held does not assume full-time positions. DOL analysis reveals a trend toward part-time work and the fact that many individuals either choose or are forced to hold several part-time jobs. One of every two jobs for dental hygienists is part time; one in four for physical therapists; and three in 10 for registered nurses (RNs). The most

■ EXHIBIT 8–1. Employment in Health Care by Select Industry Segment 2008 and Projected Change, 2008–2018 (Employment in Thousands)		
Industry Segment	2008 Employment	2008–2018 Percent Change
Health care, total	14,336.0	22.5
Hospitals, public and private	5,667.2	10.1
Nursing and residential care facilities	3,008.0	21.2
Offices of physicians	2,265.7	34.1
Home health care services	958.0	46.1
Offices of other health practitioners	628.8	41.3
Outpatient care centers	532.5	38.6
Other ambulatory health care services	238.5	6.8
Medical and diagnostic laboratories	218.5	39.8

Source: Adapted from the Bureau of Labor Statistics. Occupational Outlook Handbook, 2010–2011 edition. http://www.bls.gov/oco/ocos327. htm. Retrieved April 18, 2010.

recent figures on salaries and the number of jobs held by health care workers can be found in Exhibit 8–2.

When health care is equated with medical care, a functional structure emerges, consisting of independent practitioners, dependent practitioners, and supporting staff. Independent practitioners are those permitted by law to provide a delimited range of services (physicians, nurses, dentists, chiropractors, optometrists, social workers, and podiatrists); dependent practitioners are those permitted by law to provide a delimited range of services under the supervision or authorization of independent practitioners (dental hygienists, physician assistants [PAs], and various therapists); and supporting staff are those carrying out specific tasks authorized by and under the supervision of independent and dependent practitioners, frequently without specific legal delineation of tasks or authority. In certain situations, many in the dependent group can assume the role of independent practitioner. The scope of practice and autonomy of the dependent practitioners are great sources of conflict, particularly because many have an area of expertise not within the knowledge and skills of the independent practitioner. Moreover, the gray areas of overlapping practice are becoming greater: What a particular practitioner does may be legitimately within his or her scope of practice in certain circumstances and just as legitimately within that of another in other circumstances. Or it may be that there are some independent and some dependent activities expected of a practitioner. Nursing, social work, and pharmacy are three examples of this independent/dependent schizophrenia. The legal lines drawn also waver when it comes to supportive workers. There are tasks done by nurse's aides or practical nurses that are part of a nurse's responsibility, but in times and places where there is a nurse shortage, these tasks are often done with almost no supervision. The independent/dependent status concept of health practitioners will undoubtedly undergo considerable reinterpretation with the increasing acceptance of medical care as only one component of total health care.

Credentialing of health care providers and their educational programs is under a variety of auspices: the state, a single professional organization, or a coalition of professional organizations. The Commission on Accreditation of Allied Health Educational Programs (CAAHEP) accredits a total of 1900 allied health educational programs in 18 disciplines. CAAHEP began under the auspices of the American Medical Association (AMA), but it became an independent entity in 1994. Completion of a CAAHEP-accredited educational program is usually required to sit for the certification exam in these practice areas.

Practitioners who are not licensed may often become certified or registered on a voluntary basis by the occupation's national organization or a parent medical group. The inconsistency of these various processes is the focus of some of the complaints about health care credentialing and is discussed later in this book.

■ **EXHIBIT 8–2.** Salaries and Number of Jobs Held by Selected Health Care Personnel, 2008

Occupation	Number of Jobs	Median Salary (Annual, in US Dollars)
Chiropractors	49,100	66,490
Clinical laboratory technicians and technologists	328,100	53,500 (technologists)
		35,380 (technicians)
Dentists	141,900	142,870
Dieticians/nutritionists	60,300	50,590
EMTs and paramedics	210,700	14.10/hour
Home health aides	1.7 million	9.22/hour
Medical assistants	483,600	28,300
Medical record technicians	172,500	30,610
Nuclear medicine technician	21,800	66,660
Nursing and psychiatric aides	1.4 million	11.46/hour
Occupational therapists	104,500	66,780
Pharmacist	269,900	106,410
Physicians	661,400	186,044 (primary care)
		339,738 (specialists)
Physician assistants	74,800	81,230
Physical therapists	185,500	72,790
Podiatrists	12,200	113,560
Psychologists	170,200	64,140
Radiation therapists	15,200	72,910
Recreational therapists	23,300	38,370
Registered nurse	2.6 million	62,450
Respiratory therapists	105,900	52,200
Speech and language pathologists	119,300	62,930

Source: Adapted from the Bureau of Labor Statistics. Occupational Outlook Handbook, 2010–2012 edition. http://www.bls.gov/oco/ocos327.htm. Retrieved April 18, 2010.

Compared to other nations, the United States has a more than ample supply of health workers, even in terms of the physician: population ratio, which has been estimated by the DHHS to be about 260 to every 100,000 in population. (In most countries, nurses are in shortest supply.) The types of American health workers are also considerably more diverse; other nations have experimented more with such physician substitutes as the Russian *feldsher* or Chinese *barefoot doctor*.

The largest groups of health workers, in order, are nurses (all types, as well as aides), physicians, dentists and their allied health workers, clinical laboratory personnel, pharmacists, and radiological technicians. Between 75 and 85 percent of health workers are women. However, women are, or have been, concentrated in the lower-paid and less powerful positions. Physicians, dentists, administrators, and other policy-making roles are male dominated. This may change over time; women currently constitute over half of medical school graduates, and the number is slowly but consistently increasing.[2]

It would be unrealistic to attempt to describe all the professional and technical workers with whom nurses work or interact. However, an introduction to the most prevalent health occupations should provide a better understanding of the complex relationships in health care.

The organization of this chapter is primarily alphabetical, although on occasion two closely related groups may be described in logical succession, with general issues and trends identified at the end of the chapter. The education of RNs and practical nurses and the practice of nursing are described in later chapters. Good sources of information about health careers are the National Health Council in Washington, DC, and the DOL's *Occupational Outlook Handbook*.

■ CHIROPRACTIC

Practitioners in this area may be designated as *Doctors of Chiropractic, Chiropractic Physician,* or *Chiropractor.* They treat problems of the body's structural and neurologic systems.

All states and the District of Columbia regulate the practice of chiropractic and grant licenses to chiropractors who meet educational and examination requirements established by the state. Chiropractors can only practice in states where they are licensed. Some states have agreements permitting chiropractors licensed in one state to obtain a license without further examination, provided that educational, examination, and practice credentials meet state specifications. For licensure, most state boards recognize either all or part of the four-part test administered by the National Board of Chiropractic Examiners. State examinations may supplement the National Board tests, depending on state requirements.

To maintain licensure, almost all states require completion of a specified number of hours of continuing education each year. Continuing education programs are offered by accredited chiropractic programs and institutions as well as chiropractic associations. Specialty councils within some chiropractic associations also offer programs leading to clinical specialty certification, called *diplomate certification,* in areas such as orthopedics, neurology, sports injuries, occupational and industrial health, nutrition, diagnostic imaging, thermography, and internal disorders.

In 2009, there were 16 chiropractic programs and institutions in the United States accredited by the Council on Chiropractic Education. Successful completion of a minimum of 4 years of academic study in the sciences, public health, clinical disciplines, and chiropractic principles and practice, preceded by at least 2 years of college education, results in a Doctor of Chiropractic credential.

There have been 80,000 chiropractor licenses awarded in the United States, including those with more than one license and others who may not practice.

All 50 states and the District of Columbia and Puerto Rico recognize chiropractic as a health profession and authorize chiropractic services as part of their workers' compensation program, as do many federal health benefits programs; services are also reimbursable under Medicare and Medicaid. Virtually all major commercial health insurance carriers include chiropractic in their private policies. Based on their order of size, number of practitioners, and public utilization, chiropractic ranks second after medicine as a primary health care provider.

■ CLINICAL LABORATORY SCIENCES

There are a number of technicians or technologists working in the clinical laboratories in such specialties as immunohematology, hematology, clinical chemistry, serology, microbiology, blood banking, and histology. The work involves analysis of human blood, tissues, and fluids to determine the absence, presence, or extent of a disease. A physician who is a pathologist is usually in charge, although technologists may have specific responsibilities for technicians. Medical technologists' preparation includes 3 years of college science plus 1 year of professional course work in a CAAHEP-accredited school covering all phases of clinical laboratory work. The Board of Registry of Medical Technologists of the American Society of Clinical Pathologists (ASCP) grants certification, after successful completion of a board examination. The initials MT (ASCP) may then be used. Most states do not require licensure. Additional appropriate education and experience qualify a medical technologist for specialist certification in blood banking, chemistry, microbiology, cytotechnology, or nuclear technology.

Certified laboratory technicians, who perform routine laboratory tests, usually complete a 2-year associate degree in medical laboratory technology. Histologic technicians, who prepare body tissues for microscopic examination by pathologists, are usually prepared in 1-year programs given by hospitals or laboratory centers that are also CAAHEP-accredited. Certification is granted after passing an ASCP examination.

■ DENTISTRY

Dentists treat oral diseases and disorders. They may fill cavities, extract teeth, and provide dentures for patients. Recognized dental specialties are oral surgery and orthodontics (correction of irregularities of teeth and jaws), which together make up 60 percent of specialist practice; endodontics (root canal therapy); pedodontics (children's dentistry); periodontology or periodontics (treatment of gums, bone, and other surrounding tissue); prosthodontics (replacement of missing teeth); oral pathology (study of diseased oral tissues); and public health dentistry.

Dental school is preceded by 2 to 4 years of college with specific science courses; most entering students, however, are college graduates. The dental school curriculum is a 3- to 4-year course leading to a Doctor of Dental Surgery (DDS) or a Doctor of Dental Medicine (DDM) degree. The American Dental Association (ADA) must approve all dental schools. Dentists are licensed in all states by taking a state board examination or a National Board of Dental Examiners exam. Currently, about 17 states require dentists to obtain a specialty license before practicing as a specialist. Requirements include 2 to 4 years of postgraduate education and, in some cases, completion of a special state examination.

Most dentists are in private practice; the others practice in institutions, the armed forces, and health agencies, or teach or conduct research. Most are located in large cities. An increasing number of minorities and women are entering the field.

In recent years, there has been concern about the increasing cost of dental education and a perceived oversupply of dentists. Some dental schools are in severe financial difficulties and are threatened by closure. Legislators maintain that although there are many underserved areas of dental need, the production of more dentists does not solve the problem, because few dentists practice in those areas; most prefer a more lucrative practice.

The provision of comprehensive dental care for elementary school children and the aged, and the anticipation of the need for more periodontal and endodontic treatment as preventive dentistry grows in popularity are indicators of a need for more and different types of dental services in the future.

One frustration is that although there continues to be significant concern about dental health in this country, how do you do manpower projections when so many people still choose to ignore their personal needs in this area?

Dental hygienists, almost all of who are women, provide dental services under a dentist's supervision. They examine, scale, and polish teeth; give fluoride treatments; take x-rays; monitor patients' medical and oral health; and educate patients about proper care of the teeth and gums. In many states, hygienists' responsibilities have been expanded to include duties traditionally performed by dentists, such as giving local anesthetics, and it has been said that their training includes much more than they are permitted to do by most dentist employers. Hygienists are licensed in all states and are the only ancillary personnel permitted by law to clean teeth. The registered dental hygienist (RDH) designation is awarded after passing a written and practical certification examination.

Education may consist of 2-, 3-, or 4-year programs leading to a certificate or an associate or baccalaureate degree at vocational-technical institutes, community colleges, and universities. Those dental hygienists with master's degrees may be teachers or administrators. The vast majority of dental hygienists practice with dentists in offices. However, in recent years, a few have set up separate private practices—a move that is strongly opposed by dentists but is approved in some states by court decision or attorney general rulings. A degree of resistance to dentist domination over their practice is emerging. The demand for RDH services is growing rapidly. One of every two dental hygienists is involved in a part-time job, although their work life may consist of several of these.[3]

Dental assistants maintain supplies, keep dental records, schedule appointments, prepare patients for examinations, process x-rays, and assist the dentist chairside, but their functions are also expanding. Most assistants complete a 1- or 2-year program at a community college or vocational-technical school. These programs award a certificate, diploma, or associate degree.

Dental technicians or *denturists* make and repair dentures, crowns, bridges, and other appliances, usually according to dentists' prescriptions. Denturists are lobbying to work directly with patients, saying that they not only charge less, but also are faster and better at fitting dentures. The ADA is fighting this move, insisting that dentists must have total jurisdiction over all oral disorders because they alone are trained to diagnose and treat them. However, several states have already licensed denturists to provide direct service, and the services are proliferating (if illegally) in other states. Most Canadian provinces have had licensed denturists for many years.

The education of denturists usually consists of a 2-year certificate or associate degree program, although some prepare by working for 3 to 4 years as trainees in dental laboratories. The military also offers training.[4]

■ DIETETICS AND NUTRITION

Nutritionist is a general occupational title for health professionals concerned with food science and human nutrition. They include dietitians, home economists, and food technologists. There is no required standard for use of the title, but a baccalaureate degree in the area of home economics or nutrition is usual. A master's degree may be required for certain positions, especially in public health. And it is becoming more common to find nutritionists with doctoral degrees in corporate positions or as university faculty. The research agenda of the nutrition and dietetics field is impressive. You are referred to the *Journal of the American Dietetics Association.*

Dietitians may have a general dietary background or preparation in medical dietetics. *Medical* or *therapeutic dietitians* are responsible for the selection of appropriate foods for special diets, patient counseling, and sometimes management of the dietary service. They may manage a food service, where they are responsible for personnel, purchasing, budgeting, and planning menus. With appropriate education, they may also do research or teach students.

Clinical dietitians work with patients not only in the hospital, but also in clinics, neighborhood health centers, or in the patient's own home. These patients include pregnant women, diabetics, and those with other nutritional problems.

A baccalaureate program with majors in food, nutrition, and food management is usually basic, with the possible addition of a dietetic internship program approved by the American Dietetic Association. Certification is granted by the American Dietetic Association, after which the individual may use the RD after her name (most are female). New career opportunities include corporate positions in hotel and other chains with food service, corporate wellness programs, and management companies providing food service in long-term care (LTC) facilities.

Among the actions being considered by the American Dietetic Association is third-party reimbursement and licensure. The latter is considered a necessary step for securing third-party reimbursement. In 1983, Texas became the first state to license dietitians, albeit on a voluntary basis. Licensure as the American Dietetic Association proposes it does not protect the scope of practice of nutrition/dietetics for licensed or registered dietitians; however, it does protect those titles against unauthorized use.

Another trend is the delegation of functions to assisting personnel. Dietetic technicians graduate from one of two kinds of American Dietetic Association–approved technical programs with an associate degree. A program with a food service management emphasis allows the individual to serve as a technical assistant to a food service director and, with experience, to become a director. The program with a nutritional care emphasis enables the individual to become a technical assistant to the clinical dietitian. Both programs require clinical practice. Passing the Registration Examination for Dietetic Technicians enables the technician to use the credentials dietetic technician, registered (DTR).

A dietetic assistant is a graduate of a 1-year academic program in dietetics requiring classroom instruction coordinated with clinical practice. Included are food preparation, basic nutrition, and menu planning; purchasing; storage, safety, and sanitation; personnel supervision; and cost control. These programs may also be approved by the American Dietetic Association. Most dietetic assistants serve as food service supervisors in hospitals, schools, and nursing homes. However, a number of food service supervisors currently functioning in that position lack such preparation.

■ HEALTH EDUCATORS

Community health educators help to identify the health learning needs of the community, particularly in terms of prevention of disease and injury. They may then plan, organize, and implement appropriate programs, for example, screening programs, health fairs, classes, and self-help groups. Some health educators are employed by the state as consultants, others by insurance companies, voluntary health organizations such as the American Heart Association, the school system (school health educators), and, occasionally, industry. Unfortunately, as government funding fluctuates, programs may expand or contract, and health educators may be eliminated or spread thin, as has happened in school health.

A number of hospitals are employing *patient educators* or *health educators* to develop and direct programs of both patient education and community health education. Frequently, these people are nurses with or without training in health education and administration. Health educators usually have baccalaureate or master's degrees in health education, public health, or community health education. Master's degrees may include an administration component.

Educational therapists provide services that are part of a formal rehabilitation program for the physically or mentally ill. It is a form of teaching, but the major focus of the work is to stimulate interest and confidence, and to reconnect with life and the world. The educational therapist functions as part of the rehabilitation team and works with individual patients. A baccalaureate degree is required with a major in education or physical education. No licensure or certification is required, but the American Association for Rehabilitation Therapy offers a registration after adequate experience.

In a few states, health educators are registered or certified. Some state health educator groups are working on plans for voluntary certification.

■ HEALTH SERVICES MANAGEMENT

Health services administrators or *executives* manage multiunit systems, health care networks, organizations, agencies, institutions, programs, and services within the health care delivery system. They may work in any setting, but are probably more visible in hospitals, managed care plans, nursing homes, neighborhood health centers, and community health agencies. The principles of management can be applied to any setting, and the role of the hospital administrator is a reasonable example of that role and its functions (see Chapter 7). Nurses usually manage nursing services, but a number also hold positions as top executives, particularly in home care agencies and community health centers. Although they may retain their nursing identity, they should be functioning as administrators and be equipped with the necessary educational background. Usually, the appropriate credential is a master's degree in health services management, public health, hospital administration, or more recently, business or public administration. Other positions in the operation of health facilities and plants are the usual business positions—financial management, information systems, clinical data systems, human resources, materials management, and professional services—with all types of specific assignments and educational expectations.

For many years, controversy in health management education was centered on the proper educational credentials. There were those who believed that health services administrators should be prepared in business schools so managers could deal effectively with increasing economic pressure. Others felt that the distinctive nature of health care organizations required managers prepared in programs concentrating on health services administration. With the current complexity in health care, it is apparent that the knowledge and skills for success will best be acquired in educational settings focusing on health services management. A continuing issue, however, is the proper balance between managerial skills and practical knowledge of the health care delivery environment because, at the same time that post-master's residencies in health care administration are being recommended, economic pressures in the field are lessening the opportunities for such employer-funded education.

Currently, considerable career opportunities are to be found in managerial roles in the evolving world of managed care. The nature of managed care was discussed in Chapter 7. Although there are no managerial functions unique to managed care settings, they do place a high priority on such managerial activities as strategic planning, marketing, sales and services, integrating professionals into the organization, managing costs, controlling utilization, and ensuring quality.

■ MEDICAL RECORDS

Medical record administrators (MRAs) are responsible for the preparation, collation, and organization of patient records; maintaining an efficient filing system; and making records available to those concerned with the patient's subsequent care. Other duties include designing health information systems and providing information for reimbursement by third-party payers. They may also classify and compile data for review committees and researchers, and they must have knowledge and skills in health care databases and systems, medical classification systems, and the relationship of financial information to clinical data. CAAHEP accredits both 4-year baccalaureate programs and 1-year hospital-based programs preceded by a baccalaureate degree. After completion of these programs the candidate qualifies for certification administered by the American Association of Medical Record Librarians. Successful completion leads to designation as Registered Record Administrator (RRA).

Medical record technicians assist the physician and the MRA in preparing reports and transcribing histories and physicals, and work closely with others using patient records. In a large institution, they may specialize; in a small one, they may have full responsibility for the department. CAAHEP-accredited programs are usually 2-year associate degree programs and include theoretical instruction and practical hospital experience. A national exam leads to the title Accredited Record Technician (ART).

Advances in computerization are creating major changes in the medical records field, and a shortage is predicted. Opportunities are available in every conceivable health care setting because medical record keeping is a system-wide requirement.

The field of health information management is gaining in importance, and there is already a shortage of prepared personnel. The *health information management specialist* collects, analyzes, and manages the information that steers the health care industry. Particularly because of computers, the individual must balance patients' privacy rights with legitimate uses of aggregate data. Knowledge of medical legal systems, security systems, and the uses and users of health care information is of vital importance. This is a modern-day role that focuses on systems and the analytic use of data.

■ MEDICINE

Doctors of medicine and osteopathy practice prevention, diagnosis, and treatment of disease and injury. Doctor of Medicine (MD) degrees are awarded in 129 allopathic medical schools in the United States and are considered the first professional degree. The Doctor of Osteopathy is awarded in 25 schools in 31 locations in the United States. Some physicians may later decide to acquire advanced degrees (master's or doctorates) in a science or public health. Admission into medical schools after 4, or occasionally 3, years of preprofessional college work is considered highly selective. Programs are usually 4 years in length, with required basic sciences and clinical studies. In the last 2 years, students have clinical clerkships, usually in hospitals, but also in clinics or doctors' offices. In this first contact with patients, they are usually supervised and taught by attending physicians or residents as they apply their clinical and scientific knowledge. Generally, physicians and professors of science are the teachers in medical schools, although others include ethicists, sociologists, and occasionally, a nurse (not usually on a full-time basis). In some medical schools, nurse instructors have responsibility for teaching medical students in the clinical clerkship. In most cases, medical education has little interdisciplinary focus, and contacts with other health profession students are seldom formalized, although sometimes students in a multidisciplinary setting develop interactional opportunities of their own.

The number of women entering medicine has gradually been increasing. In 2009, medical school enrollments— once largely male—had an even gender split.[2] Preparation for the role of physician requires about 11 years: 3 to 4 years of undergraduate education, 4 years of medical school, and 3 years or more of residency.

The formalized program of education after the MD degree is titled *graduate medical education* (GME) and consists primarily of a residency, which is preparation for specialization, for a period of 2 to 5 years. At one time, a 1-year internship, usually rotating through the various clinical services, was the norm, but after years of debate and two major reports, in the mid-1960s several changes occurred. Family practice was recognized as a specialty, the internship (almost a general working apprenticeship) was abolished, and residencies in hospitals with at least minimal university affiliations were developed. A 1-year general residency is still required for licensure. Almost all residency programs now are in such hospitals, but there is a continuing conflict—education on the one hand and a functional hospital apprenticeship on the other, and the need for both. GME has been financed primarily by third-party payers, including Medicare and Medicaid, indirectly through higher payment for patient care provided in teaching hospitals and direct support for the cost of residency programs. This financing is being gradually eliminated, and many hospitals are terminating their residency programs. Residencies seem to have three distinct components: acquisition of knowledge, skills, and professional behavior. On completion of the specified years of residency, the physician may take certification exams in the specialty and is board certified; if exams are not taken (or failed), he or she is still "board eligible." In some cases, continuing medical education is required for recertification.

For a number of years, there were more first-year residency openings than American medical school graduates. Graduates from foreign medical schools, including Americans, filled these positions. In some states, the vast majority were foreign medical graduates (FMGs). Because of differences in the quality of education and language and cultural differences, problems often occurred. Legislation has drastically cut the number of FMGs. Recently the term *international medical graduate* (IMG) is being used and includes Americans graduating from non–US medical schools. The prevailing sentiment is to limit the number of residencies to the number of US medical school graduates for the year plus 10 percent.

When the number of FMGs who stay in the United States after residencies and fellowships are added to the number of US medical residents finishing their training, estimates are that 19,500 new physicians enter patient care each year.[3] In 1950, there were 142.2 physicians per 100,000 people. By 2000, this number had grown to 260.7. It has been estimated that the United States needs between 145 and 185 physicians per 100,000 people.[4] This is an important observation for the practice of advanced practice nurses (APNs).

Although most American physicians choose specialties as their field of practice, the need for more general practitioners is being met by the designation of the field of family practice (thus the residency) as a specialty and heavy federal funding for those selecting that field. Thirty-five percent of all practicing physicians in the United States are in primary care areas (medicine, family practice, and pediatrics), and 65 percent are in specialties. This is in contrast to other industrialized countries, where more than 50 percent are in primary care specialties.[5] Determination of what constitutes too many or too few physicians in a specialty, or even in primary care, seems to be constantly debatable. Whether there is a surplus or a shortage of physicians will depend on the evolving delivery system, not on the patterns of practice physicians would prefer. Current predictions of shortages in primary care may be retracted if managed care programs see the requirement for a primary care provider as distasteful to the American public, or costing more than direct access to the generalist or specialist of the patient's choice. Such is the most recent talk; however, there is no doubt a glaring need in some areas such as preventive medicine (including public health) and geriatrics.

In medical centers, a *fellow* is a post-residency physician who enters even more advanced, highly specialized, or research-oriented programs, although presumably still being involved in teaching and patient care. GME is under the direction of medical school faculty recognized as specialists or subspecialists.

A relatively new issue in graduate education is the unionization of residents (with varied success) to obtain better conditions of work, especially reduction of the long hours that may threaten competence. In those states where shorter hours and on-call time are now required, the cause was usually a well-publicized patient's death or injury attributed to decreased competence of exhausted house staff. Many teaching hospitals have developed a residents' hours policy voluntarily. But these are piecemeal solutions. The excessive work hours forced upon residents, though a historic fact, have recently aroused national attention. Sleep research has proven that excessive work hours lead to cognitive impairment, mistakes, and ultimately harm to both patients and the residents themselves. Further, the Institute of Medicine (IOM) has reported that as many as 100,000 people die every year as a result of preventable medical error. The medical community has had decades to solve this problem, but has preferred to ignore it. In July 2002, and again in 2005, federal legislation was before both the House and the Senate (the Patient and Physician Safety and Protection Act) to impose limits on work hours of residents. In both instances it failed to gain support.[6]

Physician licensure is mandatory in every state, some of which require continuing education for relicensure. The single licensure exam, called the US Medical Licensure Exam (USMLE), has three components (steps). The first two are taken in medical school and the third no later than completion of the first year of an approved residency. The Federation Licensure Examination (FLEX), authorized by the Federation of State Medical Boards and accepted in all jurisdictions, is an alternative to the third step of the USMLE. The exam may now be taken anywhere in the world by IMGs after graduation from medical school, but first they must usually be certified by the Educational Commission for Foreign Medical Graduates, which involves other testing and credentials review. No individual is fully licensed until all parts of the USMLE or USMLE/FLEX are passed; before that, practice is covered by a temporary license or is on a student basis, just as it is with nurses until they have passed state boards. These licensing exams may be repeated if failed with no restriction on the number of times they are retaken. Although the National Board of Medical Examiners (NBME) suggests a passing score, each state board sets its own score for awarding licensure in that state, and there are some states that do not recognize the third part of the USMLE exam at all.[7]

Although the public generally still holds MDs in high regard, they have become the target of much criticism, and it appears that they often have difficulty coping with the radical changes in health care and society. For instance, although they have been criticized for the use of expensive diagnostics, they claim they are responding to litigious patients who potentially drive up their malpractice premiums. At the same time, there are allegations of peer cover-up of incompetent practitioners instead of peer review and removal from practice. Now there are more deliberate efforts by medicine to identify "impaired" physicians and give them appropriate help until they are safe to practice. Continuing medical education has also been strongly supported for maintaining competence.

With economic pressures, changes in health care delivery and reimbursement, and oversupply, some physicians are finding it necessary to market their services actively (advertising is now acceptable); others are moving into salaried positions where they need not manage the business aspects of a practice. The projected oversupply may also be responsible for increased aggressiveness in opposing the practice of nonphysician providers such as certified nurse midwives (CNMs) and nurse practitioners (NPs). This can be interpreted as restraint of trade and does not only involve APNs. The Federal Trade Commission has ruled against the AMA several times on this issue.

Still another issue is the maldistribution of physicians. National Health Corps physicians do seem to select rural areas for practice more than other physicians (or are assigned there), but these areas, unattractive and isolated places, and big city ghettoes still lack even a minimally satisfactory presence of physicians. Meanwhile, more affluent areas have unnecessarily high physician-to-population ratios. Even National Health Corps physicians often do not stay after their required time of payback for their medical education. Given the maldistribution and cost problems, and the new aggressiveness of other health professionals, there is a frequent reiteration of the question, "Why should the physician be the gatekeeper to health care?"

Over the last several years, a great deal has been seen in the media and in the professional literature about problems, changes, and predictions concerning the field of medicine, usually referring to allopathic medicine. For instance, with an ongoing prediction of physician oversupply, frequent public criticism of their practice and lack of humanistic qualities, a loss of considerable autonomy and some income because of governmental and insurer programs of cost containment, as well as an increase in malpractice suits, physicians themselves have expressed discontent with their profession. An unusually large number are retiring early, changing to fields such as research and administration, or leaving medicine altogether. Moreover, they are said to discourage potential students from entering the field. College students, whether influenced or not by such attitudes, were choosing the more lucrative business fields, which do not saddle them with immense debt and an educational and practice period of long hours, much stress, and relatively poor pay. It has been predicted that, as opposed to past trends, the demography of the medical profession will change to include considerably more women and nonwhite males (a trend also evident in the overall employment picture in the United States). Some think this may lead to less resistance to radical changes in practice patterns, because those entering the profession have more moderate expectations and a greater commitment to primary care specialties. Yet, there is still concern that too many medical students continue to choose high-technology specialties over primary care areas, in part because of the potential for better income and quicker retirement of their educational debt, and the higher status of certain specialists in the medical community. (Anesthesiologists, surgeons, and radiologists have the highest incomes; general practitioners and psychiatrists the lowest.) From another perspective, escalating malpractice premiums and the reduction of surgical fees under Medicare might deter some from selecting surgery.

There is a trend for newly licensed physicians, especially women, to choose a salaried position instead of private practice. Health maintenance organizations (HMOs) provide such opportunities. A number of reasons are given for this: the cost of setting up a private practice and the struggle for success; the fact that employers often pay for malpractice insurance; more regular hours and time for self and family; a guaranteed income; and the availability of peer stimulation. Another major reason is that more physicians in solo or group practice are losing their patients, as the latter choose, or are almost forced, to join HMOs. In fact, in some instances, physicians have found that if they did not join an HMO early, they were no longer wanted by the HMO, which had enough physicians. Some experts predict that most physicians will become employees as we move further into the twenty-first century. Such positions, however, are not without problems: Employed physicians in certain HMOs have been seriously considering unionizing because of discontent about their salaries, autonomy, and conditions of work.

There are still major criticisms of physicians by the public, even when those surveyed are generally satisfied with their own physicians. Much discontent is related to physicians' lack of communication with patients and their perceived lack of interest in patients as individuals or in the broader problems of society. Physicians claim that patients are now more aggressive consumers, primed to distrust. They maintain that the potential of any patient suing when the health outcome is not as expected (because they expect perfection), even if the physician has made no error, drives a wedge in the physician-patient relationship. A number of physicians will not accept patients that they think might create a problem. Yet, there is also evidence that in the absence of a long-term and personal relationship, physician and patient never get to know one another or develop trust. Therefore, it becomes easy to criticize and attack through the courts. All of this has had some impact on the medical curriculum and even the entrance examinations. The Medical College Admission Test (MCAT) has come to emphasize critical thinking, problem solving, and communications rather than rote learning of scientific facts. Some very distinguished medical schools have revised their curricula so that students will have contact with patients within the first few weeks of their first year, instead of the third. Directed by a preceptor-physician who stays with a particular student throughout the 4 years, the student learns humanistic values through both patient contact and problem-based tutorials. Whether the approach of emphasizing human values will become widespread remains to be seen.

Doctors of osteopathy (DO) are qualified to be licensed as physicians and to practice all branches of medicine and surgery. DO schools are accredited by the Bureau of Professional Education of the American Osteopathic Association (AOA). Admission to the colleges requires at least 3 years of preprofessional education at an accredited college or university. Applicants also take a qualifying exam. The DO degree involves 4 academic years of education. Required basic sciences, anatomy, physiology, biochemistry, pathology, microbiology, and pharmacology are much the same as those in allopathic medical schools, as are the clinical courses of medicine, surgery, pediatrics, obstetrics, gynecology, radiology, and preventive medicine. After graduation, all DOs serve a 12-month rotating internship in an approved osteopathic hospital, with primary emphasis on medicine, obstetrics/gynecology, and surgery. They are then eligible for most of the same specialty residencies as allopathic graduates. The AOA requires continuing education for all DOs in practice.

Osteopathic physicians are considered separate but equal in American medicine; they are licensed in all states and have the same rights and obligations as allopathic (MD) physicians. The "something extra" they claim is the integration of osteopathic principles. These deal with the interrelationship of all body systems in health and disease and emphasize the musculoskeletal system and manipulative therapy. Holistic medicine, proper nutrition, and environment are a major focus in practice. DOs prescribe drugs, use routine diagnostic measures, and perform surgery. They comprise about 5 percent of all physicians. They are younger than their allopathic counterparts. More women are attracted to the field. Most choose primary care areas, and only 25 percent have traditionally moved into specialty practice, but there does seem to be some recent increase in these numbers. Four out of five are practicing in 16 states, with Michigan having the most.[8] The 190 or so osteopathic hospitals, located in 28 states, usually offer a full range of services. Nursing in osteopathic hospitals is comparable to that in any other hospital.

■ PHYSICIAN ASSISTANTS

In 1965, Dr. Eugene A. Stead, Jr., of Duke University inaugurated a program for PAs designed to assist physicians in their practice, either to enable them to expand their practice or to give them time to pursue continuing education or to devote to themselves and their families. The students in the Duke program came from a variety of backgrounds and included nurses and former military corpsmen. Shortly afterward, a series of programs, called MEDEX and developed specifically for ex-corpsmen, was funded by the federal government.

In the early years of these programs, there was a great deal of confusion about the education, role, legality, and scope of practice of the PA. Educational programs ran the gamut from a few months of on-the-job training to 5 years. Formalized programs prepared assistants to the primary care physician as well as specialists. Continued federal funding after 1972 not only encouraged the growth of programs, but also required a certain focus: training for delivery of primary care in ambulatory settings, placement of graduates in medically underserved areas, and recruitment of residents from these areas as well as minority groups and women. In the early 1970s, the AMA took a position requiring PA educational programs to standardize their curriculum to qualify for accreditation. (For a more detailed description of the early developments in PA education and practice, see the fifth edition of this book.)

As defined in Health Resources and Services Administration (HRSA) reports, PAs are skilled members of the health care team who, working dependently with physicians and under their supervision, provide diagnostic and therapeutic patient care. They take patient histories, perform physical examinations, and order laboratory tests. When medical problems are diagnosed, PAs develop treatment plans and explain them to patients. They are also permitted to diagnose illnesses. PAs are recognized in all states, the District of Columbia, and Guam. The requirement for physician supervision to practice varies greatly in interpretation. In 42 states, including the District of Columbia, physicians may supervise PAs without being on the premises. If PAs are necessary in underserved areas, this latitude is essential, and now supervision from a distance using electronic technology is also considered satisfactory. All 50 states, the District of Columbia, and Guam and the Commonwealth of the Northern Mariana Islands have enacted laws that authorize PA prescribing.[9] In addition to specific technical procedures that PAs perform, which vary with the practice setting, they carry out a variety of minor surgical procedures. They may also provide pre- and postoperative care. PAs with surgical training often act as first or second assistants in major surgery.

As of 2010, the Accreditation Review Commission on Education for the Physician Assistant (ARC-PA) accredited 140 programs. The typical PA program is 24 to 25 months long and requires at least 2 years of college and some health care experience prior to admission. The majority of students have a bachelor of arts or science degree and 45 months of health care experience before admission to a PA program. Of the 140 accredited PA programs, 113 award master's degrees, 21 award bachelor's degrees, 3 award associate degrees, and 5 award certificates. (Some programs offer more than one option.)[10] The trend is toward graduate education.

The curriculum includes basic natural, behavioral, and medical sciences; an introduction to clinical medicine; and 1 year of supervised clinical practice. The focus is on broadly based primary care training. Postgraduate programs (PA residencies) offer additional clinical and structured learning experiences in specialties to graduate PAs.

PAs receive their national certification from the National Commission on Certification of Physician Assistants (NCCPA). Only graduates of an accredited PA program are eligible to take the Physician Assistant National Certifying Examination (PANCE). Once certified, a PA must complete a continuous 6-year cycle to keep her or his certificate current. Every 2 years, PAs must complete 100 continuing education hours and reregister their certificate with the NCCPA (second and fourth years), and by the end of the sixth year recertify by examination or documented experience. All states require passage of the PANCE for state licensure. Forty-seven states make provisions to license new PA program graduates prior to the availability of PANCE results.[11] The Federation of State Medical Boards' Model Medical Practice Act speaks to the regulation of PAs.

Most PAs are employed in one of three specialty areas: family medicine; surgery, including subspecialties; and internal medicine. Surgery is increasingly favored. Although about 35 percent work with physicians in private or group offices and another 30 percent in a variety of clinics, there seems to be a trend in some cities for employment by hospitals. One reason for the interest of hospitals is that medical residents' hours are being limited or residency programs eliminated, and PAs are hired to fill in the gap, especially in the emergency room and assisting the doctor in the operating room (OR), where they are reimbursed as second assistants. About 40 percent of PAs practice in towns having fewer than 50,000 people.

Results of the 2001 American Academy of Physician Assistants (AAPA) salary survey indicate that salaries differ with specialty, setting, and geographic location. Women consistently make less than men, even when they have the same education, experience, and credentials. Medicare and Medicaid policies governing coverage for PA services in hospitals and other institutions encourage the hiring of PAs. PAs are reimbursed through their supervising physician or they are salaried. It is expected that the demand for PAs will exceed the supply.

The AAPA estimates that there were approximately 85,345 people eligible to practice as PAs and 73,893 people in clinical practice as PAs at the beginning of 2009. The number of new graduates in 2007 was approximately 4600.[12] PA education is not a stepping stone to medical school, but some PAs enroll in nursing school or receive degrees in public health, which offer additional opportunities.

There are still many unresolved issues related to PA practice, particularly in relation to role and functions. The AHA published a statement on PAs in hospitals, which recommends that the medical staff and administration formulate guidelines under which the PA can operate, and that any request for PA practice in hospitals should be handled by the medical staff credentials committee. Emphasis is on medical supervision; however, current reality has shown that PAs go unsupervised in busy urban hospitals where they handle many emergency and other ambulatory patients.

This has created a problem for nurses, for the authority of the PA vis-à-vis the nurse is frequently not clear. Although the nurses' associations, some state boards, some courts, and attorneys general have indicated that nurses do not take PA orders, in about 17 states the rulings are the reverse. Because the PA may function according to a protocol specified by the supervisor/physician, there may be an operational agreement reached similar to the basis on which a nurse carries out standing orders or some verbal orders from the physician. Nevertheless, there is frequently interdisciplinary conflict when roles are not clarified. Yet, there seems to be an accommodation reached when both work together cooperatively.

Concern about the relative status of APNs and PAs was, and is, an issue in certain situations. Although APNs can offer services to the public beyond any that a PA can offer, frequently nurse and PA may be competing for the same job. For a number of reasons, the PA not only may be the one employed, but will also receive a higher salary than that offered to the APN. Despite the fact that most physicians tend to say that they prefer nurses to PAs, the truth is that too often doctors have inadequate or no knowledge about APNs' capabilities. What doctors are saying is that they want the nurse as a PA. A number of nurses have sought additional credentials to qualify for status as a PA. This has caused some negative reaction from other nurses and nursing associations.

■ MEDICAL ASSISTANTS

Medical assistants (MAs) are usually employed in physicians' offices, where they perform a variety of administrative and clinical tasks to facilitate the work of the doctor; however, some do work in hospitals and clinics. They perform tasks required by the doctor, in accordance with specific state laws, and are supervised by the doctor.

The MA, among other things, answers the telephone; greets patients and other callers; makes appointments; handles correspondence and filing; arranges for diagnostic tests, hospital admissions, and surgery; handles patients' accounts and other billings; processes insurance claims, including Medicare; maintains patient records; prepares patients for examinations or treatment; takes temperatures, height, and weight; sterilizes instruments; assists the physician in examining or treating patients; and if trained, performs laboratory procedures. Most medical assistants train in 1-year certificate or 2-year associate degree programs given by community colleges, universities, and vocational-technical schools. CAAHEP accreditation is available.

■ EMERGENCY MEDICAL CARE

Emergency medical technicians-ambulance (EMT-A) respond to medical emergencies and provide immediate care to the critically ill or injured. They may administer cardiac resuscitation, treat shock, provide initial care to poison or burn victims, and transport patients to a health facility. EMT-As do not determine the extent of illness, but set priorities in emergency care at the scene of the emergency and monitor victims on the way to a hospital, often functioning under doctor or nurse voice directions or protocols. They are also responsible for the ambulance and

supplies. The basic course of 110 hours and courses for other ratings may be given by hospitals, community colleges, or fire, health, and police departments. A few 2-year associate degree programs do exist. Those certified may apply to a CAAHEP-accredited program for EMT paramedic training of 600 to 1000 hours plus an internship. EMT-A paramedics are competent in assessing an emergency situation and managing the care, initiating appropriate treatment, and assessing its effect. They are responsible for exercising personal judgment when communication failures interrupt contact with medical direction or in life-threatening situations. EMT-A paramedics are employed by community fire and police departments, private ambulance services, and hospital emergency departments. Questions of authority and scope of practice can strain the relationship between the EMT and the specialist in emergency nursing or even the RN working in emergency and trauma.

■ NURSING SUPPORT PERSONNEL

Nursing assistants, nurse's aides, orderlies, and *attendants* functioning under the direction of nurses are all part of the group of ancillary workers prepared to assist in nursing care, performing many of the simple nursing tasks, as well as other helping activities besides nursing. Usually training is on the job and geared to the needs of the particular employing institution, but there has been some increase in programs within vocational high schools, public adult education centers, and community colleges. The program may vary in length from 6 to 8 weeks or more and costs little or nothing. A high school diploma is often required and is generally preferred for employment. Commercial programs usually cost the student an unreasonable amount, make unrealistic promises of jobs, and frequently give no clinical experience; therefore, these "graduates" are seldom employed. Sometimes students who drop out of certain practical nurse programs after 6 weeks receive a certificate as aides. In-service education during employment is relatively common. It should be remembered that the difference in training, patient care assignment, and ability might be enormous on both an individual and an institutional basis. These workers are not licensed or certified as a rule, although there is a move to do so.

This is particularly true of nursing assistants in LTC facilities. Under a change in the Medicare law, assistants employed in LTC nursing facilities participating in Medicare and Medicaid programs must become certified by completing 75 hours of training and passing a competency exam. They are then awarded the title of certified nursing assistant (CAN). There is considerable concern that these chronic care workers, usually middle aged, the sole support of a family, and disproportionately minority, are underpaid, with few benefits available. The turnover is great because of these reasons, as well as their low status, few opportunities for advancement, and the stressful nature of the work. These working conditions also create a tendency to seek union representation.

The major concern over the use of *unlicensed assistive personnel* (UAP) seems to come from hospitals. In recent years, many hospitals substituted UAPs for more costly professional staff. Often, there are no consistent criteria for training or utilization, nor are RNs given authority to properly delegate or assign. Staff nurses say that they need more help, yet UAPs generate fear, distrust, and a suspicion of inadequate preparation. The question is whether certification will solve these problems or create more.

Community health aides of various kinds are found in ambulatory care settings. Indigenous health aides evolved because not enough physicians or public health nurses were available to help families described as disadvantaged to identify and correct their multiple, related medical and social problems. In addition, professionals do not always communicate effectively with disadvantaged minority clientele. Therefore, in those areas of service, community people are sometimes recruited and trained as health aides. Many are women not previously trained as vocational nurses or hospital aides. There is usually a limited didactic period with ongoing supervision and on-the-job instruction. Certain technical skills are learned, such as auditory and visual screening, but the primary purpose is to identify health problems or deficiencies, including lack of immunization, poor oral hygiene, dermatologic problems, and child development problems, and to assist and encourage families to seek and continue necessary medical, nursing, and other services. Although specific changes in the health status of the community are difficult to measure, on an anecdotal basis, evaluation seems to be positive. These workers may be based in a clinic, neighborhood health center, or other ambulatory care facility, and may also go into the community to do case finding rather than wait for the client to appear in the formal health facility.

As more attention is focused on keeping people at home rather than in institutions, the services of *homemaker–home health aides* have become reimbursable by Medicaid, Medicare, and some state or local government agencies, under certain circumstances. The term *home health aide*, introduced in the Medicare Act in 1965, was added to the older term *homemaker*. The first homemaker services were made available in 1923 to substitute for a hospitalized mother. During the Depression, the government subsidized housekeeping aides to provide work for needy women. They were assigned to assist families with children, the aged, or the chronically ill.

Today's worker is a trained, supervised person who works as a full-fledged member of a team of professional and allied workers providing health or social services. The aide is assigned to the home of a family or individual when home life is disrupted by illness, disability, or social disadvantage, or if the family unit is in danger of breakdown because of stress. Specific tasks include parenting skill enhancement, performing or helping in household tasks, providing personal care such as bed baths, helping with prescribed exercises, and providing emotional support. Educational programs are usually developed by the employing agency. An approved program specifies a minimum number of hours of classroom and laboratory instruction to prepare the individual for on-the-job functioning. Most are women who already have housekeeping skills; even so, there is some question as to how effectively they can really be prepared in the limited time suggested. New Jersey was the first state to certify this group (in 1989) and place them under the jurisdiction of the Board of Nursing.

Although there is evidence that a well-trained, conscientious home health aide can be extremely helpful to a sick person or disrupted family, there are also some serious problems in the selection of workers, the quality of training, and supervision. There are also some reimbursement problems when the homemaking part of the aide's function is reimbursable and the health part is not, or vice versa. Most often, the client needs a combination of services. So the homemaker–home health aide will respond to the situation by doing whatever is necessary regardless of the reimbursement. The result is a shortfall in revenue, creating a deficit that is absorbed by the agency. Ongoing assessment by health professionals is required to determine the client's need for specific services and the appropriate skill level of the providers. The lack of reimbursement often prevents the use of homemaker–home health aides, because this can cost hundreds of dollars a month. Still, it is often less costly than institutional care, which may be the only other option.

Surgical technicians, or *surgical technologists*, function in the OR and sometimes the delivery room. Under the direction of the OR supervisor, an RN, they perform required tasks, such as setting up for surgery, preparing instruments and other equipment before surgery, scrubbing in for surgery (assisting the surgeons by handling instruments, sutures, and so on), and otherwise assisting in the OR.

Educational programs are most frequently offered by hospitals and some community colleges. Even if educational programs are accredited by CAAHEP, they may vary in length from 9 to 20 months, depending on student selection criteria and the program's educational objectives. The curriculum has both didactic and supervised practice components, but does not prepare the student for complicated surgical procedures.

The *psychiatric–mental health technician* works in psychiatric and general hospitals, community mental health centers, and the home, working with the mentally disturbed, disabled, or retarded under the direction of a physician or nurse. In hospitals, the psychiatric–mental health technician is concerned with the patient's daily life as it affects the patient's physical, mental, and emotional well-being, including eating, sleeping, recreation, development of work skills, adjustment, and individual and social relations. In the community, the focus is on social relationships and adjustments. In the hospital, psychiatric technicians are expected to give some routine and emergency physical nursing care, but their close contact with patients makes observation and reporting of the patients' behavior particularly important. In some institutions, psychiatric technicians function almost independently in group therapy and counseling, seeking consultation as necessary. They may be skilled in nursing, communication techniques, counseling, and various types of activity and therapy groups. An educational program is generally 1 year long, but an emerging standard seems to be a 2-year associate degree program, which includes social and physical sciences, health education, laboratory work in group and interpersonal processes, and clinical experience. In some states psychiatric technicians have the opportunity to become licensed, sometimes under the nursing board.

Ward (unit) clerks or *ward (unit) secretaries* are usually trained on the job in an in-service program to assist in the clerical duties involved in the administration of a nursing unit. Ward clerks order supplies, keep certain records, answer telephones, take messages, attend to the massive amount of routine paperwork, and, in some cases, transcribe doctors' orders. This relieves the charge nurse to concentrate on the administration of patient care instead of paperwork. In more progressive hospitals, unit clerks are on the day and evening shifts and sometimes at night.

Unit managers undertake even broader responsibilities in the management of a patient unit (usually in a larger institution) and may report directly to hospital administration instead of nursing service administration. Unit clerks often function under the direction of unit managers. In some institutions, unit management is an early step in an administrative career, and managers have full administrative responsibilities.

■ PHARMACY

Pharmacists are specialists in the science of drugs and have a thorough knowledge of chemistry and physiology. They may dispense prescription and nonprescription drugs, compound special preparations of dosage forms, serve as consultants, and advise physicians on selection and effects of drugs.

With the increase of prepackaged drugs and the use of pharmacy assistants, pharmacists in hospitals and clinics are particularly interested in a more patient-oriented approach to their practice. They may be involved in patient rounds, patient teaching, and consultation with nurses and physicians. Pharmacists working in (or owning) drugstores have also been encouraged to increase their patient or client education efforts in terms of explaining medications. Many keep a medication profile, a computerized record of the customer's drug therapy, to ensure that harmful drug interactions do not occur.

In 2009, there were 116 accredited pharmacy schools in the United States, and six of these schools offered "accelerated" 3-year Doctor of Pharmacy (PharmD) programs by attending school almost year round—with fewer breaks for summer and holidays. There is also one fully accredited "distance/online" 4-year PharmD program offered by Creighton University in Omaha, Nebraska. Pharmacy programs grant the degree of PharmD, which requires at least 6 years of postsecondary study and the passing of the licensure examination of a state board of pharmacy. The PharmD is a 4-year program that requires at least 2 years of college study prior to admittance. This degree has replaced the Bachelor of Science degree, which ceased to be awarded after 2005.

Sixty-four colleges of pharmacy award the Master of Science or Doctor of Philosophy (PhD) degree. Both the master's and PhD degrees are awarded after completion of a PharmD degree. These degrees are designed for those who want more laboratory and research experience. Many master's and PhD holders work in research for a drug company or teach at a university. Other options for pharmacy graduates who are interested in further training include 1- or 2-year residency programs or fellowships. Pharmacy residencies are postgraduate training programs in pharmacy practice. Pharmacy fellowships are highly individualized programs designed to prepare participants to work in research laboratories. Some pharmacists who run their own pharmacy obtain a master's degree in business administration (MBA).

Besides the traditional responsibilities of pharmacists, the PharmD or clinical pharmacist provides consultation with the physician, maintains patient drug histories and reviews the total drug regimen of patients, monitors patient charts in LTC facilities, recommends drug therapy, makes patient rounds, and provides individualized dosage regimens. Pharmacists are also increasingly assuming a role in home care, particularly in relation to infusion therapy. In some states such as California, clinical pharmacists may also prescribe (as do APNs and PAs), with certain limitations. This new role is well accepted by some physicians, usually those who have worked with PharmDs; others consider it an infringement on medical territory.

Trends in the field favor the PharmD, which the American Council on Pharmaceutical Education sees as the basic degree. There is also increased interest in postgraduate training such as research fellowships or residencies in a defined area of pharmacy as an option to advanced degrees. Three specialties are recognized and certified: nuclear pharmacy, pharmacotherapy, and nutrition support. Enrollment for the first professional degree has been increasing after a period of decline. There has been an increase in the enrollment of women and a much smaller increase in minorities. As arguments have been advanced for the PharmD as the first professional degree, a growing number of pharmacists are taking part-time and off-campus courses toward a PharmD. Continuing education is required by a number of states for relicensure. Pharmacists are licensed in all states and have reciprocity (simultaneous recognition) among all states, with the exception of California and Florida. Most work in chain or independent pharmacies or hospitals. Although projections for future need are seen as rather doubtful as to accuracy, a shortage is anticipated.

The *pharmacy technician*, who is probably certified, and for whom the pharmacist is responsible, assists with dispensing tasks and is now considered a valuable adjunct to pharmacy practice.

Pharmacologists specialize in the research and development of drugs to prevent or treat disease or prolong life. A medical degree or a 4- to 5-year PhD program in pharmacology is usually required.

■ PODIATRY

Podiatrists, Doctors of Podiatric Medicine (DPMs) (once called *chiropodists*), are professionally trained foot care specialists who diagnose, treat, and try to prevent diseases, injuries, and deformities of the feet. Treatment may include surgery, medication, physical therapy, setting fractures, and preparing orthoses (supporting devices that mechanically rearrange the weight-bearing structures of the foot). Podiatrists may note symptoms of diseases manifested in the feet and legs and refer the patient to a physician.

Podiatrists complete a 4-year program of classroom and clinical work in a college of podiatry after a minimum of 2 years of college, but the majority already have an undergraduate degree. Although they are permitted to practice immediately after graduation in most states, almost all apply for 1 or 2 years of residency training. Enrollment in colleges of podiatry has been increasing, owing largely to federal support and the podiatric needs of the aging population. There has been an increase in women and minorities enrolled in podiatry programs. A unique aspect of podiatric medical education is the attempt to develop a system-wide, competency-based curriculum. The National Board of Podiatry Examiners gives examinations that satisfy the requirements for licensure in more than 40 states. Other states use their own examinations; some require a residency, and an increasing number require continuing education.

Most podiatrists are in private practice; others practice in institutions, agencies, the military, education, and research. As a group, they are eager to expand their scope of practice, but are being strongly resisted by physicians. Yet, podiatrists who have had surgical residencies and the requisite 5 years of practice, and have passed the exacting certification examination of the American Board of Podiatric Surgery, maintain that these physicians are unfamiliar with current podiatric education and practice or are protective of their own economic well-being.

■ PSYCHOLOGY, PSYCHOTHERAPY, AND MENTAL HEALTH

Psychology is the scientific study of mental processes and behavior, and *psychotherapy* refers generally to techniques for treating mental illness by psychological means, primarily through establishing communication between the therapist and the patient as a means of understanding and modifying behavior. In the field of mental health, there is a great overlapping of therapists treating patients with various kinds of mental and emotional problems. Besides the physician (the psychiatrist), clinical psychologists, psychotherapists, nurses, social workers, and a variety of semiprofessionals trained in mental health participate in individual and group therapy. *Psychologists* may also give and interpret various personality and behavioral tests, as might a *psychometrician*, who is skilled in the testing and measuring of mental and psychological ability, efficiency, potentials, and functions. An area of dissension in the field is the fact that various mental health therapists are fighting to have prescription privileges and are strongly opposed by psychiatrists. The latter are also complaining that preferred provider organizations (PPOs) are demanding that psychiatrists cut their fees considerably because the other practitioners do not charge as much. Education for psychologists and psychotherapists is often at the master's or doctoral level. Clinical psychologists have training in a clinical setting.

■ PUBLIC HEALTH—ENVIRONMENT

Industrial hygienists deal with the effects on workers' health of noise, dust, vapor radiation, and other hazards common to industry. They are usually employed by industry, laboratories, insurance companies, or government to detect and correct these hazards. Their education may include a baccalaureate in environmental health, engineering, or physical or biological science.

Sanitarians, sometimes called *environmentalists*, apply technical knowledge to solve problems of sanitation in a community. They develop and implement methods to control those factors in the environment that affect health and safety, such as rodent control and sanitary conditions in schools, hotels, restaurants, areas of food production, and sales. Most sanitarians work in government under the direction of a health officer or administrator. Education is generally a baccalaureate in environmental health, public health, or the physical or biological sciences. Advanced positions require a master's degree. Registration is required in most states; national certification is also available.

Also educated in schools of public health, as well as elsewhere, are *biostatisticians*, who apply mathematics

and statistics to research problems related to health, and *epidemiologists*, who study the factors that influence the occurrence and course of human health problems, including not only acute and chronic diseases, but also accidents, addictions, and suicides. Epidemiologists attempt to establish the history of health problems by focusing on the biological, social, and behavioral factors affecting health, illness, and premature death. They use investigative, analytical, and descriptive techniques. A specialized graduate degree is necessary for both biostatisticians and epidemiologists.

■ RADIOLOGY

Radiologists are physicians dealing with all forms of radiant energy, from x-rays to radioactive isotopes; they interpret radiographic studies and prescribe therapy for diseases, particularly malignancies. A number of technicians work under the direction of a radiologist in radiology departments.

The *radiologic technologist*, sometimes called *x-ray technician*, *radiology technician*, or *radiographer*, is concerned with the proper operation of x-ray equipment, preparation of patients for x-rays and therapy, developing of film, and some clerical work. Programs are usually 2-year CAAHEP-accredited hospital certificate programs, sometimes affiliated with a college or university. However, they vary from 1 to 4 years, depending on the program. The graduate may become registered [RT-(R)] after passing an examination given by the American Registry of Radiologic Technicians. A few states license radiology technicians and technologists.

Radiation therapy technicians or *technologists* assist the radiologist in the treatment of disease by exposing affected areas of the patient's body to prescribed doses of radiation, operating and controlling complex equipment and devices, and maintaining records. A 1- or 2-year program in radiation therapy given by community colleges or hospitals is required. There are some baccalaureate programs.

A *nuclear medicine technologist* works with radioactive isotopes administered to patients for diagnosis and treatment. He or she positions and attends to patients, abstracts data from records, assists in the operation of scanning devices using isotopes, and has responsibility for the safe storage of radioactive materials and disposal of wastes. CAAHEP accredits both associate and baccalaureate programs; the technical portion for each is 1 year.

Related careers are *sonographers* or *ultrasound technologists* and the *diagnostic medical sonographer*, who assists the physician in gathering sonographic data, records and processes these data, and makes pertinent observations. Programs of 1- to 4-years' duration may be accredited by CAAHEP. With advanced training, any of these technologists may work with computerized tomography (CT) scans and magnetic resonance imaging (MRI). A major trend is to identify this overall group as *diagnostic imaging personnel.*

■ REHABILITATION SERVICES

Occupational therapy is concerned with the use of purposeful activity in the promotion and maintenance of health, prevention of disability, evaluation of behavior, and as treatment of persons with physical or psychosocial dysfunction, using a wide spectrum of treatment procedures based on activities of a creative, social, independent, educational, and vocational nature. One important responsibility is helping patients with activities of daily living. Adaptive tools such as aids for eating or dressing may also be provided.

Occupational therapists (OTs), the professional workers, and *occupational therapy assistants* and *aides* work in rehabilitation facilities, hospitals, private practice, nursing homes, and community agencies. They are valuable in working with the elderly. Professional education for the occupational therapist is a baccalaureate program or a 2-year master's degree program for those with another type of baccalaureate; the program may be CAAHEP accredited.

The American Occupational Therapy Association certifies for the professional entry-level *occupational therapist registered* (OTR) or *certified occupational therapy assistant* (COTA). In some institutions, professional occupational therapists are assisted by *OT assistants* or *aides*, who may be trained in a 1-year certificate program or in 2- or 4-year colleges and vocational-technical institutes. They participate directly in the patient's activities.

Physical therapy (PT) is concerned with the restoration of function and the prevention of disability following disease, injury, or loss of a body part; sometimes PT is concerned with diagnosis. The goal is to improve circulation, strengthen muscles, encourage return of motion, and train or retrain the patient with the use of prosthetics, crutches, walkers, exercise, heat, cold, electricity, ultrasound, and massage. Most *physical therapists*, *PT assistants*, and *PT aides* work in setting similar to OTs. They are also very

prominent in home care. The physical therapist designs the patient's program of treatment, based on the physician's stated objectives. He or she may participate in giving the therapy or evaluate the patient's needs and capacities and provide psychological support. PT aides work directly under the physical therapist's supervision, with limited participation in the therapeutic program. As in OT, education for the PT is in a baccalaureate or post-baccalaureate program leading to a certificate or master's degree. Registration is possible through the American Registry of Physical Therapists, and all states now license PTs. There has been some limited effort to require licensure of PT assistants, whose education is usually at the associate degree level. This level of PT worker may be certified or registered; PT aides require no special credential.

Prosthetists make artificial limb substitutes. *Orthotists* make and fit braces. Both work with a variety of provider professionals and have direct patient contact to promote total rehabilitation services. A baccalaureate in prosthetics or orthotics plus 1900 hours of supervised clinical experience is usual; for those with a baccalaureate, special 8- to 16-month programs plus 1900 hours of supervised clinical experience are necessary. *Orthotic/prosthetic technicians* make and repair devices, but usually have no patient contact. Education is primarily in vocational-technical schools with formal training in orthotics and prosthetics. An alternative is 2 years of supervised clinical experience, but either way, a high school diploma or GED is required.

Rehabilitation counselors help people with physical, mental, or social disabilities begin or return to satisfying life, including an appropriate job. They may counsel about job opportunities and training, assist in job placement, and help the person to adjust to a new work situation. The usual requirement is a master's degree. Others assisting in patient rehabilitation include *art therapists*, *dance therapists*, *horticulture therapists*, *manual arts therapists*, *corrective therapists*, and *music therapists* who work primarily with the emotionally disturbed, mentally retarded, or physically handicapped. Their educational requirements are not firmly established and vary a great deal. *Recreation therapists* or therapeutic *recreationists* may plan and supervise recreation programs that include athletics, arts and crafts, parties, gardening, or camping. Professional status usually requires a master's degree, although some therapists only have a baccalaureate degree; assistants are generally prepared at the associate degree level. RTs require licensure or certification in a few states.

RESPIRATORY THERAPY

Respiratory therapy personnel perform procedures essential to maintaining life in seriously ill patients with respiratory problems and assist in the treatment of heart and lung ailments. Under the supervision of a doctor or respiratory therapist, the *respiratory therapy technician* administers various types of gas, aerosol, and breathing treatments; assists with long-term continuous artificial ventilation; cleans, sterilizes, and maintains equipment; and keeps patient records. *Respiratory therapists* may be engaged in similar tasks, but their more extensive knowledge of the sciences and clinical medicine allows for the exercise of more judgment and acceptance of greater responsibility in performing therapeutic procedures. Respiratory therapy personnel work in the range of health care settings.

A CAAHEP-accredited program for technicians is 1 year long; certification is available. A therapist program, also CAAHEP-accredited, may culminate in an associate or baccalaureate degree, with a minimum of 2 years required. The baccalaureate programs sometimes build on the associate program and prepare for supervision and teaching. Respiratory therapists may be registered, but are not usually licensed. Certification (RRT) may be required for administrative positions.

SOCIAL WORK

The *social worker* attempts to help individuals and their families resolve their social problems, utilizing community and governmental resources as necessary. Community and governmental agencies as well as hospitals, clinics, and nursing homes employ social workers. If the social worker's focus is on patients and families, he or she may be called a *medical* or *psychiatric social worker*. A master's degree (MSW) is required for advanced and specialized social work. There are also accredited baccalaureate programs in social work (BSW). College graduates with degrees in other areas may qualify as social workers by completing an MSW. Membership in the National Association of Social Workers is open only to social workers graduated from, or students of, accredited schools of social work. The Academy of Certified Social Workers grants certification after other criteria are met. A doctoral degree is usually required for teaching, advanced practice, and administration.

Social workers also have assistants, who sometimes carry a client load in certain agencies. There may be only on-the-job training available for these workers, but to advance they must acquire additional education. Some employers prefer a 2-year associate degree in human or social services, even for this assisting level.

One professional issue cited by social workers is related to identity. Because social work was identified as a career only in the 1930s, there is still some preoccupation with defining the field.

Like nurses, social workers are concerned with the distribution, effectiveness, and cost of their service, as well as clarification of responsibilities of each educational level of practitioners. Some also admit to concern for their professional survival, particularly because of role overlap with other health professionals. One particularly competitive area is case management, especially for the elderly. Case management can be defined as "a systematic approach to coordination of services to suitable clients through the efforts of assessing providers, treatments, and developing treatment plans which improve quality and efficacy while controlling costs and monitoring outcomes." Nurses and social workers, as well as others, both perform these activities, but each may claim ownership of the role.

SPEECH–LANGUAGE PATHOLOGY AND AUDIOLOGY

Speech–language pathologists and audiologists are specialists in communication disorders. Speech pathologists or therapists diagnose and treat speech and language disorders that may stem from a variety of causes. Speech therapists are particularly valuable in assisting patients whose speech has been affected by a cerebrovascular accident or patients with laryngectomies. Audiologists often work with children and may detect and assist with the hearing disorder of a child who has been mistakenly labeled retarded. Education for both specialties is at a master's level, after a baccalaureate in human communication science. There has been some attempt to require state licensure. The American Speech and Hearing Association offers a Certificate of Clinical Competence after specific criteria are fulfilled.

VISION CARE

Ophthalmologists are physicians who treat diseases of the eye and perform surgery, but they may also examine eyes and prescribe corrective glasses and exercises. *Optometrists*, doctors of optometry (ODs), considered independent primary health care providers, are educated and clinically trained to examine, diagnose, and treat conditions of the vision system, but they refer clients with eye diseases and other health problems to physicians. After a variety of diagnostic tests, they may prescribe corrective lenses, contact lenses, and special optical aids as well as corrective eye exercises to optimize vision. Some may specialize in such areas as prescribing and fitting contact lenses.

A minimum of 7 years' education is required, with 3 years of college before optometry school and 4 years of specialized professional education and clinical training. The programs are accredited by the American Optometric Association Council. There are also postgraduate clinical residencies for specialization. All states require licensure by state board examinations; most states accept the National Board of Optometry examinations. Continuing education is required for relicensure in most states. One trend is the increase of women and minorities in the field. In addition, optometrists are increasingly younger.

The majority of optometrists are in private office practice; others are in group practice, hospitals, public health agencies, HMOs, research institutions, manufacturing organizations, the military, and other government agencies. Others are teaching and conducting research in colleges and universities (which requires an academic doctorate or master's). About 90 percent are involved in direct patient care activities.

Given the overlap in roles with ophthalmologists in the area of vision analysis, the increasing number of optometrists, and their complaint that their income is below acceptable levels, it is not unexpected to find conflict between the groups on their scope of practice. Optometrists are permitted to prescribe drugs in many states and are authorized to use drugs to diagnose eye problems or disease in all 50 states, but may not perform surgery. These activities are strongly opposed by ophthalmologists. The Federal Trade Commission overturn of bans on professional advertising has also aided optometrists, making them more competitive in providing those services that can be rendered by both groups of professionals. It is predicted that optometrists will continue to fight for expansion of their scope of practice.

Optometric assistants assist optometrists by performing simple office and patient care duties. Technicians may also assist in office tasks, but usually assist in vision training and testing. Assistants complete a 1-year certificate or diploma program; technicians, a 2-year associate degree offered by 2- and 4-year colleges, colleges of optometry, hospitals, and the military.

Opticians grind lenses, make eyeglasses, and fit and adjust them. Both associate degree programs and on-the-job apprenticeship qualify individuals for this job. Optical laboratory technicians and mechanics may be involved in polishing and grinding lenses.

Orthoptists, working under an ophthalmologist's supervision, correct crossed eyes in adults and children through special exercises. They may also aid with visual field and glaucoma testing. Two years of college or a baccalaureate degree plus a 24-month training program given in medical schools, vision clinics, or hospitals are required.

■ OTHER HEALTH WORKERS

There are a number of other health workers not described in this chapter, such as those in science and engineering—anatomists, biologists, biomedical engineers (who design patient care equipment such as dialysis machines, pacemakers, and heart-lung machines), and biomedical technicians (who maintain and repair the equipment); technicians dealing with instrumentation—clinical perfusionists (who operate equipment to support or temporarily replace a patient's circulatory or respiratory functions); electrocardiograph (EKG/ECG) technicians; electroencephalographic (EEG) technologists and technicians; specialists in dealing with the visually handicapped; biological photographers; and medical illustrators; many of whom attended CAAHEP-accredited programs, as well as patient advocates, acupuncturists, health science librarians, and computer specialists, to name just a few. In addition, volunteers provide many useful services. That this list is not complete and is expanding may help to explain why, no matter how valuable individual services may be, the public often becomes angered by the fragmentation of services. Even health professionals may be unsure about who does what or when for the client's well-being. Yet, this list is not exaggerated; all these specialties are part of what the federal government calls health manpower and allied health manpower, for which federal funds are often distributed for educational programs. It is clear that if the public is to receive the services it requires, expects, and deserves, there must be assistance in negotiating one's way through the health care maze.

KEY POINTS

1. The health care industry is labor intensive.
2. The first step in formalizing a field of work has become certification, followed by some form of government regulation.
3. What we have observed is not proliferation of a workforce, but specialization to complement a highly complex health care system.
4. As it matures, every discipline develops its areas of specialization and its assertive or associate workers.
5. Decisions on whether to expand or contract, either educational programs or health services, frequently depend on uncontrollable external factors, such as the economy, the progress of science, and the course of health and illness.
6. Undereducated, poorly paid, non–cost-effective workers are unmotivated and angry.
7. Unions have targeted health care workers because of their generally poor working conditions.
8. To recruit and retain workers, employers must look to them as the internal consumer.
9. The responsibility that society has to educate caregivers remains to be defined.
10. Legally clear distinctions of each area of work would be helpful; practically it is impossible.
11. To accomplish the most with the least and accommodate an unpredictable future, the roles of health care workers will have to expand and contract, blur and overlap.
12. True interdisciplinary education would serve a delivery system of this complexity well.
13. The consumer will eventually be intolerant of the turf battles taking precedence over their welfare.
14. Who should be the gatekeeper to control the flow of patients in and out of the system is an important issue; it remains to be seen if many different providers should share this responsibility, or if it is the exclusive right of a single discipline.
15. The trend to increase the educational requirements for practice will be unrelenting.
16. Everyone needs to get the message that they are doing useful, decent work and that it is valued.
17. Nurses always made the decisions about the proper use of unskilled assistants to whom they delegated. Why change it if it works?
18. Coordination and continuity are essential to offset the fragmentation and confusion that the consumer is guaranteed to experience.
19. Our workforce projections may be greatly understated if services expand to cover the entire population of the United States.
20. The untapped resource is to develop the consumer's capacity for self-care.

REFERENCES

1. Bureau of Labor Statistics. Career Guide to Industries, 2010-2011 edition. Health Care. http://www.bls.gov/oco/ocos074.htm#emply. Retrieved April 18, 2010.
2. Inside Higher Ed. The Second Shift in Academic Medicine. http://www.insidehighered.com/news/2009/01/02/medwomen. Retrieved April 18, 2010.
3. Sultz H, Young K. *Health Care USA*, 6th ed. Sudbury, MA: 2008.
4. Shi L, Singh D. *Delivering Health Care in America*. Sudbury, MA: 2007.
5. Sultz and Young, loc cit.
6. H.R. 1228. Patient and Physician Protection and Safety Act of 2005. http://www.govtrack.us/congress/bill.xpd?bill=h109-1228. Retrieved April 18, 2010.
7. Bureau of Labor Statistics, loc cit.
8. Stanfield P, Hui Y. *Introduction to the Health Professions*, 5th ed. Boston: Jones and Bartlett, 2008.
9. American Academy of Physician Assistants. Frequently Asked Questions. http://www.aapa.org/about-pas/faq-about-pas. Retrieved April 18, 2010.
10. Ibid.
11. Ibid.
12. Ibid.

Updates can be found at **www.kellysnursing.com**

HELPFUL WEBSITES FOR PART II

Agency for Healthcare Research and Quality: http://www.ahrq.gov

American Academy of Physician Assistants: http://www.aapa.org

American Association of Colleges of Nursing: http://aacn.nche.edu

American Association of Colleges of Osteopathic Medicine: http://www.aacom.org

American Association of Colleges of Pharmacy: http://www.aacp.org

American Association of Homes for the Aging: http://aahsa.org

American Cancer Society: http://www.cancer.org

American Chiropractic Association: http://www.amer-chiro.org

American Dental Association: http://www.ada.org

American Dietetic Association: http://www.eatright.org

American Health Care Association: http://ahca.org

American Hospital Association: http://aha.org

American Medical Association: http://www.ama-assn.org

American Nurses Association: http://www.nursingworld.org

American Occupational Therapy Association: http://www.aota.org

American Optometric Association: http://www.aoanet.org

American Pharmaceutical Association: http://www.aphanet.org

American Physical Therapy Association: http://www.apta.org

American Public Health Association: http://www.apha.org

Association of American Medical Colleges: http://aamc.org

Bureau of Health Professions, National Center for Health Workforce Information and Analysis: http://bhpr.hrsa.gov

Children's Defense Fund: http://childrensdefense.org

Chronicle of Higher Education: http://chronicle.com

Commission on Accreditation of Allied Health Education Programs: http://www.caahep.org

Elder Care Issues: http://www.elderweb.com

Information Please (repository of general education): http://www.infoplease.com

Institute of Medicine: http://www.iom.edu

International Council of Nurses: http://cn.ch

National Center for Education Statistics (IPEDS): http://www.nces.ed.gov/ipeds

National Center for Health Statistics: http://www.cdc.gov/nchs

National League for Nursing: http://www.nln.org

Nursing Spectrum: http://www.nursingspectrum.com

US Bureau of the Census: http://census.gov

US Bureau of Labor Statistics: http://bls.gov

US Department of Education, Educational Research and Improvement Center (ERIC): http://www.ed.gov

US Department of Health and Human Services (gateway to consumer information on health and health services): http://www.healthfinder.gov

US Department of Health and Human Services, Healthy People: http://www.cdc.gov/nchs/about/otheract/hp2010

US Government Printing Office: http://www.access.gpo.gov

Nursing in the Health Care Setting

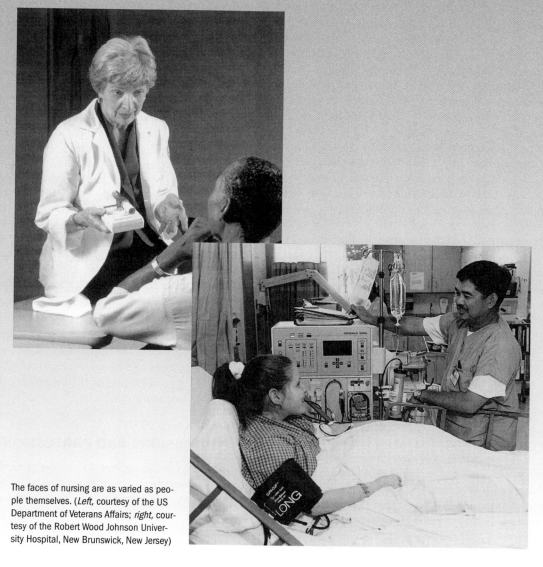

The faces of nursing are as varied as people themselves. (*Left,* courtesy of the US Department of Veterans Affairs; *right,* courtesy of the Robert Wood Johnson University Hospital, New Brunswick, New Jersey)

Nursing as a Profession

■ DEFINITIONS OF NURSING

The word *nurse* has certain cultural connotations and, for most of us, emotional attachment. Further, there are well-established public images of nursing. Add to this the fact that the discipline of nursing is moving through a period of rapid change, and you can be assured that there exists a range of contradictory and frequently inaccurate perspectives on what nursing is and should be. Schulman, in his historical analysis, sees nursing as being rooted in the contradictory roles of mother surrogate and healer: one denoting constancy, affection, intimacy, and physical closeness; the other conveying a spirit of the discontinuous, fragmented, and dynamic.[1] This same dichotomy can be observed in nursing as many contemporary theorists describe it. Lydia Hall spoke of care and cure,[2] and Leininger, Benner, and Watson seize the concept of caring and develop it with a precision that makes it the dynamic equal of curing.[3]

There seems to be a public tendency to equate nursing with illness. Current dictionaries still define a nurse as someone trained to care for the sick. Moreover, because of the proliferation of nurse's aides and practical nurses, the public is even more confused as to who the nurse is. It is not unusual for patients to consider a nurse to be anyone in a uniform who gives them personal care. Perhaps life was simpler when it was protocol for only the registered nurse (RN) to wear a white long-sleeved uniform, white shoes and stockings, and most important, the starched white cap and special pin of the nursing school, or, as an option, the easily identified navy blue of the public health nurse. It was a symbol, a tradition, an image that came packaged with preconceived notions of what that uniformed figure could do. (Never mind that, years ago, one key nursing figure described the uniform as a house-dress and the cap as a dust cap.)

It has been pointed out that, in some ways, nurses tend to cherish a traditional image, even as they move into new roles and live uncomfortably with a blurred self-image. Many nursing students enter schools with the concept that "real" nursing is bedside care. Still, surveys indicate that now more people realize that nurses also engage in research, deliver babies, teach health, provide psychotherapy, administer anesthesia, practice independently, and diagnose patients and treat their illnesses; nurses work not only in hospitals, but in jails, homes, clinics, colleges, schools, industry, their own practices, and in the most rural as well as the most urban areas. Most of all, with the complexity of nursing care today, it is clear that nurses need intelligence as well as stamina.

There are many interpretations of nursing. Why not? There are many facets to nursing, and perhaps it is not logical or accurate to settle on one point of view. All nurses must eventually determine their own philosophies of nursing, whether or not these are formalized. The public and others outside nursing will probably continue to adopt a concept or image that is nurtured by contact, hearsay, or media presentations of the profession, and the first may be the most powerful determinant. This chapter seeks to present an overview of the components of nursing, examined in the light of professionalism, legal and other definitions, nursing process, nursing theory, nursing diagnosis, and nursing standards.

■ PROFESSIONS AND PROFESSIONALISM

Almost everyone talks about the *nursing profession* in the sense of an organized group of persons, all of whom are engaged in nursing. However, another question discussed both within and without the ranks of nursing is whether or not nursing as a whole is an occupation rather than a profession, in the same sense that medicine, theology, and law have been called professions since the Middle Ages.

Professions have been historically linked with universities or other institutions of learning, implying a certain high level of scholarship and study, including research. Further, there is fairly general agreement that professionalism centers on specialized expertise, autonomy, and service. Based on Flexner's classic criteria,[4] and deriving from the thinking of many others, including the author, the following delineate the qualities of a profession in a useful manner:

1. A profession utilizes in its practice a well-defined and well-organized body of knowledge that is intellectual in nature and describes its phenomena of concern.[5]

2. A profession constantly enlarges the body of knowledge it uses and subsequently imposes on its members the lifelong obligation to remain current in order to do no harm.

3. A profession entrusts the education of its practitioners to institutions of higher education.

4. A profession applies its body of knowledge in practical services that are vital to human welfare, and are especially suited to the tradition of seasoned practitioners shaping the skills of newcomers to the role.

5. A profession functions autonomously (with authority) in the formulation of professional policy and in the monitoring of its practice and practitioners.[6]

6. A Code of Ethics that regulates the relationship between professional and client guides a profession.

7. A profession is distinguished by the presence of a specific culture, norms, and values that are common among its members.[7]

8. A profession has a clear standard of educational preparation for entry into practice.[8]

9. A profession attracts individuals of intellectual and personal qualities who exalt service above personal gain and who recognize their chosen occupation as a life's work.

10. A profession strives to compensate its practitioners by providing freedom of action, opportunity for continuous professional growth, and economic security.

Looking at these criteria objectively, it is clear that nursing does not totally fulfill all of them. It has been pointed out that nursing's theory base is still developing, the public does not always see the nurse as a professional, not all nurses are educated in institutions of higher learning, not all nurses consider nursing a lifetime career, and in many practice settings, nursing does not control its own policies and activities, nor do nurses always want to invest their time and effort in students and new graduates.

The lack of autonomy is considered the most serious weakness. Sociologists have long contended that an occupation does not become a profession unless the members of that occupation are the ones who make the final decisions about the services they provide. Autonomy is addressed again in Chapter 16. In recent years, there has been progress in both achieving autonomy and, perhaps more importantly, nurses' recognition that this is important to both the profession and to them in terms of how they practice. This mental turnaround has something to do with the fact that more nurses are seeking higher education and that more are planning nursing careers as opposed to taking nursing jobs. A scholarly corps has emerged that is committed to research and theory development. Nurses are also becoming more aggressive about getting recognition for what they have accomplished. Both nurses and others are convinced that the fact that nursing is predominantly female is also a factor in the reason why nurses have had difficulty achieving high professional status. However, with changes in society, including the effect of the women's movement, that have had at least some impact on the stereotyping of women as well as the progress of nurses themselves, this is seen as a time to move the profession forward. If nursing is not considered a profession in the strictest sense of the word, it is well on the way to becoming so. One author commented thoughtfully, "On the continuum of professionalization, qualitatively nursing and many individual nurses excel far beyond contemporary recognized professions in many areas. Quantitatively, the road ahead is very long."[9]

Another way to assess nursing's professional status is to review the manner in which public policy is constructed and applied to its issues. Nursing has had a history of being on the short end of a double standard. In 1992, a new system of Medicare reimbursement was implemented that linked the fee schedule to the service delivered as opposed to the provider. At implementation, the government recanted and proposed that nonphysician providers should receive fewer dollars because of a lesser investment in education and training. The hypocrisy continues when nurse practitioners (NPs) are compensated only 85 percent of the physician's customary rate, but can receive the full fee if their practice is "incident to" the physician and billed through that physician as part of the physician's practice. In the end, whether or not (and when) nursing will become a full profession depends on its practitioners. Will they consciously choose to fight for this demanding status and honor the inherent obligations once it has been achieved?

It should be noted that the term *profession* is essentially a social concept and has no meaning apart from its social context. Society decides that it needs the service of a group of individuals with specialized skills, and because their work is extremely complex and extremely necessary, they are allowed special privileges. The social contract that exists with the public assumes that these individuals will honor their obligation and continually evaluate the appropriateness of their role and competence of their practice. Should they renege on this obligation or value their privileged status more than the work it rewards, the public is brutal in their retribution. Unfortunately, the behavior of a few can jeopardize the reputation of everyone involved.

Professionals are expected to monitor one another. A profession is seen as a body of individuals voluntarily subordinating themselves to a standard of morality and ethics that is above the general population, and is articulated and imposed by their peers. Classically, the public has deferred to the profession to establish its code of ethics and standards, define its work, delineate its scope of practice, specify appropriate academic credentials, and establish systems for peer review. These are some of the courtesies given to professionals because they exercise unquestioned integrity and respect the client-provider relationship above all others. This tradition of autonomy has seriously eroded in recent years.

Surveys tell us that Americans have developed a suspicion about professionals (nurses have been the exception, as reported in Chapter 11). Feeling out of control when pitted against these authority figures in their lives, it was natural for the American people to look to government to provide more oversight. There are many examples: increased consumer presence on professional boards, setting of fee schedules for reimbursement, the development of guidelines for the management of certain disease conditions, and the government requirement to advise patients of their right to execute final directives.

Autonomy and immunity from governmental intrusion has always been the strongest in areas of specialty practice, where consumers feel least qualified to challenge the judgment of professionals. The recent movement to license nurses in advanced or specialty practice is both an example of eroding autonomy and a cue that we are arriving too late. In some instances, physicians have been awarded a limited license when applying to a new state after many years of specialty practice.

Declining autonomy may well be associated with the changing client-provider relationship. For nurses, that relationship is further challenged by the recurrent debate over whether nurses are statutory supervisors just because they monitor the work of assistive personnel. Supervisory status could rob nurses of the employee protection and autonomy that has enabled them to be patient advocates rather than instruments of management.

Another cautionary area is associated with the uniqueness of the services that professionals provide. The service of any group of providers must be timely, relevant, and offered with an appreciation of what complementary disciplines can contribute. Resistance to change and refusal to move with the times is not only counterproductive, but also a violation of the public trust. Examples abound as professionals strive to protect their turf. The very public and negative response of the American Medical Association (AMA) to the role of nurses as primary care providers is one instance. In contrast, the Centers for Medicare and Medicaid Services (CMS) and the Joint Commission support definitions of professional or medical staff organizations that allow nurse membership.

The stereotype of idealized professionals who are guaranteed economic security by the public in exchange for a lifetime of dedicated service to their work has become a rarity. This does not make these individuals any less, but only a product of their times. First, economic security is a relative term and open to a range of definitions. No group will have a guaranteed income, most especially those in health care, as we move into models of managed care and providers are employees more commonly than entrepreneurs.

Despite the prestige of professionalism, many other stereotypes are fading. For instance, professionals who are employed have gradually accepted collective bargaining, unionism, and strikes, once seen as the antithesis of professionalism, as legitimate activities. Physicians, nurses, teachers, social workers, and others have chosen that route as the only means left to gain certain concessions from employers. Obviously, the very fact that more professionals are employed, and thus lack a degree of autonomy, has precipitated this change.

In addition, there is an increasing tendency to use the term *professional* in another context to describe one who has an ensured competence in a particular field or occupation, such as a hairdresser or someone who participates in an activity for pay as opposed to an amateur—a musician, artist, or baseball player. It is particularly interesting to note the changes in dictionary definitions over the years to include the last two concepts. Looking at it in the pure sense, however, the idea of professionalism has been called the most important and powerful in the belief system of nursing. Yet, nurses do not hold any common view on professionalism, just as many cannot often agree on what nursing should be doing as we move deeper into this millennium.

Too small a percentage of nurses have "bought" professionalism as a way of life. The larger segment "mouth" the philosophy, go through the outward rituals, all the while digging deeper ruts from which to be extracted later by another "concerned" generation of truly professional nurses. These are the nurses who find status in the status quo. They are not progressive; they have just transferred their hardcore traditionalism to other settings and labeled it progress. These are the nurses who demand professional recognition from others, but are reluctant to assume professional responsibilities. They may get caught up in the intellectual ferment around them, but they are not seriously engaged in the professional dialogue. They may be troubled about nursing's professional role, but for self-serving reasons. To the observer, there is serious imbalance between their professional commitment and their personal ambitions. They court professionalism but balk at the price. They command higher salaries, but avoid spending their own money on professional growth—if they can use someone else's, namely, their employer's or the government's. Professionalism as a way of life implies responsibility and commitment.

We should judge ourselves more kindly; nurses are credible professionals doing an incredible job. Perhaps by accepting other American professions as its standard, nursing has deprived itself of its unique identity—once nurses did not doubt that they were professionals, but they have since allowed themselves to be intimidated.

The Nature of Nursing: Some Definitions

In *Notes on Nursing: What It Is and What It Is Not*, Florence Nightingale states in the most basic terms that the goal of nursing is to "put the patient in the best condition for nature to act upon him."[10] Since that time, a number of other definitions have evolved, but the emphasis on care has not diminished, even in the scientific era. Definitions of nursing vary according to the philosophy of an individual or group, and interpretations of roles and functions follow suit. Many have become classics.

A definition used by nurses internationally is that of Virginia Henderson, a distinguished American nursing educator and writer, frequently referred to as the "American Nightingale."

> The unique function of the nurse is to assist the individual, sick or well, in the performance of those activities contributing to health or its recovery (or to peaceful death) that he would perform unaided if he had the necessary strength, will, or knowledge. And to do this in such a way as to help gain independence as rapidly as possible. This aspect of her work, this part of her function, she initiates and controls; of this she is master. In addition she helps the patient to carry out the therapeutic plan as initiated by the physician. She also, as a member of a medical team, helps other members, as they in turn help her, to plan and carry out the total program whether it be for the improvement of health, or the recovery from illness or support in death. . . .[11]

In the 1965 American Nurses Association (ANA) position paper on entry into practice, the terms *care*, *cure*, and *coordination* were first included in the definition of professional practice, and this phrase has been used numerous times since, with the individual components often subject to differing interpretation (see Chapter 12).

As nurses expanded their functions into the NP role, *cure* acquired a different meaning for them, to include aspects of what had been medical diagnosis and treatment. Some nurses, like Rogers, felt that such medical (not nursing) diagnosis and treatment diminishes the role of the nurse as a nurse. (The same opponents also usually reject the NP designation.) However, Ford, a pioneer of the NP movement, immediately responding, called this "semantic roulette" and added, "I'm not so concerned about the words. I'm convinced that nursing can take on that level of accountability of professional practice that involves the consumer in decision-making in his care and also demands sophisticated clinical judgment to determine levels of illness and wellness and design a plan of management."[12] Indeed, the NP role represented a very appropriate readjustment of the boundaries between medicine and nursing.

Coordination and integration of the therapeutic regimen have historically been the province of nursing. It was done in the home and community within the early models of practice, and these traditions were taken into hospitals.

Nursing's 24-hour presence and holistic philosophy suited it well to this responsibility. Although assuming new prominence in case management models, active coordination on behalf of its patients has always been a nursing hallmark and is more critical today because nurses are often the only human link between patients and an intimidating experience in the health care delivery system.

Care is also translated in a number of ways, sometimes as a physical activity, such as in giving care, but it is considered by nursing experts as much more. The concept has been given considerable attention in the last several years, with research exploring the meaning and entire curricula based on related theory. Watson, who has written extensively on caring, says, "Caring is a normal ideal that guides and directs human actions, not just as a means but a human end in and of itself that is of intrinsic value to human civilization . . . human caring values and actions contribute to the health and healing of individuals."[13]

Caring is also seen as invisible or hidden, and therefore often undervalued. Says Roberts, "It is necessary that we 'uncover' more of the characteristics of this caring practice, so that it can be recognized, rewarded, and taught to students of nursing."[14] In a much praised book that presents an analysis of expert nursing, based on vivid examples of actual nursing practice, Benner remarks on "the nature of the power associated with the caring provided by nurses" and concludes, "One thing is clear: Almost no intervention will work if the nurse-patient relationship is not based on mutual respect and genuine caring."[15]

One concern that has been voiced about emphasizing caring as a major part of nursing is that people will revert to the old notion that nursing is not intellectually demanding and just requires kindness and the desire to do for patients. Therefore, although the National Commission on Nursing Implementation Project (NCNIP) nursing image campaign of 1990 emphasized caring, posters also carried the tag line, "If caring were enough, anyone could be a nurse." The other side of the coin is presented by a distinguished historian who contends that nursing's problem is being "ordered to care" in a society that refuses to value caring.[16]

Although, over the years, nursing has been defined according to the functions of nurses or the clinical fields in which they practice or the specific job titles they may hold, there is a theme running throughout the definitions that indicates that the focus of nursing is the health of whole human beings in interaction with their environment—a holistic, humanistic focus closely associated with caring. (The term *holistic* seems to have been coined to refer to care related to the "whole" patient, physical and psychosocial. Holistic once referred to paranormal healing, but is now frequently used in the same sense as wholistic.)

An extremely significant step in the definition of nursing occurred in 1980 when the ANA published *Nursing: A Social Policy Statement.* The work of a taskforce appointed by the ANA Congress for Nursing Practice was to answer the question, "What is nursing?" and further, to make explicit the nature of nursing's public commitment. Included there is a definition intended to maintain the historical orientation of Nightingale and Henderson, yet reflect the evolution that had occurred in the intervening years. The Policy Statement claims, "Nursing is the diagnosis and treatment of human responses to actual or potential health problems."[17]

The revised *Social Policy Statement: The Essence of the Profession,* published in 2010, begs the issue of any precise definition. It reaffirms nursing's roots within the tradition of Nightingale and Henderson, and seems to give liberty to alternative definitions expecting that they will acknowledge four essential features of contemporary practice:

1. Attention to the full range of human experiences and responses to health and illness without restriction to a problem-focused orientation.

2. Integration of objective data with an understanding of the subjective experience of the patient.

3. Application of scientific knowledge to the processes of diagnosis and treatment.

4. Provision of a caring relationship that facilitates health and healing.

These statements allow flexibility and confer many liberties. They

1. Remove any restriction to a problem-focused relationship (nursing may involve intervening in a good situation to make it better).

2. Recognize subjective experience as a valid source of information on which to design care (a critical admission as we enter a multicultural era, and additionally open the door to give credibility to intuition as a quality in nursing practice).

3. Use language that returns the profession to a recognition of nursing's caring relationship, and link that caring to outcomes, building a case for a science of caring.

4. Talk of diagnosis and treatment without the modifier *nursing,* thereby recognizing that as we bridge the boundaries of other professions, new role functions are not only valid, but also required.

When we speak of definitions, we are also looking for guidance in identifying our scope of practice. How does nursing fit into health care? There are four concepts that help us to do that. They may sound simple, but they are the constant cause of disagreement among health disciplines.

1. *Boundary*: Where does nurses' work end and another discipline's begin? As areas of work mature, they begin to expand these boundaries outward.
2. *Intersections*: Points in practice where two or more disciplines interface and extend their practice into someone else's scope.
3. *Core*: The phenomena of concern unique to a field.
4. *Dimensions*: Other characteristics that fall within the scope and make it unique: philosophy, ethics, functions, roles, and skills.[18]

Despite its somewhat obscure language at certain points (professions do have their own private jargon that, incidentally, can shut out others), which makes it less than totally understandable to some nurses, much less nonnurses, the social policy statements are considered a major step in defining contemporary nursing and formalizing its contract with the public.

■ NURSING FUNCTIONS

Nursing functions can be described in broad or specific terms. For instance, classically, the common elements have included maintaining or restoring normal life function; observing and reporting signs of actual or potential change in physiologic or psychosocial status; formulating and carrying out a plan for the provision of nursing care consistent with the regimen of other treating disciplines; counseling families in relation to health-related concerns; and teaching. These are referred to in the social policy statements.

Of course, some nurses (and administrators) see nurses more as managers of nursing care than as direct caregivers—in other words, they are responsible for nursing care, supervising and coordinating the work of others, but not personally giving care. This issue always emerges when nursing shortages and higher salaries are discussed. The idea that nurses are too expensive to give bedside care assumes that patients do not need expert care—which is clearly a fallacy in these times.

The degree of expertise with which a nurse carries out these functions depends on the nurse's level of knowledge and skills, but the profession has the responsibility of setting standards for its practitioners. In its 2010 revision of *Nursing: Scope and Standards of Practice, 2nd Edition*, the ANA continues to distinguish between *Standards of Practice* (patient/client centered), a *competent level of care* as demonstrated by nursing services to the patient, and *Standards of Professional Performance* (provider centered), a competent level of behavior in the professional role.[19] These standards serve as the basis for specialty standards as they are developed or updated and are recognized by 33 specialty associations.

The point has been made repeatedly that the profession is responsible for developing and disseminating statements on scope, standards, ethics, titling, and the like. However, there are also definitions authored by government and health care institutions (employers). These may not be consistent or compatible with one another, and consequently they are a major source of stress.

The Nursing Process

The term *nursing process* was not dominant in the nursing literature until the mid-1960s. Orlando was one of the earliest authors to use the term, but it was slow to be adopted. In the 1960s, models of the activities in which nurses engaged were developed, and in 1967, a faculty group at the Catholic University of America specifically identified the phases of the nursing process as assessing, planning, implementing, and evaluating. In fact, the nursing process adheres to the steps in logical thinking or problem solving. That it is used in nursing has gained it the label of the nursing process.

At this point, there is considerable information in the nursing literature about the use of the nursing process, and many schools of nursing use it as a framework for teaching. However, there are those who feel that other approaches are more suitable to today's complex care. More specifically, the abandonment of logical thought is not being proposed, but rather the incorporation into nursing's educational systems and practice of the most cutting edge of cognitive techniques. There has been an emphasis on critical and creative thinking, diagnostic reasoning, and evidence-based practice.

■ A NURSING MINIMUM DATA SET

The *nursing minimum data set* (NMDS) is defined as those essential core items of information that describe nursing practice that could ideally be recorded on a regular basis by most nurses across all settings in the delivery of nursing care. The NMDS enhances communication; allows comparisons between clinical populations across time and place; and makes it possible for nurses to identify what they treat, how they treat it, and what difference it makes. Such information is invaluable to support policy formation, program planning, management, and the evaluation of nursing in the American health care system. These data are ideally suited for collection at the national level, but less ambitious undertakings could occur regionally, by state, or locally.

The NMDS consists of 16 elements, many of which are already present in some facet of health care data collection, and most are not specific to nursing. Examples are identifying characteristics of the patient and the health care setting, discharge date, and disposition of the patient (to nursing home, home care). The nursing care elements are *nursing diagnosis*, *nursing intervention*, *nursing outcome*, and *intensity of nursing care*. The intensity factor could be derived from acuity systems that are in fairly common use in health care settings to approximate the number of hours of nursing care required by a patient and the skill level of the personnel who are needed to deliver that care. Although it may not be easy to gather this information given the size and complexity of the delivery system, at least some mechanism exists.

The challenge was more formidable with diagnosis, interventions, and outcome. After generations of pioneering efforts, NANDA International (formerly the North Atlantic Nursing Diagnosis Association) has succeeded in generating a scientifically based and tested taxonomy or classification system (a collection of labels that are ordered and arranged on the basis of a single principle or set of principles) that has gained relatively broad acceptance in the profession. A nursing diagnosis is

> a clinical judgment about individual, family or community responses to actual and potential health problems/life processes. Nursing diagnoses provide the basis for selection of nursing interventions to achieve outcomes for which the nurse is accountable.[20]

This definition establishes diagnosis as the linchpin in the diagnosis, intervention, outcome triad. The NANDA diagnoses are organized under nine broad concepts or patterns: exchanging, communicating, relating, valuing, choosing, moving, perceiving, knowing, and feeling. There are currently 172 diagnoses, each including the label itself, a definition, defining characteristics, and related factors. Because the process of developing, validating, and reaching

consensus on a diagnosis has evolved over more than 40 years, not all the diagnoses are developed to the same extent. Some diagnoses have major and minor defining characteristics, major being the indicators that are present in 80 to 100 percent of clients with the diagnosis, and minor appearing in 50 to 79 percent of situations; others do not.[21] Exhibit 9–1 presents a diagnosis.

The Nursing Intervention Classification (NIC) and the Nursing Outcome Classification (NOC) are of more recent origin and are the products of the Center for Nursing Classification at the University of Iowa College of Nursing, which has excelled in this work under the leadership of Joanne McCloskey Dochterman and Gloria Bulechek. Both NIC and NOC are organized at the broadest level of abstraction into six domains. These domains are subdivided into 24 to 27 classes or categories, under which are clustered 330 outcomes or 514 interventions.[22] Although the domains are slightly different from one classification to the other, each gives credibility to the holistic orientation of nursing. NIC and NOC not only enable the nursing community to respond to the challenge of the NMDS, but they are developed in a form ideally suited for computerization. Each NOC outcome is accompanied by a five-point scale to measure patient status for indicators specific to that outcome and collectively for the outcome as a whole. Work is under way to determine the clinical usefulness and psychometric capabilities of NOC.

None of these systems will ever be complete. They will continue to evolve with the growing sophistication of nursing science. Examples from NIC and NOC are presented in Exhibits 9–2 and 9–3, respectively. It is easy for the reader to see the natural linkages between these systems as well as their usefulness in both education and prompting clinical decision making. NANDA diagnoses and NICs are labels, whereas NOC incorporates the capacity to indicate the direction and extent of change in the patient's condition. Students are referred to the primary works on diagnosis, intervention, and outcomes, both to understand their own practice better and to appreciate the precision with which nursing treats its stewardship to the public.

Such a monumental work is not without its critics. It remains to be seen whether the NMDS movement has been a strategy to bring maturity to nursing as a profession or is a sign of our immaturity. The trends in health care restructuring move us toward interdisciplinary practice. Should our language also reflect a unity of practice? There

■ **EXHIBIT 9–1. One Example of a NANDA Diagnosis**

Anxiety

Definition	A state in which the individual/group experiences feelings of uneasiness (apprehension) and activation of the autonomic nervous system in response to a vague, nonspecific threat.

Defining Characteristics

Physiologic	Increased heart rate, elevated blood pressure, increased respiratory rate, diaphoresis, dilated pupils, voice tremors/pitch changes, trembling/twitching, palpitations, nausea or vomiting, frequent urination, diarrhea, insomnia, fatigue and weakness, flushing or pallor, dry mouth, body aches and pains (especially back, neck, chest), restlessness, faintness/dizziness, paresthesias, hot and cold flashes, anorexia.
Emotional	Patient states he/she has feelings of apprehension, helplessness, nervousness, lack of self-confidence, losing control, tension or being "keyed up," inability to relax, anticipation of misfortune.
Cognitive	Inability to concentrate, lack of awareness of surroundings, diminished learning ability, confusion, forgetfulness, rumination, orientation to past as opposed to present or future, blocking of thoughts (inability to remember), preoccupation, hyperattentiveness.

Related Factors

Exposure to toxins; threat to or change in role status; related to unconscious conflict about essential goals and values of life; familial association/heredity; unmet needs; interpersonal transmission/contagion; situational/maturational crisis; threat of death; threat to or change in health status; threat to or change in interaction patterns; threat to or change in role function; threat to self-concept; unconscious conflict about essential values/goals of life; threat to or change in environment; threat to change in economic status; substance abuse

Source: Adapted from Carpenito-Movet L. *Nursing Diagnosis: Application to Clinical Practice*, 13th ed. Philadelphia: Lippincott Williams & Wilkins, 2009.

are those who believe that our own classification systems are requisite for autonomy and must be well developed before any move to a consolidated language is made.

In the late 1980s, the ANA initiated an era dedicated to recognition of the work nurses do as reflected in their classification systems. The diagnostic labels of NANDA, NIC, and NOC were accepted by the National Library of Medicine and incorporated into their metathesaurus. A formal appeal to the World Health Organization (WHO) asked for the NANDA classification to be included in the next revision of the International Classification of Diseases (ICD). This request was denied based on the opinion that this language was not internationally useful, understandable, or relevant. Rejection provided the challenge to claim our practice internationally. This gave birth to the expanded presence of the North American Nursing Diagnosis Association and its transition to officially become NANDA International.

The need to move nursing out of the shadows and formalize its presence proved to be a common cause that transcended national borders. Although Americans contributed the most advanced work in this area, they were not alone. There had been significant progress in other countries. Profiting from the mistakes of others and generous funding from the Kellogg Foundation, the International Classification of Nursing Practice (ICNP) moved forward under the leadership of the International Council of Nurses (ICN).

An international constituency presented new problems. There was a need to search for the most agreeable language if these labels were to be useful and to avoid any negative cultural connotations. There was common agreement that the language must originate at the bedside. Local area work in Europe, South America, Asia, and Africa has allowed the ICNP to forge ahead.[23] Both alpha and beta versions of the ICNP are available on the ICN website. Nurses are invited to browse these sites, personally review the classifications, and propose revisions to diagnosis, intervention, and outcomes language.

■ **EXHIBIT 9–2. One Example of an NIC Intervention**

Anxiety Reduction

Definition	Minimizing apprehension, dread, foreboding, or uneasiness related to an unidentified source of anticipated danger
Suggested/Optional Interventions	
Use a calm, reassuring approach	Active listening: listen attentively
Clearly state expectations for patient's behavior (anticipatory guidance)	Reinforce behavior, as appropriate
Explain all procedures, including sensations likely to be experienced during the procedure	Create an atmosphere that facilitates trust
	Encourage verbalization of feelings, perceptions, and fears
Seek to understand the patient's perspective of a stressful situation	Identify to patient when level of anxiety changes
Provide factual information concerning diagnosis, treatment, and prognosis	Provide diversional activities geared toward the reduction of tension
Provide presence for safety	Help patient identify situations that precipitate or increase anxiety
	Support the use of appropriate defense mechanism(s)
Encourage patient to stay with child, as appropriate	Assist patient in articulating a realistic description of an upcoming event
Provide objects that symbolize safeness	
Administer back rub/neck rub, as appropriate	Determine patient's decision-making ability
Encourage noncompetitive activities, as appropriate	Instruct patient on the use of relaxation techniques
Keep treatment equipment out of sight	Administer medications to reduce anxiety, as appropriate

Source: Adapted from Bulechek G, Butcher H, Dochterman J. *Nursing Interventions Classification (NIC)*, 5th ed. St. Louis, MO: Mosby, 2008.

■ NURSING THEORIES AND CONCEPTUAL MODELS

As nursing has grown in professionalism, nursing scholars have given us a theoretical body of knowledge, and the science of nursing has come of age. A theoretical base of practice defines nursing's uniqueness; that is, it has a science of its own and is not simply an extension of another profession. In scientific inquiry, observations of seemingly unrelated phenomena are organized into intelligible systems that show relationships among the phenomena and a linking of truths. Nursing research enables us to describe, understand, and predict the life processes of humans, to the end of effectively intervening (prescribing) to promote the health of the well and the ill as individuals and social groups. Nursing science is the umbrella over research, theory, and practice. As eloquently put by Greenwood,

Science may be defined as an internally consistent system of propositions (theory) that are descriptive generalizations

about some aspect of nature (practice) and have been derived from observations conducted and analyzed according to standardized procedures (research).[24]

To put it another way, nursing theory is an internally consistent set of interrelated concepts linked to form propositions. These propositions, or relational statements, specify connections among variables derived from the concepts and provide a systematic view of phenomena of interest to nursing. Theory allows intelligent practice; practice provides the questions for research; and research exists to expand theory. And so the cycle continues.

The shift in nursing education from the practice setting of the hospital to the academic setting of the university brought with it a keen interest in identifying and developing a scientific body of knowledge unique to nursing. Theories were formulated and tested that would distinguish nursing from medicine, whose models of disease and dysfunction historically had dominated nursing education and practice, and from the common caretaking principles

■ EXHIBIT 9–3. One Example of an NOC Outcome

Anxiety Control

Definition	Personal actions to eliminate or reduce feelings of apprehension and tension from an unidentifiable source				
Anxiety Control	**Never Demonstrated 1**	**Rarely Demonstrated 2**	**Sometimes Demonstrated 3**	**Often Demonstrated 4**	**Demonstrated Consistently 5**
Monitors intensity of anxiety	1	2	3	4	5
Eliminates precursors of anxiety	1	2	3	4	5
Decreases environmental stimuli when anxious	1	2	3	4	5
Seeks information to reduce anxiety	1	2	3	4	5
Plans coping strategies for stressful situations	1	2	3	4	5
Uses effective coping strategies	1	2	3	4	5
Uses relaxation techniques to reduce anxiety	1	2	3	4	5
Reports decreased duration of episodes	1	2	3	4	5
Reports increased length of time between episodes	1	2	3	4	5
Maintains role performance	1	2	3	4	5
Maintains social relationships	1	2	3	4	5
Maintains concentration	1	2	3	4	5
Reports absence of sensory perceptual distortions	1	2	3	4	5
Reports adequate sleep	1	2	3	4	5
Reports absence of physical manifestations of anxiety	1	2	3	4	5
Behavioral manifestations of anxiety absent	1	2	3	4	5
Controls anxiety response	1	2	3	4	5
Other _____ (Specify)	1	2	3	4	5

Source: Adapted from Moorhead S, Johnson M, Maas M. *Nursing Outcomes Classification (NOC)*, 3rd ed. St. Louis, MO: Mosby, 2004.

and practices of helping, protecting, and mothering found in the lay public. Without research and theory building, nursing scholars argued, nursing would be unable to carve out a role in the future health care system, and would thus allow itself to be defined, instructed, and controlled by other disciplines.

Although the 1950s and 1960s witnessed a proliferation of conceptual models and theories for nursing, the question of a body of knowledge specific to the discipline probably began with Florence Nightingale. Among her other achievements, she identified the relationship between patient and environment as a major focus for nursing intervention and provided hints that would guide nurses in providing comfort, speeding recovery, and preventing disease. Like theories, her hints were derived from systematic observation of patients and their responses. Nightingale submitted that by using these hints, nurses could teach themselves. Although her work was groundbreaking for nursing science, the immaturity and transitional nature of nursing at that point in history is evident in her reference to the importance of precise observations, on the one hand, and to "common sense," for which she had no clarifying definition, on the other. Accordingly, she explicitly distinguished nursing knowledge, "which everyone ought to have," from medical knowledge. Nevertheless, the seeds were sown for the development of a science of nursing that began to flower over 100 years later.

The question of the uniqueness of nursing knowledge continues to be a thorny issue among nursing theorists, particularly because nursing is said to borrow so much of its knowledge from other disciplines. Although many nursing scholars find this excessive borrowing troublesome as they seek to identify what is unique to nursing, others argue that the uniqueness of nursing lies in its very reliance on many disciplines—that in fact, because it synthesizes knowledge from so many disciplines, nursing provides a more comprehensive, holistic approach to patient care than any of the other health professions.

Theory in nursing takes several forms and has several purposes. *Philosophical theory* gives meaning to situations requiring nursing. This is accomplished through the cognitive skills of analysis, reasoning, and often divergent thinking. *Mid-level theory* has a narrower focus, is more concrete, and targets practice specialty questions. *Grand theory* is the most comprehensive, applying to the entire domain of nursing. It attempts to explain and define nursing—what it is, what it does, why it is important, how it differs from other health professions—and exposes to critical examination such concepts as patient, nurse, illness, health, support, care, and comfort, which are each theories in their own right. Every theory or conceptual model for nursing has its own concepts, definitions, and assumptions and derives from different basic scientific models and theories. Exhibit 9–4 provides an overview of select nursing theorists and their work. The common theme of holism and patient/client empowerment through the nurse-patient relationship to achieve quality of life or death is noteworthy. Essentially the goal of each theoretical view is the same, but the route to that goal may differ. Further, each theory is organized around its view of man (human beings), health, society (environment), and nursing. These are the meta-paradigm elements that, when defined and viewed as a whole, create an individualized view of nursing.

Exhibit 9–4 provides a representative sample of philosophical, grand, and midrange nursing theories. The information contained is only a limited glimpse. A concept, definition, or assumption has been chosen to depict the distinctiveness of each theorist's work. In some instances, they are very subtle variations on a theme. There are other observations that are even more telling. Chronologically the earliest theorists were more philosophical, searching to give form and meaning to nursing, and they were successful. In many contemporary situations, we go back to the work of these early theorists for a clarity that has been lost over the years. Later, theorists became highly abstract, applying behavioral, systems, and developmental models to nursing. For all the difficulty in sometimes translating their work into practice, they have given us credibility as scholars. Swept away as we have been in the allure of high technology and the search for precise scientific explanations for our practice, the humanness of nursing often became lost. Our most recent theorists bring us full circle to our roots, reminding us that health and illness are personal experiences, and that nurses serve the public best by their commitment to caring.

Most grand theories, including the ones presented here, do not begin with observation of empirical phenomena (what nursing is) but rather from a philosophical position on what nursing should be in the best of all possible worlds to be most effective or therapeutic. As such, they contain a significant value component that profoundly influences the development, acceptance, and utility of each theory. Philosophical unity at some level is essential for the development of the science. Theory is the means to the end, but often tells us very little about the end itself. The end of improving the human condition is the same for all nurses. Nursing's diversity demands a wide range of theoretical orientations to allow each of us to choose what is most comfortable. Restated, science builds from the foundation of philosophy. Because philosophy is abstract, it needs the concepts and relationships of theory to be operational. Theory provides the means to the end that is consistent for all of us. Under each grand theory there is a philosophy, and midrange theory can be traced to grander theories that lend philosophical underpinnings. Careful analysis convinces us that there is more consensus about what nursing hopes to accomplish than ever before.

From the scientific perspective, nursing is an observational science, sharing with astronomy, zoology, anthropology, medicine, public health, and others a method for formulating its theories by chronicling and analyzing systematic observations. Unlike these other disciplines, however, nursing is still in the early stages of describing the phenomena with which it deals. From medical theory, we

Theorist, Theory/ Conceptual Model and Date of Early Work[a]	Concepts/Definitions/ Assumptions	Influential Models or Sciences	Nursing Role	Theory Type	Major Contribution
Florence Nightingale: Patient-Environmental, 1859	• Disease is a reparative process • Rejected germ theory • Imbalance between patient and physical environment frustrates energy conservation and decreases the capacity for health • Focus on pure air, pure water, efficient drainage, cleanliness, noise, diet, and light • Patients are one with their environment	Environment/sanitation	• Manipulation of the external environment, such as ventilation, warmth, light, diet, cleanliness, and noise contributes to well-being and the reparative process • Patient is relatively passive • Nursing places patients in the best condition for nature to act on him or her • Saw nursing role in health as well as illness • Stressed nurses' use of observation	Philosophical	• Pioneered nursing's domain as the patient/environment relationship • Statistical analysis for health and nursing
Hildegard Peplau, The Theory of Interpersonal Relations, 1952[a]	• Psychodynamic nursing • Experiential learning • Four phases of the nurse-patient relationship: orientation, identification, exploitation, resolution • Nursing roles: stranger, resource, teacher, leader, surrogate, counselor	Maslow Sullivan Freud Fromm	• Patient relives (hypothetically) stressful experiences, with nurse as an objective presence; old conclusions are reassessed and often corrected • The nurse and patient form a mutually therapeutic relationship • Fostering personality development toward maturity is a function of nursing	Midrange (psychiatric nursing)	• Ended ambiguity surrounding the nurse-patient relationship

(Continued)

■ **EXHIBIT 9–4. Select Nursing Theorists and Their Work**

Theorist, Theory/ Conceptual Model and Date of Early Work[a]	Concepts/Definitions/ Assumptions	Influential Models or Sciences	Nursing Role	Theory Type	Major Contribution
Dorothy Johnson: Behavioral Systems Model, 1959	• Seven behavioral subsystems that can be analyzed in terms of structure and function • Structure includes the elements of drive (motivation), set (predisposition to act), choice (behavioral repertoire), and action (behavior) • Functional requirements are protection, nurturance, and stimulation • Attachment, or the affiliation subsystem is the cornerstone of social organization	Ethological systems	• Maintain or restore balance and equilibrium, or • Help person achieve a more optimum structure if possible or desirable	Grand	• Strong philosophical statements related to model • Strong influence on Roy, Neuman, and others
Dorothea Orem: Self-Care Model, 1959	• Constituted from three related theories: self-care, self-care deficit, and nursing systems • People have a need for the provision and management of self-care actions on a continuing basis to sustain life and health and to recover from disease	Henderson	• Self-care deficit is the target of nursing • The nursing system is designed as wholly or partially compensatory or supportive—educative as dictated by the agency of the patient	Grand	• Pragmatic and comfortable concepts

Theorist/Model	Assumptions	Theoretical Sources	Concepts	Type	Contributions
Virginia Henderson: Developmental Model, 1961	• When an individual's self-care agency is not adequate to their requirement or that of their dependents, deficit is created • The patient is a person who requires help toward independence	Thorndike Rehabilitation principles Orlando Maslow	• Acts on patients' behalf to do those things that patients would do for themselves, assuming the strength, knowledge, or willingness to do so • Identifies 14 components of basic nursing care corresponding to Maslow's hierarchy of needs • Three levels of the NPR: substituting, helping, and partnering • Use of empathic understanding • Interdependence with other providers	Philosophical	• Delineates autonomous functions • Stresses goals of interdependence with the patient • Self-care concepts that influenced later theorists
Ida Jean Orlando: Theory of Deliberative Nursing Process, 1961	• Distinguishes automatic from deliberate actions • Perceptions, thoughts, and feelings are not explored in automatic actions	Eclectic	• A nursing situation consists of patient behavior, nurse reaction, and nursing actions • Nurse provides assistance to patients to deal with helplessness	Midrange (psychiatric nursing)	• Advanced nursing to a disciplined practice

(Continued)

■ **EXHIBIT 9-4. Select Nursing Theorists and Their Work**

Theorist, Theory/ Conceptual Model and Date of Early Work[a]	Concepts/Definitions/ Assumptions	Influential Models or Sciences	Nursing Role	Theory Type	Major Contribution
	• Deliberate actions yield solutions and prevention of problems		• Physician's orders directed to patient, and nurse helps patient comply or decide not to comply		
Imogene King: General Systems Model, 1964	• The dynamic nature of life assumes continuous adjustment to life's stressors • The self is a person's total subjective environment and is a distinctive center of experience and significance for each • Adjustment entails three open systems interacting with the environment: personal, interpersonal, and social	Highly eclectic Piaget Erikson Etzioni Bennis (among others)	• Nursing's goal is to help individuals maintain their health so that they can function in their roles • The nurse enters the situation when the client can no longer perform the usual daily activities, yet . . . • The domain of nursing includes health promotion and maintenance • Nursing is a process of human interaction with a patient based on communication, to set goals and a means for achievement	Grand	• The Theory of Goal Attainment is a product of this model, and describes the nature of the nurse-client encounter • Emphasis on the derivation of nursing knowledge from other disciplines
Myra Levine: Conservation Model, 1966	• Focuses on holism, integrity, and conservation	Borrowed from a range of natural and behavioral sciences	• The goal of nursing is promotion of wholeness	Grand	• Distinctive and extensive vocabulary that makes it complex

Theorist	Assumptions	Propositions	Category	Importance
	• The life process is characterized by unceasing change that has direction, purpose, and meaning • The organism retains integrity through adaptive capability • Loss of balance causes fear, inflammation, stress, or sensory response	• Nursing intervention provides help in adaptation based on the principles of conservation of energy and structural, personal, and social integrity		• Logically consistent and wholistic • Great influence on later theorists
Joyce Travelbee: Human-to-Human Relationship, 1966	• The self-actualization aspect of illness is a natural and commonplace life experience • Healing is based on empathy, sympathy, and emotional bonding	• A major goal of nursing is helping the patient find meaning in illness through building a mutually therapeutic relationship	Peplau Orlando Midrange (psychiatric nursing)	• Early emphasis on caring
Lydia Hall: Core, Care, and Cure Model, 1969 (clinical work dates to 1950s)	• Illness and rehabilitation are learning experiences	• Stressed the autonomous function of nurses • The nurse guides and teaches in the process of personal caregiving • The nursing role consists of therapeutic use of self (core), the treatment regimen within the health care team (cure), and nurturing and intimate bodily care (care)	Carl Rogers Philosophical	• The eventual base for primary nursing • Applied to practice in a large metropolitan setting

(Continued)

Theorist, Theory/ Conceptual Model and Date of Early Work[a]	Concepts/Definitions/ Assumptions	Influential Models or Sciences	Nursing Role	Theory Type	Major Contribution
Martha Rogers: Science of Unitary Human Beings, 1970	• The person is a unified energy field continually interacting and exchanging matter and energy with the environment • This exchange results in increased complexity and innovativeness of the person • Well-being is reflected in pattern and organization	Systems Electromagnetic Theory	• Acts to promote symphonic interaction between man and environment • Achieve maximum health potential by repatterning the human and environmental fields	Grand	• Strong voice for the development of nursing as a basic science
Sister Callista Roy: Adaptation Model, 1970	• Individual adapts behavior to cope with stimuli from environment that are stressors • Stressors disrupt dynamic state of equilibrium and illness results • Adaptive modes focus on physiological needs, self-concept, role function, and interdependent relations • A positive response to stress is determined by whether the simulation exceeds the level that can be accommodated by the individual	Systems Stress Helson's Adaptation Theory	• Nurse assesses the adequacy of the patient's coping, and if needed changes the patient's response potential by holding the stimuli to the point where positive response is possible	Grand	• Excellent example of how knowledge can become unique in nursing; an eclectic view including stress, systems, and adaptation

| Betty Neuman: Systems Model, 1972 | • Stressors as well as reaction and reconstitution can be viewed as intra-, inter-, and extrapersonal
 • Each individual has a usual range of responses to stress that maintains equilibrium and is called the normal line of defense
 • A flexible line of defense also exists to protect against unusual stress
 • Should a stressor break through the normal line of defense, lines of resistance attempt to stabilize the situation | Gestalt Theory
 Levels of Prevention
 Systems Theory
 Stress Theory | • Nursing aims at the reduction of stress factors and adverse conditions that threaten optimal functioning in a given situation
 • This is accomplished by identifying stress factors and assisting individuals to respond by strengthening their normal and flexible lines of defense
 • Purposeful intervention with a total person approach | Grand | • Potentially useful in a variety of health care disciplines
 • Produced two separate theories: Optimal Patient Stability and Prevention as Intervention |
| Jean Watson: Theory of Human Caring, 1979 | • Caring is a universal social behavior
 • Care for the self is necessary before care for others
 • Care and love are the cornerstones of humanness | Leininger
 Existential phenomenology | • Emphasizes the humanistic dimension of nursing that can only be practiced interpersonally | Philosophical | • Makes the humanism in nursing scientific and credible |

(Continued)

EXHIBIT 9-4. Select Nursing Theorists and Their Work

Theorist, Theory/ Conceptual Model and Date of Early Work[a]	Concepts/Definitions/ Assumptions	Influential Models or Sciences	Nursing Role	Theory Type	Major Contribution
Patricia Benner: Caring, 1984	• Describes caring as a common human bond	Dreyfus Model of Skill Acquisition	• Primary focus of the model is nursing • Through a qualitative process describes five stages of competency development: novice, advanced beginner, competent, proficient, and expert • A phenomenological theory describing caring	Philosophical	• Recognizes the value of experience in a practice discipline • Gives credibility to the role played by intuition in practice

[a]As determined by published work.

have a sophisticated set of classifications for describing disease, but we do not as yet have a very well developed description of persons in need of nursing. The closest nursing has come is the classification of nursing diagnoses, as mentioned. The process of developing such a compilation of diagnostic categories is in many ways the first (descriptive) stage of theory development. These are our empirical observations of human responses to birth, death, illness, parenting, aging, stress, and other factors. Nursing, perhaps more than any other discipline, is in a position to observe and record these events and develop theories that shift clinical practice from a disease to a patient orientation.

Levels of theory, such as grand, middle-range, and philosophical, are linked together and inform each other. However, midrange theories are the most testable and lend themselves to the research process, and eventually the incorporation of research-based changes into practice. The establishment of the National Institute for Nursing Research (NINR) within the National Institutes of Health (NIH) has encouraged the progress of midrange theories to focus research on both the refinement of grand theories and the development of practice innovations grounded in theory-based research.

The growth of the NMDS and nursing theories has been the major development in nursing over the last 70 years, and they complement one another. It is imperative to continue and strengthen clinical research so that nursing theories may flourish, guide practice, and measure the extent to which nursing action attains its goals in terms of patient behavior.

Whether nursing emerges as a mature discipline as well as a profession depends to a great extent on the direction that its theory building will take. For instance, constructing explanations of the connection between nursing phenomena that can be tested against experience; developing its technology, policies, and procedures; clarifying its concepts and relationships; and reconfirming its philosophy and ideological base are each part of theory building. Ultimately, the most important test of any theory is its applicability and utility in clinical practice.

Nursing practice has become very complex, and the information encountered in order to make a therapeutic decision is often intimidating. A theoretical orientation helps the nurse to progress in an orderly manner with assessing, planning, intervening, and predicting outcomes, while considering options at each turn. Even where nurses claim to practice without a clearly defined theoretical orientation, they have one. Their beliefs about care will reveal them. In many cases their orientation is eclectic, borrowing pieces from many great minds to undergird their practice.

■ WHAT IS NURSING?

It can easily be seen that there may not be a single definition of nursing. Perhaps there never will be, because nursing is such a multifaceted profession. This is one problem legislators have had in writing a nursing practice act, which is, after all, the legal definition of nursing. (These definitions, along with other aspects of licensure, are discussed in Chapter 20.) Nevertheless, at some point, every nurse has to decide what nursing is to him or her and how to interpret it to others. This chapter, its references, and its bibliography may provide a basis for working out your own definition, but the final determination is yours.

KEY POINTS

1. The basic criteria for professionalism include the qualities of autonomy, a defined body of knowledge that is constantly expanding, and social value.

2. The ANA's *Social Policy Statements* of 1980, 1995, and 2010 were major steps in defining contemporary nursing and formalizing nursing's contract with the public.

3. A profession has a responsibility to monitor its practitioners and develop and disseminate standards and its code of ethics.

4. There are often situations where the profession, the government, and health care institutions each author policies on the same subject; they can be inconsistent or incompatible with one another, and thus become a major source of stress.

5. The mental processes required to design and deliver care go well beyond the nursing process and include critical and creative thinking, diagnostic reasoning, evidence-based practice, and more.

KEY POINTS

6. The NMDS provides an exceptional data source for nursing to prove its value.

7. NANDA diagnoses, NIC, and NOC provide useful linkages for both teaching and direct care.

8. The metaparadigm is the most abstract level of knowledge; for nursing it consists of the concepts of person, health, environment, and nursing.

9. Philosophy must be translated into theory to be operational.

10. Nursing conceptual models provide a broad frame of reference for understanding the phenomena with which the discipline is concerned.

11. Most nursing models have a range of theories from which they have been developed.

12. Nursing theory is a group of related concepts that derive from conceptual models; theories are testable, whereas models are not.

13. Midrange theories have a narrower view than grand theories, focusing on a specific condition or population.

14. All nurses are committed to improving the human condition; one theory or another just helps nurses to get there through a different route.

REFERENCES

1. Schulman S. Basic functional roles in nursing: Mother surrogate and healer. In Jaco EG (Ed.): *Patients, Physicians and Illness: Behavioral Sciences and Medicine.* Glencoe, IL: Free Press, 1963.

2. Wiggins L. Lydia Hall's place in the development of theory in nursing. *Image* 12:10–12, February 1980.

3. Watson J, Smith M. Caring science and the science of unitary human beings. *J Adv Nurs* 37:452–461, March 2002.

4. Flexner A. Is social work a profession? *Proceedings of the National Conference of Charities and Correction.* New York: New York School of Philanthropy, 1915.

5. Greenwood E. Attributes of a profession. In Fuszard B (Ed.): *Self-actualization for Nurses.* Rockville, MD: Aspen, 1984, pp 13–26.

6. American Nurses Association. *Nursing's Social Policy Statement.* Washington, DC: American Nurses Publishing, 2010.

7. Brint S. *In an Age of Experts: The Changing Role of Professionals in Politics and Public Life.* Princeton, NJ: Princeton University Press, 1994.

8. Ibid.

9. Beletz E. Professionalism—A license is not enough. In Chaska N (Ed.): *The Nursing Profession: Turning Points.* St. Louis, MO: Mosby, 1990.

10. Nightingale F. *Notes on Nursing.* London: Lippincott, facsimile of 1859 edition.

11. Henderson V. *ICN Basic Principles of Nursing Care.* London: International Council of Nurses, 1961. Expanded in Henderson V. The Nature of Nursing. New York: Macmillan, 1967.

12. The nurse practitioner question. *Am J Nurs* 74:2188, December 1974.

13. Watson J. The moral failure of the patriarchy. *Nurs Outlook* 38:62–66, March–April 1990.

14. Roberts J. Uncovering hidden caring. *Nurs Outlook* 38:67–69, March–April 1990.

15. Benner P. *From Novice to Expert.* Menlo Park, CA: Addison-Wesley, 1984.

16. Reverby S. *Ordered to Care: The Dilemma of American Nursing.* New York: Basic Books, 1987.

17. *Nursing: A Social Policy Statement.* Kansas City, MO: American Nurses' Association, 1980, p 1.

18. *Nursing: A Social Policy Statement,* 1980, loc cit.

19. *Nursing: Scope and Standards of Practice,* 2nd ed. Washington, DC: American Nurses Publishing, 2010.

20. Carpenito-Movet, L. *Nursing Diagnosis: Application to Clinical Practice,* 13th ed. Philadelphia: Lippincott Williams & Wilkins, 2009.

21. Ibid.

22. Ibid.

23. International Council of Nurses. International Classification for Nursing Practice (ICNP). http//www.icn.ch/icnp_def.htm. Retrieved April 20, 2010.

24. Greenwood E. *Lectures in Research Methodology for Social Welfare Students.* Berkeley, CA: University of California Press, 1962.

Updates can be found at **www.kellysnursing.com**

Professional Ethics and the Nurse

CHAPTER 10

■ WHO CARES ABOUT ETHICS?

Facing ethical issues is a daily part of a nurse's practice. The sheer complexity of the health care system, the focus on cost containment, and the scientific advances available or not available to people are only a part of what all health care professionals must deal with. Moreover, the changes in society, including changes in the mores of an increasingly diverse population, may well conflict with the nurse's own beliefs. Add to this, the nurse's interaction with people in various stages of illness, their significant others, and other health professionals, all of whom have their own moral and ethical beliefs and all of whom are functioning in some sort of bureaucracy that is itself hedged in by rapidly changing rules, regulations, laws, and economic pressures, and it is no small wonder that nurses look for help to practice ethically. Often, they are up against more powerful individuals; at times their colleagues are reluctant to provide support. Worse yet, there simply does not seem to be a "right" answer to so many ethical dilemmas; at best, decisions are never easy. Nor are these issues always wrapped in the drama of life or death; sometimes the issues are part of the day-to-day practice and lack an ethical environment.

There are many examples of ethical dilemmas in the health care setting. Consider these not uncommon situations.

1. An 86-year-old man is comatose and has an inoperable brain tumor. He had indicated to friends and family that he did not wish to be kept alive by artificial means if he was hospitalized, but had no written advance directive. Despite the family explaining this to the physician, she intubates the patient when he has respiratory problems.

2. A 38-year-old woman with terminal cancer whose severe pain is not relieved by the maximum dose of ordered medication asks the doctor to give her something stronger, even if it means the dose would kill her. He obliges, and she dies.

3. Twin babies, joined at the waist and sharing one digestive tract and three legs, are born in the hospital. Experts say that they cannot be separated. The orders on the chart say, "Do not feed according to family's wishes." Some nurses do feed the babies and report the order to the legal authorities. The parents are arrested.

4. A 35-year-old woman with two children is admitted for a lung biopsy. The test results show a very aggressive carcinoma with inevitable metastasis. The physician tells the patient that everything is all right, saying to the nurse, "Nothing can be done; there's no use upsetting her."

5. A well-liked nurse seems to be having mood swings, but always volunteers to work the evening or night shift and take care of the sickest patients. However, her patients often complain of unrelieved pain, although the narcotic record shows frequent narcotic administration.

6. A young woman has been in a persistent vegetative state (PVS) for a month after a serious accident. Although the medical team tells the family that further medical care is futile, the family says that they believe God will heal her and refuse withdrawal of ventilator support. They have no money or health insurance.

7. A medical center nurse faculty member has had surgery at his home hospital. A clinical instructor sees that the medical chart information has been brought

up on the computer screen, and a group of students start talking about the patient.

8. An 80-year-old man with diabetes is brought to the hospital with gangrene of both feet. He does not always seem lucid and has no family, but when told by the physician that he must have the feet amputated or die, he shouts loudly, "Leave my feet alone." The physician goes ahead with the amputation to save the man's life, stating that the man clearly did not understand the situation.

9. A patient infected with human immunodeficiency virus (HIV), who is a drug abuser and often homeless, demands the multiple medications that might keep him from developing acquired immunodeficiency syndrome (AIDS). However, the staff doubts that he will be able to follow the complex regimen required by the drugs and is reluctant to give the drugs. He threatens to sue.

10. Two men in the same hospital room have cardiac arrests within moments of each other. There is only one crash cart available. The nurses and residents resuscitate the respected family man, as opposed to the elderly Mexican janitor.

11. A pregnant woman with three boys has an amniocentesis that reveals that the baby is another boy. She and her husband decide on an abortion because they want a girl and prefer to try again.

12. A 10-year-old girl is sexually abused by her alcoholic father and becomes pregnant. She is not sure about what is happening to her body, but the school nurse, in talking to her, discovers what has happened. She reports it to child welfare, but the girl is early in her third trimester, and her parents, denying incest, say they have religious objections to abortion.

13. A psychiatric patient refuses more electro-shock therapy, even though it has been helping him. His family cannot manage his erratic behavior, and after having him declared incompetent, they approve the therapy, which is done.

14. A retarded boy refuses kidney dialysis because he fears it. No effort is made to relieve his anxiety. He dies shortly thereafter.

15. A couple discovers, through genetic testing, that they are carriers of a serious hereditary disease. Their teenage daughter does not yet show signs of the disease, but the parents decide not to have her tested or tell her of her potential carrier status so as not to upset her.

16. A famous sports figure, who is a known alcoholic and drug abuser, is in immediate need of a liver transplant. When a suitable one becomes available, he is moved to the top of the waiting list and receives the transplant.

17. An obstetrician in a community hospital spends little time with his Spanish-speaking patients. He is called three times by the nurse to see a patient who she fears is in trouble. He is at a dinner party and says he will be there shortly, but does not come until hours later. The patient almost dies.

18. A patient with AIDS is ordered an experimental drug by phone. The nurse knows that he has not had the treatment explained and hesitates to give it. Her supervisor tells her to go ahead, even though it is against hospital policy.

19. In speaking with a patient scheduled for surgery, the nurse realizes that the patient really does not understand what is to be done and what alternatives are available. She tells the doctor, who sarcastically replies that she should stick to nursing and let him decide what's best for the patient.

20. A top-level administrator has a habit of touching young nurses inappropriately. They are afraid of him and of losing their jobs and ask for help from a nurse manager. She speaks to him and he replies, "Jealous?" She reports him to the chief executive, who tells her to relax. "No harm done."

If you were the nurse involved in any of these situations, what would you do? Whose rights are or might be violated? The patient's? The family's? The nurse's? The doctor's? Society's? Nobody's? How much would you be affected by your own moral beliefs? If your action were contrary to what the hospital administrators, the physicians involved, or even some of your colleagues thought best (for whatever reason), would you be willing to face the consequences? What if your concept of "right" collided with a legal ruling? What if the patient or family asked you to help them and you agree with them, not the doctors or administrators? What if the case goes to court?

All the cases cited are real; a nurse somewhere faced one of these difficult situations (and probably others) and had to make a decision to act or not to act. How that decision was arrived at is the essence of ethics. As you read the sections on morality and the various theories of ethics, as well as the nursing code of ethics, consider the ethical problems given as examples, and note how your decisions depend on your ethical, or perhaps moral, beliefs. You may have also noted how many of these cases relate to patients' rights. It is very difficult to separate many ethical issues from patients' rights.

Does it matter? *Moral distress*, sometimes called *ethical distress* and eventually transformed into *moral outrage* if the situation remains unresolved, is a serious problem for nurses. Rushton and Scanlon say,

> When nurses are unable to translate their moral choices into action, moral distress occurs. Acting in a manner that is contrary to nurses' personal and professional values is an attack on their individuality, authenticity, and integrity.... If their moral distress is unrelieved, their self-worth is jeopardized; personal and professional relationships may be affected; and psychological, behavioral, and physical symptoms may occur. Ultimately the quality of patient care suffers.[1]

Nurses in moral distress reported anger, sadness, frustration, and anxiety. Some coped by going along with the situation. Others avoided the patient involved, and just did not deal with the ethical issue at all.[2] In one study of critical care nurses, fully 25 percent of the sample ($N = 106$) had left a position because of moral distress. An earlier study by the same researcher showed 18 percent with this response—a disturbing indication that this problem is increasing.[3]

To a great extent, the environment in which many nurses function is not an ethical environment—a positive setting in which to provide health care services. In an ethical environment, practice "reflects the understanding of the values in that milieu regarding ethical behavior . . . there is concern for health care practice that recognizes the rights of patients."[4] There are three ingredients that reflect positive ethical environments:

1. The ability to engage in deliberations regarding their practice as it pertained to ethics;
2. The presence of an administrator who supported them in their practice, especially concerns of an ethical nature; and
3. The presence of policies and procedures regarding the care given in that organization that was consistent with their care practice.[5]

In a similar manner, it has been suggested that health care organizations should look critically at how professed institutional values can best be realized in day-to-day interactions within the institutions and with the wider community. Contradictions between what institutions teach (or say) and what they do encourages undesirable behavior and cynicism, because what they really value is picked up and internalized as standards and passed on to students and workers. This institutional dissonance also influences society. Certain values desirable for institutions include the following:

1. *Humaneness*: A sense of benevolence to people and compassion for those in need
2. *Reciprocal benefit*: Refraining from actions that harm some to benefit others
3. *Trust*: Confidence in the integrity and reliability of individuals
4. *Fairness*: Impartiality in judgments about advantages given and benefit gained
5. *Dignity*: Respect for the person and the views of individuals
6. *Gratitude*: Appreciation of benefits received, relationships sustained, and obligations met
7. *Service*: Recognition that learning about treating disease transcends the usual requirements of reward for labor
8. *Stewardship*: Obligation for appropriate oversight and husbanding of resources.[6]

But talk to identify such values and goals simply is not enough. Put life in your rhetoric by creating documents stating these values, holding administrative rounds that bring together the diverse constituencies to discuss specific cases that cut across administrative units, and sponsoring value-based staff education.

■ MORALS, ETHICS, AND THE LAW: A DIFFERENTIATION

There has been a tendency to use the words *moral* and *ethical* interchangeably in some of the health profession's literature. However, they are not the same. *Morality* refers to a personal standard of what is right and wrong, good and bad in a situation. This opinion derives from the conventions and norms of society as conveyed through custom, tradition, religion, and your reference groups. In comparison, *ethics* is the reasoned analysis and disciplined inquiry of relationships underlying the moral code of a particular group.[7] Ethics seeks to answer the question, "What, all things considered, ought to be done in a given situation?" With this completely unrestricted frame of reference, it is impossible to proceed with your moral course on "automatic pilot."[8] In this context, the nine tenets of the American Nurses Association (ANA) Code of Ethics (see Exhibit 10–1) are the moral code of the profession, whereas the interpretative statements are the ethical principles that give additional substance to the code. People can be moral, but they must aspire to be ethical.

Bioethics is the application of ethical theories and principles to situations in health care.

Legal questions often play an important part in ethical decision making, since legal and ethical standards often develop within the same historical, cultural, and philosophical climates. Both relate to rights, and the law may

---

■ EXHIBIT 10–1. First ANA Suggested Code of Ethics (1926)

The Relation of the Nurse to the Patient

The nurse should bring to the care of the patient all of the knowledge, skill, and devotion that she may possess. To do this, she must appreciate the relationship of the patient to his family and to his community.

Therefore, the nurse must broaden her thoughtful consideration of the patient so that it will include his whole family and his friends, for only in surroundings harmonious and peaceful for the patient can the nurse give her utmost of the skill, devotion, and knowledge, which shall include the safeguarding of the health of those about the patient and the protection of property.

The Relation of the Nurse to the Medical Profession

The term "medicine" should be understood to refer to scientific medicine, and the desirable relationship between the two should be one of mutual respect. The nurse should be fully informed on the provisions of the medical practice act of her own state in order that she may not unconsciously support quackery and actual infringement of the law. The key to the situation lies in the mutuality of aim of medicine and nursing; the aims, to cure and prevent disease and promote positive health, are identical; the techniques of the two are different and neither profession can secure complete results without the other. The nurse should respect the physician as the person legally and professionally responsible for the medical and surgical treatment of the sick. She should endeavor to give such intelligent and skilled nursing service that she will be looked upon as a co-worker of the doctor in the whole field of health.

Under no circumstances, except in an emergency, is the nurse justified in instituting treatment.

The Relation of the Nurse to the Allied Professions

The health of the public has come to demand many services other than nursing. Without the closest interrelation of workers and appreciation of the ethical standards of all groups, and a clear understanding of the limitations of her own group, the best results in building positive health in the community cannot be obtained.

Relation of Nurse to Nurse

The "Golden Rule" embodies all that could be written in many pages on the relation of nurse to nurse. This should be one of fine loyalty, of appreciation for work conscientiously done, and of respect for positions of authority. On the other hand, loyalty to the motive which inspires nursing should make the nurse fearless to bring to light any serious violation to the ideals herein expressed; the larger loyalty is that to the community, for loyalty to an ideal is higher than any personal loyalty.

Relation of the Nurse to Her Profession

The nurse has a definite responsibility to her profession as a whole. The contribution of individual service is not enough. She should, in addition, give a reasonable portion of her time to the furtherance of such advancements of the profession as are only possible through action of the group as a whole. This involves attendance at meetings and the acquisition of information, at least sufficient for intelligent participation in such matters as organization and legislation.

The supreme responsibility of the nurse in relation to her profession is to keep alight that spiritual flame which has illumined the work of the great nurses of all time.

Source: Lyndia Flanagan, One Strong Voice: The Story of the American Nurses Association. Kansas City, MO: American Nurses Association, 1976, pp 89–91. Reprinted with permission.

codify these rights, but often the law takes a while to catch up with the need for certain kinds of ethical decisions, for example, disconnection of a ventilator when medical care is futile. Laws are rules of social conduct made by man to protect society and are chiefly concerned with fairness and justice.

The Subject Matter of Ethics

Ethics has several areas of inquiry: descriptive, normative, and metaethics. *Descriptive ethics* identifies, describes, and explains the phenomena of moral beliefs and behavior. The works of Kohlberg, Gilligan, and Notting on moral development are an example. Corley focuses on the ethical decision making of nurses in critical care. When does a situation qualify as a moral dilemma? Descriptive ethics is content.

Metaethics examines the nature of ethical inquiry itself. It gives us theories about ethics rather than theories for ethical conduct. Questions about the moral language of nursing would be well placed here. What is the meaning of advocacy, accountability, and cooperation? What is the relationship among ethical principles? Do we say an act is "right" because our society says so, or do we believe the act is right even if many members of society do not agree? Metaethics is process.

Normative ethics examines the standard of right and wrong. Theories and principles for human conduct are used to support one position or the other.

The coalescing of these forms of ethics inquiry yield a system of applied ethics.

> One might first use descriptive ethics to describe a moral phenomena (such as the protection of the patient from harm), then use normative ethics to argue for the moral accountability of the nurse . . . and finally use metaethics to explain the meaning of accountability within nursing practice. The results of this process could then be applied to a particular patient care situation.[9]

Moral Development

Kohlberg, structuring a theory of moral development, used the term stages for individual phases of moral thinking. In the 0, or premoral, stage, the individual does not understand the rules or feel a sense of obligation to them, acting only to experience that which is pleasant (good) or avoiding that which is painful (bad). In the preconventional level, stages 1 and 2, the individual's moral reasoning is based on reward and punishment

from those in authority. In the conventional level, stages 3 and 4, the expectations of the social group (family, community, nation) are supported and maintained. In the postconventional level, stages 5 and 6, the individual considers universal moral principles, which supersede the authority of groups. Kohlberg believes that most American adults function at stages 3 to 5, but moral maturity is gained at stage 6, when the individual makes up his or her own mind about what is right and wrong. Although the term *moral* is used in this analysis, there are those who interpret stage 6 as an "ethical orientation" because

> at this stage, morality is based on decisions of conscience, made in accordance with self-chosen principles of justice, which are comprehensive, universal, and consistent. These principles are abstract and ethical, rather than concrete moral rules.[10]

Although Kohlberg's theory is still used when discussing moral development, there is some disagreement with his approach, in part because

1. Actual actions of the subjects in the real world were not studied. They were asked to respond to hypothetical situations.

2. The moral dilemmas presented were limited, dealing with justice and fairness in terms of competition, property rights, right to life, and obligations.

3. His study was originally based on a sample of 50 men, but assumes that both men and women develop in the same way. Women were left at the third or fourth stage; men progressed to higher levels.

Gilligan was particularly disturbed that Kohlberg did not acknowledge the concerns and experience of women in moral development. She carried out a study designed to clarify the nature of women's moral judgment as they faced a real moral dilemma of whether to continue or abort a pregnancy. Results showed women do progress to the postconventional level, but that their moral judgment differs from that of men. For women, the worst problem was defined in terms of exercising care and avoiding hurt. The infliction of hurt was seen as selfish and immoral. "Women's moral judgment proceeded from initial concern for survival, to focus on goodness, to a principled understanding of care."[11]

Noddings' model, building on the work of Gilligan, is more recent and has been given considerable attention in nursing. She centers her ideas on the value of care and caring, stressing that caring is a relationship, not a unilateral activity. "The choice to enter a relationship as one caring . . . is grounded in a vision that we hold of our best selves," our "ethical ideal."[12] Noddings' moral theory would be well placed in the nursing curriculum to prepare nurses as more than "applied scientists."

Caring has been getting increased attention as a "value" on which nursing practice is based—a moral-ethical concept. It cannot be said to be only feminine, because men in nursing (and other fields) certainly embrace this concept as much or as little as women in the so-called caring professions. In one study, nurses seemed to feel that caring behaviors were their most important acts, whereas patients considered the technical aspects of their care more important. However, there is strong support for caring as an important value that is a constituent of moral reasoning.

Ethical Thinking

All ethical dilemmas are not solvable, but they are resolvable. Even where the choice is between two equally undesirable alternatives, taking no action may be worse than making a choice. With this in mind, there are three levels of decision making in solving ethical problems: (1) the immediate level, in which there is no time for reflection (the two men in cardiac arrest); (2) the intermediate level, in which there is some time for explanation and reflection (the woman with metastatic cancer); and (3) the deliberate level, in which there is enough time to get information and to think and consult to make a rational decision (the parents with the hereditary disease). The deliberate level of decision making is probably the most common.

Nurses involved in decision making need all the help they can get, because even the ethical problems that seem most easily resolved seldom are. The examples given earlier are indicative of the difficulties. There are a number of aids available. From a practical point of view, the guidance of an ethics consultant or ethics committee can help nurses think out the alternatives, along with others involved. A decision-making model also helps clarify thinking. The nursing code of ethics and its interpretive statements put the focus on the nurse's responsibility. Ethical theories and principles provide an overall background. There are many detailed descriptions of these approaches in the nursing and health care literature—ethics books and articles by the hundreds, some more readable than others. Interested nurses may find it useful to assemble an ethical library to which current articles can be added. The principles do remain the same, but discussions

of new problems and approaches (and there is always something new) can make a nurse more secure in her decision making.

■ THEORIES OF ETHICS

This section on the theories is only a brief overview. It is also important to remember that these are Western-oriented theories/principles.

One way to classify theories of ethics is as *consequential* or *nonconsequential*. The former claims that an action is right to the degree that it produces a good outcome and wrong when the consequences are poor. The latter maintains that certain acts are inherently right or wrong. *Utilitarianism* and *deontology* are common examples. Finally, *cultural relativism/pluralism* is presented because of our ethnic diversity in the United States where people draw on multiple value systems and varied ethical theories.

Utilitarianism (situational ethics) aims to produce the greatest balance of value over disvalue. It is based on the principles, "the greatest good for the greatest number" and "the ends justify the means." Utilitarianism may be further divided into act and rule utilitarianism. In rule, decisions on rightness are based on previous experience. With act, the rightness or wrongness of an act is determined by the presenting situation. In fact, the true utilitarian does not look to any rules, since each situation has to be judged on its merits. Utilitarianism is one example of a consequential theory.

Deontology (formalistic system) is ethical decision making based on unchanging rules and principles. The moral rightness or wrongness of an action is absolute and separated from any consequences of the decision. The deontological system is further divided into *rule* and *act*. Rule suggests that there are unchanging rules or standards for judging morally. Patients' Bill of Rights statements can take this tone. Whereas in act, the individual has great liberty to choose, but must decide in the same way for each similar situation. If it is expected that the nurse will discuss final directives with the patient immediately on admission, that would be done with every patient regardless of the patient's anxiety over the hospitalization. There would be no latitude for making exceptions in consideration of the atypical nature of this admission. Deontology is an example of a nonconsequential theory.

In *social or cultural relativism* what is ethical and what is unethical is determined by the customs, beliefs, and practices of a society or culture. In a clash between the requirements of a patient and the demands of one's culture, a nurse would choose the sentiments of the culture. In *pluralism*, there is recognition of the difficulty in making moral judgments across cultures. Culturally diverse societies reflect multiple moral standards, which may result in conflicting moral truths. Cultural pluralism does not rule out the possibility that a consensus on moral standards could emerge across cultures, even if no compatibility among those standards exists on the surface. It is important to note that ideas about what is moral are not arbitrary or subjective; they must be justified to be considered.[13]

■ ETHICAL PRINCIPLES

In every ethical dilemma there are one or more key principles that stand in the way of a decision—sometimes in conflict, at other times waiting to be appeased. The analytic work starts with identifying and understanding these relationships. Determining how these principles relate also allows the nurse and patient to interact on the basis of shared goals.[14] These are the resources without which no interpersonal agreement would be possible.

- *Autonomy* is the responsibility placed on the health care professional to accept the uniqueness of the person. It is recognition of the fact that a person's purposes cannot be abridged because the person does not agree with a certain social norm or clashes with those of the health care professional. There are times when a health care professional must act for a patient, but in these emergency situations, the patient has tacitly agreed to limited intervention. Health care professionals do nothing wrong if they remember that the situation is not a permanent emergency.

- *Justice* is the obligation to be fair to all people, to treat each equally regardless of race, sex, marital status, medical diagnosis, social standing, economic level, religious belief, or sexual preference. Another interpretation takes this a step further to define justice as equal rights for everyone and the greatest benefit given to the least advantaged. With this latter reasoning, people would be treated preferentially according to their need. This expanded interpretation is called *distributive justice*.

- *Freedom* derives directly from the standard of autonomy. A patient does not have to deliver the agency of his or her will to the doctor or nurse. Freedom not only recognizes an individual's right to be told about what will happen to him or her, but to consent, and further to take independent action based on the individual's evaluation of the present situation.

- *Veracity* means to deal with truth; to allow yourself to know the true nature of your patient; to be confronted with true ideas and to have freedom to choose to deal with them; to tell and be told the truth. The restriction would be when the telling of truth would harm the patient (*nonmalfeasance*).

- *Privacy* involves the right to be protected against intrusive contact from others.

- *Confidentiality* is the duty of health care providers to protect the secrecy of a patient's information, no matter how it is obtained. This is not to be confused with the legal standard of privileged communication, and there will be times when the law would have us break confidentiality.

- *Beneficence* speaks to the quality of interaction with the patient; the constant attitude of doing good toward those under your care; not demeaning the human status of your patients by violating their rights.

- *Nonmalfeasance* is in many ways the opposite of beneficence; the intent is to do no harm to your patients and to protect from harm those who cannot protect themselves (*justified paternalism*). From another perspective, it tells us to do no harm to our patients, either intentionally or unintentionally.

- *Fidelity* is faithfulness or loyalty to responsibility accepted as part of the practice of nursing. It is the basis for accountability.

- The *ideal observer* principle requires that a decision be made from a disinterested, dispassionate, consistent viewpoint, with full information available and consideration of future consequences. Although this approach can theoretically be applied to any ethical situation, the probable impossibility of any one person being able to do so might necessitate the involvement of other people, perhaps an ethics committee.

- *Standard of best interest/substituted judgment* involves making decisions on a patient's behalf when the patient is unable to participate. It is very important that you consider an individual's wishes, expressed either formally or informally. Unilateral decisions that disregard the patient's wishes are examples of paternalism.

- *Obligations* are demands made on all sectors of society to honor the rights of others. Obligations may be legal or moral.

- *Rights* are things due an individual according to just claims. One may claim something as a right that is really a privilege, a concession, or a freedom.

These principles, which have been presented very briefly, and others are often complex and sometimes appear more philosophical than practical. However, they provide a beginning framework for ethical decision making, whether the underlying theoretical orientation is relative or absolute.

■ CODES OF ETHICS

Another guide to ethical behavior is a professional *code of ethics*. In recent years, ethical behavior has been increasingly a topic of discussion in almost every field—business, politics, law, the academe, and perhaps most of all, health care. One symbol of this focus might be the new interest in codes of ethics. Codes of ethics, by whatever name, have been common in professions for some time. It is generally conceded that medicine was the first profession in the United States to adopt a code of ethics, but law, pharmacy, and veterinary medicine were also early comers. However, in the last several decades, one interesting phenomenon has occurred: ethics has become fashionable and codes have been newly adopted by organizations representing business and industry.

Both business journals and the popular literature have been commenting on business and industry's burgeoning acceptance of the need for ethical behavior (code or no code). In fact, they are being advised to police themselves before the government does it for them. Possibly the new outlook is at least partly a reaction to political and other scandals involving respectable people. Legislators, stimulated by public pressure, have increasingly incorporated aspects of ethical behavior into legislation, with legal penalties for violations.

In the history of ethical codes, there is almost no literature on how they should be written. There are striking differences in both the format and the content of various codes, and even more dramatic changes in the revisions dictated by social changes. Not just the American Medical Association (AMA) code, but also the ANA code, described later, are excellent examples of these contrasts. Moreover, in some fields, the codes are a highly important document; in others, the practitioners seem unaware of them.

Nevertheless, a code of ethics is considered an essential characteristic of a profession, providing one means whereby professional standards may be established, maintained, and

improved. It indicates the profession's acceptance of the trust and responsibility with which society has invested it. The public has granted the professionals certain privileges, with certain expectations in return.

In that context, professionals today need to look at their ethical codes in terms of whether they are focused on the consumer or are more inclined to emphasize professional etiquette—relationships within or across professional lines. For instance, in a previous AMA code, a statement about not associating professionally with anyone who does not practice a method of healing founded on a scientific basis was aimed at preventing, among other things, medical referrals to chiropractors. The Federal Trade Commission deemed this restraint of trade and no such statement is found in the current code. In fact, the most recent revision of the Code of Medical Ethics in 1995 was called "feisty, ornery, and even courageous" by bioethicist Arthur Caplan in an April 1995 article in *JAMA*. Among the points mentioned is "futile care": Patients should not be given treatments simply because they demand them if such treatment would be futile. The topics reviewed ranged from euthanasia and surrogacy to confidentiality, and were expected to raise some hackles in the medical community.

It is perhaps because of the influence of changing times that the self-serving aspects of ethical codes have diminished considerably over the last few years and recent revisions of most codes are beginning to show more concern for protecting society than protecting the profession.

Fry cites five objectives or purposes generally accepted for codes of ethics, all of which seem relevant to nursing codes:

1. To inspire members of the professional group to be ethical in their conduct

2. To sensitize members of the group to the moral aspects of their work

3. To enforce certain rules on the members of the group, thus defining the group's integrity and protecting its ethical standards of practice

4. To offer advice on resolving moral conflict

5. To indicate what the public might expect from a member of the professional group[15]

■ NURSING CODES OF ETHICS

The ANA Code of Ethics

Although Isabel Hampton Robb wrote a book on ethics and nursing practice at the turn of the twentieth century, and although there were columns on ethics in nursing journals, there was no formal code in early American nursing. In the early nursing literature, ethics appears to have been defined as Christian morality. There is some feeling that this was owed in part to the authoritarian milieu in which nursing existed. Nursing education valued obedience, submission to rules, social etiquette, and loyalty to the physician, instead of judgment, responsibility, and humanitarianism. What might have been a substitute for an ethical code, Lystra Gretter's Florence Nightingale Pledge (quoted in Chapter 3) illustrates the mixture of contemporary morality, ethics, and loyalty expected in 1893. In 1935, Mrs. Gretter revised the last paragraph of the pledge to read, "With loyalty will I aid the physician in his work, and as a 'missioner of health' I will dedicate myself to devoted service to human welfare." The Alumnae Association, Harper Hospital School of Nursing, Detroit, Michigan, copyrighted the 1935 version; the original is not copyrighted. It also appears to be based on the Hippocratic Oath, which was associated with physicians and supposedly drawn up at the time of Hippocrates to express the commitments of healing practitioners. You may be familiar with some of that oath's precepts:

> The regimen that I adopt shall be for the benefit of my patients according to my ability and judgment. . . . I will give no deadly drug to any. . . . Whatsoever things I see or hear concerning the life of men, in my attendance on the sick or even apart there from, which ought not be noised abroad, I will keep silence thereon, counting such things to be as sacred secrets.

The Nightingale Pledge is still recited or sung (as the *Nightingale Hymn*) by some graduating students of nursing, as some graduating physicians recite the Hippocratic Oath.

After several years of trying to decide between a pledge of conduct and a statement on the ideals of the nursing profession, in 1926, the ANA's relatively new Committee on Ethical Standards presented to the ANA House of Delegates a suggested code of ethics (Exhibit 10–1). The purpose was not to provide specific rules of conduct, but to create an awareness of ethical considerations. The code is a realistic reflection of the times, and comparison with succeeding codes illustrates that although certain basic precepts of ethical behavior may persist, codes are altered by the demands of the times and changing concepts of an emerging profession by the professionals. For instance, in the next decade, nurses' ethical concerns encompassed such diverse topics as "uniform requirements and outlining diabetic diets to a patient in the absence of a physician."[16] In 1940, a "Tentative Code," published in *AJN*, was not much different from the 1926 version. Even the more modern and first official Code for Nurses (1950) has been revised a number of times (1956, 1960, 1968, 1976, 2001, 2010) and shows the influence of societal changes. For instance, the 1950 code emphasized respect for the religious beliefs of patients; then, with the civil rights movement, the same statement was broadened to include "race, creed, color, or status"; and then it was enhanced further to stress human dignity and the "uniqueness of the client unrestricted by considerations of social or economic status, personal attributes, or the nature of health problems." (See Exhibit 10–2.) There is also decreasing emphasis on relationships with physicians and professional etiquette. The focus is on protection of the patient/client, and in this sense, it represents a transition to a real ethical code.

The interpretative statements to the Code are especially valuable because they not only enlarge on and explain the code in more detail, but also provide more focus and direction on how the nurse can carry out the code. The interpretative statements were revised in 1985, when the following statement was included that recognizes the changing tone of the nurse/client relationship:

> Clients should be as fully involved as possible in the planning and implementation of their own health care. Clients have the moral right to determine what will be done with their own person.[17]

The 2001 revision of the *Interpretative Statements* includes under each statement in the code a clinical or professional situation that is of particular relevance. Given the ethical pressures of the times, the Committee on Ethics has also felt the need to develop position papers and guidelines to address particular ethical situations with more specificity. The reader is referred to Exhibit 10–3 for a partial list. The position papers are quite detailed, with referral to ethical principles and past actions of the ANA. They include a definition of terms and references that are quite helpful in discussion of these issues. The full Code with interpretative statements and position statements are available through the ANA, including the ANA website, http://www. nursingworld.org.

Although the ANA code is, more or less, the basic nursing code of ethics, other nursing organizations have similar statements, somewhat more specific to the purpose of that organization, such as the specialty groups.

■ EXHIBIT 10–2. Code of Ethics for Nurses—American Nurses Association

1. The nurse, in all professional relationships, practices with compassion and respect for the inherent dignity, worth, and uniqueness of every individual, unrestricted by considerations of social or economic status, personal attributes, or the nature of health problems.

2. The nurse's primary commitment is to the patient, whether an individual, family, group, or community.

3. The nurse promotes, advocates for, and strives to protect the health, safety, and rights of the patient.

4. The nurse is responsible and accountable for individual nursing practice and determines the appropriate delegation of tasks consistent with the nurse's obligation to provide optimum patient care.

5. The nurse owes the same duties to self as to others, including the responsibility to preserve integrity and safety, to maintain competence, and to continue personal and professional growth.

6. The nurse participates in establishing, maintaining, and improving health care environments and conditions of employment conducive to the provision of quality health care and consistent with the values of the profession through individual and collective action.

7. The nurse participates in the advancement of the profession through contributions to practice, education, administration, and knowledge development.

8. The nurse collaborates with other health professionals and the public in promoting community, national, and international efforts to meet health needs.

9. The profession of nursing, as represented by associations and their members, is responsible for articulating nursing values, for maintaining the integrity of the profession and its practice, and for shaping social policy.

Source: American Nurses Association. *Code of Ethics for Nurses with Interpretive Statements*. Washington, DC: American Nurses Publishing, American Nurses Foundation/American Nurses Association, 2001.

■ EXHIBIT 10–3. Supportive Material for Ethical Decision Making, American Nurses Association

Ethical Issues Included in Interpretative Statement of the Code, 2001	Ethical Position Papers from the ANA
Right to self-determination	Promotion of comfort and relief of pain in dying patients
Primacy of patients' interests	Cultural diversity
Confidentiality	Foregoing artificial nutrition and hydration
Protecting participants in research	Nursing and do not resuscitate decisions
Addressing the impaired nurse	Nurses' participation in capital punishment
Delegating nursing activities	Nurses and patient self-determination acts
Moral self-respect	Risk versus responsibility in giving care
Environmental influences on ethical obligations	Using placebos for pain management in patients with cancer
Responsibility to the public	Assisted suicide
Intraprofessional integrity	Human cloning

Source: Fowler, M. *Guide to the Code of Ethics for Nurses*. Silver Springs, MD: ANA, 2010.

The ICN Code of Ethics for Nurses

In 1933, the International Council of Nurses (ICN) established an Ethics of Nursing Committee to study the method of teaching ethics in nursing, survey activities by national organizations relative to ethics, and collect data on ethical problems. From this evolved an ICN Code of Nursing Ethics that, after a long delay partially caused by World War II, was adopted in 1953 at a Grand Council meeting in Brazil. As might be expected, there was a major emphasis on nurses, not the nursing profession. Nurses were expected to recognize the limitations as well as the responsibilities of their roles, especially when it came to obeying doctors' orders. With slight revisions in 1965 at Frankfurt, the code was re-titled the Code of Ethics as Applied to Nursing, underlining the commonalities in all codes. Finally, at the 1973 meeting in Mexico City, the Council of National Representatives accepted some drastic revisions. It was considerably shorter than the 1965 code, and many of the statements appeared to be combined and reworded. It was presented to the ICN congress in an effort to enunciate concepts that would be clear, concise, universal, and broad enough to be useful to nurses in many cultures, but also able to stand the tests of time and social change.

The most recent revision of the ICN Code of Ethics was in 2006. (See Exhibit 10–4.) There are striking contrasts with earlier versions. Over the years, language has appeared that makes explicit the nurse's responsibility and accountability for nursing care, and statements have been deleted that ignored the nurse's judgment and showed dependency on the physician that nurses worldwide no longer see as appropriate.

Ethical Guidelines for Managed Care

A recent development is the publication of Ethical Guidelines for Professional Care and Services in a Managed Care Environment by the National Academies of Practice (NAP) in late 1998. The NAP includes academies of practice in dentistry, medicine, nursing, optometry, osteopathic medicine, pharmacy, pediatric medicine, psychology, social work, and veterinary medicine. The guidelines were presented to the President's (Clinton) Advisory Commission on Consumer Protection and Quality in the Health Care Industry, which subsequently authored *The Consumer Bill of Rights and Responsibilities*. This bill was never passed. The NAP Guidelines proclaim that "it is unethical to compromise a patient's needs and quality care concerns to satisfy financial objectives," "that the practitioner has an ethical obligation to present reasonably considered clinical options for care and services" regardless of economic restrictions, and that the "values of teaching and research, which are enduring in the advancement of science, must not be lost."[18]

Research Guidelines

When the ANA code was revised in 1968, the major change was the addition of a statement on the responsibilities of a nurse in research activities. Specific guidelines were delineated in the ANA publication, *The Nurse in Research: ANA Guidelines on Ethical Values*. The increasing participation of nurses in medical research as well as nurse-initiated research made this a timely statement. Among the points made, which are still pertinent, are that the nurse is expected to participate in a research or experimental activity only with the assurance that the project has the official sanction of a legally constituted research committee or other appropriate authority within the institutional or agency settings, and he or she must have sufficient knowledge of the research design to allow participation in an informed, effective, and ethical fashion. If the nurse sees conflicts or questions related to the well-being and safety of the patient, this concern must be voiced to the appropriate person in the institution. At all times, nurses remain responsible for their own acts and judgments.

The most recent ANA statement on the ethical issues of research, *Ethical Guidelines in the Conduct, Dissemination, and Implementation of Nursing Research*, published in 1995, is quite detailed. It delineates nine ethical principles that cover the classic ethical concerns in research. These include informed consent by subjects; prevention of harm; respect for the "personhood" of subjects and their families; ensuring that benefits and burdens of research are equitably distributed in the selection of subjects; protection of privacy; ensuring the ethical integrity of the research process; reporting scientific misconduct; maintaining competency in the subject matter and methodologies; and, if engaged in animal research, maximizing research benefits with the least possible harm to the animals.[19] The application of these principles is discussed in Chapter 22.

There have been a number of scandals that involve universities, physicians, and even governmental agencies concerning research done on prisoners, members of the military, the mentally retarded, or others who simply were not properly informed. Some caused serious harm; all violated patients' rights. When discovered, there was public outrage, usually followed by congressional hearings and

■ **EXHIBIT 10–4. International Council of Nurses' Code of Ethics for Nurses (2006)**

Preamble

Nurses have four fundamental responsibilities: to promote health, to prevent illness, to restore health, and to alleviate suffering. The need for nursing is universal.

Inherent in nursing is respect for human rights, including the right to life, to dignity, and to be treated with respect. Nursing care is unrestricted by considerations of age, color, creed, culture, disability or illness, gender, nationality, politics, race, or social status.

Nurses render health services to the individual, the family, and the community and coordinate their services with those of related groups.

The ICN Code

The ICN Code of Ethics for Nurses has four principal elements that outline the standards of ethical conduct.

1. *Nurses and people*

The nurse's primary professional responsibility is to people requiring nursing care. In providing care, the nurse promotes an environment in which the human rights, values, customs, and spiritual beliefs of the individual, family, and community are respected.

The nurse ensures that the individual receives sufficient information on which to base consent for care and related treatment.

The nurse holds in confidence personal information and uses judgment in sharing this information.

The nurse shares with society the responsibility for initiating and supporting actions to meet the health and social needs of the public, in particular those of vulnerable populations. The nurse also shares responsibility to sustain and protect the natural environment from depletion, pollution, degradation, and destruction.

2. *Nurses and practice*

The nurse carries personal responsibility and accountability for nursing practice, and for maintaining competence by continued learning.

The nurse maintains a standard of personal health care such that the ability to provide care is not compromised.

The nurse uses judgment regarding individual competence when accepting and delegating responsibility.

The nurse at all times maintains standards of personal conduct which reflect well on the profession and enhance public confidence.

The nurse, in providing care, ensures that the use of technology and scientific advances are compatible with the safety, dignity, and rights of people.

3. *Nurses and the profession*

The nurse assumes the major role in determining and implementing acceptable standards of clinical nursing practice, management, research, and education.

The nurse is active in developing a core of research-based professional knowledge.

The nurse, acting through the professional organization, participates in creating and maintaining equitable social and economic working conditions in nursing.

4. *Nurses and co-workers*

The nurse sustains a cooperative relationship with co-workers in nursing and other fields. The nurse takes appropriate action to safeguard individuals when their care is endangered by a co-worker or any other person.

The *ICN Code of Ethics for Nurses* is a guide for action based on social values and needs. It will have meaning only as a living document if applied to the realities of nursing and health care in a changing society.

Source: International Council of Nurses. http://www.icn.ch/icncode.pdf. Retrieved April 21, 2010.

legislation. Because nurses are also involved in research by physicians, they should be aware of changes in the rules regarding medical or drug research. For instance, the Food and Drug Administration (FDA) and National Institutes of Health (NIH) have released final rules that make it easier for promising experimental drugs and medical devices to be used on people in life-threatening situations who are unable to give informed consent or who do not have a legal representative present. The people (patients) may be enrolled in clinical trials without their consent, but there are a number of measures that must be fulfilled first, including that it must be agreed that the clinical trial addresses a life-threatening situation and other available treatments are not satisfactory.[20] Some ethicists strongly disapprove of these rules.

ETHICAL ISSUES IN NURSING

A recent study with a large sample of staff nurses asked, "What were your most frequently experienced ethical issues," and, "What are the ethical issues most personally disturbing to you?" The answers were as follows.

Those most frequently experienced are

- Protecting the patient's rights and human dignity
- Informed consent
- Providing care with possible risk to the nurse's health
- Staffing patterns that limit patient access to nursing care

Those ethical issues that are the most disturbing are

- Patients/families who are uninformed
- Prolonging the dying process with inappropriate measures
- Not considering the quality of the patient's life
- Implementing managed care policies that threaten the quality of care
- Working with unethical/impaired colleagues[21]

Increasingly, these issues have become subjects of legislation or court decisions but even this does not lessen potential conflicts in which nurses may find themselves. Not only must they confront the distinct possibility that their personal value systems may be different from that of the profession, but they are also caught in the value systems of their employing institutions.

Nurses have responsibilities to their patients regardless of their personal beliefs. For instance, nurses today are faced constantly with the need to make decisions about their roles in euthanasia or abortion. The decision for action may not be easy. However, one of the rights that health professionals have is to be free to choose not to participate in a procedure or activity against one's moral principles, provided that the patient is not abandoned. What is never allowable is to neglect or abuse (mentally, if not physically) patients about whom you have moral reservations,

such as homosexuals, criminals, alcoholics, or women having abortions. Clearly, this situation is intolerable and violates any professional code of ethics.

These actions, however, are taken on a personal level, and grossly unethical behavior is probably relatively rare. The conflicts nurses face often come from another source. Historically, nurses were seen as servants of physicians and were expected to be obedient and loyal to them (note the Nightingale Pledge). Even as times changed and ethical guides for nurses became less blatant in demanding loyalty at the price of harming the patient, the health care system still fostered the notion of loyalty to the employer and physician first. Thus, in some cases, when the nurse's ethical beliefs and standards conflict with the decisions made by physicians and/or administration, a way must be found to resolve the problem. Hamric writes about nurses occupying a unique position in the health care system. They are frequently in "the middle." This is both a resourceful and often a contentious place to be, in the middle between doctor and patient, family and patient, administration and patient, and so on. It is also a position that can hold some serious ethical challenges. Keep fidelity in mind when confronted with nurse-in-the-middle problems. Where does your allegiance lie?[22] One example is to provide a liaison between family and caregivers to clarify the patient's wishes, possibly in conjunction with a multidisciplinary ethics conference (discussed later).

Because so many ethical issues in health care have become legal issues, sometimes resulting in precedent-setting court decisions or in state or federal legislation, it is sometimes difficult to differentiate legal from ethical issues. In Chapter 22, the trail from ethics to law is made clear. However, both nurses and physicians are sometimes unclear as to whether certain actions are illegal, even if they themselves believe that the actions are ethical. Therefore, they may choose the more conservative path. This is particularly true in so-called right-to-die issues. In the case of contemporary health care, one person rarely makes decisions. The problem is not that health care professionals are insensitive, unfeeling, or driven by a "technological imperative," at least not most of them. Rather, the complexity of our systems can frustrate their ability to be as sensitive and compassionate as they would like to be.

End-of-Life Ethical Decisions: An Application

Ethics is plagued by misinformation and the inability to hear as well as listen. One of the surprising findings is the confusion of both house officers and nurses about the ethics and legalities of certain end-of-life decisions. Although most agreed that a patient could choose to refuse treatment, they felt that, once started, withdrawing treatment was unethical and probably illegal. Many also thought that nutritional support and hydration must always be given. These beliefs are in direct contradiction to most national and legal guidelines, including those published by their own professional organizations (see Chapter 22).

In relation to pain control, the vast majority believed "sometimes it is appropriate to give pain medication to relieve the patient's suffering even if it may hasten a patient's death," and that large quantities of narcotic analgesics may be given when the purpose is not to shorten patients' lives but to alleviate their suffering. Yet, many nurses believe that physicians give inadequate pain medication because they fear hastening a patient's death. Actually, both the medical and nursing literature find that inadequate pain management is a major issue in patient care, often because of insufficient knowledge about appropriate pain management and poor communication about pain between patients and providers.[23]

Some of these issues that seem to be creating confusion can be clarified when the patient makes a "living will," or as it is more commonly called now, an advance directive, which has legal approval in every state (see Chapter 22). However, most people, including health care providers, still do not have a living will, so if they are not able to speak for themselves, their unwritten wishes about terminating treatment, whatever that may be, could become a legal case, as the institution or physician attempts to get court permission to treat what they think is necessary.

It is true that sometimes the care provider or institution fears a lawsuit from family or even the patient, if the patient changes his or her mind, but more often, it is simply that years of medical education have trained physicians more to save lives than to consider the quality of life. Physicians, nurses, judges, and others may also have a moral belief that life is sacred, no matter what kind of life, so that fatally deformed newborns, the very old, and those with illnesses or accidents that are totally devastating to them are victims of someone else's moral beliefs. It is possible that, once more, the sheer visibility of such situations, often through the media, is making people more aware of the problems and forcing them to think through the issue for themselves and their loved ones. This is equally true of health professionals.

The do not resuscitate (DNR) order is another end-of-life decision. DNR means that "in event of cardiac or respiratory failure, no resuscitative efforts should be instituted," but that does not mean that any other care or interventions should be lessened.[24] The DNR should be a shared decision by the patient or surrogate and the physician, with the patient's decision being the ultimate determinant. The order should be written clearly and promptly by the physician, supported in the progress notes, and reviewed as needed. The Joint Commission requires an institutional policy to that effect.

Although this should be clearly understood, nurses cite DNR as a major problem for them. Why? Physicians and others do not like to speak about negative truths, and after all, a DNR implies that death will follow. Some patients and families also avoid the topic, although fewer than health providers think. Therefore, a variety of subterfuges are used. Unwritten orders are a special problem for the nurse. Some physicians believe, wrongly, that not writing a DNR or cloaking the intent with words such as "comfort nursing measures only" dispels any potential liability. Sometimes a slow code is understood or carried out by nurses when a terminally ill patient is not put on DNR. This means that a half-hearted effort at resuscitation is made. None of these approaches is ethically justified. They undermine the right patients have to be involved in their clinical decisions and violate the trust patients have in us to give our full effort. Again, the fear is that the doctor or hospital would be sued. Yet, this is completely unreasonable, because guidelines published by the AMA; the Hastings Center, which deals with ethical issues; and the ANA are clear about what is involved, including the fact that the patient's choices must be given priority or, if the patient is not competent, that of the surrogate. The DNR must be clearly ordered by the physician, documented, reviewed, and updated periodically (also a Joint Commission requirement). Other necessary care must continue to be given, and there must be mechanisms in place, preferably including the ethics committee, for resolution of disputes among health care professionals, patients, and/or families. If there is continuing disagreement about resuscitation, the case should be brought to court.[25]

It is also recommended that nurses be educated about various advance directives and themselves educate the family, and that they should be involved in developing DNR policies. Nurses who are morally opposed to carrying out DNRs should see about transferring the responsibility for that patient to another nurse.

One issue that is receiving considerable attention is the implementation of DNR orders in the operating room (OR). Because cardio-pulmonary resuscitation (CPR) was originally developed for use in the OR, carrying out a DNR order there may present an ethical difficulty for some. Many types of surgery provide palliative benefits to patients who either will not survive long term, or do not wish resuscitation in the OR. A patient with an esophageal obstruction from cancer might benefit from gastrostomy placement through reduced pain and improved nutritional status, yet not want CPR if cardiac arrest happens in the OR. Requiring such a patient to suspend their DNR orders to be a candidate for surgery uses their discomfort, pain, and desire to benefit from surgery to coerce them into accepting medical care (CPR) they do not want. Because arrests in the OR are often due to hemorrhage or medication effects rather than the patient's underlying disease, physicians may feel that their actions caused the arrest, and that they are ethically obliged to resuscitate the patient, even if the patient has clearly expressed wishes to the contrary. But competent patients, or their appropriate surrogates, have the right to refuse medical procedures and care, even if the care is to counteract the effects of previous medical intervention. Patient refusal of some medical therapy, such as CPR, does not ethically justify physicians denying them other medical therapy, such as surgery, that might benefit them.[26]

Because DNRs were originally intended for direction when an individual is in an institution, problems have arisen when, for instance, an emergency medical team has been called to a home because a person has stopped breathing. Varied out-of-hospital DNR orders exist from state to state. In some places, it is understood that these medics must make an attempt to resuscitate, because the DNR is not in effect outside the hospital. A nonhospital DNR has been developed. A physician must complete a form indicating that the person does not want to be resuscitated. That person may wear a bracelet or carry some sort of card that gives the DNR information and should also post the form prominently in the home. More than half of the states have enacted laws to provide for nonhospital DNR orders.

AIDS

AIDS, the modern world's new plague, has brought on new ethical dilemmas. One survey showed that AIDS patients were much more likely to have DNR orders than other patients with equally serious diseases. Some health professionals refuse to treat them or even interact with them. Although nurses have been applauded for the quality of personalized care they have given to AIDS patients, some studies have shown that the majority of nurses feel that nurses should have a right to refuse to care for AIDS patients, especially if the nurse is pregnant. The majority, also given the choice, would prefer not to care for AIDS patients. However, the reason appears to be fear of infection and death, not matters of morality or prejudice.[27] One of the ANA position papers on ethics states that in certain cases, the risk of harm to the nurse may outweigh the nurse's responsibility to patients; in other words, the nurse is not obligated to care for a patient who may endanger her or him, but the patient does get care from another nurse. Realistically, you have to question what value you are to an employer if you are ethically or physically unable to care for many categories of patients. The nurse might refuse an assignment because of safety considerations associated with pregnancy or personal health problems, but in most cases would be obligated to give care even when there is a dangerous disease condition.[28]

In addition, the issue of confidentiality is at the forefront here. It should be noted that AIDS is currently a reportable diagnosis in all 50 states. HIV positivity without the diagnosis of AIDS is reportable in 30 of 50 states.[29]

■ GUIDANCE IN ETHICAL DECISION MAKING

To make ethical decisions it is sometimes useful to use a structured format. A number of bioethical decision models have been presented over the years, and each ethics expert has a favorite, but most include the following steps or variations of them:

1. Identify the health problem.
2. List the relevant facts needed to understand the situation.
3. Identify the ethical problem or issues.
4. Determine who is involved in making the decision (the nurse, the doctor, the patient, the patient's family).
5. Identify your own role (quite possibly, your role may not require a decision at all).
6. Define your own moral/ethical position, the profession's (code of ethics), and, as much as possible, that of the key individuals involved.

7. Consider as many possible alternative decisions as you can.

8. Try to identify value conflicts.

9. Consider the long- and short-range consequences of each alternative decision.

10. Reach your decision and act on it.

11. Follow the situation until you can see the actual results of your decision and then evaluate it.

12. Use this information to help in making future decisions.

Referring to the ANA Code of Ethics will help you to understand how the philosophical concept is related to reality. No single model is appropriate for everyone, but they can help the decision-maker answer the questions needed for ethical decision making in specific situations. Having some educational background on the issues, including a course in which these frameworks are explained and used, is also important. Other aids in facing ethical dilemmas are consultation with an ethicist or ethical consultant; ethical rounds, which allows nurses to routinely review clinical questions and evaluate the presence of ethical concerns; and use of and/or involvement with multidisciplinary ethics committees. A particularly helpful resource is the Nursing Ethics Network, an online inquiry service of the World Wide Web. The address is

http://www.nursingethicsnetwork.org

Using the Nursing Code

The ANA Code of Ethics, like other professional codes, has no legal force, as opposed to the licensure laws promulgated by state boards of nursing (not the nurses' associations). However, the requirements of the code often exceed, but are never less than, the requirements of the law. Violations of the law may, of course, subject the nurse to civil or criminal penalties. Violations of the code should be reported to constituent member associations (CMAs) of the ANA, which may reprimand, censure, suspend, or expel members. Most CMAs have a procedure for considering reported violations that also gives the accused due process, and the ANA has a policy statement regarding methods. Even if the nurse is not a member of a CMA, an ethical violation, at the least, results in the loss of respect of colleagues and the public, which is a serious sanction. All nurses, whether or not they are CMA members, should be familiar with the profession's ethical code; there is a

professional obligation to uphold and adhere to the code and ensure that nursing colleagues do likewise.

Implementation of the code occurs at two levels. Nurses may be involved in resolving ethical issues on a broad policy level, participating with other groups in decision making to formulate guidelines or laws. But the more common situation is ethical decision making in daily practice, on a one-to-one basis, on issues that are probably not a matter of life and death but must be resolved on the spot by the nurse who faces them. Still, in clinical areas, such as intensive care units, there are life-and-death ethical issues that require decisions, and collaborating with colleagues in other disciplines is important.

The code, and particularly its interpretations, is useful as a guideline here, but nurses must recognize that in specific incidents, the reaction will be both intellectual and emotional, and will be strongly influenced by the nurse's cultural background, education, values, cognitive ability, and experience.

Ethics Committees

Ethics committees in one form or another have been in existence for about 35 years. In 1976, a New Jersey Supreme Court judge ordered a sort of internal ethics committee (actually more of a prognosis committee) to help institutions and physicians make decisions about situations such as the Karen Quinlan case, over which he presided. Karen had been in a PVS for some years and her family wanted to remove her respirator (this case is discussed further in Chapter 22). Although it was thought that such a mechanism would be quickly adopted, in 1983 a survey showed that less than 1 percent of all hospitals nationwide had established an ethics committee. Today, the majority has one, as well as an increasing number of long-term care (LTC) facilities. In 1991, the Joint Commission began to require that institutions have "a mechanism for the consideration of ethical issues arising in the care of patients and to provide education to caregivers and patients on ethical issues in health care." In 1993, the Joint Commission mandated the same for home health agencies.

The institution-wide ethics committee may or may not be integrated into the hospital's administrative structure, but the members usually include one or more nurse managers and staff nurses, one or more physicians, a therapist, a social worker, a member of the clergy, an attorney, an ethicist, and one or more representatives from the community. This multidisciplinary group, usually volunteers, forms a "community of concern" whose primary purpose is to serve patients and protect their interests. The functions of most committees are generally within the framework of those suggested by the prestigious President's Commission for the Study of Ethical Problems in Medicine and Biomedical and Behavioral Research in 1983. These are as follows:

1. They can review the case to confirm the responsible physician's diagnosis and prognosis of a patient's medical condition.

2. They can provide a forum for discussing broader social and ethical concerns raised by a particular case; such bodies may also have an educational role, especially by teaching all professional staff how to identify, frame, and resolve ethical problems. They can be a means for formulating policy and guidelines regarding such decisions.

3. Finally, they can review decisions made by others (such as physicians and surrogates) about the treatment of specific patients or make such decisions themselves.[30]

The commission noted that ethics committees have an important role in educating professionals about issues relevant to life support, but heads of these committees felt that this was not a particularly successful activity, perhaps because of the difficulty in getting staff, especially physicians, to attend lectures on this topic. The committees were also seen as providing a setting for people within medical institutions to become knowledgeable and comfortable about relating specific ethical principles to specific decisions, especially when real cases in the hospital were used as examples. There was also some concern that the case review function, that is, reviewing certain decisions made by the family of an incapacitated person and his or her practitioner, would be overutilized.[31] However, generally this is not so. Ethics committees have stayed away from these topics for several observable reasons: political (infringing on the authority of the physician), psychological (the difficulty a group might have in making life-and-death decisions), and cultural or intellectual (the differences in attitudes about certain ethical dilemmas).

From a practical point of view, the members of the committee, most of whom do not have training in ethics, should be educated themselves, perhaps by the ethicist or external experts. They are then in a better position to recommend or set policies for the institution (depending on what authority the committee is given). They will also be more knowledgeable when called on for consultation. One role that seems to be helpful is to provide a neutral forum for the discussion of difficult cases in which the nurses and others involved can talk out their concerns. The emotional support provided seems to be very helpful in alleviating the stress that usually accompanies difficult ethical situations. One important point is that staff nurses should be on the committee, because they are on the firing line. Unfortunately, there is some indication that this is not a given, and consequently there may be major disagreement between nurses and the committee about issues considered important. Some committees are seen as inadequate to address ethical issues. Too medically oriented, too theoretical, not knowledgeable, and too inactive are some of the complaints about them. Nevertheless, nurses are becoming more aggressive about their right to be on ethics committees, and their value as participants is quickly acknowledged when they are members. A good ethics committee has an important role in working out ethical problems. This is the "ideal observer" in some very complex situations.

However, because daily nursing practice problems, which may have ethical components, are not usually suitable for discussion in the institutional ethics committees, nursing ethics committees (NECs) have been established by a number of nursing departments. The functions of these committees include identifying, explaining, and resolving ethical issues in nursing practice; educating nurses in bioethics and nursing ethics; preparing nurses for interdisciplinary decision making regarding ethical issues; serving as a resource group; reviewing nursing ethics materials; reviewing departmental policies related to ethics; encouraging nursing ethics research; and preparing nurses to serve on institutional ethics committees.

■ THE ETHICS OF ACCESS AND QUALITY

Nurses have indicated that access to care is a concern, but this is not a problem that fits neatly into a decision-making model or ethics committee, although many have labeled it an ethical issue.

Experts in health care and health policy generally agree that ethical decision making will be of increasing concern in the coming years, and access to health care is already a major problem. Most of these experts may look with pride at the new technology, surgery, and drugs that can prolong life, but they are also forced to look at the cost and, sometimes, simple lack of availability. For instance, new technology has made possible heart, liver, and kidney transplants and new drugs that fight against organ rejection, but the organs are not readily available and surgery, aftercare, and drugs may run into the hundreds of thousands of dollars during a lifetime, if there even is an extended lifetime. Some people can afford it; health insurance covers others, at least partially, and still others get the attention of the media or powerful figures and receive donations and priority. What of the person who can do none of this? Should the public, through some sort of governmental subsidy, pay for extraordinary treatment if an individual cannot afford it? Or is it extraordinary? Under what circumstances should it be paid? Should age, potential quality of life, possibility of good outcome, ability of the individual and significant others to give proper follow-through care, or "worthiness" be considered? What of the simple primary care or any care that vast numbers of Americans cannot access?

If we say everyone should have equal access in an era of limited resources that will probably never change, what other funding should be cut? Education? Environment? Housing? Social service? Transportation? Civil rights? Drug enforcement? Police? Defense? Not only is the decision not a simple one, it is highly political. Every one of the other areas that exists primarily through public funding is important one way or another to the public's well-being. Every legislator has one or more constituencies that demand attention to their needs or wishes. Therefore, it is not surprising that legislative action is slow in coming, seldom satisfactory, and, unfortunately, hardly in effect before it is evident that the action taken does not go far enough or is already out of date. Moreover, the cost factor will undoubtedly increase, not decrease, as new, more expensive technology continues to develop.

So what happens? Except in rare instances, limits are set by default. In the case of health care, silent or not so silent, rationing is and has been in effect. Surveys have been taken that reveal primarily what people think they should say: Everyone should have equal access to the best possible health care. But when it comes down to how this would be paid for, there is considerable hesitation about making personal sacrifices. And, of course, the political ramifications are tremendous. An attempt early in the Clinton administration that looked toward a one-payment system that covered just about everyone, imperfect though it was, fell to political squabbling and a powerful advertising campaign by the insurance industry. Now, there are considerable data that the number of uninsured and underinsured, mostly the working poor, is growing—this despite patchwork legislative efforts.

Unequal access to health care is not a new phenomenon, so its current visibility may be owing to the unrelenting voices of advocates for the have nots, the slight possibility of the public having more of a social conscience, or the simple fact that it is quite evident that there are many who do not receive even basic care. (The reader is referred to Chapter 6.) Nevertheless, visibility does not guarantee solutions. What standards should be used to determine who gets what? There has been considerable discussion about age as a criterion, especially in terms of prolonging the life of an elderly patient. In part, this is because a large percentage of Medicare funds are used for life-prolonging care in the last few months of an elderly patient's life. (The fact that such a person may not wish such care, but is given no choice, is another issue.) Clearly it is not easy to use age as an indicator, particularly because of the changing demographics of the elderly. There was quite a furor when, in the late 1980s, Callahan, a director of the Hasting Center, suggested some background principles concerning care of the aged (those in their late 70s and 80s)—that medical care should no longer be oriented to resisting death.[32] However, there were some arguments that probably the majority of the aged preferred such a plan; what they feared was helplessness, pain, disability, and loss of mental alertness, that is, a deteriorating quality of life. Actually, there is some evidence that the suicide rate of the elderly is increasing, but also that some kind of rationing is already silently in effect as technology expands. For instance, there is the question of trauma care for the elderly. Trauma from accidents and falls is quite common, and care often does not have a good outcome. Does that mean that the expensive diagnostic and therapeutic activities that seem necessary should be eliminated?

But age is not the only factor in rationing care. A study covering 282 US metropolitan areas showed that income inequality was associated with increased mortality levels for almost all conditions, but especially in infant mortality.[33] Over the years, there have been similar reports regarding discrimination against minorities and women in relation to expensive treatments.

Other access issues involve transplants: who gets them when; when are risks to a healthy donor acceptable; should an irrevocably damaged newborn be kept alive artificially to harvest organs; should untried animal transplants be used on anyone; what about the use of tissues of an aborted fetus? Needless to say, feelings run high, and rational discussion is difficult.

One approach to managing scarce resources is managed care, sometimes defined as almost any alternative to traditional fee-for-service plans. Although the philosophy of managed care, often health maintenance organization (HMOs), is encouraging wellness, preventing illness, and eliminating unnecessary treatment, particularly expensive technology, the reality has turned out differently. There are complaints that individuals are denied needed diagnostic tests and treatments if they involve expensive drugs or equipment. Physicians often complain that the insurance company employees have taken over medical decision making. One major complaint is that high-priced and effective advertising entice people to join HMOs without full knowledge of what is involved, thus violating the ethical principle of informed consent. On the other hand, there is no question that the traditional fee-for-service system that reimbursed for just about anything, and the competition among hospitals that included providing expensive services and equipment, were fiscally out of control. Some major complaints seem to point at the for-profit sector, where there has been evidence of dumping patients, patient abuse, gag rules, and other manifestations of "dirty hands" that also drag in nurses who are afraid of losing their jobs. Piece by piece, each of these inadequacies in our system have been addressed by state and federal legislation.

What can be done? The anger of the public, as usual, has stirred talk, if not effective action in the Congress. In 1998, there was much discussion of a proposed Patient Bill of Rights aimed at managed care, which should guarantee appropriate care and benefits and access to specialists as necessary. However, as noted, the expected wrangling between Democrats and Republicans, not to mention the lobbying by those threatened by such a law, has prevented any finalization. The good news is that similar legislation has been passed in many states. The most vigorous activity for reform will occur at the state level. And on March 23, 2010, the president signed into law the Patient Protection and Affordable Care Act, as amended by the Health Care and Education Reconciliation Act of 2010 (together, the "Act"). The Act gives direction for federally mandated health care reform and aims for a veritable overhaul of the present system. (See Chapter 19 for specifics.) There are many good things in the bill, and others that are suspect to the public. The details of the Act will be worked out in the rule-making process.

Managed care, at first portrayed very negatively, has generated some positive responses and some real advantages to people, if properly implemented. The greater emphasis on low-tech care–oriented treatments is often a better approach, and, without question, rationing of care has always existed. Every time a unit is short staffed, nurses must make a decision about who gets how much care, and that, too, is rationing. Although all nurses may be affected to some extent, primary care nurses, especially advanced practice nurses (APNs), responsible to patients, physicians, and employers, are under particular pressure. But at the least, patients need to be fully informed of their options, including risks, benefits, and financial constraints, so that there is "justice with integrity." Still another concern, especially for nurse executives, is the reduction of professional staff to a level that might endanger patient care, but certainly limits high-quality care. However, the executive also has a responsibility to the institution to keep down costs. The ANA has long voiced concerns about the use of unlicensed personnel as a cost-savings mechanism that endangers quality care. Case managers who perhaps must limit services face similar ethical dilemmas.

There are also other service problems related to quality. Fraud and abuse have been given considerable attention in the media and by the federal government. This follows the Health Insurance Portability and Accountability Act (HIPAA) of 1996, which changed how the government investigates and punishes fraud and abuse in health care. In fact, there have been intensive governmental investigations and penalties involving some respected institutions. The Joint Commission has also moved toward action, requiring a "corporate compliance program" to detect, correct, and prevent fraud and abuse for those institutions and agencies seeking accreditation. There are many aspects to this, and nurses are involved in working with the new "compliance officer" to prevent and detect criminal activities.

All the points discussed, however briefly, are aspects of organizational ethics. As long as nurses work in organizations, they must be aware of the ethical issues that are an inevitable part of health care today. One of the major trends, health care mergers, which boards and executives may consider a necessary tactic for market advantage, indeed sometimes even survival, also raise questions of quality and safety. Unfortunately, nurses who may see themselves as powerless in these business decisions that cause them moral distress are not given easy answers. Perhaps one of the best approaches is to try to work out a way of dealing with the ethical/moral dilemmas. First of all, though, nurses must deal with ethical issues among their own colleagues.

■ NURSES AS PATIENT ADVOCATES

Over time, it appears that more and more often, nurses themselves, and others, have come to see nurses as natural patient advocates. In a sense, this has been manifested by the fact that long before the American Hospital Association (AHA) published its Patient's Bill of Rights (see Chapter 22), the National League for Nursing (NLN) drafted a statement on what the patient might expect from the nurse. (This was done at a time when no one told patients what their caregivers should be doing.) The statement coincided closely with the statements in the ANA Code for Nurses. Then in 1977, the NLN released a new document on patients' rights. Again, this clearly delineated nursing's support for patients' rights. Many of these statements are now law.

Patient advocate could be an employment position or simply individual action. Just what does it mean to be an advocate on an individual basis, officially or unofficially? In general, it means acting on behalf of a patient/client. It also includes the role of mediator, coordinating services and clarifying communication, and trying to resolve conflicting interests of patient and provider. The nurse advocate is also a protector of the patient's right to be actively involved in decision making related to his or her health. This means informing clients adequately so that they can make knowledgeable decisions and supporting their decisions even if you disagree. To do this job well, nurses need to understand the role and competing loyalties (the doctor and the employer), be recognized by others as an advocate (including the patient), have sufficient power, and recognize and be willing to deal with the fact that advocacy in a bureaucracy is bound to be controversial. The informal, often invisible coercion of the group, that the nurse or other employees face, is seen as a serious inhibition to whistle-blowing. It is not likely to be an easy role. Pointing a finger at nursing colleagues is not so simple.

A serious issue is the number of nurses impaired by dependence on drugs or other addictions. In the last few years, both state nurses' associations and individual employers have developed plans for helping these nurses, but also for protecting the public from them. In addition, responsibility is being taken in dealing with incompetent nurses.

The Nursing Practice Act lists substance abuse under unprofessional conduct, which are grounds for disciplinary action. However, the trend now is to try to help the nurse. Journal articles describe behaviors indicative of substance abuse, including alcohol. The need to report such behavior, going up the institution's communication chain as necessary, is mandated; however, there are options for the addicted nurse. A program is generally available, sometimes through the institution or the SNA, and the nurse is assisted in overcoming the addiction.

Those who choose not to be helped must be reported to the nursing board. There are also peer assistance programs that are generally seen as successful for the majority of impaired nurses. Unfortunately, drinking and other substance abuse problems seem to be prevalent among nursing students as well, and faculty must follow a similar process to get the students help and protect the public. The process of recovery is devastating to the nurses, but it is also important to public safety.

Equally significant to the public is the issue of academic dishonesty, which is considered a serious problem with students today in both the classroom and the clinical setting. With students, there is particular concern because lack of academic integrity might also be a prediction of behavior as a graduate. Would students who lie about the care they did or did not provide to a patient because of how the incident would affect their grade also continue to lie about errors made as an RN to avoid a problem—errors that might endanger a patient's life? There is speculation that the increase in student dishonesty in higher education is owed in part to changing mores and a less honest society, but in a helping profession, dishonesty is dangerous, not just unethical. It might be that there is also academic or professional dishonesty among highly educated health professionals in their reported research and publications— not good role models for younger colleagues.

In all of these situations, as well as situations where other health professions or the employing institution are engaged in unethical conduct, the question arises: Should you be the whistle-blower? Unfortunately, the whistle-blower may suffer consequences—for instance, loosing a job, even with built-in legislative protection. This is particularly likely if the ethical issue has to do with unsafe care, perhaps owing to insufficient staffing. Still, this is a matter of patient advocacy. A suggested procedure is

1. Be personally above reproach.

2. Document the act of misconduct and seek support from others who have witnessed it.

3. Follow the identified hierarchy for communication concerns about misconduct and maintain documentation of communications.

4. Be open to advice and be persistent while exhausting all possible institutional options.

5. At this point, make a public complaint if no action has been taken. Complaints may be made to state professional regulatory boards or professional groups. Go to newspapers if necessary for the public's safety.

There *should* be a work environment that is willing to follow through on legitimate complaints. That may be one aspect of the corporate compliance officer's responsibility. Many states protect whistle-blowers. Still, it is risky to go public: If at all possible, the best and most collegial approach is to work within the institution. If this reaches a dead end, perhaps the next question the nurse faces is, "Do I really want to work in such an environment?"

Unlike personal ethical conflicts, these are real dilemmas that may have serious economic repercussions for the nurse, and it is quite possible that a nurse cannot resolve them alone. Instead, nursing must develop a support system for individual nurses who experience conflict in the employment setting with respect to implementation of the Code of Ethics. The precepts of the code must be widely publicized so that not only nurses, but also the public and others in health care, understand the ethical basis of nursing practice. Nurses may also turn to the ANA's Center for Ethics and Human Rights, which provides practical guidance. With the power of the profession behind them, nurses are in a much better position to face and resolve ethical issues.

7. Cultural pluralism does not rule out the possibility that a consensus on moral standards could emerge across cultures, even if no compatibility among those standards exists on face value.

8. Ethical principles are the underpinnings of every ethical dilemma regardless of theoretical orientation: autonomy, justice, freedom, veracity, privacy, confidentiality, beneficence, nonmalfeasance, fidelity, the ideal observer, best interest, obligations, and rights.

9. The ANA and ICN codes of ethics have changed over the years to reflect the increasing autonomy of the consumer and the growing professionalism of nursing.

10. Ethical decision making is a skill that can be learned through study and practice.

11. It is important to use an ethical decision-making framework in patient care situations.

12. Great ethical controversy is associated with end-of-life decisions.

13. Virtually all hospitals and many nursing homes have ethics committees.

KEY POINTS

1. Morality is a personal standard of conduct, whereas ethics is the reasoned analysis and disciplined inquiry of relationships underlying the moral code.

2. The ANA Code of Ethics is the moral code of the profession; Interpretative Statements are the ethical principles that give additional substance.

3. Kohlberg, Gilligan, and Noddings give us different perspectives on moral development.

4. Most of our ethical decision making is deliberate, allowing enough time for rational, measured decisions.

5. Three common theories of ethics are utilitarianism, deontology, and cultural relativism/pluralism.

6. Utilitarianism is oriented to consequences without any established rules; deontology is based on established rules without consideration of the consequences.

REFERENCES

1. Rushton C, Scanlon C. When values conflict with obligations: Safeguards for nurses. *Ped Nurs* 21:260, May–June 1995.

2. Fry S, Riley J. *Ethical Issues in Clinical Practice: A Multi-State Study of Practicing Registered Nurses.* http://www.nursingethicsnetwork.org. Retrieved June 15, 2002.

3. Corley M. Ethical work environment, nurse moral distress, and patient satisfaction with participation in treatment decision-making (poster presentation). *Proceedings of the Academy for Health Services Research Annual Meeting.* San Francisco, CA, June 26, 2000.

4. Dinkins C, Sorrell J. Ethics: The expanding circle of environmental ethics. *On-line Journal of Issues in Nursing.* November 30, 2007. http://www.nursingworld.org/MainMenuCategories/ANAMarketplace/ANAPeriodicals/OJIN/Columns/Ethics/EnvironmentalEthics.aspx. Retrieved April 20, 2010.

5. Fox E, Crigger B, Bottrell M, Bauck P. Ethical Leadership: Fostering an Ethical Environment and Culture. Washington, DC: The Veteran's Administration, 2008. www.ethics.va.gov/IntegratedEthics. Retrieved April 10, 2010.

6. Ibid.

7. Oermann M. *Professional Nursing Practice*. Stamford, CT: Appleton & Lange, 1997.

8. Benjamin M, Curtis J. *Ethics in Nursing*, 2nd ed. New York: Oxford University Press, 1986, p 11.

9. Fry S. *Ethics in Nursing Practice*. Geneva: The International Council of Nurses, 1994, pp 22–23.

10. Krowczyk R, Kudzma E. Ethics: A matter of moral development. *Nurs Outlook* 26:255, April 1978.

11. Gilligan C. *In a Different Voice*. Cambridge, MA: Harvard University Press, 1982.

12. Noddings N. *Caring, A Feminine Approach to Ethics and Moral Development*. Berkeley: University of California Press, 1984, p 45.

13. Volbrecht R. *Nursing Ethics*. Upper Saddle River, NJ: Prentice Hall, 2002, pp 12–13.

14. Husted J, Husted G. *Ethical Decision-Making in Nursing and Health Care*. New York: Springer, 2007.

15. Fry, op cit, p 70.

16. Flanagan L. *One Strong Voice*. Kansas City, MO: American Nurses Association, 1976, pp 88-91.

17. *Code of Ethics with Interpretative Statements*. Washington, DC: American Nurses Publishing, 1985.

18. President's Advisory Commission on Consumer Protection and Quality in the Health Care Industry. Consumer Bill of Rights and Responsibilities. http://www.hcquality commission.gov. Retrieved November 1, 2002.

19. Silva M. *Ethical Guidelines in the Conduct, Dissemination, and Implementation of Nursing Research*. Washington, DC: American Nurses Publishing, 1995.

20. Minkoff H, Marshall M. Government-Scripted Consent: When Medical Ethics and Law Collide. *The Hasting Center Report*, 40:2, March–April 2010. http://www.the-hastingscenter.org/Publications/HCR/Detail.aspx?id= 3878&terms=human+consent+and+%23filename+*.htm l. Retrieved April 20, 2010.

21. Fry S, Riley J. Ethical Issues in Clinical Practice. http://www.nursingethicsnetwork.org. Retrieved June 20, 2002.

22. Hamric A. Reflections on being in the middle. *Nurs Outlook* 49:254–256, November–December 2001.

23. Fohr S. The double effect of pain medication: Separating myth from reality. *International Association for Hospice and Palliative Care*. http://www.hospicecare.com/Ethics/fohrdoc.htm. Retrieved April 10, 2010.

24. University of Washington School of Medicine. Do Not Resuscitate Orders. http://depts.washington.edu/bioethx/topics/dnr.html#nobene. Retrieved April 10, 2010.

25. Ibid.

26. University of Washington School of Medicine. Do Not Resuscitate Orders during Anesthesia and Urgent Procedures. http://depts.washington.edu/bioethx/topics/dnrau.html. Retrieved April 2, 2010.

27. Demmer C. AIDS attitudes and attitudes toward caring for dying patients. *Death Stud* 23(5):433–442, July–August 1999.

28. Kearney R. *Advancing Your Career*, 2nd ed. Philadelphia: FA Davis, 2001, p 313.

29. *HIV and AIDS. Ethics in Medicine*. University of Washington, February 17, 2000. http://depts.washington.edu/bioethx/topics/dnrau.html. Retrieved April 10, 2010.

30. President's Commission for the Study of Ethical Problems in Medicine and Biomedical Research. *Deciding to Forego Life-Sustaining Treatment*. Washington, DC: The Commission, 1983, pp 160–161.

31. Ibid.

32. Callahan D. *Setting Limits: Medical Goals in an Aging Society*. New York: Simon & Schuster, 1987.

33. The Office of Minority Health. African American Profile. http://minorityhealth.hhs.gov/templates/browse.aspx?lvl=2&lvlID=51. Retrieved April 18, 2010.

Updates can be found at **www.kellysnursing.com**

CHAPTER 11

Profile of the Modern Nurse

Who are today's nurses? Where do they work? How do they differ from the nurses of 10 or 20 years ago? What are their personality characteristics and attitudes? What is the public image of the nurse? Unfortunately, many studies on these topics have been based on small sample sizes, been conducted by graduate students, or are limited in scope. Thus, comparisons were difficult. Recently, the image issue has received renewed attention. This is partially owing to the concern over the nursing shortage, and the notion that problems in recruitment stemmed from nursing's poor public image.

The oldest continuing study on the characteristics of nursing is the *National Sample Survey of Registered Nurses* (NSSRN) conducted by the Division of Nursing of the US Department of Health and Human Services (DHHS). The sample survey was first conducted in September 1977, and was repeated in November 1980 and 1984, and in March 1988, 1992, 1996, 2000, 2004, and 2008. Nursing is also included in a periodic report to Congress by the DHHS on the status of *Health Personnel in the United States.* In contrast to the sample survey, the report to Congress deals with supply, distribution, and future projections for health personnel.

National nursing associations provide other useful information. The National League for Nursing (NLN), American Association of Colleges of Nursing (AACN), National Council of State Board of Nursing (NCSBN), and the American Nurses Association (ANA) are particularly rich in the databases they share. Industry interest groups regularly conduct surveys on the presence of nurses in specific health care settings. One example is the *Hospital Nursing Personnel Survey* conducted annually by the American Hospital Association (AHA). A variety of opinion polls and surveys of nurses have also been done around topics such as employment conditions, job satisfaction, wage and salary trends, and attitudes on public policy, most especially health care reform.

A very significant trend, beginning in earnest in 1985, has been the effort to identify consumer attitudes toward nurses and monitor these sentiments over time. Between 1985 and 2010, several well-conceived and well-executed public opinion surveys were completed. There are also noteworthy differences between the public image of the nurse and reality. This has always been true. When Dickens wrote about the slovenly Sairey Gamp, dedicated women were functioning as nurses. Even the British newspapers' glowing reports of Florence Nightingale as the gentle lady with the lamp overlooked her tough and efficient administrative stance, which had a large part in providing better care for soldiers in the Crimean War. Indeed, major national nursing organizations found the public image of the nurse so detrimental that in 1989, the National Commission on Nursing Implementation Project (NCNIP) and the Ad Council launched a 3-year public service campaign aimed at improving the image of the nurse. The Johnson and Johnson Corporation funded another such initiative in 2002 in an effort to increase recruitment and retention to the profession. This has resulted in a very rich website with links to many other nursing organizations. Salary information and basics about the work of nursing can be accessed there at

http://www.discovernursing.com

This chapter, in building a profile of the modern nurse (and student), will deal with three major areas: demographic data, attitudes of and about nurses, and the nurse as seen by the public. Comparisons to previous data are made when useful. Obviously, it is necessary to present only a synopsis of the available data, but both the references and the bibliography will provide useful follow-up. Additional data about today's nurses are also incorporated into Chapters 5, 9, and 15.

■ GENERAL DEMOGRAPHIC DATA

The most current, general, comprehensive demographic data about nurses come out of the Division of Nursing of the DHHS. The most recent published report was released in March 2010 and reports data from the National Sample Survey of Registered Nurses conducted in 2008. Exhibit 11–1 summarizes data from the 2008 sample survey and includes comparisons with the 1980, 1988, 1992, 1996, 2000, and 2004 surveys. There are easily discernible trends. In March 2008, an estimated 3,063,163 individuals were licensed to practice nursing in this country, 5.3 percent more than in 2004, and over 68 percent more than in 1980. This produced a ratio of 854 registered nurses (RNs) for every 100,000 people, although there were state-to-state variations. Utah has the fewest with 598 RNs for every 100,000 people; the District of Columbia has the most with 1868 per 100,000. Most RNs are actively practicing nursing (84.8 percent—the highest in the history of the survey) and most are working full time (63.2 percent vs. 58.4 percent in 2004—the first increase since 1996).[1]

White, non-Hispanics are 65.6 percent of the US population, yet comprise 83.2 percent of licensed RNs, a decrease of 4.3 percent since 2004. The next largest group is Asians, Native Hawaiians, and Pacific Islanders (non-Hispanic) who are 5.8 percent of the RN population and 4.5 percent of the US population. African Americans (non-Hispanic) are 5.4 percent of RNs and 12.2 percent of the US population, and Hispanics/Latinos of any race are 3.6 percent of RNs and 15.4 percent of the US population. Women outnumber men by more than 15 to 1 in the overall number of RNs, but among those who became RNs after 1990, there is one male RN for every 10 women.

The "aging" of the RN population continues. In 2008, the average age of RNs was 47, as compared with 46.8 in 2004. This represents some stabilization after many years of increasing average age. However, almost 45 percent of RNs were 50 years of age or older in 2008, a dramatic increase from 33 percent in 2000 and 25 percent in 1980.

In contrast, the number of RNs younger than 40 showed an increase, comprising 29.5 percent of all RNs in 2008. This may indicate a growing appeal for the field from young career choosers, or an outreach for security through a field that has proven to be relatively recession-proof. From a less optimistic viewpoint, the aging trend among RNs raises concerns that future retirements could substantially reduce the size of the US nursing workforce at the same time that the general population is growing and the proportion who are elderly is increasing, raising the demand for health care and nursing services across the nation.

In 2008, half of the RN population had a baccalaureate or higher degree in nursing or a nursing-related field, while the other half's highest education level was a diploma or associate degree. Over 45 percent of RNs claimed that their initial nursing program was an associate degree, an increase from 2004; 33.7 percent claimed baccalaureate entry preparation, and 20.4 percent identified diploma entry into practice. However, 32 percent of RNs with a baccalaureate or higher degree reported that their initial RN education was a diploma or associate degree. Nurses are recognizing the need for education as a vehicle to upward mobility in the profession. For many, the associate degree has become a stepladder to higher education. The decline of diploma education continues, the ongoing trend having begun in 1980.

Nurses with advanced degrees, the master's and doctorate, comprised 13.2 percent of all licensed RNs in 2008, a 46.9 percent increase from 2004. The estimated 28,369 RNs with a doctoral degree in 2008 represented a 64.4 percent increase over 2000. The functional roles of teaching, administration, and management are no longer the primary focus of graduate education. The science of nursing has developed to the point where there is growing public recognition for advanced practice. Further, the salaries in advanced practice have outpaced teaching. Schools of medicine and law have retained faculty by basing their salaries on the market and supplementing their earnings through faculty practice opportunities. Nursing has not followed suit. But nurses are recognizing that doctoral preparation is necessary for credibility in higher education, and there is a growing market for nurse researchers in business and industry, health care organizations, and more. Our educational pathways and preferences are a sign of our maturation as a profession. More negatively, 9500 qualified applicants to master's and doctoral degree programs had to be turned away in 2009 due to shortages in resources.[2]

	2008	2004	2000	1996	1992	1988	1980
Total RN population	3 million	2.9 million	2.7 million	2.5 million	2.2 million	2.0 million	1.7 million
Employed in nursing[a]	84.8%	83%	81.7%	82.7%	82.7%	80.0%	76.6%
	(about 21.5 part-time)	(about 24% part-time)	(about 28.4% part-time)	(about 23.7% part-time)	(about 25.7% part-time)	(about 26% part-time)	(about 24.6% part-time)
Sex (%)							
Female	94.4	94.2	94.6	95.1	96.0	96.6	96.1
Male	6.6	5.8	5.4	4.9	4.0	3.3	3.0
Ethnic/racial background (%)							
White/non-Hispanic	83.2	81.8	86.6	89.7	91.1	91.7	90.4
Black/African American	5.4	4.2	4.9	4.2	4.0	3.6	4.3
Asian/Pacific Islander	5.5	3.1	3.7	3.4	3.4	2.3	2.4
Hispanic	3.6	1.7	2.0	1.6	1.4	1.3	1.4
American Indian/Alaskan native	0.8	0.3	0.5	0.5	0.4	0.4	0.28
Age (%)							
Under 25	2.6	2.1	2.5	2.3	2.1	3.9	9.6
25–34	16	14.3	15.8	18.3	23.6	29.8	36.2
35–44	22.2	24.0	30.6	34.4	34.7	29.5	23.3
45–54	30.6	33.4	29.9	25.1	20.6	19.1	17.2
55–64	21.1	18.8	14.6	13.7	12.7	12.3	15.7
65 or over	7.5	6.4	5.7	5.7	5.6	5.0	4.5
Marital status (%)							
Married	74.0	70.5	71.5	72.3	71.5	70.6	70.6
Divorced, separated, widowed		18.1	17.9	17.6	16.5	15.4	13.8
Never married		9.2	9.9	9.8	11.1	13.0	14.8
Places of employment (%)							
Hospital	62.2	56.2	59.1	60.1	66.5	67.9	65.6
Nursing home	5.3	6.3	6.9	8.1	7.0	6.6	8.0
Public/community health/home health	14.4	10.7 (14.8) (includes occupational & student health)	12.8	13.1	9.7	6.8	6.6

EXHIBIT 11–1. Who Are the Nurses?[a]

	2008	2004	2000	1996	1992	1988	1980
Ambulatory care (including physician's offices)	10.5	11.5	9.5	8.5	7.8	7.7	5.7[b]
Nursing education	3.8	2.6	2.1	2.3	2.0	1.8	3.7
Student health service			4.7	3.0	2.7	2.9	3.5
Occupational health			2.1	1.0	1.9	1.3	2.3
Private duty				N/A	0.6	1.2	1.6
Public/community health (includes occupational and school health)	7.8		18.2				
Type of position (%)							
Staff nurse	66.3	59.1	61.6	61.9	61.6	66.9	65.0
Head nurse/supervisor	14.6 (includes admin.)	9.2	8.4	10.3	9.6	10.9	13.1
Administration (service and education)		5.2	5.7	5.3	6.2	6.6	4.8
Instructor	2.6	2.6	2.1	3.5	3.5	3.8	4.7
Clinical specialist/clinician	1.2		2.0	3.1	1.9	2.9	2.1
Nurse practitioner/midwife							
Midwife	3.8	0.3	3.6	2.1	1.4	1.5	1.3
Nurse anesthetist	1.1	1.1	1.1	1.0	1.0	1.0	1.1
Nurse practitioner/clinical nurse specialist		6.0					
Nurse practitioner		3.5	0.54				
Clinical nurse specialist		1.2					
Other				10.0	6.5	6.6	6.8
Highest level of education (%)							
Doctorate	13.2 (masters and doctorates)	13.0	10.2 (masters and doctorates)	0.6	0.5	0.3	0.2
Master's				9.1	7.5	6.2	5.1
Bachelors in nursing	36.8	34.2	32.7	28.8	27.3	25.1	20.7
Other bachelors				2.5	2.6	2.3	2.6
Diploma	13.9	17.5	22.3	27.2	33.7	40.4	50.7
Associate degree	36.1	33.7	34.3	31.7	28.2	25.2	20.1

[a]Data refer to employed nurses. Some figures do not total 100% because of no response and rounding of figures.
[b]Refers to physician's office only.
Source: DHHS Division of Nursing. *National Sample Survey of Registered Nurses, 1980, 1988, 1992, 1996, 2000, 2004, 2008.*

Hospitals remain the most common employment setting for RNs in the United States, with 62.2 percent of employed RNs reporting that they worked in hospitals in 2008. In 2004, 56.2 percent of RNs worked in hospitals. An estimated 10.8 percent of hospital-employed RNs worked in outpatient clinics or medical practices in community or specialty hospitals, while 1.5 percent worked in long-term hospitals, and 2 percent in psychiatric hospitals. The increase in the share of RNs working in hospitals between 2004 and 2008 is the first increase since 1984, when 68.1 percent of RNs worked in hospitals. The growth in the number of RNs estimated to be hospital employees is 17.7 percent and is consistent with data reported by the American Hospital Association (AHA), which reported that between 2004 and 2008, RN full-time equivalent (FTE) employment increased 16.6 percent.[3] It is interesting to speculate whether this increase is due to a growing public awareness that patient safety and efficacy in hospitals is associated with the level of RN staffing.[4] There also was a modest increase in the number of RNs working in home health agencies. The increase in home health nurses was from 3.8 percent in 2004 to 6.4 percent in 2008. Other changes in employment settings were negligible. It is difficult to interpret these statistics given that the workplace categories in the Sample Survey have been modified and reorganized on several occasions. Additionally, the frequency of health care services and consequently the employment of nurses are driven by reimbursement. Home care is a good example. Home care nursing services have been predicted to skyrocket given the portability of technology and pressure for early discharge from hospitals, but growth has been nominal. A recent edition of the *Wall Street Journal* shows an overall decline in home visits to Medicare recipients of 32 percent from 1998 to 2008. This reflects a decline of 16 percent for skilled nursing visits and a 57 percent decrease in social work visits, while occupational therapy (OT) and physical therapy (PT) visits have increased 74 and 51 percent, respectively. Both OT and PT have been allocated special fee incentives for therapy visits under PPS.[5]

Average annual earnings for RNs employed full-time were $66,973 in 2008, rising 15.9 percent since the 2004 average of $57,785. When annual earnings are adjusted for inflation using the Consumer Price Index (CPI), earnings in 2008 were $26,826, which is only a 1.7 percent increase from average real (inflation-adjusted) 2004 earnings of $26,366. Thus, growth in earnings of full-time RNs between 2004 and 2008 only slightly outpaced inflation.

In 2008, an estimated 170,235 RNs living in the United States received their initial nursing education in another country or a US territory, comprising 5.6 percent of the US nursing population compared with 3.7 percent in 2004. About half of internationally educated RNs living in the United States in 2008 were from the Philippines (48.7 percent). The other half were predominately from Canada (11.5 percent), India (9.3 percent), the United Kingdom (5.8 percent), US Territories (2.8 percent), Korea (2.6 percent), and Nigeria (2.0 percent). This is in keeping with the US immigration laws to provide access to employment opportunities to nurses from the global community. The continued access for graduates of foreign nursing schools will depend on the future nature of immigration policies, which are stalled in Congress.

The advanced specialties reported through the NSSRN include nurse practitioners, nurse midwives, nurse anesthetists, and clinical nurse specialists. Requirements to practice vary from state to state and over time. Most states require recognition by either a state regulatory agency or national certifying organization for a nurse to function in advanced practice. This analysis focused on nurses who have ever been prepared in an advanced specialty, regardless of whether they presently hold a certification. In 2008, an estimated 250,527 RNs reported that they were prepared as an advanced practice nurse in one or more advanced specialties or practice areas, an increase of 4.2 percent over 2004, when there were 240,460 prepared for advanced practice. Nurse practitioners comprised 63.2 percent of nurses in advanced practice in 2008. The number of nurse practitioners grew 12.1 percent since 2004. Of these nurse practitioners, over 19,000 were prepared as both a nurse practitioner and either a clinical nurse specialist or a nurse midwife. There were an estimated 18,492 nurses prepared as nurse midwives in 2008, representing a 35.1 percent increase from the 13,684 in 2004. There was a modest 7.1 percent growth in the number of nurse anesthetists between 2004 and 2008, from 32,523 to 34,821. There was a decline among the ranks of clinical nurse specialists between the two surveys, from an estimated 59,242 compared with 72,521 in 2004—a drop of 22.4 percent.

■ MINORITY GROUPS IN NURSING

Studies on the general population of nursing students and graduates are inevitably influenced by the fact that the majority of nurses are both women and white. There is increasing interest in nursing among minority groups, such as blacks, Native Americans, Hispanics, and men.

Nursing recruitment for all ethnic minorities has gradually become more successful, stimulated particularly by federal grants available since 1965. However, despite these efforts, and although there has been an increase in the number of ethnic minorities, their proportion among employed RNs has not shown remarkable gain (see Exhibit 11–1). White/non-Hispanics were 83.2 percent of the RN population in 2008. There are many real and perceived financial and cultural barriers that impede recruitment and retention of minority students to nursing. One of the most serious may be the shortage of role models among faculty and leaders in nursing service for minority students to emulate.

There has been a slow and arduous increase in minority enrollment in basic nursing education programs over the past years. Minority enrollment accounted for 18 percent of students in 2002, 18.2 in 2003, 20.6 in 2004, 24.1 in 2006, 25.2 in 2008, and 26.3 in 2009. In 2008, the minority enrollment in entry-level education programs was 11.1 percent for black/African Americans (non-Hispanic), 8 percent for Asian/Pacific Islander/Native Hawaiians (non-Hispanic), 6.5 percent for Hispanic/Latino, and 0.7 percent for American Indians/Alaskan Natives. This is at odds with national census data that shows a black presence of 12.3 percent, Hispanic 15 percent, American Indian 0.8 percent, Asian 4.4 percent, and Pacific Islander 0.1 percent.

There are implications here for a nursing workforce that must be prepared to minister to a population in which the minority presence is rapidly growing. A serious imbalance is noted among faculty, with 8.7 percent of nursing faculty being ethnic and racial minorities. This is less than the 19.8 percent minority faculty representation in American medical schools.[6] Yet, Asian as well as black RNs were more likely than either Hispanic or white RNs to attain at least baccalaureate preparation. And black (14.2 percent) and white nurses (13.2 percent) were the racial/ethnic groups with the highest percentages of master's and doctoral degrees.[7]

Men have been neglected as potential sources of nurse power, although male nurses have existed almost as long as female nurses in the United States. By 1910, about 7 percent of all student and graduate nurses were men, but in succeeding years the percentage declined until by 1940 it had dropped to 2 percent. Most men were graduates of hospital schools connected with mental institutions; not

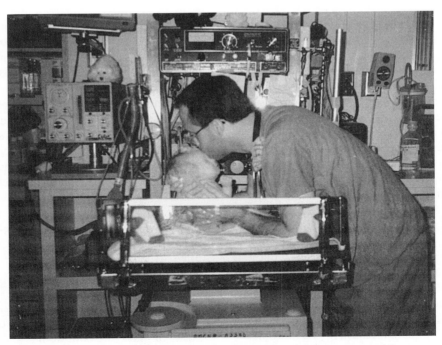

EXHIBIT 11–2. Nursing requires intellectual ability, technical competence, and the capacity to continue to care. (Courtesy of US Army Center of Military History)

many schools (for men) were affiliated with general hospitals, and few coeducational ones existed (see Chapter 3). By 1960, male nurses (not including students) comprised 0.91 percent of the nursing workforce. The current 6.6 percent reflects a slight increase in the number of male nurses, from 5.4 percent in 2000. In 1996, the enrollment of men in basic RN programs reached 12.1 percent and they represented 12.5 percent of graduates. There is little variation in this pattern based on the nature of the program (diploma, associate, baccalaureate). This trend has been attributed to a variety of circumstances, including the general economic recession, employment opportunities in nursing, and the good salary gains achieved during the period of a recent nursing shortage.

Men suffered the same discrimination in nursing that women encountered in male-dominated fields, although this was not always the fault of nursing. For instance, male nurses were kept in the enlisted ranks in the regular armed services until 1966 when, with the continuous pressure of the ANA, commissions were finally available to them in the Regular Nurse Corps. During World War II, male nursing students were not exempt from the draft, although the need for nurses was critical. Therefore, nursing enrollment for men dropped drastically to fewer than 200. After the war, enrollment began to climb slowly until in the 1971–1972 academic year, a total of 5170 men—about 6 percent—were admitted to basic RN programs, nearly twice the proportion that enrolled over the previous 3 years.

Male nurses also find themselves subject to other preconceptions and biases. Their service has sometimes been rejected in obstetrics and gynecology, and many female nurses believe that men in nursing are apt to dominate the upper echelons. These attitudes often create role strain. The response from a preeminently successful male nurse exudes common sense. He described how the fact that nursing is composed of mainly white women "poses both a social and an ethical problem for the profession." He contended that women, when they are in power, are just as reluctant to share power with men as men have been accused of doing in their relationships with women. He added that "the recruitment of men into the profession is not a panacea. Men candidates range from exceptional competence to borderline ability. They bring with them all the positive and negative variables that are indigenous to all humans."[8]

Men in allied health roles or with other health care experience represent a major recruitment pool for nursing.

They should not be expected to choose traditional male specialties, such as emergency, anesthesia, or intensive care, but should be urged to consider a whole range of career choices. They should be supported in career mapping to build a future in the profession.

When looking at the issues regarding the role of minorities in nursing, it is important to remember that cultural differences stem from a myriad of components in all our backgrounds—gender, religion, ethnicity, and even geography. The same insensitivities that thwart our attempts to increase the ethnic, racial, gender, and religious diversity among the ranks of nurses hamper our ability to minister to those who are different from us. Thus, it is important to be aware of and sensitive to minority issues in nursing, but not to give them greater weight than the human issues that affect all people and are the mainstay of nursing care.

■ ATTITUDES OF NURSES AND ABOUT NURSES

Studies of the personality characteristics of nurses vary a great deal and therefore are probably more interesting than useful. Most involve only a small sample and are not applicable to the total population. Which personality traits are studied depends on both the overall purpose of the researcher and the type of test used. Small studies have been done on the personalities of nurses in various specialty areas, with inconsistent findings. All these studies, although of interest, should be regarded with some caution.

The lack of consistent findings creates some questions of overall usefulness, although the heterogeneity of nurses is undoubtedly a key factor in their diverse results. The variety in nursing guarantees that all nurses can find an area of practice that complements their personality and style. Those that like fast-paced action and the unpredictable may gravitate toward emergency or trauma. Others who prefer healing the mind and can use their interpersonal skills to advantage may find the most satisfaction in psychiatric nursing. Order and precision are constants in operating room or special care units. Work with substance abusers or AIDS patients requires the ability to be accepting while refusing to condone antisocial behavior. The danger is to prejudge a person's suitability for an area of practice.

The last nursing shortage, which came to an abrupt halt in the early 1990s, prompted a series of studies about nurses and their job satisfaction. It became obvious that those factors that were dissatisfying to nurses in their work did not create job satisfaction when reversed. Nurses were dissatisfied because of low pay and poor working conditions. Job satisfaction hinged on things such as status, respect, pride in their work, and career mobility. Whether the technique was a summit meeting of nursing organizations, focus groups, or direct mail survey, nurses have consistently expressed the same priorities. The reason for choosing nursing as a career has not changed over the years; it continues to be a desire to help people and an interest in health care.

During career choice, nursing has been seen as a route to professionalism, a vehicle for upward mobility, and a provider of good job opportunities. However, patient care and professional issues dominate workplace concerns. Examples are fear over quality, safety of patients, adequate staffing, the ability of support personnel who relieve nurses of non-nursing duties, nursing representation on committees that make patient care policy, opportunities for maintaining competence in practice, and a safe working environment.

Nurses have reiterated these same priorities over the decades as they have suffered through surpluses, shortages, restructuring, job redesign, and downsizing. The *American Journal of Nursing* partnering with Boston College in 1996 conducted the largest survey of nurses, almost 7500. Again the quality of the nurses' work life was much more closely associated with pride in their work than salary and benefits. Pride in work means pride in patient care: feelings of personal competency, the ability to control the environment on behalf of your patients, and the absence of any "moral compromise."[9]

The ethic of nursing has remained constant. Nurses see their work as stressful, but they anticipate the stress and are willing to live with it given a certain modicum of respect and support.

The workplace stresses most mentioned by nurses are inadequate staffing, interruptions that keep them from their patients, paperwork, lack of support from peers, unattractive and disorganized work areas, high noise levels, lack of supplies, absence of information or directions, no voice in decisions that affect them, lack of respect, conflict between the business orientation of the industry and the service orientation of the profession, and the death of "my" patient. Put eloquently by someone whose name I cannot remember, "Nurses love their work, but hate their job."

The changing health care system, the expectation that nurses take on increased responsibility within any restructured system, and the emphasis on consumer satisfaction have prompted a series of consumer surveys that provide some interesting public opinions about nurses. These surveys and studies span a period of 25 years and provide a great deal of consistency about the relationship between nursing and its public. In 1985, public opinion supported an expanded role for nurses and saw nurses as an untapped resource for decreasing the cost of health care. A 1990 survey conducted by Peter Hart Associates for the Tri-Council Organizations (ANA, NLN, American Organization of Nurse Executives [AONE], and the American Association of Colleges of Nursing [AACN]) and funded by the Pew Charitable Trusts found similar public sentiment. The public saw nurses as respected, trustworthy, and underutilized. A poll conducted by the Gallup Organization in 1993 found the public supporting the use of nurses as primary care providers; 86 percent of the respondents would personally use a nurse for these purposes, and over half of the respondents were very willing. A Kellogg Foundation poll in 1994 found that half of their sample had been treated by a nurse practitioner (NP) in the last year, and in a Gallup poll of the same year respondents identified reductions in RN staffing as the most dangerous strategy for cutting costs in hospitals. In 1996, motivated by the continued displacement of RNs from hospitals in favor of assistive personnel, ANA began the public information campaign, "Every Patient Needs a Nurse." That campaign included a survey conducted by the Princeton Survey Research Associates to gauge the true opinion of the American public. The public saw nurses as a vital ingredient in hospital care and was apprehensive about their decreased presence at the bedside. The public supported the right of nurses to take action if they observed unsafe conditions, and most were interested in knowing how hospital units were staffed and details about patient satisfaction surveys and morbidity and infection rates. In 1997, the AHA partnered with the Picker Institute to conduct a study with both qualitative and quantitative dimensions on the public's perceptions of health care and hospitals. To the American public, the key measure of quality in their hospital care was the nurse. They fear for their safety in hospitals because, in their opinion, poorly paid and ill-prepared nonprofessionals were replacing skilled nurses.[10] Again in 2001, a Gallup poll showed that nurses have a significant edge over doctors in public opinion. Eighty-four percent of American adults rated nurses' honesty and ethical standards as "high" or "very high," second only to firefighters.[11] Gallup polls conducted in 2005 and 2010 revealed similar opinions. Nurses were dominant for ethics, honesty, and compassion when compared to other professionals, among them doctors and elected public officials.[12] This series of public surveys gave a consistent message about the public's trust in nurses and strongly influenced ANA's media strategy and governmental agenda. To summarize the public attitude, consumers see nurses as advocates for their welfare and safety and as an untapped resource for the nation's health.

■ THE MEDIA IMAGE OF NURSING

Set apart from public opinion on nurses as provider professionals is the media image, which often remains as a deadly undercurrent, being laden with all the stereotypes of generations. The thoughtfulness consumers have demonstrated in giving opinions on the value of expanded services delivered by nurses and of the RN as their advocates should eventually filter down and reshape the media image. To effect that change, a healthy dose of intolerance is necessary from the profession, and vigilance on our own behalf, to discourage destructive portrayals of the nurse. Interestingly, a cultural comparison of images of nurses and physicians in 30 geopolitical areas of the world found that cross-culturally, nurses were viewed as positive, active, and kind, but not associated with power, independence, and knowledge. This was in contrast to physicians, who were viewed as powerful and strong. Clearly, the image problem is not confined to this country.

The rest of this chapter discusses nursing's image by focusing on current and past solutions to the image problem. Topics to be covered include contemporary notions of nursing's image, studies on the public's image of nursing, the role of the media, and collective and individual strategies for improving the professional image of the nurse. Although the topic is enormous, only major themes and strategies will be covered.

Presently, nurses are at a critical stage in changing this image. Periodic shortages have forced organized nursing to admit that nursing's public image can be a hindrance in the recruitment of talented individuals to the field. In response, many organizations and health care professionals have been motivated to take a new look at the image issue. Typically, when many laypeople think of a nurse, the crisp, white uniform comes to mind. Nursing's mandate with regard to its image is to educate the public that nurses make serious decisions about their health, and a career in nursing requires intellectual talent, stamina, and dedication, but provides rewards commensurate with that investment. The image of the nurse is highly variable, depending

on the respondent's personal experiences. This is to be expected, because if there is no one typical nurse, how can we expect the image of the nurse to be the same across groups? Few, however, would doubt the power of the media in forming the public's image of many professions, not just nursing. Interviews and research articles or news programs generally portray the nurse in a reasonably accurate way when nursing is singled out to be in the limelight. As a rule, however, in fiction, the media have not, and still do not, correct a distorted image. Comic strips, novels, and television tend to portray the nurse (almost always female) either as a very sweet or sexy young girl, playing obedient handmaiden to the doctors, or as a tough, starched older woman, efficient and brusque. The popularity of medically oriented television series is supposedly a reflection of the public's intense interest in the field. However, the images of the nurses portrayed have been notoriously inaccurate, and even nursing advisers to the shows seldom get the script changed. On the screen, Nurse Rachet in the award-winning movie, *One Flew Over the Cuckoo's Nest*, which was also a book and a play, was probably thoroughly hated by millions of people.

It is important that the image of a careerist become associated with nursing in the entertainment media. Careerists are intelligent and sophisticated and defined largely by their work. They are assertive on behalf of their commitment to the public and hold to high ethical and practice standards. Our silence has contributed to the perpetuation of dysfunctional stereotypes. There are many strong reasons for nurses to persuade the public (as well as other nurses) that the status given to nurses in the media is much lower than what it is and ought to be. One of the most important reasons is recruitment. A mindless, subservient image of nurses will hold little attraction for the best and the brightest that are making career choices. A 1999 survey showed that the supply of nurses is definitely negatively influenced by the inaccurate media images of nursing, decreasing the selection of nursing as a career option by many young people.[13]

In the late 1980s, nurses did take a proactive stand against the NBC-TV show *Nightingales*, which portrayed nurses as well meaning, if promiscuous, and having no real stake in the care of patients. Nursing organizations and individuals offered to provide script consultation and were turned down. The surge of protest against the show from nurses across the country led many of its commercial sponsors to back out, and eventually the show was canceled. Yet, not all TV programs portray nurses in a negative manner. *China Beach* managed to depict the challenges of nursing during the Vietnam War realistically and sensitively. The more recent, award-winning *ER* includes nurses who show the profession positively. Several documentaries on nursing and health care have also been favorable.

The power of the media and the numerous shows that continue to portray nurses in a negative and unrealistic manner led to the organizing of a group called Nurses of America (NOA) and their publication, *Media Watch*. NOA was sponsored by the Tri-Council organizations. It was funded by a grant from the Pew Charitable Trusts and administered by the NLN. NOA worked with a variety of media, ranging from newspapers and magazines to TV and community forums. A large component of their activities included monitoring the media for health-related issues and the portrayal of nurses and nursing practice, and developing a speaker's bureau of nurses who were media prepared and had newsworthy stories to tell about their work. Suzanne Gordon provided important leadership for the NOA. She is not a nurse, but a journalist who was astounded at the invisibility of nursing given their powerful impact on the human condition. She has used the power of the pen to bring vivid descriptions of our work to public attention. Gordon has continued to be an eloquent spokesperson for nursing, and in her book, *Life Support*, she shares her observations on the practice of three nurses that she followed for a 3-year period. She describes their "tapestry of care" that is woven with such intimacy ". . . that many would choose to forget the weaver."[14]

This same phenomenon of invisibility is described in the final report of the Woodhull *Study on Nursing and the Media*, completed under the sponsorship of Sigma Theta Tau. The study was designed to

> . . . document popular cultural attitudes, as reflected by the news media, about nurses and the nursing profession, and the relationship of nurses and nursing to American health care.[15]

Although nurses are a critical mass in health care—the front-line caregivers—and trends in health care verify that their roles are expanding and increasing, they are relatively invisible to the media. The Woodhull recommendations are explicit and reiterate all that has been suggested before.

In addition to media images, nurses are significantly impacted by how physicians perceive them and their profession. Historically, the perception is of an inferior, with the awareness that nurses are necessary to the success of their practice. If physicians' current image of the nursing profession can be equated with their image of the nurse, it is clear that their perceptions are as confused as they were 100 years ago (see Chapters 3 and 4). Now, as then, there are physicians and leaders in organized medicine who see and applaud the changes in nursing toward full professionalism; others find this trend either threatening, incongruent with what they think a nurse's role should be, or just plain unacceptable. As more nurses and physicians engage in collaborative practice and we move toward interdisciplinary educational experiences, the image of the nurse among physicians should improve.

Other strategies to improve the image of nursing are discussed in articles on how to handle the media and be interviewed. Nurses can also improve their image by being involved in community services and organizations. At the worksite, nurses can improve their image by being more visible and serving on various committees. Most importantly, within the profession, nurses need to educate each other about their own subspecialties. It would benefit the image of the profession if more nurses could converse easily on a wide range of issues, including those of colleagues in areas such as nurse anesthesia, nurse midwifery, occupational health, critical care, and more.

One of the most widely applauded strategies to improve nursing's image was the advertising campaign launched between 1989 and 1992 by the NCNIP and the Advertising Council of New York. The Ad Council guaranteed a minimum of $20 million in creative development and media exposure over a 3-year period. The idea was to portray nursing as a "discipline that offers excitement, clinical substance, and authority and responsibility, all tied up in the richness of interpersonal closeness with patients."[16] A more recent event is the Johnson & Johnson *Discover Nursing Campaign*, with much the same purpose.[17]

Obviously, there is no one profile of the modern nurse, particularly in these dynamic times. However, the information obtained from these various studies tells us a great deal about the practitioners of nursing. Resources being allocated to improve the image of nursing have already demonstrated that with work, the image can be changed to one that is more positive and realistic than it has been in the past. Nursing's image has already begun to change in the mass media, among physicians, and most importantly, for members of the profession itself.

KEY POINTS

1. Changes in the growing RN population include an older average age for working nurses and a higher level of education.

2. Because nursing is a large profession made up of a diverse population, information about the background and attitudes of subgroups, as well as the majority, helps nurses understand one another better.

3. The public sees nurses as vital to their safety, their advocates in the health care delivery system, and a resource for curtailing escalating costs.

4. Those factors that are dissatisfying to nurses in their work do not create job satisfaction when reversed.

5. Nurses are dissatisfied because of low pay and poor working conditions, and satisfaction hinges on status, respect, pride in their work, and career mobility.

6. The image of nursing in the media is often distorted, but the public may also form a more lasting image, whether positive or negative, through direct contact.

7. Each nurse must take personal responsibility for creating a true, positive image of nursing and challenging dysfunctional stereotypes.

REFERENCES

1. USDHHS, HRSA. The Health Professions. Initial Findings: 2008 National Sample Survey of Registered Nurses. (3/17/10). http://bhpr.hrsa.gov/healthworkforce/rnsurvey/. Retrieved April 20, 2010.

2. American Association of Colleges of Nursing (AACN). Amid Calls for More Highly Educated Nurses: New AACN Data Show Impressive Growth in Doctoral Nursing programs. March 4, 2010. http://www.aacn.nche.edu/media/newsreleases/2010/enrollchanges.html. Retrieved April 10, 2010.

3. American Hospital Association. Trendwatch Chartbook 2009. http://www.aha.org/aha/research-and-trends/chartbook/index.html. Retrieved April 20, 2010.

4. Aiken H, Clarke SP, Sloane DM, Lake ET, Cheney T. Effects of hospital care environment on patient mortality and nurse outcomes. *J Nurs Admin* 39 (7–8 Suppl):S45–51, 2009.

5. Martinez B. Home care yields Medicare bounty. *The Wall Street Journal.* April 27, 2010. CCLV (97). Pp. A1, A14.

6. Association of American Medical College. Minorities in Medical Education. https://services.aamc.org/publications/showfile.cfm?file=version53.pdf&prd_id=133&prv_id=154&pdf_id=53. Retrieved April 26, 2010.

7. USDHHS, HRSA. The Registered Nurse Population: Findings from the 2004 National Sample Survey of Registered Nurses. http://bhpr.hrsa.gov/healthworkforce/rnsurvey04/3.htm. Retrieved April 20, 2010.

8. Christman L. Men in nursing. *Imprint* 35:75, September 1988.

9. Shindul-Rothschild J, Long-Middleton E, Berry D. 10 keys to quality care. *Am J Nurs* 97:35–43, November 1997.

10. American Hospital Association. *Reality Check: Public Perceptions of Health Care and Hospitals.* Chicago: The Association, 1997.

11. The Gallup Organization. Shift Change: Where Did All the Nurses Go? http://www.gallup.com. Retrieved July 10, 2002.

12. The Gallup Organization. Nurses Tops for Ethics and Honesty. December 10, 2007. http://www.gallup.com/video/103117/Nurses-Top-Ethics-Honesty.aspx. Retrieved April 25, 2010.

13. William M. Mercer, Inc. *Attracting and Retaining Registered Nurses: Survey Results.* Chicago, IL: Author, 1999.

14. Gordon S. *Life Support.* Boston: Little, Brown, 1997.

15. Woodhull Study on Nursing and the Media. *Health Care's Invisible Partner.* Indianapolis: Center for Nursing Press Sigma Theta Tau International, 1998.

16. Joel L. NCNIP/Advertising Council campaign challenges resistant stereotypes. *Am J Nurs* 22:13, February 1990; *Am J Nurs* 97:7, May 1997.

17. Johnson & Johnson. *Discover Nursing Campaign.* http://www.discovernursing.com/jandj.aspx. Retrieved April 26, 2010.

Updates can be found at **www.kellysnursing.com**

HELPFUL WEBSITES FOR PART II, SECTION TWO

Alzheimer's Association: http://www.alz.org

American Association of Retired People: http://www.aarp.org/index.html

American Medical Association: http://www.ama-assn.org

American Society of Bioethics and Humanities (ASBH): http://www.asbh.org

Bioethics Center of the University at Buffalo: http://www.freenet.buffalo.edu/sigs/links/bioethic

Careers in Bioethics: http://www.ethics.ubc.ca/byrnw/jobs.html

The Center for Bioethics at the University of Pennsylvania: http://www.med.upenn.edu/~bioethic

Center for Civilian Biodefense Studies: http://www.hopkins-biodefense.org

The Center for Health Ethics and Law at the West Virginia University: www.hsc.wvu.edu/chel

Compassion in Dying: http://www.thebody.com/cid/cidpage.html

DeathNet: http://www.islandnet.com/deathnet

Dying Well Network: http://www.ior.com/~jeffw/homepage.htm

Eldercare Web: http://www.elderweb.com

Euthanasia Research and Guidance Organization (ERGO): http://www.islandnet.com/~deathnet

Growth House: http://www.growthhouse.org

Hospice Foundation of America: http://www. hospicefoundation.org

Hospice Web: http://www.teleport.com/~hospice

Interfaith Volunteer Caregivers: http://www.nfivc.org

International Anti-Euthanasia Task Force: http://www.iaetf.org

Kennedy Institute of Ethics, Georgetown University: adminweb.georgetown.edu/research/kie

Last Acts: http://www.lastacts.org

Lawrence Berkeley National Laboratories ELSI in Science (Ethical, Legal, and Social Issues in Science): www.lbl.gov/education/ELSI/ELSI.html

MacLean Center for Clinical Medical Ethics at the University of Chicago: ccme-mac4.bsd.uchicago.edu/CCME.html

Midwest Bioethics Center: http://www.midbio.org, http://www.midbio.com

NANDA International: http://www.nanda.org

National Catholic Bioethics Center: http://www.ncbcenter.org

National Family Caregivers Association: http://www.nfcacares.org

National Hospice Organization: http://www.nho.org

National Institute on Aging: http://www.nih.gov/nia

National Reference Center for Bioethics Literature: http://www.bioethics.georgetown.edu

National Association for Home Care: http://www.nahc.org

Not Dead Yet: http://www.acils.com/NotDeadYet

Nuffield Council of Bioethics: http://www.nuffieldfoundation.org/bioethics

Project Nightlight: http://www.nightlight.org

Project on Death in America: http://www.soros.org/death/

Robert Wood Johnson Foundation: http://www.rwjf.org

The San Francisco Examiner—The Caregivers: http://www.sfgate.com/examiner/caregivers/

Seniors-Site: http://www.seniors-site.com

University of Iowa, Center for Nursing Classifications. Nursing Intervention and Outcomes Classification: http://www.nursing.uiowa.edu/excellence/nursing

Nursing Education and Research

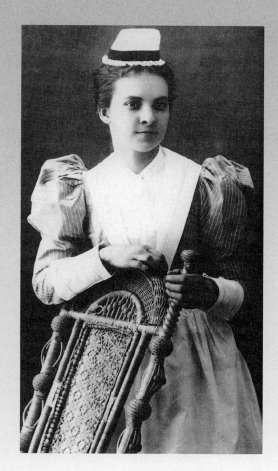

The typical student nurse from the mid-nineteenth century in starched uniform and cap. The past is prologue. (From the private collection of Lucie Young Kelly.)

Major Issues and Trends in Nursing Education

Unlike most professions, nursing has a variety of programs for entry into practice (also called basic, preservice, or generic education). This situation confuses the public, some nurses, and employers. The three major educational routes that lead to registered nurse (RN) licensure are the diploma programs operated by hospitals, the baccalaureate degree programs offered by 4-year colleges and universities, and the associate degree (AD) programs usually offered by junior (or community) colleges. Some states have permitted hospital programs to "award" associate or baccalaureate degrees, usually in cooperation with an institution of higher education and fulfillment of specific criteria, but there are only a few of these. For the most part, diploma programs do not award an academic degree and are rapidly declining. A master's degree program for beginning practice is also available at a few universities. These entry-level master's programs admit students with baccalaureate or higher degrees in fields other than nursing.

Although at one time diploma schools educated the largest number of nurses (more than 72 percent of the total number of schools in 1964 were diploma schools), the movement of nursing programs into institutions of higher education has been consistent. In 2010, there were fewer than 100 schools awarding the diploma, 974 awarding the associate degree in nursing, 621 the baccalaureate in nursing, 70 an entry-level master's degree, and 228 an accelerated bachelor's degree in nursing to candidates with a prior non-nursing degree. This is a total of 1993 basic nursing education programs. In 2008, 59 percent of all new graduates were prepared in 2-year associate degree programs; slightly over one-third (38 percent) graduated from baccalaureate nursing programs; and 8 percent graduated from diploma programs.[1]

■ NEW AND OLD ISSUES

Statistics on admissions, enrollments, and graduations are interesting but provide limited sensitivity to trends without understanding the environment within which these things happen. Recruitment to nursing has been at the mercy of circumstances that repeat themselves with relative frequency, but they are never totally the same. Some of them were unpredictable, but more often nursing should have been able to anticipate the sequence of events and consequences.

Government funding in terms of its students and programs has significantly influenced nursing education. The Nursing Education Act (NEA), as the largest single source of federal dollars for nursing, provided significant support from 1972 to 1994. The years of generous versus meager funding generally paralleled federal administrations that were allies or adversaries of nursing. Some critics question the wisdom of concentrating nursing's educational funding agenda in one major piece of legislation. Also, there are those who oppose becoming so dependent on government funding in the first place, preferring to develop alternate sources of dollars, such as philanthropy, business, industry, and so on. In every sense the trends follow the money, and legislation that is too categorical reshapes the profession, even if the members of that profession would have made different choices. After the expiration of the NEA in October 1994, funding for nursing education was bundled with the dollars for other health professions. Although politically strategic in the mid-1990s, this model ultimately slowed our momentum in moving the nursing education agenda. Organized nursing has secured legislation that sets us apart once again and provides more flexibility through less categorical funding, only singling out the broad areas of advanced nursing education, basic nursing education, and workforce diversity.

Despite the current easing of the nursing shortage due to the recession, the US need is projected to grow to 260,000 RN positions by 2025. A shortage of this magnitude would be twice as large as any nursing shortage experienced in this country since the mid-1960s. A cyclical nursing shortage has also had a significant impact on the decision to choose nursing as a field of work. There was a shortage of nurses in both the late 1970s, and 1980s, and then again in the early 2000s. Each shortage was preceded by a period of oversupply. Aiken describes this cyclical pattern. Nurses' salaries are held artificially low both because of a perceived oversupply and because they are not usually militant on their own behalf. Salary gains of less sophisticated workers who provide some aspect of nursing service outpace the RN's gains. Health care organizations see the value of the RN, given their excellent work ethic, potential for cross training, capacity to expand and contract based on the demands of the moment, and reasonable cost. Consequently, RNs replace nonprofessionals, and a nursing shortage ensues. The shortage prompts all sorts of activity aimed at recruitment to educational programs and the workplace. An essential aspect of enhancing recruitment is securing better salaries and benefits. However, then, once nurses are paid more fairly, they are used more cautiously and often sparingly. Using nurses (now a costly commodity) more judiciously "kicks in" the oversupply phenomenon.[2] The field becomes less attractive to recruitment for fear that one might not be able to secure employment after a long and expensive period of educational preparation. The cycle repeats, and market forces produce corrections in a manner that is more or less predictable. The difference in the shortage of early 2000 was the presence of an aging nurse workforce, and additionally the consumer preference for RNs had been documented, and consumer satisfaction is potent leverage in a competitive health care environment (see Chapter 11).

In November 2007, the US Bureau of Labor Statistics claimed that more than one million new and replacement nurses will be needed by 2016. Additionally, government analysts project that more than 587,000 new nursing positions will be created through 2016 (a 23.5 percent increase).[3] The graying of the population, the complexity of people's needs when they enter the delivery system, the expansion of the delivery system into new markets, and the continuing growth of technology speak for themselves. This is an opinion contrary to the assumptions of the Pew Commission, which predicted a surplus of 200,000 to 300,000 nurses by the turn of the century based on patterns of hospital closures and downsizing.[4] (See the discussion on the Pew Health Professions Commission in Chapter 5.)

The arguments about supply and demand are continuing, and organized nursing has had little success in bringing these factors into balance. In response to much the same observations, the Robert Wood Johnson Foundation conceived the Colleagues in Caring (CIC) program. The goal is to build regional consensus about the future needs for a nurse workforce, its numbers, and skill level. Bringing the major stakeholders to the table is intended to create a synergy that will lead to creative solutions and cooperation (voluntary or mandatory) with a master plan. Discussions will inevitably get to the issue of competency and the utilization of graduates from the three major kinds of basic RN programs.

The future of nursing will depend on recruiting students in numbers great enough to satisfy public need. This responsibility falls to the profession, and is all the more difficult because nursing is an aging profession. The secret seems to be how to attract a younger student group, and yet those are not the individuals who are attracted to nursing. Nursing promises the ability to earn a good living with the minimum of a 2-year educational investment (AD). This is an appealing prospect to the more mature learner: the mid- or later-life career change, single moms entering or reentering the workforce, and individuals with degrees in other areas that hold little promise of employment. To break that mold will mean reshaping our image to appeal to a younger generation and competing with the broad range of career options available to today's youth. For women, who are a major recruitment pool, it will mean creating appeal in the presence of many career choices that were unavailable to them generations ago. With the stereotype of mediocre pay at best, hard work, and often unsafe working conditions, there is hardly much of a choice. And so nursing must choose where best to invest its effort, continuing to focus on the more mature learner with only a limited number of years to give to nursing or make the younger learner a priority. The other associated question is whether students should be recruited to AD programs as an expedient. Should education for practice be promoted as a ladder, building from the AD in a planned and orderly fashion, one layer as a foundation for the next? These are serious questions and involve the choice of allowing circumstances to take us where they please, or seizing control and directing change in the best interests of the public. Speaking in support of the mature learner, they seem uniquely suited to the complexity and stress of modern nursing.

Organized nursing's response to earlier shortages proves that we can recruit. One response was the collaboration of nursing organizations in the NCNIP/Ad Council media campaign, as discussed in earlier chapters. More recently, we have the "Discover Nursing" Campaign funded by Johnson & Johnson and sponsored by organized nursing to increase recruitment to the field. Individual schools also used many new techniques to recruit students to their own programs. Among these are building relationships with liberal arts programs or schools to funnel students directly into nursing education more easily; adopting a high school or even middle school, or mentoring specific students in these schools to orient them to nursing careers; and working with unions to encourage and assist LPNs or aides to move on to RN education. One well-funded program united the forces of over 100 hospitals, long-term care (LTC) facilities, and nursing programs into a consortia to provide educational advancement opportunities for aides and practical nurses, with the expectation that because they had already chosen nursing, they would, as RNs, stay on the job. Included in their package of benefits were accelerated training, loan/service payback programs, and support services such as remedial help, and counseling.[5] Launching a new Cadet Nurse Corps, which had increased nursing enrollment dramatically during World War II, has also been suggested. Some hospitals provide scholarships or make arrangements with potential students to pay back funding by promising to work in that institution for a specific period of time. One school recruits students in Ireland and other foreign countries, granting them full scholarships and maintenance in return for a promise to work in the hospital for 3 years after graduation.

The problem of minority underrepresentation in the profession is not new, but is a serious concern with the changing demographics in the United States. There are five issues to be considered, all of which are tied to nursing education: recruitment and graduation of more ethnic/racial minority students in basic RN programs, an increase in the number of ethnic/racial minorities who complete graduate degrees, the presence of faculty who are suitable role models, and the assurance that all practitioners of nursing are qualified to give culturally competent care.

In basic RN programs, the minority problem has always been more with retention than recruitment. This problem is particularly pronounced for black students. However, recent years have produced some gains in these areas. Baccalaureate programs have seen a jump in minority representation from 16.6 percent of the student body in 1990 to 21.5 percent in 2001. The percentage of graduating minority students from both programs is currently close, 20 percent from baccalaureate and 21.5 from AD programs.[6] Dr. Hattie Bessent, Director Emerita of the ANA Ethnic/Racial Minority Fellowship Program, eloquently presents the qualities for successful recruitment, retention, and graduation of minority students.

- Present the nature of nursing and career options clearly and completely.
- Involve both faculty and administrators in recruitment.
- Be aware of, assess, and accommodate different learning styles.
- Aim for recruiters and faculty from minority backgrounds.
- Support and showcase cultural diversity.
- Collaborate actively with the community of the targeted minority population.
- Elicit the help of an advisory group of representatives of the targeted population.
- Recognize the influence of families on the recruit.
- Have explicit expectations of students and communicate them clearly.
- Commit to leadership development of minority students.
- Provide emotional, educational, and financial support.
- Involve both internal and external mentors.
- Admit only those students that will succeed.
- Ensure interaction between majority and minority faculty and students without either losing their cultural distinctiveness.
- Resocialize faculty to create a milieu that guarantees success.[7]

This list is not all-inclusive, nor are these points exclusive to the minority student, but they have more urgency with this cohort. And most are equally critical for success in graduate education, where our low numbers are of even more concern. The absence of minorities who complete master's and doctoral degrees translates into the absence of minority faculty and mentors for leadership in the profession.

Aiming at cultural competence in practicing nurses presents other challenges. Development of sensitivity to our own biases and the ability to do no harm is probably a good starting point. The best environment for cultivating this insight is multicultural. Therefore, it is to our advantage to establish a varied student population for many reasons. It is personal associations that help us know people very unlike ourselves.

■ PROGRAM OVERVIEW

There are certain similarities that all basic nursing programs share, in part because all are affected by the same societal changes.

- Nursing is very *expensive*, and although some financial support is trickling in because of the current shortage, the amount is not great and much is in the form of scholarships rather than programmatic support. Much of the cost of nursing is associated with the mandatory low student-to-faculty ratios required for clinical instruction. There is also the obligation to be supportive of young faculty as they begin to develop their scholarly work. This is more a concern at the university level than in AD/diploma programs, where this expectation does not exist. Without accomplishments in research and scholarship, university faculty have trouble competing for higher rank or tenure. And in the end, the status of the educational program they are associated with suffers. Appreciating this situation, administrators may try to give a lighter teaching load to new faculty members, allowing time for them to develop their scholarly work.

- The student population is very *heterogeneous*. Although there are still students of the traditional college age, many are older. It is not unusual to have a grandparent in class as more mature individuals look for a new or better career. Many students bring other academic credentials and previous success in fields that are both related and unrelated to nursing. All programs are including more men, by a small but definite percentage. The percentage of minority students has increased. The profession sees the development of minority leadership as a priority.

- Educational programs are generally more *flexible* than ever. This is a response to more students who are dependent on personal and spousal income for support, but also the general trend in higher education. Students should be able to expect flexible class hours, convenient clinical placements, and the ability to extend the course of studies beyond the originally planned 2, 3, or 4 years. Most programs have also incorporated the opportunities for distance education, self-paced learning, proficiency and equivalency testing, and the like. The popularity of the external degree program is testimony to this trend.

- The nursing community has a history of *supporting upward mobility* through education. Although it is still true that the shortest distance between two points is a straight line, many find it impossible to take that route. The classic example are those students who begin as an LPN/LVN (Licensed Practical/Vocational Nurse), move on to the AD, sit for the RN licensing exam, and subsequently complete a baccalaureate in nursing. Most programs recognize the earlier educational experience and give credit toward the next credential.

- *State approval* is required and national accreditation is expected of all nursing education programs. Every basic RN program, as well as practical nurse programs, must meet the standards of the legally constituted body authorized to regulate nursing education and practice within that state. These agencies are usually called *state boards of nursing* or some similar title. Without the approval of these boards, a school cannot really operate, because the graduates would be ineligible to take the licensing examination. In addition, most schools of nursing also seek accreditation by either the Commission on Collegiate Nursing Education (CCNE), a subsidiary of the AACN, or the National League for Nursing Accrediting Commission (NLNAC). Accreditation is voluntary and not required by law. Most schools seek it, however, because it represents nationally determined standards of excellence and the absence of accreditation may affect the school's eligibility for outside funding or hamper the graduates' entrance into baccalaureate or graduate programs in nursing, or their ability to obtain grants and loans.

- Just as the government and national accreditors scrutinize programs of nursing education, individual nurses are examined by the state and awarded a *license* as verification of their *competence*. The public has a legitimate right to demand competence, and the school has a responsibility to ensure that competence in their graduates. Nursing is highly demanding work, and those who cannot successfully complete the course of studies should not be admitted or allowed to continue.

- *Clinical facilities* are at a premium. There is a need to be more flexible and use nontraditional clinical placements, such as community nursing centers, hospice, and nurse entrepreneurs. Distance methods for postconferences may increase the options where the best placements involve much travel. Having practicing nurses participate more actively in the education of students bears merit. Physicians have been doing this for years. Additionally, the faculty responsible for clinical instruction must be clinically skilled themselves.

- If we are to solve the nursing shortage by attracting increasing numbers of men and women to the field, we must have adequate numbers of qualified faculty to teach them. There are currently schools of nursing who have to turn away students because of a lack of faculty. A survey of 16 southern states and the District of Columbia revealed
  - More than 425 unfilled faculty positions.
  - 86 institutions reporting that they did not have enough faculty to cover their undergraduate and graduate programs for the forthcoming semester.
  - 144 faculty members retiring in the current academic year.
  - More than 550 resignations either experienced in that academic year or expected over the next 2 years.
  - Most of the remaining 6322 nurse educators had a master's degree in nursing as their highest credential.

This scenario is not unusual. Service positions are much more lucrative than faculty positions. Additionally, the argument has always raged in nursing as to whether you had to be academically prepared to teach or you had to be an expert in practice, or both. Faculty practice arrangements have allowed schools of medicine to supplement faculty salaries. There are many issues here.

- There is a slow but perceptible trend toward involving *students in curriculum* development, policy-making, and program evaluation. Social trends and the maturity of students, with their demands to have an active role in maintaining the quality of the educational program, are making some inroads on faculty and the administrative control of schools.

- All nursing students have *experience in clinical settings*. Somewhere a myth arose that only practical nursing and diploma students give "real" patient care in their educational programs; that AD students barely saw patients; and that baccalaureate students rarely focused on "doing." In fact, the time in the clinical area differs as much among programs that award the same academic credential as it does among various types of programs. In all good programs, students care for patients to gain skills and apply theoretical knowledge. There should also be experience in caring for larger numbers of patients. This opportunity can diffuse some of the inevitable "shock" that comes with graduation and your first job.

- Students should be encouraged to get involved in the work of nursing, particularly through access to employment with clinical affiliates of the school. *Summer externships and work/study opportunities* are an asset. Nursing is a practice discipline: The more you apply the science the more artful you get.

■ ENTRY INTO PRACTICE

With five types of basic educational programs in nursing, the uncertainty of both the public and the profession as to the differences among these practitioners has appeared to escalate. To add to the confusion, graduates of all programs are eligible to take the same licensing examination and have the same passing score. There have been arguments that no one could expect the public and employers to differentiate among nursing graduates when all are designated as RNs on licensure. Often, RNs are employed in the same capacity, with the same assignments, expectations, and salary. Are they all professional nurses? If so, what justification is there for all these separate educational programs?

An important function of ANA is that of setting standards and policies for nursing education. A major action taken in 1965 by the Committee on Education resulted in the ANA position that nursing education should take place within the higher education system. Reaction to *Educational Preparation for Nurse Practitioners and Assistants to Nurses—A Position Paper* was decidedly mixed. Although the concept underlying the paper had been enunciated by leaders in nursing since the profession's inception, reiterated through the years, and accepted as a goal by the 1960 House of Delegates, many nurses misunderstood the paper's intent and considered it a threat to them personally. Probably the greatest area of misinterpretation lay in the separation of nursing education and practice into professional, technical, and assisting components. Minimum preparation for professional nursing practice was designated at the baccalaureate level, technical nursing practice at the AD level, and education for assistants in health service occupations was to be in short, intensive preservice programs in vocational education settings, rather than in on-the-job training. An obvious omission in the position paper, and perhaps purposeful, was the place of diploma and practical nurse education. A large number of hospital-based diploma graduates, students, faculty, and hospital administrators were angered by the omission. A major source of resentment was that the term *professional nurse* was reserved for the baccalaureate graduate.

Even in this period of confusion, many realized that the largest system of nursing education, the hospital school, could not be eliminated or wished away by the writing of a position paper. Later, both ANA and NLN prepared statements that advocated careful planning for phasing diploma programs into institutions of higher education. Others also pointed out that as practical nursing programs improved and increased their course content, their length became close to that of the AD program. Nevertheless, the storm has raged and periodically subsided for almost 40 years, although repeated attempts were made to clarify the content and intent of the position paper. It was felt that ANA suffered a membership loss through the alienation of some diploma nurses. As expected, social and economic trends gradually brought about many of the changes suggested by the position paper, and the definitions of *professional nurse* and *technical nurse* were widely used in the literature (although there was no major indication that employers were assigning nurses according to technical or professional responsibilities).

In June 1973, in what some considered a belated effort to placate diploma nurses, assure them of their importance to ANA, and encourage unity in the profession, a *Statement on Diploma Graduates* was issued. In essence, the statement asked all units of ANA to give special attention to the needs and interests of diploma graduates, particularly in relation to continuing education and upward mobility. In addition, a taskforce was appointed to examine the contemporary relevance of the terms professional and technical, to distinguish basic preparation for nursing practice and recognize all RNs as professionals. Although there appeared to be no major reaction from diploma nurses to this statement, some nurses considered it a step backward, because it seemed to reject the concept that professional nursing was different from technical nursing.

In February 1974, the Commission on Nursing Education approved a report on the contemporary relevance of the terms professional and technical. Meanwhile, the NLN's AD group rejected the term technical, but others continued to use it.

In 1976, the New York State Nurses' Association's voting body overwhelmingly approved introduction of a "1985 Proposal" in the 1977 state legislative session. Although variations of the proposal evolved over the years, the basic purpose of the legislation was to establish licensure for two kinds of nursing. The professional nurse would require a baccalaureate degree, and the other, whose title changed with various objections, would require an AD. The target date for full implementation was 1985; currently licensed nurses would be covered by the traditional grandfather clause, which would allow them to retain their existing title and status (RN). The bill did not pass but was consistently reintroduced during each legislative session. Later, other nurses' associations introduced similar legislation without success. Immediately, the 1985 Proposal became both a term symbolizing statutory recognition of baccalaureate education as the entry level into professional nursing and a rallying point for nurses who opposed this change. There was, and is, considerable opposition from some diploma and AD nurses and faculty, some hospital administrators, and some physicians. Nursing organizations were formed whose major focus was opposition to such proposals. They were primarily made up of diploma nurses, and were supported by hospital organizations and administrators. Nevertheless, an increasing number of ANA's constituent state organizations, primarily made up of diploma nurses, voted in convention to work toward the goal of baccalaureate education for professional nursing. In 1978, the ANA House of Delegates passed such a resolution, as did the National Student Nurses' Association. The ANA resolution had emerged from an ANA-sponsored "Entry into Practice" conference held earlier that year. The 400 or so participants included representatives from various nurses' associations, the federal government, all types of schools of nursing, as well as administrators and staff nurses from all types of employment settings. The major recommendations, supporting the concept of two categories or types of practitioners in nursing (although they could not agree on titles), were that competencies be developed for those levels, statutory distinctions be established, and career mobility opportunities be increased, including the use of innovative and flexible educational programs. All these recommendations were incorporated into resolutions that the ANA House of Delegates also approved in 1978. Where once ANA conventions were consumed with entry into practice debates, gradually the question in education became, how do we facilitate the transition? (See the reports of ANA conventions in *Nursing Outlook* and the *American Journal of Nursing* in the even years.) The 1980

Social Policy Statement, which clearly stated that baccalaureate education was the basis of professional nursing practice, was accepted, and the Cabinet on Nursing Education continued to work toward this goal.

The reader should note that the "entry into practice" controversy consists of three separate issues: the intent of bringing preparation for nursing into the educational mainstream, distinction between two (or more) categories of nurses, and linking these distinctive categories to statutory requirements that include different competencies and title protection. The idea of establishing licenses for two categories of nurses originated in New York in 1976, was introduced and supported at the ANA House of Delegates in 1978, but was never vigorously pursued until 1983. In 1983, ANA provided grants to several of its constituent member states to implement their plans to establish the baccalaureate as the minimum educational qualification for professional nursing. Further, ANA set its own timetable for implementation in all states before the end of the century. The final report of the interdisciplinary National Commission for Nursing saw pursuit of the baccalaureate as an "achievable goal." A 3-year project funded by the W. K. Kellogg Foundation in late 1984 (NCNIP) to carry out selected Commission recommendations included the objective, ". . . to outline the common body of knowledge and skills essential for basic nursing practice, the curriculum content that supports it, and a credentialing process that reinforces it." (See Chapter 5 for more details on both the Commission and NCNIP.) In later meetings, the ANA House of Delegates became involved in trying to agree on how the two types of nurses could be accommodated as members. Eventually, this was more or less resolved by changes in the bylaws (see Chapter 25).

The NLN has played an interesting role in the entry into practice debate. In 1979, it supported all pathways (baccalaureate, associate, diploma, and practical nursing). Given the structure of the NLN and its historic position as the accrediting body for all levels of nursing education, this statement is understandable. In 1982, however, the NLN Board of Directors endorsed the baccalaureate degree as the criterion for professional practice. This position was affirmed when the voting body met in June 1983. (See the convention reports published in *Nursing Outlook* in the odd years between 1979 and 1983.)

Later, reaffirmations by the board that also called for two separate licensing exams infuriated the AD programs and community college presidents, who threatened to pull out of NLN membership. There was a demand for clarification and objections that this action downgraded AD nurses for the sake of elevating BSN nurses. (From all this agitation came a number of organizations whose purpose was basically to support AD nursing and to protect AD nurses and programs from ANA and NLN actions they saw as detrimental.) The LPNs were not happy either. What resulted was a compromise statement that seemed reasonably acceptable. An interesting nonaction occurred at the next NLN convention when the issue was tabled indefinitely.

Entry into practice and its possible corollary, changes in nurse licensure, continue to be major issues in nursing. Most nursing organizations, at the state and national levels, have taken a stand supporting baccalaureate education as the appropriate education for the professional nurse. After that, there is still disagreement as to whether the "other" nurse would be the technical or AD nurse with separate licensing and if the LPN/LVN would remain the same. Some think that AD education should be required for the practical nurse, leaving only two levels of nursing. Because this means a major change in nurse licensure, which is always a political as well as legal risk, only one state has taken that big step. The North Dakota Board of Nursing changed its administrative rules, so that since 1987 the baccalaureate degree is the educational credential for those wishing to take the RN licensure exam, and an AD is required for practical nursing (see Chapter 20). Although there was a legal attempt by several hospitals to prevent this from happening, the North Dakota attorney general ruled that this decision was within the purview of the board, and so change came about through administrative rule making. No other states were successful in their plans for legislation, rules and regulations, or administrative statements to move the "entry" debate, probably because of a more pressing issue, the nursing shortage. Opponents seized on the shortage to maintain that this was not the time to make such changes because all types of nursing education programs were needed. Even when some study reports recognized the need for baccalaureate nurses, the approach suggested was most often to encourage educational mobility, as opposed to direct entry to professional practice (see Chapter 5). This opened the door to the articulation of diploma and AD programs with those awarding baccalaureate or higher degrees, as well as more high-quality external degree programs and flexible campus-based instructional programs for nurses who want baccalaureate education.

In the long debate about the nature of education for practice, opinion varies. It is not surprising that there are those who think that the system should stay as it is. Others opt for changing the baccalaureate nurse's title and license to set them apart. A few anticipate the time when a professional nurse doctorate, like the MD and DDS of physicians and dentists, will be the entry level to the profession. Still others see certification for the baccalaureate nurse as the additional credential to distinguish professional nursing.

Some natural fears of nonbaccalaureate nurses are to be expected: that they will lose status and job opportunities despite the grandfather clause, and that those who desire baccalaureate education will find it too expensive, unavailable, or rigidly repetitive. As to the first issue, there has been and is already some selectiveness in the workplace. There is also slow but definite progress in making RN/BSN programs accessible, affordable, and challenging. These issues will not be quickly resolved, but inevitable societal and professional changes, such as the decrease in diploma schools and the expectations of professional practice, will be major factors in the final outcome. (Nursing is the only health profession for which entry is less than a baccalaureate.) During the periods of a nursing workforce surplus, baccalaureate graduates have been preferentially hired by service agencies.

The times and the complexity of health care are gradually making this issue less debatable and more resolvable. Because nursing loses power every time its practitioners battle internally, it is essential that nurses work together toward a satisfactory conclusion, one that includes appreciation and respect for all competent nurses and focuses on providing the best possible nursing care to the public. The step ladder approach to nursing education has fueled a movement to legally require AD graduates to move on to complete a baccalaureate in nursing within 10 years of graduation. "The BSN in 10" has garnered significant attention and support, but has not become law in any state as of yet.

In the meantime, there has been a quiet revolution, one that may end the recurrence of the entry into practice issue that has followed nursing throughout its history. Although many RNs are not convinced that baccalaureate education necessarily means professionalism, others are, and back to school they go.

■ OPEN CURRICULUM PRACTICES

The *open curriculum* concept became a reality for nursing in the early 1970s and provided the opportunity to exit and enter a course of studies and achieve recognition for previous learning and experience. The philosophy to support this concept emerged gradually, but was inevitable. The poor and ethnic minorities, often guided into lower-level nursing positions, and the middle-class nurses who had chosen diploma or AD education, as well as service corpsmen returning to the civilian workforce, became irritated at the difficulty of achieving any upward mobility in nursing through education. All became increasingly hostile toward a system that offered no credit for previous study and experience, or, at most, recognized a few liberal arts courses. Unions included in their contracts provisions for organized programs of education that facilitated upward mobility for nonprofessionals. Others turned to the legislatures. The result was evident in such states as California, which enacted laws to force schools of nursing to give credit to prospective students with previous experience in health care.

Today, almost all programs accept transfer credit as a means of advanced placement. Innovative programs have been designed that feature new methods for measurement of knowledge and competency. Other programs have made flexibility their mantra. The *ladder approach* provides direct articulation between programs, moving an individual from nursing assistant to practical nurse to AD or diploma nurse to baccalaureate status. For some, this means the ability to begin at a basic level and move one step at a time to the highest achievable level. For others, it means that one can aim at a particular level but be able to exit at distinct points, become licensed, and earn a living if necessary before carrying on. In 2009, 621 RN-to-BSN programs were available nationwide, including more than 390 offered at least partially online. Program length varied between 1 and 2 years depending on the school's requirements, program type, and the student's previous academic achievement. "Concerns about the limited availability of RN-to-BSN programs are unfounded. In fact, there are more RN to BSN programs available than 4-year nursing programs or accelerated baccalaureate programs for non-nursing college graduates. Access to RN-to-BSN programs is further enhanced since many programs are offered completely online or on site at various health care facilities."[8] To provide even more opportunity, there are a variety of programs that fast-track RNs and second-degree candidates to a master's and specialization. There are 160 programs available nationwide to move RNs with diplomas and associate degrees to the master's level.[9]

There are still nurse educators who do not agree that the ladder is a viable concept. They believe that each program in nursing has its own uniqueness and that one cannot be based on the other. Further, they believe that the ladder tends to denigrate the role of workers at each level, implying the necessity of moving upward. One solution seems to be the utilization of standardized and teacher-made tests to measure the individual's knowledge, according to a clear delineation of the achievement expectations of the program. There are a number of standardized tests available in both the liberal arts and nursing, but there is still some question as to how to test for clinical competency.

Another approach is to allow students to proceed with a course at their own pace through testing, self-study, the use of media, and computers. These techniques are very suited to distance education. A number of schools offer self-pacing and self-learning, and reports indicate that students find these stimulating and satisfying, but motivation and self-discipline are essential.

Other ways of giving students opportunities are to offer courses more frequently, during evening hours, weekends, and in summer, and to have class sessions off the main campus in areas convenient to students living in communities that are not easily accessible. Interactive television (ITV) is also helpful in these distance situations.

Another variation on the open curriculum is the *external degree* or "virtual" university. It confers credentials based on independent study validated by testing, an approach used in other countries as early as 1836. In the United States, Excelsior College of Albany, New York (formerly Regents College), pioneered this approach for nursing education. Excelsior shares many goals and activities with conventional campus-based programs. However, it differs significantly in the ways students learn and the methods used to recognize and credential that learning. Sources of college credit that can be used toward an Excelsior College degree program include Excelsior College distance learning courses, courses from other regionally accredited institutions, college-level subject-matter examinations (including CLEP exams, GRE subject exams, and DSST/DANTES exams), noncollegiate training (including corporate, governmental, and military training) that has been evaluated for college-level credit by the American Council on Education (ACE), and assessments of prior learning portfolios. Unlike most colleges, Excelsior College sets no limitations on the amount of allowable transfer credit. Excelsior College also offers Excelsior College Examinations (ECE), which are comparable to CLEP and DSST exams and are accepted as a source of credits by many (but not all) colleges in the United States.[10]

Since 1972, Excelsior has developed associate, baccalaureate, and master's degree programs in nursing. All degrees are accredited. AD graduates, who are typically LPN/LVNs, are eligible for licensure in all states. Since 1974, the pass rate on the licensure examination has averaged 94 percent, with scores higher than those for New York State as a whole. Master's degree programs are available in three areas: education, informatics, and clinical systems management. Additionally, two certificate programs are offered: a post-baccalaureate certificate in nursing management and a post-master's certificate in nursing education, each requiring 12 credits in specified course areas.[11]

AD nursing students must complete 35 credits of general education, six nationally standardized nursing written examinations, and a $2^1/_2$-day clinical performance examination. The arts, sciences, and nursing content are equivalent to those expected in conventional AD programs. The baccalaureate nursing degree program was completed in 1979, and following a 2-year series of meetings and appeals, the NLN accredited this most innovative of nursing programs and included all of its graduates retroactively. The content of degree requirements, in general education and nursing, is consistent with conventional BSN programs. A total of 120 semester credits must be earned with 72 in the typical categories of arts and sciences, 20 credits in theory for nursing documented by five nationally standardized written examinations, and 28 credits in clinical nursing documented through four criterion-referenced performance examinations. For the RN student there is the option to waive the performance examinations and substitute portfolio development. This is a process of committing to paper a very rigorous analysis of your personal practice experiences.

In March 2005, there were more than 17,000 students enrolled at Excelsior, about 16,000 in the AD program, 1242 in the BSN, and 319 in the master's program. Retention of students continues to be a problem. Overall, about 25 percent of Excelsior students withdraw over time. Nearly 80 percent of the BSN candidates are RNs from diploma or AD programs with an average of 10 years of experience in nursing and an average age of 40. Many BSN students have baccalaureate, master's, or doctoral degrees in other fields. Approximately three-fourths of the graduates state intentions of continuing with graduate school.[12]

Some 250 nurse faculty members, all of whom have completed the extensive training developed and administered by Excelsior, conduct the performance examinations. Nursing performance examinations are administered on weekends throughout the year at the national network of Regional

Performance Assessment Centers created and established by Excelsior. The written nursing examinations are administered by the American College Testing Program (ACT PEP tests) at some 160 locations throughout the country and in embassies and military bases throughout the world. Excelsior is no longer the only "external degree" option. Others exist and can be identified through the NLN or AACN.

■ GRADUATE EDUCATION

The demand for innovation and fresh approaches, or at least an open mind, has not excluded graduate education. The issues are much the same. The need is to be consumer friendly yet maintain the integrity of education for advanced practice. Much of the controversy focuses around the term *advanced practice*. Health care reform has catapulted nurses with advanced practice education into prominent roles. The nature of the preparation has become the topic of debate, with slowly growing consensus. Should clinical nurse specialists and nurse practitioners be educated as advanced practice nurses with the subsequent abandonment of the distinctions between the two roles? And should the terminal degree for practice be the Doctor of Nursing Practice (DNP), which has begun to dominate the mainstream of graduate education, leaving the master's degree behind?

A second issue, with less current controversy, is whether nurse executives require joint degrees in both business and nursing to serve the profession, given the complexities of today's health care system, and to claim educational equality with other system executives. And where does the Clinical Nurse Leader (CNL) master's degree fit in this paradigm of roles to serve an increasingly complex health care delivery system?

Neither does preparation for teaching escape scrutiny. Can you teach it, if you can do it? And who should teach clinical nursing in the new millennium? How do you infuse adequate clinical knowledge and skills into a preparation program for teachers? The challenges of teaching in ADN programs or an integrated curriculum are unique. Faculty may not find assignments that conform to traditional specialty areas.

■ DISTANCE EDUCATION

Distance education is as old as correspondence courses, but has taken on a new meaning, with the consumer outcry for easy access to education, the knowledge explosion, and technology making it possible to transcend time and distance. It is both an instrument of social change and a response to that change. Distance education involves the geographic separation of learner and instructor, the use of technology for communication that allows us to transcend time and distance, the capacity for bidirectional interaction, and sometimes the absence of a peer group.

Distance education involves both synchronous and asynchronous technology. Synchronous technology allows students and instructor to be together in real time, whereas asynchronous technology allows the scheduling of course responsibilities according to your personal preference. Synchronous technologies include ITV, chat rooms, and teleconferencing. Some asynchronous approaches are threaded discussions (students placing responses to a discussion topic on an Internet site, but not simultaneously), the Internet, e-mail queries of the instructor and transmission of assignments, accessing course materials, and testing using a course-specific website, videotapes, faxes, and computer disks, as well as textbooks and study guides. The distance experience is strange and uncomfortable for many students, but it makes it possible to offer smaller, more specialized courses and convenience.

In choosing a distance course, it is important to be an informed consumer. Inquiry about some of the following points would be wise.

- Has the instructor taught by distance before? (The learning curve is often steep for faculty.)
- What is the variety of teaching/learning strategies used? (Variety and a combination of synchronous/asynchronous techniques make for quality.)
- How quickly can you expect to receive feedback from your instructors when you direct a question to them? (Immediate gratification is one positive of distance.)
- How many students are there in a course, and how many sites are connected electronically with what number of students at each site? (It is often possible to create your own peer group.)
- In the case of ITV, will there be a facilitator and/or technician at each site? (Equipment failure can be a big problem, and an academic presence of some sort is common in many ITV sites.)
- What equipment do I need to participate? If I do not personally own suitable equipment, how can I participate? (Equipment is often available to you through public libraries, elementary and secondary schools, or your workplace.)

Distance education is a guaranteed growth area. If you have not experienced learning in this mode, you will eventually.

■ ACCREDITATION

The major accrediting organization for diploma, AD, and practical nursing education programs is the National League for Nursing Accrediting Commission (NLNAC). Baccalaureate and graduate programs in nursing are accredited by both the NLNAC and the Commission on Collegiate Nursing Education (CCNE). The issues involved here relate in part to the accrediting process and in part to who should do the accrediting.

Accreditation is defined as the process by which an agency or organization evaluates and recognizes an institution or program of study as meeting certain predetermined criteria or standards. As noted, educational accreditation is a voluntary process, but it presumably indicates excellence in program and resources, thereby attracting students and faculty. It is often a requirement for external funding.

Standards are set by the profession, and the degree to which a program or institution conforms to these standards is determined through the accreditation process, which includes significant consumer input. By way of example, standards for nursing practice are established by ANA, but the American Nurses Credentialing Center (ANCC) in the process of awarding certification applies them to the practice of an individual nurse. It is required that the accrediting agency be autonomous and those who make credentialing decisions be free of conflict of interest and protected from any external coercion that might affect those decisions.

In most situations, the accreditor maintains a close relationship with the professional association that created it. There are philosophical and power issues: Should the NLN (and NLNAC), which was given the responsibility at the reorganization of the major nursing organizations in 1952, continue to be a major force in educational standard setting and accreditation in nursing? Should the AACN, which represents the interests of the academic deans and directors and is associated with the CCNE, become the major force?

There is also the obvious matter of control and income. Considerable income is derived from activities related to accreditation: organizational memberships, consulting, and the accreditation process itself. These resources provide attractive incentives to enter the business of accreditation or to participate in an allied association that drives standards. A final issue is the fact that the NLNAC offers a comprehensive service with all programs having the ability to seek accreditation under the same auspices. The CCNE is only associated with baccalaureate and higher degree programs, thus sacrificing this consolidation.

Another factor, which is not to be discounted, is the bias or belief system of the accreditation agency. Rejection of programs or denial of accreditation can be attributed to organizational or reviewer bias rather than application of criteria or standards. Negative responses to decisions about accreditation have in many ways perpetuated the who-shall-accredit debate.

■ RISING TO THE OCCASION OF THE FUTURE

The recurrent problems and issues of the profession should not distract us from taking charge of our future in an era of inevitable health care reform. There are challenges to nursing education that must be addressed from within, even though that has not always been our tradition. Nursing has rather chosen to respond, and often simultaneously, to contradictory messages. Respecting that education prepares for the future and not the past, there is a clear mandate for education to

- Broaden its clinical emphasis to prepare graduates for immediate entry into community-based practice.
- Stress delivery of care as a seamless fabric with the nurse either handing-off patients to colleagues or moving with patients across the continuum.
- Be cautious not to abandon our traditional venues and populations—the sick, the hospital, the nursing home, and home care.
- Believe in empowerment of the consumer and practice what you believe.
- Convey the expectation from the outset that students are accountable for their practice, including cost and quality implications.
- Expect that students will come to you literate in the use of computers.
- Include educational experiences to prepare for practice in a multicultural society. Realistically, this may be no more than becoming aware of one's own biases and

accepting others as they are, including their personal definitions of health and wellness.

- Establish true interdisciplinary education in the form of required courses, electives, and joint practice opportunities.

- Take equal care to provide intradisciplinary experiences so that the students will see the advanced practice nurse as a resource and become comfortable with nurses prepared at different educational levels.

- Realize that it is impossible to teach everything, so make process your content. Focus on creative and critical thinking, evidence-based practice, collaboration, shared decision making, a social epidemiological viewpoint, and analyses at the systems and aggregate level.

- Remember it will be a luxury to just be responsible for your practice; students must be equipped with the skills to delegate and to evaluate the performance of assistive personnel.

- Demand faculty-to-faculty and faculty-to-student relationships that are more egalitarian and characterized by cooperation and community building.

- Ensure that the faculty teaching clinical nursing are certified and have the skills to practice at an advanced level.

- Involve employers in curriculum design, so that nursing education is truly preparing individuals suited to the realities of practice.

- Target recruitment and retention efforts toward individuals of diverse racial, cultural, and ethnic backgrounds, especially faculty and graduate students.

- Shift the emphasis for research toward studies concerned with health promotion and disease prevention at the aggregate and community levels.

- Seek more balance between the traditional definitions of scholarship and the scholarship of application, so that faculty can establish their projects within delivery systems as part of their teaching.

- Become actively involved in the placement of your graduates, so that nurses will begin to claim their place in new markets.

- Commit to increasing the numbers of advanced practice nurses, so that as a profession we can both move forward to fill the primary care gap and continue to show strength in specialization.

KEY POINTS

1. Nursing education programs share certain concerns: escalating cost, recruitment challenges, a change in student mix, scarce clinical resources, and consumer demands for flexibility in education, among others.

2. Nursing education programs differ in many ways, particularly in the expected competencies of their graduates.

3. The number of minority students admitted and graduating from schools of nursing has increased, but there is still a great need for minority faculty who can serve as role models.

4. RNs seeking baccalaureate education have many more choices than they did a generation ago, including self-directed learning activities, distance education, and external degrees.

5. Educational programs for preparation for entry into nursing practice must reflect health care as it is delivered in the twenty-first century.

6. Issues about education for entry into practice focus on whether baccalaureate education should be required for the professional nurse and AD education for the technical or associate nurse, how and where this should be accomplished, and whether it should be legally required.

7. Beginning with the ANA position paper on education in 1965, the actions of the various nursing organizations have tended to support baccalaureate education for professional practice.

REFERENCES

1. All Nursing Schools. Entry Level Nursing Programs, 2008. http://www.allnursingschools.com/faqs/programs. Retrieved April 20, 2010.

2. Aiken LH. Economics of nursing. *Policy, Politics, & Nursing Practice* 9(2):73–79, 2008.

3. American Association of College of Nursing. *Fact Sheet: The Nursing Shortage.* September 2009. http://www.aacn.nche.edu/Media/FactSheets/NursingShortage.htm. Retrieved April 25, 2010.

4. Pew Health Professions Commission. *Critical Challenges: Revitalizing the Health Care Professions for the Twenty-First Century.* San Francisco: University of California, 1995, pp 48–51.

5. Johns Hopkins Medicine. Project LINC (Ladders in Nursing Careers). http://www.hopkinsmedicine.org/jhhr/Community/linc.html. Retrieved April 10, 2010.

6. American Association of Colleges of Nursing (AACN). Associate Degree in Nursing Programs and AACN's Support for Articulation. http://www.aacn.nche.edu/Media/Backgrounders/ADNFacts.htm. Retrieved July 10, 2002.

7. Bessent H (ed). *Strategies for Recruitment, Retention and Graduation of Minority Nurses in Colleges of Nursing*. Washington, DC: American Nurses Publishing, 1997.

8. AACN. Degree Completion Programs for Registered Nurses. February 2009. http://www.aacn.nche.edu/Media/FactSheets/DegreeCompletionProg.htm. Retrieved April 5, 2010.

9. Ibid.

10. Excelsior College. School of Nursing. https://www.excelsior.edu/Excelsior_College/School_Of_Nursing. Retrieved April 20, 2010.

11. Ibid.

12. Interview. Todd Thomas, Director, Institutional Research, Excelsior College, Albany, New York, March 10, 2005.

Updates can be found at **www.kellysnursing**.

Programs in Nursing Education

Educational preparation for licensure as a registered nurse (RN) takes place primarily in associate degree (AD) programs and baccalaureate in nursing (BSN) programs (BSN is used here for simplicity, although some institutions may grant a BS or a BA in nursing). A few remaining diploma schools continue educating nurses, but they are rapidly declining. This chapter gives an overview of these educational options, as well as graduate education and continuing education (CE).

■ DIPLOMA PROGRAMS

The *diploma* or *hospital school of nursing* was the first type of nursing school in the United States. Prior to the opening of the first hospital schools in the late 1800s, there was no formal preparation for nursing. But after Florence Nightingale established the first school of nursing at St. Thomas's Hospital in England in 1860, the idea spread quickly to the United States.

Hospitals, of course, welcomed the idea of training schools because, in the early years, such schools represented an almost free supply of nurse power. With some outstanding exceptions, the education offered was largely of the apprenticeship type. There was some theory and formal classroom work, but for the most part students learned by doing, providing the bulk of the nursing care for the hospitals' patients in the process.

This is no longer true. Today, to meet standards set in each state for the operation of a nursing school and to prepare students to pass the licensing examinations, diploma schools must offer their students a true educational program, not just an apprenticeship. Hospitals conducting such schools employ qualified nurse faculty, offer students a balanced mixture of coursework (in nursing and related subjects in the physical and social sciences), and supervised practice, and look to their nursing staff, not their students, to provide the nursing service needed by patients. The educational program has been generally 3 years in length, although most diploma schools have now adopted a shortened program. On satisfactory completion of the program, the student is awarded a diploma by the school. This diploma is not an academic degree. Because most hospitals operating schools of nursing are not chartered to grant degrees, no academic credit can be given for courses taught by the school's faculty. For this and economic and educational reasons, large numbers of diploma schools enter into cooperative relations with colleges or universities for educational courses or services. It is not uncommon for diploma students to take physical and social science courses and, occasionally, liberal arts courses at a college. Then, credit may be transferable if the nursing student decides to transfer to a college or continue later with further education. Diploma schools usually provide other necessary educational resources, facilities, and services to students and faculty, such as libraries, classrooms, audiovisual materials, and practice laboratories. At one time, it was taken for granted that students would be housed, and the school had dormitory and recreational space as well as educational facilities. Although the physical setup may still be the same, such housing must usually be paid for and may also be used by others educated in or involved with the hospital. The primary clinical facility is the hospital, although the school may contract with other hospitals or agencies for additional educational experiences. Advocates of diploma education usually say that early and substantial experiences with patients seem to foster a strong identification with nursing, particularly hospital nursing, and thus graduates are expected to adjust to the employee role without difficulty.

Admission requirements to diploma schools usually call for a college preparatory curriculum in high school, with standing in the upper half, third, or quarter (depending on the school) of the graduating class. Personal characteristics and health are also assessed.

The proportion of the total RN population who claimed the diploma as their highest educational credential declined from 63 percent in 1980 to only 13.9 percent in 2008, and the number of practicing RNs who identify the diploma as their initial preparation was 20.4 percent.[1] The perceptible shift away from diploma school preparation for nursing can be explained (in an oversimplified way) by three factors.

1. The expense of maintaining a school is substantial, and patients and their insurers have often absorbed that cost. This practice has become unacceptable, resulting in inadequate funding and difficulty maintaining standards, including attracting qualified faculty.

2. Increasing numbers of high school graduates are seeking some kind of collegiate education with the assurance that credits earned will be accepted for transfer.

3. The nursing profession is becoming ever more committed to the belief that preparation for nursing, as for other professions, should take place in institutions of higher education.

The vast majority of current diploma programs are accredited by the National League of Nursing (NLN), and many were "phased into" AD or BSN programs over the years. The 1970 National Commission study recommended that strong, vital schools be encouraged to seek regional accreditation and degree-granting status, but only a few have done so. Another recommendation—that other hospital schools move to effect interinstitutional arrangements with collegiate institutions—has been acted on more readily.

Although hospitals are less likely to operate schools, they continue as a major clinical laboratory for nursing education programs. In communities where new AD or BSN degree programs have opened, there was often planning for new programs to evolve as diploma programs closed—a phasing-in process. This cooperation enabled prospective candidates for the diploma program to be directed to the new program, a qualified diploma faculty to be employed by the college, and arrangements made to use space in the hospital previously occupied by the diploma school.

Cooperative planning provided for continuity in the output of nurses to meet the needs of the community. The diploma schools were the professional schools of another era, and we owe them much for their contribution.

■ ASSOCIATE DEGREE PROGRAMS

By far the greatest increase in programs and students has been at the AD level. These programs are 2 years in length and are offered by junior or community colleges, and occasionally by 4-year colleges. The first three programs were started in 1952; by 1965 there were more than 130 such programs, and in 2008 there were at least 1050 AD programs.[2] Over 45.4 percent of the current RN population received their basic nursing education in an AD program, and for 36.1 percent it was their highest educational preparation.[3] More than half of AD programs are NLN accredited, and regional accrediting groups accredit most of the others as part of their college's accreditation.

The AD program is the first nursing education program to be developed under a systematic plan and with carefully controlled experimentation. In her doctoral dissertation, published as a book in 1951, Mildred Montag conceived of a nursing technician able to perform nursing functions smaller in scope than those of the professional nurse and broader than those of the practical nurse. This nurse was intended to be a "bedside nurse" who was not burdened with administrative responsibilities.

Montag listed the functions as (1) assisting in the planning of nursing care for patients, (2) giving general nursing care with supervision, and (3) assisting in the evaluation of the nursing care given.[4] The emerging community college was seen as a suitable setting for this education. Nursing education would be in the mainstream of education, and the burden of cost would be on the public in general, not on patients. The curriculum was to be an integrated one, half general education and half nursing, with careful selection of educational and clinical experiences. An AD would be awarded at the end of the 2 years. The program was considered to be comprehensive and complete in itself (terminal) and not a first step toward the BSN.

At the end of 1951, the 5-year Cooperative Research Project in Junior and Community College Education for Nursing was funded, and seven junior colleges and one hospital school were selected to participate in the project; each had complete autonomy in the development and conduct of its pilot program, but had free access to consultation from the project staff (see Chapter 5).

The results of the project showed that AD nurses could perform the intended nursing functions, that the program could be suitably set up in community colleges with the use of clinical facilities in the community, and that the programs attracted students. The success of the experiment plus the rapid growth of community colleges combined to give impetus to these new programs.

Over the years, as Montag predicted, the AD curricula have varied and changed; for instance, when college policies permit, there is a tendency to put a heavier emphasis and more time on the nursing subjects and clinical experiences, sometimes through the addition of summer sessions. Most programs have also added managerial principles because their graduates are put in positions requiring these skills. Today, most AD programs are between 18 and 24 months in length, but some require that all science and general education courses be completed before the nursing program is begun, which may lengthen the AD program to over 2 years.

The entire concept of the AD nursing program as terminal has changed over the last 20 years. Obviously, no educational program should be dead-ended in the sense that graduates cannot continue their education toward another degree. Whether or not they get full or only partial credit for their previous education depends on the philosophy and policies of the BSN program they select. However, articulation programs with baccalaureate programs are common, and it has become usual to receive full credit for the AD experience.

Because AD nursing is often described as *technical nursing practice*, the description of technical practice as differentiated from professional practice in the controversial ANA position paper on nursing education may be helpful.

Technical nursing practice is carrying out nursing measures as well as medically delegated techniques with a high degree of skill, using principles from an ever-expanding body of science. It is understanding the physics of machines as well as the physiologic reactions of patients. It is using all treatment modalities with knowledge and precision.

Technical nursing practice is evaluating patients' immediate physical and emotional reactions to therapy and taking measures to alleviate distress. It is knowing when to act and when to seek more expert guidance.

Technical nursing practice involves working with professional nurse practitioners and others in planning the day-to-day care of patients. It is supervising other workers in the technical aspects of care.

Technical nursing practice is unlimited in depth but limited in scope. Its complexity and extent are tremendous. It must be rendered under the direction of professional nurse practitioners, by persons who are selected with care and educated within the system of higher education; only thus can the safety of patients be assured. Education for this practice requires attention to scientific laws and principles with emphasis on skill. It is education that is technically oriented and scientifically founded, but not primarily concerned with evolving theory.[5]

Whether the term *technical* will continue to be used is not clear. The concept of a technical worker, honored in other fields, has never been fully accepted in nursing, possibly because it is considered a step down from the professional label that has been attached to all nurses through licensing definitions and common usage over the years. Montag, noting the difficulty of choosing an appropriate term for the new type of proposed nurse, said, "It is also probable that the term 'nursing technician' will not satisfy forever, but it is proposed as one which indicates more accurately the person who has semi-professional preparation and whose functions are predominantly technical."[6] This same division of labor has prevailed in other medical fields of practice, such as respiratory technologists and technicians, laboratory technologists and technicians, and so on. It is a simple principle of occupational development that as fields of work mature, associates surface who take on some of the less complex activities of the full journeyman, and specialists become common.

The NLN Council of Associate Degree Programs in a 1976 action rejected the use of the term technical or technician, and the term *associate degree nurse* (AD nurse) was suggested.

More important than the name are the role and functions of the AD nurse. Because of nursing shortages and lack of understanding of their preparation and competencies, a tendency to use the diploma nurse of previous years as a standard, and general traditionalized concepts of nursing roles, employers have often not assigned AD nurses in the manner that best utilizes their preparation. Like nurses through the centuries, AD nurses have been placed quickly in leadership roles, such as team leader and charge nurse positions, where they are not prepared or intended to function.

There have been complaints that AD nurses are not proficient in technical skills, cannot handle large patient loads, and are slow to assume full staff-nurse responsibilities and activities. Such concerns may be less common as AD nurses increasingly have externships and similar experiences (see Chapter 12). Almost everyone agrees that AD graduates have a good grasp of basic nursing theory, have inquiring minds, and are self-directed in finding out what they do not know. It is also generally agreed that a good orientation program, sometimes combined with internships, can be the key to satisfactory acclimation to the work setting. It should be noted that the AD nurse was an idea based on the success of the Nurse Cadet Corps during World War II. To satisfy the need for nurses in the military, the usual 3-year diploma education was reduced, eliminating much clinical experience. It was assumed that graduates would be closely supervised and become clinically seasoned during their tenure in the Army Nurse Corps. The cadets were never considered to be a finished product at the completion of their basic education. Montag brought these same concepts to a peacetime America.

■ BACCALAUREATE DEGREE PROGRAMS

The first BSN program was established in 1909 under the control of the University of Minnesota through the efforts of Dr. Richard Olding Beard. Since then, these programs have become an increasingly important part of nursing education. In 2008, there were over 700 baccalaureate programs.[7] Of the total RN population, 34.2 percent held the baccalaureate as their initial nursing preparation, and for 36.8 percent it was their highest academic credential.[6]

The individual enrolled in a BSN degree program obtains both a college education culminating in a bachelor's degree and preparation for licensure and practice as a registered professional nurse.

This program, considered by ANA as minimum preparation for professional nursing, is usually 4 academic years in length. Unless the college is tax supported, with minimal tuition fees, BSN education is usually more expensive for students than other basic programs. It is also an expense to the institution. These are serious problems as funding cuts lessen student aid and public funding to higher education in general.

The BSN degree program includes courses in general education and the liberal arts, the sciences germane and related to nursing, and nursing. In most programs, the student does not begin studies in nursing until the completion of the first 2 years of college work. In other programs, nursing content is integrated throughout the 4 years.

As in the other nursing programs, BSN programs have both theoretical content and clinical experience. The BSN student who completes courses in the physical and social sciences will have great depth and breadth of knowledge because many students majoring in nursing take college courses in the sciences and humanities with students majoring in these areas of study. Nursing majors meet the same admission requirements and are held to the same academic standards as all other students. The nursing program is an integral part of the college or university as a whole.

The most notable differences between baccalaureate education and that of the other basic nursing programs are related to liberal education, development of intellectual skills, and the addition of public health, community health, teaching, and management concepts, although some of the other programs do include a limited amount of such content. Baccalaureate nurses have the opportunity to become liberally educated. Almost all programs allow free electives in the humanities and the sciences as well as nursing courses. Although technical skills are essential to nursing, learning activities that assist students to develop cognitive artfulness is a priority. Skills in recognizing and solving problems, applying general principles to particular situations, establishing a basis for making sound clinical judgments and instituting evidence-based practice are emphasized. This enables the nurse to function more easily in an unfamiliar situation or when a familiar situation takes an unexpected turn. The BSN program is the only basic program offering both theory and practice in public health and community health nursing. There is also content in administrative and teaching principles. These skills are clearly necessary when the baccalaureate nurse functions as a primary nurse or as team leader, coordinating, planning, and directing the activities of other nursing personnel.

On completion of the program, most BSN graduates select hospitals as their place of employment, but then often turn to other practice areas. The changing pattern of health care delivery has made community practice and ambulatory care centers attractive employment sites for new baccalaureate graduates. However, those hospitals that have primary nursing, which gives nurses individual responsibility for a group of patients, also seem to attract and retain baccalaureate nurses. Graduates with long-term plans for teaching, administration, or advanced practice continue into graduate study.

The number of RNs enrolled in baccalaureate programs is significant. In some nursing programs, RNs receive credit or advanced standing for their previous education through challenge examinations. In others, there is a direct articulation with full credit for the basic RN course of study. Frequently, courses and clinical experiences are individualized to meet RNs' needs and goals. Although many more educational opportunities now exist for RNs, some, because of circumstances, desire, or lack of counseling, choose non-nursing majors, which generally precludes their acceptance into a graduate program in nursing and may limit their job options (see Chapter 12).

As mentioned in Chapter 12, a noticeable trend is admission of students with baccalaureate or advanced degrees in fields other than nursing. These students complete a second baccalaureate. Depending on how many of their previous courses satisfy the BSN requirements, their program may consist primarily of the upper-division major nursing courses. A growing number of BSN programs are especially designed for the second-degree student. However, there are other alternatives for these second careerists.

An unusual study that looked at the overall education of a baccalaureate nurse should be of particular interest to those considering this educational route. Although, like other nurse faculty, those in baccalaureate education constantly review (and often revise) the curriculum, relatively little attention has been given to the liberal arts component, even though this part of the program is important in developing the unique attributes of the baccalaureate nurse as an educated person as well as a competent clinician.

In 1986, the American Association of Colleges of Nursing (AACN) released a landmark document, *Essentials of College and University Education for Professional Practice*, which defined the fundamental knowledge, skills, and values of this graduate, and was particularly pioneering and explicit in statements about the qualities derived from a liberal education. Baccalaureate programs were charged to ensure the ability of their graduates to

1. Write, read, and speak English clearly and effectively to acquire knowledge, convey and discuss ideas, evaluate information, and think critically.

2. Think analytically and reason logically using verifiable information and past experience to select or create solutions to problems.

3. Understand a second language, at least at an elementary level, to widen access to the diversity of world culture.

4. Understand other cultural traditions to gain a perspective on personal values and the similarities and differences among individuals and groups.

5. Use mathematical concepts, interpret quantitative data, and computers and other information technology to analyze problems and develop positions that depend on numbers and statistics.

6. Use concepts from the behavioral and biological sciences to understand oneself and one's relationship with other people and to comprehend the nature and function of communities.

7. Understand the physical world and its interrelationship with human activity to make decisions based on scientific evidence and be responsive to the values and interests of the individual and society.

8. Comprehend life and time from historical and contemporary perspectives, and draw from past experiences to influence the present and future.

9. Gain a perspective on social, political, and economic issues for resolving societal and professional problems.

10. Comprehend the meaning of human spirituality to recognize the relationship of beliefs to culture, behavior, health, and healing.

11. Appreciate the role of the fine and performing arts in stimulating individual creativity, expressing personal feelings and emotions, and building a sense of the commonality of human experience.

12. Understand the nature of human values and develop a personal philosophy to make ethical judgments in both personal and professional life.

Finally, the authors identified nursing faculty as responsible for integrating knowledge from the liberal arts and sciences into professional nursing education and practice. They further noted that the "liberally educated person who is prepared in this manner can responsibly challenge the status quo and anticipate and adapt to change."[8]

Essentials, which was never intended to be a finished product, was revised in 1998 and again in 2008 (retitled *Essentials for Baccalaureate Education in Professional Nursing Practice*) through a consensus-building process involving a broad cross-section of the nursing and health care community. The environment within which nurses practice has undergone profound change in the intervening years since the first *Essentials* and additional educational experiences were seen as essential. The nine essentials have been defined as follows[9]:

Essential I: Liberal Education for Baccalaureate Generalist Nursing Practice

Essential II: Basic Organizational and Systems Leadership for Quality Care and Patient Safety

Essential III: Scholarship for Evidence-Based Practice

Essential IV: Information Management and Application of Patient Care Technology

Essential V: Health Care Policy, Finance, and Regulatory Environments

Essential VI: Interprofessional Communication and Collaboration for Improving Patient Health Outcomes

Essential VII: Clinical Prevention and Population Health

Essential VIII: Professionalism and Professional Values

Essential IX: Baccalaureate Generalist Nursing Practice

A BSN degree offers many career opportunities, a fact that is widely acknowledged. Equally important is the fact that when nursing has been under particular scrutiny, experts agree that what is needed to meet the nursing needs in today's complex health care environment is more baccalaureate nurses. This point has been made loudly and often. The reader is referred to the report of the Pew Health Professions Commission in Chapter 5 and the recommendations of the National Advisory Council on Nurse Education and Practice reported in Chapter 12. All well-prepared, competent nurses are valuable, but because baccalaureate nurses are still more or less in the minority in the workforce and because the kinds of skills needed now and certainly in the future are those for which the BSN nurse is educated, the recruitment and retention of both basic RN and RN/BSN students for baccalaureate programs is important to the future.

■ CLINICAL NURSE LEADER (CNL)

The AACN together with representatives of nurse executives and nurse educators designed the CNL role (the first new role in nursing in 35 years) in response to the Institute of Medicine's (IOM) comprehensive report on medical errors, *To Err is Human: Building a Safer Health System*, released in November 1999.[10] The report, extrapolating data from two previous studies, estimated that somewhere between 44,000 and 98,000 Americans die each year as a result of medical errors.[11] This is just the tip of the iceberg; there are other incidents, accidents, and infections that escalate those numbers further. In other words, highly prepared professionals are required in these days of complex treatment to assure safety and efficacy.

In response, the CNL role was formulated. The CNL is an advanced generalist educated at the master's level (either post–high school entry or second baccalaureate degree model) who concentrates on the efficiency and effectiveness of outcomes for patients or patient populations. The CNL coordinates, delegates, and supervises care, and maintains effective flow of communication among patients, families, and the multidisciplinary health care team, thereby ensuring seamless, comprehensive service. The CNL role is not one of administration or management. The CNL is a provider and manager of care at the point of care to individuals and cohorts of clients within a unit or health care setting.[12]

The CNL role differs from that of a Clinical Nurse Specialist (**CNS**) in that the CNL is a master's-prepared RN with a focus on **generic** clinical and leadership skills. The CNL is trained in health care systems management at the clinical unit level, while the CNS has master's-level preparation in an advanced practice **specialty**.

The CNL is currently being implemented through education and practice partnerships involving more than 210 practice settings and 105 nursing schools in 38 states plus Puerto Rico.[13] Efforts are under way on many fronts to expand the integration of the CNL role in the US health system. Two successes are particularly noteworthy. In November 2008, the Joint Commission released a white paper urging the health care industry to take action to better meet the needs of patients. Titled *Health Care at the Crossroads: Guiding Principles for the Development of the Hospital of the Future*, one of the innovations spotlighted in the report to address the increase in patient acuity and complexity is to utilize the CNL.[14] In another instance, the AACN convened its first meeting with the Department of Veteran's Affairs (DVA). This liaison was formed to strengthen the collaborative relationship between the AACN and DVA for the purpose of introducing the CNL, among other innovative roles, to the DVA professional nursing workforce.[15]

■ OTHER PROGRAMS LEADING TO RN LICENSURE

There are educational programs that grant a master's degree in nursing as the basic (entry) credential. A variation on this theme is the accelerated master's for students with a non-nursing baccalaureate. The BSN is completed as an interim step, and the student moves on to specialty preparation at the master's level. A student may sit for the licensing exam after completion of the bachelor's degree, depending on state law, and then continue directly to completion of the master's. In 2008, there were 56 generic master's programs in the United States.[16]

A program for the nurse doctorate (ND) for college graduates was established at Case Western Reserve in 1979. The ND was a professional (practice-focused) degree best suited to universities with health science centers preparing several types of health professionals. The curriculum prepared the ND graduates to become proficient in the delivery of primary, episodic, and long-term nursing care, and to evaluate their own practices and the practice of those who may assist them in giving care. Graduates of this program would continue graduate study in a specialization or a functional area such as teaching or administration. As is true of medical students whose professional degree is a doctorate, they might also obtain a master's or doctor of philosophy (PhD) concurrently or after this first doctorate. There were many questions raised as to the functions, role, and job market for the graduates and the best organizational structure for the program.

It can be surmised that as a result of the initial confusion surrounding the ND, relatively few institutions (five) offered this degree. In addition, there was some, but not complete, consistency among these programs. The most problematic area of confusion is whether the degree is an entry-level or an advanced-practice degree. Of the five ND programs, three (Case Western Reserve University, Rush University, and the University of South Carolina) prepared individuals for advanced practice. The University of Colorado and Case Western Reserve University were the only institutions to offer the ND as an entry-level degree or pre-licensure option.[17] The flurry of activity around the ND and noted progress of other disciplines in establishing practice-focused doctoral preparation gave birth to the Doctor of Nursing Practice (DNP). The ND proved to be a catalyst to push us forward in our evolution. No colleges currently award the ND.

■ GRADUATE EDUCATION

Graduate education in nursing, of a kind, can be traced back to the first decades of the twentieth century. However, there was considerable confusion in those early years because what was called *graduate education* was actually education for graduate nurses beyond their basic diploma program. The first programs concentrated on public health nursing and preparation for teaching and supervision.

As late as 1951, it was finally recognized that there was little differentiation between the programs leading to a BSN degree and those leading to a master's; the master's was found to be little more than a symbol that the nurse had previously earned a bachelor's degree. This led to a series of recommendations to place graduate education for nurses on a par with other disciplines.

Over the years, various reports have been issued with recommendations that the public has a dire need for nurses with graduate education (see Chapter 5). Even with the federal funding that followed, the specified goals were not reached. For one, only a limited number of master's programs in nursing were available and even fewer nursing doctoral programs. Therefore, many nurses received their graduate degrees in other disciplines, often education. When federal funding focused on preparing nurse scientists in the late 1960s and early 1970s, these nurses who received both master's and doctoral degrees in biological or social science were hailed as fine examples who showed that nurses could indeed compete successfully with others in rigorous non-nursing disciplines. Unfortunately, in another two decades, many found the lack of a nursing master's degree unacceptable for nursing faculty positions.

Although the growth of doctoral programs has been extraordinary (from only 18 in 1977 to 241 in 2010), the number of graduates has been less impressive, partially because so many nurses find it necessary to be part-time students, and this seriously compromises their academic progress. It is well to point out that 126 of these doctoral programs are preparation for the DNP. The DNP is a practice-oriented degree, and the counterpoint to the research-focused PhD. The DNP is intended to take the place of the master's degree in advanced practice by 2015. In 2008, about 13.2 percent of the nurse population held a master's or doctoral degree.[18] The challenge is daunting; the development of our science depends on a critical mass of scholars who see nursing as their frame of reference.

Despite the rapid penetration of the educational market by the DNP, we will continue to speak of master's preparations here. The DNP will extend and strengthen master's preparation, adding a capstone project in most settings and a supervised residency in practice in addition to more coursework in systems and quality assurance. The purpose of master's/DNP education is to prepare professional nursing leaders in the areas of advanced practice, teaching, and management. Nurses with these special skills and knowledge are desperately required now and will be for the foreseeable future. In 2004, nearly 44 percent (43.8 percent) of RNs with post-RN master's degrees chose clinical practice as their field of study.

Nearly 15 percent (14.5 percent) focused on supervision/administration while 13.4 percent studied education. Post-RN doctoral degrees were frequently focused on education (21.3 percent), research (17.7 percent), or law (11.3 percent). In contrast, clinical practice was only the focus of 5.8 percent of post-RN doctoral degrees. These statistics hold strong implications for the DNP as a necessity. Details of specialization selection are presented in Exhibit 13–1. This represents a significant change from earlier history when graduate education was dominated by preparation for teaching and management/administration. In many ways the pendulum may have swung too far. It will be interesting to observe how these numbers change with the establishment of the DNP degree.

Graduate programs in nursing vary in admission requirements, organization of curriculum, length of program, and costs. Admission usually requires RN licensure, graduation from an approved (or accredited) BSN program, a satisfactory grade point average, achievement on selected tests, and sometimes nursing experience. Some programs will admit a few nurses with a non-nursing baccalaureate and assist them in making up deficiencies. Part-time study is available in almost all programs, but often certain courses must be taken in sequence, so at least some full-time study is required. Reduced federal support and fewer traineeships have stimulated faculty to develop more part-time study options and the government has become more flexible in the allocation of what traineeship monies do exist by allowing support for part-time study. Part-time study has also been made possible by flexible schedules in the workplace and improved salaries to nurses. The stipends and salaries given to research/teaching assistants or on traineeships are no competition.

Not all graduate programs offer all possible majors. The degrees granted are usually the Master of Science (MS), Master of Science in Nursing (MSN), Master of Education (MEd), Master of Arts (MA), or Master of Nursing Science (MNSc). More important than the letters is the assurance that the program will provide the content and developmental experiences that are necessary to achieve master's-level competencies in your chosen role. In *Essentials of Master's Education for Advanced Practice Nursing*, the AACN details the core competencies that each master's student in nursing is expected to achieve, and additional core competencies for advanced practice that are supplemented by specialty content. *Specialty content* is the product of a consensus-building process involving the appropriate specialty association(s).[19]

■ **EXHIBIT 13–1.** Primary Focus of Post-RN Master's and Doctoral Degree 2008

| | Master's Degree | | | Doctoral Degree | | |
| | | Estimated | | | Estimated | |
Primary Focus of Degree	Number in Sample	Number	Percent	Number in Sample	Number	Percent
Total	4,544	387,199	100.0	330	27,725	100.0
Clinical practice	2,192	190,347	49.2	42	3,133	11.3
Education	565	48,743	12.6	86	6,498	23.4
Supervision/administration	890	76,918	19.9	33	2,885	10.4
Research				67	6,129	22.1
						1.3
						.0
						.3
Public health/community health	306	22,782	5.9	12		.4
						.1
						.4

Note: Estimated numbers may not equal totals, and percents may not add to 100, because of rounding and exclusion of other varied degrees in reporting.
Source: National Sample Survey of Registered Nurses: 2008. http://bhpr.hrsa.gov/healthworkforce/rnsurvey/2008/nssrn2008.pdf. Retrieved October 19, 2010.

Most master's programs offer study of a clinical area, such as medical-surgical nursing, maternal-child nursing, community health nursing, or psychiatric nursing, including cognates in the specialty, supportive natural, or behavioral sciences and supervised clinical experience. The depth of clinical study varies in relation to the functional role selected: teaching, management, or advanced clinical practice. A practicum (planned, guided learning experiences that allow a student to function within the role) is usual for the functional role as well as the area of clinical specialization, and most often they are combined. Practice varies from program to program, from 1 day a week for a semester to almost a year's full-time residency. Acquisition of research ability is also considered essential. In general, master's education in nursing includes an introduction to research methods. Debate continues around whether a thesis or independent study project should be a degree requirement. As the terminal degree became the doctorate, the credits for the master's have decreased, and many programs have eliminated the thesis, choosing to reserve any independent research project for the dissertation (PhD) or capstone project (DNP). Contrary to this trend, the AACN also recommends some type of a capstone experience that allows integration of learning that has taken place in the master's program. One example of a capstone according to the AACN definition is a thesis or research project.

Although some nurses obtain graduate degrees outside the field of nursing, advanced positions in nursing usually require a nursing degree, preferably with a practicum. With increased emphasis on the need for interdisciplinary collaboration and new opportunities for nurses, some nursing programs now offer joint or dual degrees with graduate programs in law, business, public health, and other disciplines.

The first American nurse to earn a doctorate received her PhD in psychology and counseling in 1927, although the first doctoral program for nurses opened at Teachers College, Columbia University, in 1924, offering the EdD in nursing, which is still its hallmark. Until 1946, when two of the 46 colleges and universities offering advanced programs in nursing also initiated doctoral education for nurses, nurses who wanted doctoral studies had to attend programs outside of nursing or Teachers College. Although many nurses are still enrolled in non-nursing doctoral programs, the choice has become the doctoral degree in nursing. Theoretically, the PhD is a research degree and the PhD graduate is expected to expand theory and conduct basic research. The person with the professional doctorate,

the DNP, is supposed to use existing theory and engage in original and applied research within their functional role, which is advanced practice, teaching, or administration. The PhD is more interested in the creation of knowledge for its own sake; the DNP searches out new answers for their practical value in improving the human condition.

Whether or not the PhD conducts research of any kind depends on personal inclination or professional pressure (the publish-or-perish syndrome). The fact remains that scholarship (often narrowly interpreted as research alone) is a requirement for university faculty, and nursing faculty are expected to adhere to this standard. For those who wish to pursue a career in higher education, a postdoctoral fellowship is strongly advised after completion of their doctorate. This kind of experience should be used to provide a jumpstart on their research program and publishing.

One consistent concern is quality in doctoral programs, particularly as they proliferate. Monitoring doctoral programs is usually a university responsibility, but it is not clear how well this is done. If inadequate programs are allowed to be established and continue, nursing's doctorates, late on the academic scene, will lose credibility.

The point has already been made for the urgent need to expand the pool of doctorally prepared nurses. The reasons are many: to expand the science, to secure our status in higher education, to bring the credibility of the degree to nursing service, and to establish an active research presence in our practice sites. Currently 13.2 percent of the nurse population has post-RN master's degrees and doctorates.[20] Certainly, the availability of federal funds for programs and students will help to achieve expansion, but it will be the responsibility of nursing to see that the quality of each program is good and serves the American public.

■ CONTINUING EDUCATION

Professional practitioners of any kind must continue to learn because they are accountable to the public for high-quality service—a service that is impossible to maintain if pertinent aspects of the tremendous flow of new knowledge are not integrated and used. A thought-provoking model of the fleeting hold professionals have on what they learn was described some years ago in a journal.

Assuming that the professional life of an individual (in this example, a physician) is forty years, the amount of clinically applicable knowledge available in midcareer should be hypothetically 100 percent of what exists in the field. However, only about half the body of knowledge is available at the time of the educational program, leaving 50 percent useful. It is possible to teach only a fraction of this knowledge in any educational program, leaving 20 percent useful. Of this, a small part is erroneous, leaving 19 percent useful. Not all that is taught is learned, leaving 16 percent useful. Much of what is learned is forgotten within a few years, leaving 8 percent useful; some of what is learned is never used because of specialization, leaving 5 percent useful. Much of what is learned becomes obsolete in 20 years, leaving 3 percent of useful knowledge gained in the professional's basic educational program.[21]

Although the precision of the figures can obviously be challenged, the message is clear, even in nonquantitative terms: Ongoing learning is necessary if a professional is to function effectively.

The American Nurses Association (ANA) has defined *nursing professional development* as the "lifelong process of active participation in learning activities to enhance professional practice," and included both CE and staff development. When nurses participate in the educational process through post-basic activities, they learn to maintain or increase their competency in the ever-changing health care environment.

For nurses specifically, the need for CE is primarily to keep abreast of changes in nursing roles and functions, acquire new knowledge and skills (or renew what has been lost), and modify attitudes and understanding. To achieve these goals, various approaches to CE can be used, such as formal academic studies that might lead to a degree; short-term courses or programs given by institutions of higher learning that do not necessarily provide academic credit; and independent or informal study carried on by the practitioner, utilizing opportunities made available through professional organizations and employing agencies. CE does not mean that enrollment in a formal academic, degree-granting program is necessary, although it might be a reasonable route for a nurse who has specific career goals. On the other hand, neither does holding the highest academic degree mean an end to continued learning.

In the 1970s, a number of states enacted legislation that required evidence of CE for relicensure of nurses (and of certain other professional and occupational groups). According to a recent survey, 32 state boards of nursing now have CE requirements for renewal of licenses for the RN and/or Licensed Practical Nurse/Licensed Vocational Nurse (LPN/LVN) (Exhibit 13–2).[22] Additionally, all states currently recognize advanced practice in nursing, and most make the legal recognition of an individual contingent on

■ EXHIBIT 13–2. States/Territories with Mandatory Continuing Education for Relicensure, 2010

Alabama
Alaska
California
Delaware
District of Columbia
Florida
Illinois
Iowa
Kansas
Kentucky
Louisiana
Massachusetts
Michigan
Minnesota
Nebraska
Nevada
New Hampshire
New Jersey
New Mexico
New York
North Carolina
North Dakota
Ohio
Oregon
Pennsylvania
Rhode Island
South Carolina
Tennessee
Texas
Utah
West Virginia
Wyoming

Source: National Council of State Boards of Nursing. https://www.ncsbn.org. Retrieved May 3, 2010.

national certification that entails CE for recertification. Formalized programs are given under the auspices of educational institutions, professional organizations, and commercial for-profit groups. Either the American Nurses Credentialing Center (ANCC), a national accrediting and certifying board for nursing, or the state board of nursing has accredited most of these providers so that their programs will be acknowledged as legitimate sources of CE. Most programs use the contact hour, which is nationally accepted as the unit of measurement for all kinds of CE programs. A contact hour is the measure of 50 minutes of an approved, organized learning experience.

More nurses seem to be attending formal programs. How much CE improves practice is still debated; however, many impact evaluation studies appear to confirm that there is benefit, albeit inconsistent. It has been shown that the motivation of the learner and the opportunity to apply what is learned are key factors. Opportunities and funds to attend programs are often part of collective bargaining agreements. However, nurses, if they consider themselves professionals, should be prepared to pay for their own CE.

Is CE readily available to most nurses? Despite some justifiable complaints that formal programs are not always available in all geographic areas, there are many ways for nurses to continue professional development independently or through independent study. Examples of self-directed learning activities include self-guided, focused reading; independent learning projects; individual scientific research; informal investigation of a specific nursing problem; correspondence courses; self-contained learning packages using various media; directed reading; computer-assisted instruction; programmed instruction; study tours; and group work projects. Many nursing journals have developed self-learning programs that include evaluation for a minimal or no fee. One of the richest sources of CE is the Internet. Some of the best Internet locations are used as references throughout this book.

The opportunities for CE in nursing are considerably greater than they were some years ago. What kind of CE a nurse chooses remains, to a large extent, an individual decision. However, the necessity to be currently competent is both a legal and an ethical requirement for any professional. Equally important, nursing cannot advance unless all nurses accept the responsibility of lifelong learning.

■ PROGRAMS FOR PRACTICAL NURSES

Professional nurses work closely with *practical nurses* (PNs) in all branches of hospital and public health nursing. Moreover, in the last few years, an increasing number of PNs have been entering RN programs at either a beginning or an advanced level. It is helpful, therefore, to be informed about the educational preparation of a PN.

Practical nurses (called *vocational nurses* in Texas and California) fall into three general groups: (1) those with experience but no formal education who have taken state-approved courses to qualify them to take state board examinations and become licensed; (2) those who have been licensed through a grandfather clause; and (3) those who have graduated from approved PN schools and, by passing state board examinations, have become licensed in the state or states in which they practice. There are also a few who were enrolled in RN programs and were permitted by their state law to take the PN examination after a certain number of courses. The large majority of LPNs/LVNs are licensed by examination. Employers with a choice usually prefer graduates from approved schools that have been licensed by examination.

PNs are usually educated in 12- to 18-month programs in vocational, trade, or technical schools; hospitals; or community colleges. Very few pursue accreditation. On graduation, the student is eligible to take the licensing examination (NCLEX-PN) to become an LPN or an LVN (see Chapter 20). The licensing law is now mandatory in all states.

The growth rate of both programs and numbers of students, which had been increasing steadily over the years, leveled off and even decreased between 1983 and 1989. In other years, there has been a remarkable increase in enrollments. This was a direct response to the industry shortage of RNs.

The federal government has heavily supported PN education for some time. The desire for LPNs to reach RN status is evident in their admission to (and graduation from) basic RN programs. For some years, PN programs have seemed to attract more blacks, men, and older students than any other type of nursing program. However, many of these potential students, if qualified, now seem to choose AD or BSN programs. Some RN programs, particularly for the AD, give partial or total credit for the PN program (often only if the PN has also passed the licensing examination). Increasingly available are ladder programs in which the student can move from PN to RN status in an organized way. In this approach, a PN program serves as the first year of a 2-year AD program. A student may exit at the end of the year, become licensed, and work, or become licensed and not work and continue into the second year, becoming eligible for the RN examination.

In PN programs, many teachers have a BSN degree or less. PN programs emphasize technical skills and direct patient care, but a (usually) simple background of the physical and social sciences is often integrated into the program. Clinical experience is provided in one or more hospitals and other agencies. The number of skills that are taught increases each year, probably because of employers' demands.

As in all areas of health care, there is a need for CE programs. Employers frequently offer courses, reviews, or in-service programs for giving medications and performing new treatments, but the PN organizations and NLN have provided programs on care of geriatric patients, psychiatric patients, and others. The major employment site for LPNs has shifted again and again, based on the availability and salary expectations of the RN. During the boom years, when RN salaries were significantly depressed and hospitals were proud to claim an all-RN staff, the presence of the LPNs in acute care declined. During periods of the nursing shortage, LPNs were again hired for hospital practice. In the late 1980s, the ANA tirelessly lobbied for the 24-hour presence of an RN in nursing homes. As a governmental compromise to the economically strained nursing home industry and given the perceived shortage of RNs, the modifier *registered* was changed to *licensed*, allowing the hiring of either LPNs or RNs. It has become common practice to substitute LPNs for RNs, and often in a very arbitrary manner.

Studies on the role activities of the LPN prove a great deal of state-to-state inconsistency. There is also a tendency for LPNs to expand their practice once they become experienced. This is accomplished through a sequence of events: an educational program appropriate to the activity, supervised practice, documented competency, continued supervision, and state board approvals. However, despite the fact that many of these activities have become a usual part of LPN practice, they are not included in the basic educational program. This may be owing to the absence of a national standard on which to base the licensure examination and the political need to curtail lengthening the educational program. LPNs report administering intravenous (IV) medications, starting IVs, hemodialysis monitoring, pronouncing death, inserting gastrointestinal (GI) tubes, ventilator care, central line management, and management of total parenteral nutrition (TPN), as some examples. These situations are of great concern to the RN, who is not only legally responsible, but is bound by a code of ethics.

Because LPNs are often pressed to perform functions beyond the level of their education (such as charge nursing and certain specialty practice), there has been an increasing movement of PNs to "be paid for what we do, not what we are." However, health care economics, some earlier LPN layoffs, and the continuing trend toward two levels of nursing have brought new concerns. Some years ago, citing "concern for job safety," the National Federation of Licensed Practical Nurses (NFLPN) House of Delegates endorsed two levels of nursing (RN and LPN/LVN) and

the expansion of the LPN/LVN curriculum program to at least 18 months. An implementation date of 10 years was set. That target date was not met; however, ladder programs are becoming increasingly popular. The number of RN students who are LPNs has already been noted. It has been suggested that increasing the educational requirements for the LPN/LVN may resolve some of the entry-into-practice debate.

■ THE NURSING ASSISTANT

It has been traditional that nurses are helped in their work by individuals called nursing assistants, orderlies, nurse's aides, attendants, or more recently, unlicensed assistive personnel (UAP). This category of workers has received added attention lately because of their increased presence in hospitals, often for the purpose of reducing the number of RNs needed to provide care. The result has sometimes been an adversarial relationship between RNs and management, with UAPs caught in the middle.

This group of caregivers was traditionally prepared through on-the-job training. In 1987, the dissatisfaction with the quality of care in this nation's nursing homes resulted in a series of amendments to the Omnibus Budget Reconciliation Act (OBRA). One of these amendments required that nursing aides in facilities qualifying for Medicare reimbursement be certified and that certification be based on the successful completion of 75 hours of instruction, including an examination to verify competency in both theory and practice. Although this process is handled by the state, there are specific federal guidelines. Many states have requirements that exceed those of Medicare. By 1990, all nursing assistants in long-term care facilities were required to either have had a competency evaluation or have completed an approved course. In each state the certification is awarded by a different administrative agency, but for the most part it is the Board of Nursing, Department of Health and Human Services, or the Department of Health. Long-term care aides were singled out for this degree of scrutiny because of the vulnerability of the population they serve (the frail elderly) and the token amount of supervision from the RN. In some ways this was to compensate for unsuccessful legislative attempts to increase the numbers of RNs required in nursing homes.

There are similar certification requirement for home health aides. However, there seems to be the assumption that the homebound are more in control because they are candidates for community living. The skeptic would say that they could be even more isolated and potentially open to abuse and victimization. Although the incidents of unloving care are few, they do exist.

Although state law governs the functions of nurse's aides and there is a great deal of inconsistency, some comments are possible. Nurse's aides are generally responsible (under the direction and supervision of the RN) to maintain a safe environment, perform basic nursing tasks such as grooming, and help with feeding, elimination, and mobilization. The most important thing for RNs to remember is that the aide functions under their license. It is the RN who supervises and determines the appropriate utilization of any UAPs involved in direct care. A health care facility, high school, vocational/technical school, community college, or a privately owned program that may be run for profit and guarantees no employment may give the basic education course for this assisting role. Nursing home aides and, in some states, home health aides must have completed an approved course.

Many schools of practical nursing will award some credit for a formal nursing assistant course, thereby creating the first rung in a career ladder. Certification of assistive personnel has never been an issue for hospitals, where the assumption has been that patient contact is more limited and the RN presence is intense enough to honor the true spirit of delegation and supervision. This has not always been true in recent years. Because of increased salaries of professional nurses, and in the wake of the recent nursing shortages, considerable change has occurred. UAPs have been used more extensively in hospitals, and there are often no consistent criteria for training or responsibilities. Issues of competence, motivation, security, and supervision have been raised. Staff nurses say they need more help, yet UAPs often generate fear, distrust, and a perception of inadequate preparation. Nursing must move to clarify these issues and institute solutions.

KEY POINTS

1. Nursing has slowly, but deliberately, moved its preparation for practice into higher education.
2. Diploma education was the professional program of its day, but has since become very costly to health care institutions and awards the student no academic credit to ensure career mobility.
3. The associate degree program, modeled after the Nurse Cadet Corps of World War II, is currently producing the greatest number of nurses joining the workforce.
4. AD nurses move on to complete their BSN degrees in large numbers.
5. The debate over education for entry into practice is not settled, but has taken a temporary backseat to the shortage.
6. The mature learners that have been attracted to nursing are ideally suited to distance education and open curriculum practices.
7. Distance education is best when a combination of synchronous and asynchronous techniques is used.
8. Advanced clinical nursing has become the preferred focus for over half of the graduate students in nursing; administration and education draw about 20 percent each.
9. Mandatory CE is required for continued licensure in 32 states, but this number has not increased much in recent years.
10. Many LPNs/LVNs use this status as the beginning of an ascent into professional nursing.

REFERENCES

1. National Sample Survey of Registered Nurses: 2008. bhpr.hrsa.gov/healthworkforce/rnsurvey/initialfindings2008.pdf. Retrieved April 25, 2010.
2. National League for Nursing. Research Data. http://www.nln.org/research/slides/ndr_0708.pdf. Retrieved May 1, 2010.
3. National Sample Survey of Registered Nurses: 2008. Ibid.
4. Montag M. *The Education of Nursing Technicians.* New York: Putnam's, 1951, pp 94–100.
5. American Nurses Association. *Educational Preparation for Nurse Practitioners and Assistants to Nursing: A Position Paper.* New York: The Association, 1965, pp 7–8.
6. National Sample Survey of Registered Nurses: 2008. Ibid.
7. National League for Nursing. Research Data. Ibid.
8. Essentials of College and University Education for Professional Nursing. Washington, DC: AACN, 1986, p 5.
9. AACN. Essentials of Baccalaureate Education for Professional Nursing Practice. October 20, 2008. http://www.aacn.nche.edu/Education/pdf/BaccEssentials08.pdf. Retrieved May 1, 2010.

10. Institute of Medicine (IOM). To Err is Human: Building A Safer Health System. November 1, 1999. http://www.iom.edu/Reports/1999/To-Err-is-Human-Building-A-Safer-Health-System.aspx. Retrieved May 1, 2010.

11. Ibid.

12. AACN. White Paper on the Education and Role of the Clinical Nurse Leader. February 2007. http://www.aacn.nche.edu/Publications/WhitePapers/ClinicalNurseLeader07.pdf. Retrieved April 30, 2010.

13. AACN. Annual Report 2009, loc cit. Advancing Higher Education in Nursing. http://www.aacn.nche.edu/Media/pdf/AnnualReport09.pdf. Retrieved May 1, 2010.

14. The Joint Commission. Health Care at the Crossroads: Strategies for Addressing the Evolving Nursing Crisis. Chicago: The Joint Commission, 2005. http://www.jointcommission.org/NR/rdonlyres/5C138711-ED76-4D6F-909F-B06E0309F36D/0/health_care_at_the_crossroads.pdf. Retrieved May 1, 2010.

15. AACN. Annual Report 2009, loc cit.

16. AACN. Accelerated Programs: The Fast Track to Careers in Nursing. April 2008. http://www.aacn.nche.edu/Publications/Issues/Aug02.htm. Retrieved April 27, 2010.

17. AACN. Position Statement on the Practice Doctorate in Nursing. October 2004. from http://www.aacn.nche.edu/DNP/pdf/DNP.pdf. Retrieved May 2, 2010.

18. National Sample Survey of Registered Nurses: 2008. Ibid.

19. AACN. The Essentials of Master's Education in Nursing. February 10, 2010. http://www.aacn.nche.edu/education/mastessn.htm. Retrieved May 3, 2010.

20. Ibid.

21. West K. Influences of the scholar. *Bul Med Libr Assoc* 56:43, January 1968.

22. National Council of State Boards of Nursing. https://www.ncsbn.org. Retrieved May 2, 2010.

Updates can be found at **www.kellysnursing.com**

Nursing Research: Status, Problems, and Issues

CHAPTER 14

■ HISTORICAL OVERVIEW

Like so many beginnings in nursing, research in nursing probably had its start with Florence Nightingale, who made detailed reports on observations of both medical and nursing matters during the Crimean War, documented the evidence, and pointed out significant data, which resulted in reform. After that, there was no other published research by nurses in the early periods of nursing. This was partly because it became an apprenticeship occupation in the United States and because, in the Victorian era, females were encouraged to leave intellectual initiative to males, and nurses often epitomized Victorian females. However, nurses gradually gained more education, moved into universities, and formed professional organizations that supported a research agenda.

Early studies that might be called a form of research were primarily for the improvement of nursing education and nursing service, because the early leaders were almost always responsible for both of those areas and there were obvious knowledge gaps. At a time when medicine was only semi-scientific, it is natural that nurses, scientifically untrained, would not attempt to establish a scientific base for nursing. But there was an attempt to gather data about nursing. One of the first, if not the first, study of American nursing education was Adelaide Nutting's survey of the field, published in 1906. Lillian Wald's school nursing project in New York was probably the first demonstration project reported in the *American Journal of Nursing* (by Dock in 1902). Wald herself wrote *House on Henry Street* in 1915, about that innovative experiment in public health

nursing. (See Chapters 3 and 4 for further details.) Other studies followed.

In 1909, an American Nurses Association (ANA) committee initiated a series of studies of public health. In 1912, Adelaide Nutting's survey of nursing education was published by the US Bureau of Education, followed by the first major study of nursing, the 1923 Goldmark Report. These and succeeding studies by the Committee on the Grading of Nursing Schools, described in Chapter 5, greatly influenced the direction of nursing, and to some degree, nursing research. Although most of these studies focused on the nurse rather than nursing care, some of the nurse-teachers in universities did experiment with nursing techniques.

In the late 1920s and 1930s, a few fellowships were granted to nurses in graduate programs who showed an aptitude for research, and by 1930 nursing leadership had recognized the value of research and attempted to foster it. However, few were in positions to become involved in problems of patient care, and the nurses closest to the patient did not see themselves in a research role.[1]

Notter, as well as Simmons and Henderson, cites a handful of nurses who conducted minor studies related to clinical nursing, most often of nursing procedures, in the 1920s and 1930s.[2] However, although medical research was plunging ahead and finding new answers to disease, research in and about nursing was still related to the image, role, and functions of the nurse and was conducted as often as not by social scientists rather than nurses. Still, there was support by nurses of some of this research, such as the 5-year ANA-initiated study of nursing functions, which yielded much useful data.[3,4]

Sigma Theta Tau, the honor society for nursing, awarded the first grant for nursing research in 1936 and since then has awarded research grants to about 300 nurse scientists, often seed money to enable promising researchers to attract larger grants from major funding sources. By 1970, ANA had also established a Commission on Nursing Research, and in 1972 a Council of Nurse Researchers was started.

The growth of the university schools of nursing had a definite effect on nursing research. As better-prepared faculty and students became involved in studies, sometimes a particular school concentrated on particular problems. Some universities also developed research centers, such as the Institute of Research and Service in Nursing Education at Teachers College in 1953 and Wayne State's Center for Health Research in 1969. This trend continued through the 1970s. In addition, the launch of *Nursing Research* in 1952 and the publication of several texts on nursing research at about the same time drew nursing closer to professionalism. The American Nurses' Foundation was established by ANA specifically to further nursing research by conducting and supporting projects, as it still does today.

As might be expected, federal interest in nursing research was highly influential in its development. In 1955, a Research Grants and Fellowship Branch was set up in the Division of Nursing Resources of the US Public Health Service, providing funds that enabled many nurses to complete their doctoral studies, as well as funds for other research, faculty development, workshops, and the nurse scientist programs.[5]

In 1960, the Division of Nursing Resources combined with the Division of Public Health Nursing, and the research program became a branch within this new division of nursing. Formal support for nursing research, which had begun in 1955, focused in those years on helping nurses obtain a doctorate to prepare leaders needed to facilitate nursing scholarship. Most of these awards went to nurses obtaining doctorates in related biologic, behavioral, or allied fields because of the limited number of doctoral programs in nursing. A Department of Nursing was also established in the Walter Reed Institute (1957), and it was there that much of the early nursing research was done and where prominent nurse researchers received their training.

In 1963, the Surgeon General's report noted that research is one of the obligations of society and urged increased government funding. "The potential contributions of nursing research to better patient care are so impressive that universities, hospitals, and other health agencies should receive all possible encouragement to conduct appropriate studies."[6] Even so, funds were not available in large amounts and progress in the development of clinical nursing research was slow. Seven years later, the National Commission for the Study of Nursing and Nursing Education (NCSNNE) expressed dismay that so little research had been performed on the actual effects of nursing intervention; the profession had few definitive guides for the improvement of practice. The kinds of clinical studies completed by nurses were cited as major contributions to health, and it was again urged that funds for nursing research be increased.

Although funds were increased for a time, continued cutbacks in federal funds soon created a major problem in nursing research as well as in education.

■ WHAT IS NURSING RESEARCH?

Schlotfeldt's definition of the term *research* is classic: all systematic inquiry designed for the purpose of advancing knowledge.[7] Notter makes a useful comparison between problem solving related to patient care (sometimes also described as the *nursing process*) and scientific inquiry.[8] Both go through such steps as (1) identifying a problem, (2) analyzing its various aspects, (3) collecting facts or data, (4) determining action on the basis of analysis of the data, and (5) evaluating the result. In scientific inquiry, step 4 includes developing a hypothesis as well as setting up a study design or method.

After the analysis and evaluation of data in terms of the hypothesis, the findings of the research are reported. Despite the obvious similarities between problem solving and research, they are not the same. *Problem solving* is specific to a given situation and is designed for immediate action, whereas the results of *research* are generalizable and are designed for long-term solutions.

Research may be characterized in a number of ways. It may be designed as basic (the creation of new knowledge or theory that is not immediately applicable) or applied (the attempt to solve a practical problem). Then, it may be quantitative or qualitative. *Quantitative research* is more objective and uses data-gathering techniques that can be replicated and verified by others. It produces information that can be counted or measured using standardized instruments. The approach is deductive: identifying the question of interest and then reviewing the literature to determine what has been done to create a conceptual framework or organizational structure for ideas on which to base the study. *Qualitative research* is more subjective and focuses on questions that cannot be answered by quantitative designs. It is particularly useful in understanding perceptions and feelings and answering the question *why*. Its approach is inductive, proceeding from the careful analysis of individual situations to evolve a conceptual structure to explain the phenomenon of interest. Research may generate theory when executed with an inductive approach, or it may test theory when conducted with a deductive approach.

There are also the broad categories of design: experimental and nonexperimental. If the research influences the subject in any way, the research is *experimental*; if not, it is *nonexperimental*. There are numerous types of design in each of these categories, but the basic difference is whether the researcher manipulates or influences the subjects. In experimental research, there is preferably one controlled setting or group in which certain factors or variables are held constant, and an experimental setting or group in which one or more variables are manipulated and the results are compared. Such studies might be conducted in a laboratory, using animals, chemical or biological substances, or people. If the study involves human beings, whether in a standard laboratory, in a clinical setting, or in the field (the subject's home, school, or workplace), the ethical principles or laws related to human experimentation must be observed.

Historical or *documentary research* uses specialized methods and is more than a record of the past; because history tends to repeat itself (not totally correct, but it makes the point here), its study can prevent mistakes and help point out new directions. Real historical research requires the study of original records or documents (primary sources) to prevent the distortion that comes with interpretation by succeeding historians.

Historical research is having a resurgence in nursing. Not only are the past and its human figures being studied on the basis of new hypotheses, but there is interest in preserving the ideas and attitudes of contemporary nursing leaders—while they are still alive. One good example of a technique being used is the oral history, which involves audiotaped or videotaped interviews that may also be published, such as Gwendolyn Safier's *Contemporary American Leaders in Nursing.*[9]

Descriptive research describes what exists and analyzes the findings in terms of their significance. The purpose may be simply to get information, such as the periodic

National Sample Survey of Registered Nurses, which reports on the nurse population and factors affecting their supply, or to gather facts that might be later used as a basis of a hypothesis of another type of study. Various techniques can be used: interviews, observations, case studies, surveys, or literature review. The studies can be both clinical and nonclinical.

The controversy about who should engage in what kind of research seems rather foolish in light of the need. There are proponents of *pure* or *basic research* who feel that nursing needs a scientific base before practice can be studied. The separation is artificial. Basic research can be a foundation for applied clinical research but, given the unanswered questions in nursing care, there is no reason that there should not be research of both kinds, the abstract and the pragmatic. Equally pointless is the scientist/practitioner dichotomy. Probably all good nurses should have some configuration of practice, education, and research skills, because all are part of nursing's role. Clinicians who do not know, understand, or care about research are missing a source of knowledge that could enhance their practice, and an investigator without sound clinical knowledge is not fully prepared.

One useful definition of nursing research is "research that arises from the practice of nursing for the purpose of solving patient care problems."[10] Gortner describes nursing research as a "systematic inquiry into the problems encountered in nursing practice and into the modalities of patient care, such as support and comfort, prevention of trauma, promotion of recovery, health education, health appraisal, and coordination of health care."[11] Newman maintains that if the criterion "relevance to practice" is applied, then all nursing research is clinical research, but "the distinguishing factor between basic and clinical research is the purpose of the research: whether it is knowledge for the sake of knowledge or knowledge for a specific purpose."[12] Johnson and others have another perspective, seeing new concepts developed by the nurse researcher from the reformulation of concepts from other sciences, then leading to the development of "theories of nursing intervention which will yield predictable responses in patients when implemented in nursing care" (see Chapter 9).[13]

■ WHY NURSING RESEARCH?

Research of one kind or another has been responsible for the major advances in most fields. The notion that much of the science of nursing is derived from medicine or the social sciences probably evolved because nursing did borrow many of its concepts and practice patterns from other disciplines. Some nurses began to recognize that many of these concepts had not been tested or tested recently, and certainly had not been tested in relation to nursing practice. Others began to wonder what in nursing care made that critical difference in patient outcomes. What was the impact of nursing care, how could it affect health care, and how could it affect health care of the future?

Research is an integral factor in the development and maintenance of any professional area of service. It provides the opportunity to prove the value of your services to the public, to bring evidence-based practice to the public rather than interventions based on tradition or common practice, and to progress nursing toward full professional status as it builds its science. As the backbone of practice, research is also necessary for decisions on what nurses should be taught. Nursing is recognized as an important variable in the health system, and as such is expected to prove its value and ensure state-of-the art practice. The outcry for a greater research presence has come from a succession of commissions and studies that can be reviewed in Chapter 5.

The extent to which nursing has become research driven is primarily owing to the relentlessness of the profession's leadership. The challenge remains to develop a research attitude in the bedside nurse and systems for prompt utilization of new scientific insights. Where we have made significant progress is in the establishment of a scientific community of nurse researchers characterized by three factors: communality (sharing research ideas and findings), colleagueship (providing a supportive environment within which ideas can be challenged), and constructive competition (providing a strong motivator for creating ideas). This is the important cornerstone for building a research tradition that will touch the practice of every nurse.

■ RESEARCH INTO PRACTICE

Over the years, a major issue has been the utilization of nursing research. After all, no matter how important the findings of research studies may seem, if they are not tested in practice over a period of time and in a variety of settings, the results might still be questioned. If they are not used at all, practice may change, but it will not change as a result of research. The first step is communication. Without communication, there can be no replication,

application, utilization, or evaluation by others. Over the years, the means of reporting research and participating in peer review have improved considerably. As late as 1977, *Nursing Research* was the only journal in the United States devoted exclusively to reporting nursing research, but since that time several others have come on the scene. Because they are refereed journals, that is, the articles are reviewed and approved by a panel of experts before publication, the methodology, content, and analysis have been scrutinized by others in research and found appropriate. This may or may not be true of research articles in other nursing or non-nursing journals, but here, too, peer review is becoming more common, and such articles are increasing in number, although they are not necessarily presented in as much detail.

Other major avenues of reporting research exist: the federal government; state, regional, and national organizations; foundations, universities, and health agencies—all of which might be responsible for the publication of newsletters, abstracts, reports, articles, monographs, books, and conferences, seminars, programs (with proceedings), as well as publishing houses that produce various indexes. *Dissertation Abstracts International* carries abstracts of all doctoral dissertations, complete photocopies of which can be purchased through the publisher, University Microfilms (Ann Arbor, Michigan), or through the Internet at http://library.dialog.com/bluesheets/html/bl0035.html. In addition, there are individual and university libraries, governmental and private networks of health science libraries, and professional association libraries that use computer-based retrieval service techniques to prepare bibliographies on requested topics. Internet connection to the National Library of Medicine (NLM) allows you to search topics at no cost (see Chapter 29).

Does better communication guarantee utilization? Unfortunately, nursing has a history of ignoring the results or recommendations of research, or at least delaying action. For instance, early recommendations from studies of nursing education about the educational preparation of nurses are only now coming to fruition, after about a 75-year lag. But here, at least, social and economic factors may have been contributors to such slow action. What about the utilization of clinical findings?

For years, there have been complaints that staff nurses not only did not read research reports, but also had no interest in research. Even research results directly applicable to practice probably were not used except in the clinical setting where the research was done, if then. A number of obstacles to research utilization are still present: lack of perceived value of nursing research; lack of motivation to change on the part of both nurses and the systems within which they practice; lack of sophistication in interpreting and applying research findings to practice; lack of knowledge of these findings in the first place; lack of authority to autonomously change patient care procedures; inadequate and ineffective means for the dissemination of research information; and lack of clinician-researcher communication.

Probably in many practice sites this outlook is common. Frequently, nurses in practice today, including nurse administrators, have been socialized to a workplace where research is not part of their responsibility, and they may only be marginally educated to interpret or participate in any type of research. At best we can hope that there is some appreciation of the science of nursing and an ember of excitement about practice that can be fanned by research if it is proposed strategically. Because most hospitals are not affiliated with university programs, where research has been the tradition, and because even in programs of higher education most nurse faculty cannot claim to do substantive research, it is no small wonder that research has not been a part of nursing practice.

However, some clear trends are emerging that may turn this situation around. First, some researchers are beginning to realize that they have a responsibility for translating the research into terms and concepts understandable to the clinician and disseminating their research results in places other than research journals and conferences. Research messages that are relevant to the practicing nurse are being placed where they will be read by that audience and in a form that is friendly yet credible. Practicing nurses do not want reports of nursing research that lack substance. They have no reason to change their way of doing things without clear evidence, verified by a scientific publication, that the new way is evidence based and better. The question becomes, where do practicing nurses go for their reading? The Internet provides a unique opportunity. The effort to identify and reach out to nurses who are known as innovators is time well spent.

Basic registered nurse (RN) students, regardless of their program, are oriented to research during the educational experience, and research is not always an unfamiliar presence in clinical sites. This could take several forms. The most common has been that of university faculty establishing their program of research in a service agency. Where research is agency based, a researcher may be hired temporarily to help design or conduct a study (and then depart) or, more commonly today, be employed in a full-time, permanent position. In the latter case, staff nurses are more likely to be actively involved in defining the research problem and gathering the data. It is assumed that the staff would also be more motivated to use the findings because the research reflects their concerns and questions. A similar feeling of ownership and commitment may develop when faculty who are at a clinical site with students or hold joint appointments involve staff in their clinical research.

Some hospitals with a commitment to nursing research emphasize it in the philosophy of their nursing department and are very clear about expectations in their orientation of new employees. There may be a research committee that helps nurses understand various aspects of research and gives them ongoing support as they become curious about their practice. Networking nurses with similar research interests has proven successful. Research participation may be included in a job description and therefore be part of periodic performance appraisals. Participation in research or the planned application of research findings in your practice may be the behavior that allows a nurse to climb the clinical ladder, or may be the expectation of the next rung on that ladder. The strategies vary, but the rule is to weave a research attitude into the fabric of the organization. Many obstacles may be overcome, and staff can be motivated over time with adequate support systems and incentives, but very little is possible without administrative encouragement and support. Magnet hospitals are such settings (see Chapter 20). The American Nurses Credentialing Center's (ANCC) Magnet Recognition Program distinguishes health care organizations that are committed to nursing excellence. Evidence-based practice, outcomes measurement, and research are part of the essential nature of these organizations. Further, the participation of every nurse in these processes is expected and planned for.[14]

Natural curiosity and the longing for discovery are attributes that should be sought out and nurtured. Educators, supervisors, and advanced practice nurses (APNs) are encouraged to search for this quality in students and staff nurses, even as work pressures tend to discourage these attributes. The challenge is to identify and reduce curiosity-stifling situations on their behalf.[15]

Research utilization has been described as a systematic series of activities that can culminate in the change of a specific nursing practice. One model for research utilization includes the following:

1. Identification, assessment, and synthesis of studies and reports of research-based practice in an area relevant to the problem at hand

2. Transformation of the knowledge derived from that information into a solution/clinical protocol

3. Breakdown of the protocol into specific nursing actions that will be used with patients

4. Planning and execution of a clinical trial, including the specific outcome criteria

5. Evaluation of the practice to determine if it produced the desired result and whether to adopt, alter, or reject the innovation

6. Developing the means to extend (or diffuse) the new practice beyond the trial unit, if appropriate

7. Identifying and establishing mechanisms to maintain the innovation over time

Oddly enough, another problem in nursing research is indiscriminate or unthinking application of research findings. Nurses who become aware of research that seems to be pertinent to their field tend to use it without appropriate evaluation or validation. In some cases, this happens because most nurses currently practicing have not been taught to evaluate the quality of research, although guidelines are available in the literature. To do so, the consumer (of research) must first make a critical validation of the study, that is, question each step of the author's assumptions, findings, and conclusions. If the conclusions are weak, tentative, or contradicted by others, convincing others to apply the research becomes an ethical issue. If the settings or subjects are too different from the consumer's practice environment, the findings may not make a useful transition. If there is too much resistance or apathy in the practice environment, the attempt to implement the findings may require considerable groundwork. Nevertheless, assuming the study is valid, each attempt at consciousness raising is useful and reinforces the expectation for evidence-based practice.

The standard of evidence-based practice, of which research utilization is a component and not a synonym, is only possible if nurse researchers or APNs and staff nurses work in partnership with the goal of putting the latest science into practice at the bedside. Evidence-based practice is the integration of the best research evidence with clinical expertise and patient values.[16] The growing presence of APNs is the profession's secret weapon. The APN's core competencies in the area of research should be proficiency at the utilization of research including the evaluation of research, problem identification within the clinical practice setting, awareness of practice outcomes, and the clinical application of research. This potential is especially promising for clinical nurse specialists who traditionally work much of their magic through their impact on the practice of staff.[17] The cost and quality outcomes of evidence-based practice create the data to justify the increased presence of APNs in general and clinical specialists in particular. Exhibit 14–1 presents some research products with obvious cost and quality implications for practice.

Undoubtedly, actually carrying out all these processes in a significant number of hospitals and other health care settings will take time, but the advances that have been made in a relatively short time are impressive. General nursing journals and especially clinical journals, which staff nurses and other direct care providers are most likely to read, are publishing an increasing number of articles or even columns on research findings. Other articles pinpoint the obstacles to applying research in the work setting and make pragmatic suggestions on how to overcome them. There is also an indication that more practicing nurses are aware of, and even knowledgeable about, certain kinds of research findings, and most reported using research-based innovations at least some of the time. With the number of nursing research conferences being held locally, regionally, nationally, and even internationally, information about current research is much more readily available. It has been found that nurses who read journals, use Internet sites on research, and attend conferences are more likely to be interested in research application.[18]

Even teaching about research in nursing education programs has improved, especially if the school is research oriented and students can be involved with faculty research. Then, too, it may be useful to consider a broader definition of research utilization: "Research utilization is the process by which research knowledge is moved into the clinical arena, and it can happen in many different ways. Research utilization does not always mean implementing research findings in practice. Research can be used in education to spark additional research or to help nurses better understand clinical situations, even if practice changes do not occur. However, research utilization usually means changing practice or validating that current practice is appropriate and does not require change."[19]

■ ISSUES AND CHALLENGES

The establishment of the National Center for Nursing Research (NCNR) within the National Institutes of Health (NIH) in 1986 represented a milestone for nursing

■ **EXHIBIT 14–1. Examples of Nursing Research Products with Significant Cost and Quality Implications**

1. New ways to reduce the numbers of low-birth-weight babies
2. Shorter hospital stays and earlier discharge for low-birth-weight babies with home follow-up by APNs
3. Treatment barriers among pregnant drug-dependent women
4. Nurse-midwifery care of women at risk for low birth weight
5. Exercise intervention to reduce recurrent preeclampsia
6. Baby Boot Camp: Facilitating adaptation to motherhood
7. Reproductive decisions in carriers of genetic disease
8. Helping women decide about estrogen replacement therapy
9. Improved ability of nursing home residents to manage their daily activities without assistance
10. Enhancing Alzheimer's care giving: Cost impact
11. Type 2 diabetes: Ethnic variations in knowledge and beliefs
12. Teaching resourcefulness in chronically ill elders
13. Nurses' home follow-up care increases patient satisfaction and cost savings
14. Management of sleep-activity disruption in Alzheimer's disease
15. Reduction of the use of restraints in the institutionalized elderly
16. Promoting self-care to prevent urinary incontinence
17. Relocation appraisal of nursing home residents
18. Examining the value of special care units
19. Best practice in the use of pain-relieving drugs for women (US pain costs are $100 billion a year)
20. Beyond crying: Uncovering the cues in infant pain
21. Use of saline flush to maintain patency of peripheral intravenous locks

Source: National Institute of Nursing Research. http://www.nih.gov/ninr/news-info/resdir.html. Retrieved April 24, 2010.

research. In 1983, two major reports on nursing from the National Commission on Nursing and the Institute of Medicine (IOM) reiterated the importance of nursing research (see Chapter 5). Both recommended that a high priority be given to nurse researchers and nursing research. The IOM group specifically commented on the "remarkable dearth of research in nursing practice" and noted that the lack of adequate funding for research and the resulting scarcity of talented nurse researchers have inhibited the development of nursing research. They also made the point that because the government grants were administered at the manpower unit in the Division of Nursing at the Department of Health and Human Services (DHHS), and not at a level of visibility and scientific prestige such as the NIH, there was no encouragement for nurses to devote their careers to nursing research of patient problems. It was recommended, therefore, that the government establish an organizational entity to place nursing research in the mainstream of scientific investigation.

In what has been considered a direct response to the IOM recommendations, legislation was introduced to Congress in late 1983 to do just that—in this case, to create a National Institute of Nursing as part of NIH. Although the House and Senate passed the bill, it was killed by President Reagan's pocket veto at the end of the 1984 session. He called the creation of a nursing institute "unnecessary and expensive."

Nevertheless, at the end of 1985, our advocates in Congress managed a compromise and included authorization of the NCNR (one compromise was changing the term *institute* to *center*) under the Health Research Extension Act of 1985 (P.L. 99–158). This was a broad piece of legislation that reauthorized the NIH and included the establishment of two new research units: nursing and arthritis. The legislation was vetoed for a second time by the president. On returning to Congress, the bill became law in one of the rare overrides of a presidential veto during the Reagan Administration. There was no doubt about the support of our congressional advocates for nursing research and evidence-based practice as they delivered eloquent testimony on behalf of the NCNR. Orrin Hatch and Edward Kennedy deserve special recognition. In April 1986, the Secretary of the DHHS announced the establishment of the NCNR for the purpose of conducting a program of grants and awards supporting nursing research and research training related to patient care, the promotion of health, the prevention of disease, and the mitigation of the effects of acute and chronic illnesses and disabilities. In support of studies on nursing interventions, procedures, delivery methods, and ethics of patient care, the NCNR programs are expected to complement other biomedical research programs that are primarily concerned with the causes and treatment of disease.[20]

Research funding had originally been one of the responsibilities of the Health Resources and Services Administration (HRSA) Division of Nursing and the small research staff was moved to the NIH as a core of the NCNR. Dr. Doris Merritt, a research physician appointed as acting head, proved to be not only capable as an organizer, but also fully supportive of nurses and nursing research. She served until the appointment of the first nurse director, Dr. Ada Sue Hinshaw, a distinguished researcher. Contrary to some expectations, both the head of the NIH and the Division of Nursing, who had opposed having a nursing research unit in the NIH, were extremely helpful, as were other institute directors.

The NCNR went into action immediately, supporting research, research training, and career development in health promotion and disease prevention, acute and chronic illness, and nursing systems, which included such areas as innovative approaches to the delivery of quality nursing services, strategies to improve patient outcome, interventions to ensure the availability of resources, and bioethics research, a special initiative. The National Nursing Research Agenda (NNRA) was launched in 1987 to provide structure for selecting scientific opportunities and initiatives. Also, a number of research training awards were granted to beginning and advanced nurse researchers through individual and institutional predoctoral, postdoctoral, and senior fellowships.

At the request of the Senate Committee on Appropriations, the NIH Task Force on Nursing Research was reconvened in 1989. The taskforce commended the progress of the NCNR and made a number of recommendations on how to strengthen nursing research within the NIH. Among them were recommendations to foster an awareness of nursing research as an Area of Inquiry, to encourage collaborative and interdisciplinary research in nursing, to assist in the development of nurse researchers, to ensure access to data on nursing research, and to increase the number of nurse reviewers and advisors.[21] President Bush recommended an increase in funding following the report, and nursing research began to be integrated into the scientific community, something that had been lacking for a long time.

Although the NCNR was not an institute in the NIH as nursing leaders had wished, its mandate, structure, and activities mirrored those of an NIH institute. Therefore, the various nursing organizations worked together closely to mount a new effort for institute status. They had powerful help from people in Congress and the Executive Branch, and support from the NIH Director, but it still took over 2 years to achieve because the 1991 NIH reauthorization of which the proposal was a part was stalled by other political issues. However, the situation changed with a new administration, and on the evening of June 10, 1993, President Clinton signed the NIH Revitalization Act of 1993, which, among other things, created the National Institute of Nursing Research (NINR).

The current research priorities to guide a portion of NINR funding are as follows:

1. Health promotion/disease prevention
2. Elimination of health disparities
3. Caregiving
4. Symptom management
5. Self-management
6. Care at the end of life (NINR is the lead institute on this issue)[22]

Special emphasis is being given to research initiatives that are collaborative with other disciplines and institutes, and those that are associated with or show promise for public/private partnerships.

Although grants addressing established priorities receive funding emphasis, only about one-third of the NINR's total competing grant funds are awarded in this manner. The majority of the NINR's funds are for meritorious research proposed by investigators on topics of their choice. Some of those choices may be influenced by research priorities identified by the NINR and by the profession's associations in testimony to the Congress.

Since the advent of the NINR, an impressive cohort of nurse researchers has developed. Their research is respected not only within the profession, but also in other disciplines. Nursing research has been given recognition in the public arena and has been cited in the press. Some examples include research related to incontinence, pain, bedsores, and low-birth-weight infants. For sponsoring institutions, research may yield more cost-effective methods of delivering care or teaching, reducing staff or faculty turnover, providing answers for recruitment and publicity for the institution, as well as adding income.

For schools and colleges of nursing there is a value-added benefit. Involving undergraduate and graduate students as well as faculty who are not primarily researchers provides the opportunity to become comfortable with the research process and perhaps to publish. In nursing programs committed to research, faculty and administrators must come together to identify creative strategies for integrating research into the faculty workload. Further advances are predicted in clinical settings where nursing research is being valued for both its status and its potential impact on cost and quality. Both clinical and nonclinical topics may be studied. For instance, nurse practitioners, working with clinical specialists, can develop appropriate research projects that may provide new information on the blending of their roles.

The quality of nursing research is sometimes raised as a problem or issue. Much of the research in the past 30 or so years has been done as part of the requirements for a master's or doctoral degree. Although it may be of satisfactory quality, it is almost always limited in scope because of both monetary and time constraints. This may be true, particularly in schools that have an insufficient number of faculty prepared in research techniques. Those qualified may be overextended, and others, whose own research experience is limited, may assume some of the responsibilities.

Because education and scholarship are frequently equated, why do so few nursing faculty engage in research, and fewer invite their students to participate with them? A number of reasons are given: The high number of student contact hours assigned to many faculty allows little time for individual research; many faculty are not as clinically competent as they should be or do not have access to clinical facilities that permit clinical research (although with the increase of required faculty practice, this is changing; see Chapter 12), and there is little research money available externally and a lack of institutional support as well. Nurses have also lacked mentors in research, and research mentors have been shown to make a difference. Whatever the reason or combination of reasons, pressure is increasing for nursing faculty to conduct research, develop a program of scientific inquiry, and become scholars in their environments.

Another issue related to education is when and how to teach research. Baccalaureate programs are expected to include research in their curricula, whether as a simple introduction or to involve the students in faculty research, but there is concern as to whether some approaches actually discourage students' interest in research.

Even more controversial are the rapidly multiplying doctoral programs, which are discussed in more detail in Chapter 13. Besides questions of quality (particularly faculty and resources), there is considerable debate on what the curriculum should include in order to prepare a competent nurse researcher.

Although there are still only a fraction of the doctoral nurses needed and too few pursue research activities after their dissertations are completed, the number is growing, the kind of research done has a rich diversity, and there is good support for collaborative work with other disciplines in which the nurse is an equal partner.

Overall, the amount of research has risen considerably, the focus has shifted to clinical problems, and it has become more theoretically oriented and sophisticated in its methods. There is also reason for optimism about federal funding for nursing research, and, as has been noted, the NINR has set priorities that may also attract private sector funding. We can be proud of our progress in nursing research, but be ever mindful that there is a great distance to go.

KEY POINTS

1. Nursing research is a systematic inquiry into questions and problems arising from the practice of nursing.

2. Problems of translating the findings of nursing research into action are related to the lack of knowledge about research on the part of many practicing nurses.

3. Qualitative and quantitative approaches to research are both valid for the investigation of nursing phenomena, although each is derived from a different philosophic perspective and uses different methods of data collection and analysis.

4. For nursing to develop as a research-based discipline, the staff nurse must be a discriminating consumer of research.

5. Nurse researchers have made significant improvements in health care possible.

6. The establishment of the NINR has greatly enhanced the significance and productivity of nursing's research.

7. Evidence-based practice is the integration of research evidence with clinical expertise and patient values.

8. The APN is critical in moving research into action.

REFERENCES

1. Simmons L, Henderson V. *Nursing Research—A Survey and Assessment.* New York: Appleton-Century-Crofts, 1964, pp 7–24.

2. Notter L. *Essentials of Nursing Research,* 2nd ed. New York: Springer, 1978, pp 9–10.

3. American Nurses Association. *Nurses Invest in Patient Care.* New York: The Association, 1956.

4. Hughes E. *Twenty Thousand Nurses Tell Their Story.* Philadelphia: Lippincott, 1958.

5. Abdellah F. Overview of nursing research 1955–1968. Part I. *Nurs Res* 19:6–17, January–February 1970; Part II. *Nurs Res* 19:151–162, March–April 1970; Part III. *Nurs Res* 19: 239–252, May–June 1970.

6. Department of Health, Education, and Welfare. *Toward Quality in Nursing. Report of the Surgeon General's Consultant Group on Nursing.* Washington, DC: The Department, 1963, pp 51–53.

7. Schlotfeldt R. Research in nursing and research training for nurses: Retrospect and prospect. *Nurs Res* 24:177, May–June 1975.

8. Notter, op cit., pp 20–23.

9. Safier G. *Contemporary American Leaders in Nursing, An Oral History.* New York: McGraw-Hill, 1977.

10. Larson E. Nursing research outside academia: A panel presentation. *Image* 13:75, October 1981.

11. Gortner S. Research for a practice profession. *Nurs Res* 24:193, May–June 1975.

12. Newman M. What differentiates clinical research? *Image* 14:88, October 1982.

13. Johnson D. Development of theory: A requisite for nursing as a primary health profession. *Nurs Res* 23:373, September–October 1974.

14. ANCC. Magnet Recognition Program. http://www. nursecredentialing.org/Magnet/ProgramOverview.aspx. Retrieved May 3, 2010.

15. Redfearn MR, Lacey SR, Cox KS, Teasley SL. An infrastructure for organizational support of research. *J Nurs Adm* 34:346–353, July–August 2004.

16. Boström AM, Ehrenberg A, Gustavsson JP, Wallin L. Registered nurses' application of evidence-based practice: A national survey. *J Eval Clin Pract* 15(6):1159–1163, December 2009.

17. Kring D. Clinical nurse specialist practice domains and evidence-based practice competencies: A matrix of influence. *Clin Nurse Spec* 22(4):179–183, July–August 2008.

18. Mulvenon C, Brewer M. From the bedside to the boardroom: Resuscitating the use of nursing research. *Nurs Clin North Am* 44(1):145–152, March 2009.

19. Gennaro S. Research utilization: An overview. *JOGNN* 23:313–319, May 1994.

20. Merritt D. The National Center for Nursing Research. *Image* 18:84–85, Fall 1986.

21. *Report of the 1989 NIH Task Force on Nursing Research.* Bethesda, MD: DHHS/NIH, 1990.

22. USDHHS. *NINR.* Frequently Asked Questions. April 30, 2010. http://www.ninr.nih.gov/ResearchAndFunding/ GrantDevelopmentandManagementResources/FaqFile.htm. Retrieved May 3, 2010.

Updates can be found at **www.kellysnursing.com**

HELPFUL WEBSITES FOR PART II, SECTION THREE

American Association of Colleges of Nursing: http://www. aacn.nche.edu

American Association of Community Colleges: http://www. aacc.nche.edu/servlet/webacc

American Nurses Association: http://www.nursingworld.org

Excelsior College: http://www.excelsior.edu/nur_home.htm

Journal of Nursing Education: http://www.slackinc.com/ allied/jne/jnehome.htm

National Institute of Nursing Research: http://www.nih.gov/ ninr

National League for Nursing: http://www.nln.org

National Student Nurse Association: http://www.nsna.org

Nurse Web Search—The Nurse Directory: http://www. nursewebsearch.com

Nursing and Nursing Research, Hardin Library for Health Sciences, University of Iowa: http://www.nursewebsearch. com

Research Methods: http://isu.indstate.edu/gabanys/course341

Sigma Theta Tau: http://www.nursingsociety.org

Statistical Resources on the Web: http://www.lib.umich. edu/govdocs/sthealth.html

Yahoo Directory of Nursing Sites: http://dir.yahoo.com/ Health/nursing/

The Practice of Nursing

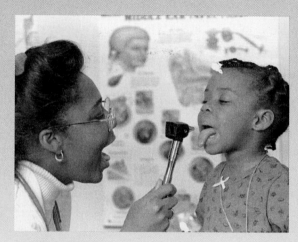

Nursing is caring. (Courtesy of the Visiting Nurse Association of Central Jersey)

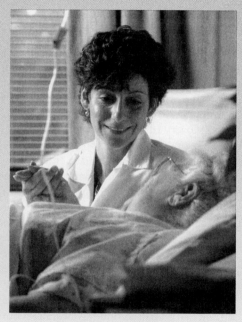

Subacute care services are being established in many hospitals and nursing homes. (Courtesy of the US Department of Veteran's Affairs)

Opportunities in Modern Nursing

One of the most exciting aspects of nursing is the variety of career opportunities available. Nurses, as generalists or specialists, work in almost every place where health care is given, and new types of positions or modes of practice seem to arise yearly. In part, this is in response to external social and scientific changes—for instance, a shift in the makeup of the population, new demands for health care, the discovery of new treatments for disease conditions, recognition of health hazards, and health legislation. In part, these roles for nurses have emerged because nurses saw a gap in health care and stepped in (nurse practitioner, nurse epidemiologist) or simply formalized a role that they had always filled (nurse thanatologist).

Usually, further education is required to practice competently in specialized areas. Sometimes, this is part of on-the-job training, but frequently it requires formal or other continuing education (CE). Practice in areas of clinical specialization will vary to some extent according to the site of practice and the level and degree of specialization. For instance, in a small community hospital, a nurse may work comfortably on a maternity unit, giving care to both mothers and babies; in a tertiary care setting, prenatal nurse specialists, psychiatric nurse specialists, and nurses specializing in the care of high-risk mothers may work together; in a neighborhood health center, the nurse-midwife may assume complete care of a normal mother and work with both the pediatric nurse practitioner and hospital nurses.

In addition, nurses hold many positions not directly related to patient care as consultants, administrators, teachers, editors, writers, patient educators, executive directors of professional organizations or state boards,

lobbyists, health planners, utilization review coordinators, nurse epidemiologists, sex educators, and even anatomic artists, airline attendants, legislators, and legislative aides. Therefore, it is difficult to find any one way to present areas of practice. In this chapter, the approach used is first to describe positions and the responsibilities and conditions of employment for each. Certain systems (armed forces, Public Health Service, and Veterans Administration) that may have different requirements or opportunities, and international nursing are treated separately.

Patterns of employment have changed over the years. The largest number of registered nurses (RNs) is still employed in hospitals, but what was once a very dominant field—private duty—has all but disappeared as an employment choice. Other changes are described in Chapter 11. One definite trend seems to be toward specialization.

Further information is available from the specialty nursing organizations, educational programs, and career articles published by various nursing journals. Career guides are published annually by the *American Journal of Nursing* (AJN), the National Student Nurses' Association (NSNA), and *Nursing Spectrum*.

◼ NURSING SUPPLY AND DEMAND

Throughout the history of nursing there have been repeated shortages and surpluses. Controversy has raged over the causes of these shortages, with less curiosity about how to deal with the periods of oversupply. The consequences to society of an inadequate number of nurses are appreciated. So, with each shortage there is an outcry, and external pressure is brought to bear on the profession to increase the nursing resources available to the public. That outcry reached a fever pitch at the beginning of the new millennium. The shortage made headline news in *The New York Times*, *Time Magazine*, and *The Wall Street Journal*. Although hospitals received the greatest attention (employing 60 percent of nurses) and much of our discussion is geared to their response, shortages and surpluses have been a concern in every segment of the health care industry, and the comments found here can be applied more broadly.

Nurse shortages have always been a response to either public need (as in wartime), or more commonly, uncontrolled consumer demand related indirectly to economics. The relatively low salaries of nurses and their readiness to take on a broad range of responsibilities have continually made them an excellent value. Regardless of the cause, each shortage has prompted organized nursing to rise to the occasion, producing greater and greater numbers of nurses, but the demand was never satisfied. Instead, demand increased salaries, and subsequently economic conditions forced more restraint in how and when the professional nurse was used . . . here comes the surplus, and history repeats itself.

The profession's reaction to every shortage in memory has been to respond blindly to external pressures, devising solutions with little thought about the long-term consequences. Nurses were the logical choice to provide continuity and caring as hospitals became commonplace for care of the sick. Inadequate numbers of nurses for both home care (which was the more usual site for the sick) and hospitals inspired the establishment of diploma schools. Nursing leadership for World War I was drawn from the ranks of college-educated women who received further concentrated education for nursing at the Vassar Camp, a program that, if protected and strengthened, would have allowed nursing to resolve its perpetual struggle for educational parity. But non-nurse influentials terminated the Vassar project once the wartime need passed. World War II created the Cadet Corps, which became the prototype for associate degree (AD) education in nursing. AD nursing was both an expeditious solution to the postwar shortage of nurses and suited to the growing community college movement.

The nursing community had done its work well and without question. By 1988, RN employment was at an all-time high, and there was one employed nurse for every 142 Americans, most of whom were well and self-sufficient.[1] Nursing services were being offered in more varied and diverse settings, but even those new markets had not decreased the concentration of nurses in hospitals. At the peak of the 1988–1990 shortage, there were over 90 nurses per 100 hospitalized patients, as opposed to 50 in the late 1970s.[2] The optimist would say that nurses were more central than ever to the care of patients. The pessimist sees that they were an exceptional value, misused, and still unappreciated for their unique role. Nursing salaries experienced little consistent growth over the years. Nurses willingly expanded and contracted their work, responding to the demands of their patients and employers. Nurses were the ultimate multipurpose workers, easily taking on the work of a variety of other providers. It became the mark of status in hospitals to boast of an all-RN staff. This theory of economic advantage is one explanation for the shortage that should justify organized nursing exercising more control in future cycles.

The shortage of the late 1980s did provide us with some new challenges and opportunities. Organized nursing was moved to a spirit of solidarity when in 1988, the American Medical Association (AMA) proposed the creation of a new caregiver, the registered care technologist (RCT), to supplement hospital nurses. Hospitals were hardest hit by the shortage. In some situations, 22 percent of nursing positions were vacant (5 percent is considered full employment). The RCT was to follow the orders of the physician but be supervised by the nurse. The proposal was illogical and insulting and moved nursing to a unity and assertiveness that has since come to characterize its management of issues.

The shortage of the late 1980s can be traced to several unique situations. In fact, in some ways it really was a different shortage, a point well established by the Secretary's Commission on Nursing.[3] An insatiable demand stemming (at least in part) from a more intensely ill hospital patient, the fact that nurses are the most versatile health care workers (and perhaps the most dedicated and docile), and increasing demands for nursing services in what had been secondary markets (home care, nursing homes, and ambulatory care) set the stage. A general disenchantment among women with nursing as a career choice (about 90 percent of nurses are women) resulted in enrollment declines of more than 28 and 19 percent in baccalaureate (BSN) and AD programs, respectively.[4] So, the demand was high and the future was bleak.

The National Commission on Nursing Implementation Project (NCNIP), jointly sponsored by the leadership of organized nursing and non-nursing groups, spearheaded a major public relations campaign directed at selecting nursing as a career (see Chapter 5). This initiative, conducted with the Ad Council in combination with a general economic recession in this country (nurses could always find work), resulted in a dramatic increase in applicants to educational programs. These enrollment trends are discussed in Chapters 12 and 13.

During this nursing shortage, organized nursing spoke out boldly and detailed what had to be done to recruit and retain nurses. The costliness of the 20 percent annual turnover rate of nurses in the workplace was graphically depicted. To attract and retain nurses, they needed fair wages and attractive benefits, emancipation from the non-nursing duties that keep them from their patients, status and prestige, and the opportunity to build a career.

Salary increases were noteworthy, at least through 1991. Although when increases were adjusted for inflation, they only amounted to 3 percent per year.[5] In 1988, the American Organization of Nurse Executives (AONE) proposed a 100-percent differential between starting salary and the most experienced individual in a job classification. That goal was finally realized in 1993. Nurses represented by the New York State Nurses Association and employed by a Manhattan medical center achieved a starting salary of $40,000 to $43,000 and guaranteed differentials that boosted many experienced staff nurses to the $80,000 to $90,000 salary bracket. Several of the most experienced would earn nearly, or over, $100,000.[6] This growth in range is particularly important. Salary compression, and the fact that in the late 1980s staff nurses would reach their maximum earning capacity in about 5 years, made it impossible to experience much economic advancement over a lifetime of work. The reader is also alerted to the often dramatic variation in salaries based on geography, practice, and employers among rural, urban, and suburban locations, with the West Coast and the Northeast being the most highly paid markets, nursing homes paying less than hospitals, and government salaries lagging behind the private sector.

The health care industry (especially hospitals and nursing homes where the shortage was greatest) took additional steps to resolve their workforce problems. An increasing number recruited nurses abroad, hired contract or traveling nurses, employed nurses from supplementary staffing agencies (creating problems of quality and continuity of care), or formed their own pool of nurses who worked per diem (generally with no benefits). Those familiar with the use of episodic personnel know it is rare that they are as productive as regular staff, but that to the nonclinical mind they are cost-efficient, providing flexibility and avoiding the cost of benefits in most cases. In-house agencies and consistency in the use of part-time workers may modify that effect somewhat, but there is still a difference. An appeal to inactive nurses to return to their work and to part-time workers to increase their hours was extremely successful. Again nurses rose to the occasion personally and professionally.

Particularly interesting were the variety of techniques used to attract and retain nurses. Most favored were increasing benefit packages, reimbursing for tuition, providing bonuses for referral and retention, and paying interview expenses. Benefits were flexible (giving choices): dental, vision, and malpractice insurance; buybacks for unused sick time; added vacation days (one hospital offered a 9-month year); free educational seminars; added conference days; child care and elder care programs; subsidized housing; a sabbatical after a number of years of service; differentials for shift, weekends, education, and certification; longevity bonuses; paid parking; purchasing discounts; health and fitness center discounts; nonmandatory float policies and frequent-floater bonuses; even maid service and a food purchasing co-op.

Although hospital administrators have been advised for decades through many studies on what it takes to retain nurses, the advice seemed to fall on deaf ears all too often (see Chapter 5). More important, the industry seemed to be blind to the value of the seasoned employee over a new hire. Nurses are aware that some hospitals are noted for their ability to attract and retain nurses, and others began to emulate them. Once salaries and benefits were competitive, attention had to turn to improving the environment and the conditions of the workplace. Some changes were elementary and cost little, but had been largely ignored, including better communication with accessibility to administrators, attitude surveys, open forums, nurse relations programs, newsletters, physician–nurse liaison programs, nurse recognition days, positive stories about nurses and ads praising nurses in local newspapers, employee-of-the-month programs, appreciation of nurses by physicians, directors' letters of commendation, and anniversary and recognition teas or receptions. There were also reward systems, including clinical ladders, clinical excellence in nursing awards, promotions from within, and liberal transfer policies.

Most important, the value of the nurse and the nurse's work was demonstrated by involving nurses in various types of planning, shared governance, and nurse empowerment. In many facilities nurses determined their own schedules, regulated their own staffing needs, and were accountable for their own productivity. Employing assistive personnel placed under the control of nursing to do the fetching, carrying, transporting, message taking, and other non-nursing tasks often left to nurses was a good use of resources.

Another common recruiting and retention approach was to offer flexibility in scheduling. There were endless variations on work schedules, but more to suit the worker than to enhance care. Some innovations were weekend 12-hour days for a full week's salary, 12-hour shifts and shorter workweeks, four 10-hour days, split hours in one work day, and top pay for unpopular shifts. Many of these scheduling concessions have come back to haunt us as we begin to question whether human stamina can tolerate some of these schedules and their effect on our capacity to be vigilant for our patients and to nurse effectively. But these scheduling exceptions had their roots in the shortage of the early 1990s, and it is hard to take back what you have given.

There were also signs of better interdisciplinary relationships between nursing and medicine. Many physicians recognized the need for more collegiality and worked in their own settings toward joint practice committees. The lack of such relationships is considered one major cause of nurses' dissatisfaction.

As noted, NCNIP's nationwide campaign for attracting potential students to nursing was in part underwritten by groups other than nursing—a sure sign that the shortage was seen as a national emergency. A second Commission on Nursing (the Commission on the National Nursing Shortage), appointed in 1990, set its goal as finding "doable defined projects" that are both "creative and realistic," and do not duplicate, but ideally build on what has already been done. The Commission, in its charge, was also urged to facilitate the establishment of public/private sector partnerships to undertake some of the specific projects that were recommended.[7] A Louisiana hospital provided money to pay nursing faculty for a school that had enough prospective students, but not enough faculty and no funds to hire more. This was an early example of forging public/private sector partnering for the common good.

Although hospitals received most of the publicity, other areas of practice, such as home care, also suffered shortages.

These agencies tried to match the salary and benefit packages of hospitals, as well as many of the workplace qualities that attracted nurses.

One practice area of particular concern is long-term care (LTC). Because of fiscal constraints, poor image, and the fact that the federal government mandates only the minimum licensed presence, nurses did not see nursing homes as an attractive career opportunity. Much discussion ensued in the industry, and some recommendations were (1) that Medicaid, the major payer in LTC, reconsider its rate structure so that salaries and benefits can be raised and become competitive with hospitals; (2) that grassroots partnerships between LTC facilities and schools of nursing be developed; (3) that LTC facilities redefine the roles for nurses and restructure staffing and compensation accordingly; and (4) that the image of LTC facilities be improved.

By 1995, the nursing shortage was history, and we were moving toward a surplus. Nursing enrollments had rebounded owing to vigorous and sophisticated recruitment. Nursing began to be seen as well paying, and our image was immensely upgraded. In fact, the public so highly valued nurses that quality judgments on hospitals were closely associated with the extent to which RNs were present and directly involved in care. See Chapter 11 for more detail on public opinion.

Our success in managing the shortage of the late 1980s and early 1990s provided no consolation, however, as a surplus moved in quickly to take its place. It is exactly this repetitive scenario that the Colleagues in Caring (CIC) Project is attempting to control (see Chapter 5). The intent of CIC is to push nursing ahead of the curve by defining the public's regional nursing service requirements and establishing a voluntary mechanism to ensure that those numbers and types of nurses are available. Instead, change moved too quickly and the solutions we created to ease the pain of the shortage were used to our disadvantage. Our recruitment efforts were successful, but not always to the right educational program.

Organized nursing proposed that one way to ensure more hours at the bedside was to unburden nurses of the tedious nonclinical duties that could just as capably be done by someone else. However, growing economic pressure in the health care industry opened the door to a much broader interpretation, and these less highly compensated workers were often substituted for RNs and assumed responsibilities that left nurses uneasy. In 1996, over 60 percent of respondents to the largest-ever survey of the nursing community claimed that within the past year they had personally observed a reduction in the number of RNs giving direct care, and almost half reported the substitution of part-time workers and agency personnel for RNs in permanent, full-time positions.[8] A 1994 survey conducted for the ANA showed similar patterns and more: Two-thirds of the respondents reported a decrease in the total number of RNs in the past 12 months (at the bedside was not specified, but may or may not be inferred), and reductions in service or staff in other areas such as housekeeping (mentioned by 40 percent of respondents), clerical (40 percent), supplies (31 percent), lab services (28 percent), and pharmacy (24 percent).[9]

As support services are cut back, more work inevitably falls on the shoulders of nurses, and in most cases we expand our capacity for work to rise to do what is expected. It is probably that general usefulness and cooperative nature that has made our frequent underutilization so acceptable to the industry. Instances have been reported where more than 70 percent of the RN's time is involved in support activities and non-nursing functions. It is also our vigorous recruitment during the shortage that aged the nursing workforce beyond where it would have been. Portions of the Ad Council Campaign targeted older students and obviously they heard our message. Nursing has become a preferred occupational choice for the mature student, mid-life career changers, and early retirees.

Meanwhile, there has been an almost 30 percent increase in hospital-based RNs between about 1986 and 1996. The numbers are misleading, however, and deserve some explanation. Where have all the nurses gone? The versatility of nurses has not gone unnoticed, and they have become the preferred choice for a broad spectrum of nonclinical roles: risk management, infection control, utilization review, discharge planning, and so on. They are not necessarily in direct care, nor are they visible to the staff nurse, but they are there. Clinically, nurses have been dispersed to new areas, with a 70 percent increase of RNs in hospital outpatient areas between 1988 and 1992. In 1996, almost 15 percent of all hospital RNs were in emergency rooms and primary care and specialty clinics. Factor in the higher acuity (sicker patients, more technology, more to be done for patients in fewer days that are allowed for care) and allegations of inadequate nurse staffing take on new meaning, even if the numbers are there. Between 1981 and 1991 alone there was a 20 percent growth in the complexity of hospital inpatients.[10]

The period of shortage and concurrent pressure to cut cost initiated a flurry of activity to restructure, redesign, and reengineer hospitals in pursuit of efficiency (see Chapter 7). These efforts were likely to take the form of some of the following:

1. Elimination of management layers and decentralization of many operations responsibilities to the patient care unit
2. New structural designs that often eliminated the traditional reporting relationships of nurses to nurses in authority positions
3. Early retirement of senior staff through the offer of buyouts
4. Introduction of nursing care models that dilute the skill mix
5. Increased use of supplementary agency and part-time nurses without benefits
6. Increased use of licensed practical nurses/licensed vocational nurses (LPNs/LVNs)
7. Cross-training of RNs to allow them to float to specialty services
8. Cross-training of ancillary personnel to allow them to assume additional clinical responsibilities
9. Elimination of preferential staffing and scheduling
10. Reduced hours of operation for clinical support services: pharmacy, lab, x-ray

Not all of these changes were bad. For instance, cross-training made nurses highly marketable. Decentralization can create a more efficient and effective work environment, and many supervisory relationships are unnecessary, and even offensive, to a licensed professional. However, the reduced presence of clinical support services increased the burden on nurses, as did the elimination of nurse managers who controlled the environment within which care was given on behalf of nurses.

Therefore, in no more than 12 to 14 years, we have run the course of a violent shortage, a more painful surplus, and have moved into another shortage. The surplus has come to an end because of public opinion (see Chapter 11). Consumers have conveyed the message that they want a nurse, and in an era of competition, hospitals have responded. Americans have not just bought a media message, the complexity and instability of the hospital population warrants rich staffing. And the thrust of public policy supports consumer choice and quality, a good fit with nurses. The decrease in graduate medical education funding will also create a demand for nurses as the most likely candidates to take on many of the activities once exclusive to medical residents. Most of all, we are still the best value in the industry.

Although there are conflicting data, the overall pattern is a 6-year stagnation of earnings for nurses (1991–1996). Buerhaus blames a health care industry reshaped by managed care where many nurses have been moved into lower-paying nonhospital jobs; the personal need for job security owing to lingering fears from the recession of the early 1990s (particularly spousal unemployment); and job uncertainty associated with industry-wide restructuring.[11] This safe haven mentality sustained a high level of employment for many years.

History does not repeat itself. We are in the midst of another shortage, the patterns are new and old solutions will not work. Ten percent of the nation's nursing jobs are empty, and one in seven hospitals are reporting a nursing vacancy rate of 20 percent. This shortage, in contrast to 1988–1990, is caused by supply, rather than demand. Admissions, enrollments, and graduations from schools of nursing have experienced 6 years of decline, with the first sign of recovery in 2002 showing a 3.7 percent increase in enrollment. Still, there are roughly 21,000 fewer students than in 1995, not enough to meet the demand for new nurses or stave off a projected shortage of 500,000 RNs by 2020. Yet, serious faculty shortages mitigate against admitting more students.[12] Additionally, the aging of the nursing workforce, general shortages in ancillary professions and support labor, and the global nature of this shortage have intensified the situation.

In the last shortage, we directed much of our educational recruitment efforts to those who were considering mid-life or retirement career changes. Another major strategy was appealing to retired or part-time employed nurses to return to the profession or increase their hours. We were successful, and now we are reaping what we sowed, a dramatically aging workforce. Moreover, less than satisfactory working conditions and a plethora of tangential jobs in the health care delivery system ideally suited for nurses also drew nurses from the bedside. The unprecedented level of employment in the early 1990s gradually saw nurses soured on their jobs as reengineering and restructuring robbed them of satisfaction.

A numerical analysis may indicate enough current numbers of nurses, but the level of expertise may be the cause of the problem. We looked to unlicensed assistive personnel (UAP) in earlier times, both to cut costs and to fill the ranks of caregiver. These people are no longer available in sufficient quality or quantity to fill the need, nor are they appropriate. Increased patient acuity, early discharge, and the extent of chronic disease and frailty demand highly skilled nurses. The clinical picture had not reached this degree of complexity in earlier years. There is growing proof that the shortage of nurses in America's hospitals is putting patients at risk.[13]

In 2009, we saw some easing of the nursing shortage, probably due to the recession. Predictions are that this is only temporary relief, but in some geographic areas there is already significant nurse unemployment. More positively, this situation could give hospitals a welcome respite and the opportunity to strengthen the practice environment, making it more attractive to nurses.[14] Earlier shortages brought creative workplace enrichments, which were lost as shortage gave way to surplus. This attitude of enhancing the workplace did not characterize the last decade of shortage. This may have been because the health care system was forced to deal with greater clinical intensity on fewer dollars. The major issues today are an outcry for still more clinical sophistication, and a workplace friendlier to older and foreign-born nurses.

The corollary challenges are in nursing education. If nurse utilization continues in its traditional model, workplace imbalances will reappear. The greatest need will be to increase student capacity. Academic nursing has done an impressive job in recent years, creating a plethora of programs to attract a variety of students. There are accelerated courses of study to serve RNs, second-degree seekers, and retirees. The Clinical Nurse Leader is an entry-level program that prepares leaders for practice within unique staffing patterns, as yet undetermined. The Doctor of Nursing Practice (DNP) provides the terminal professional degree for advanced practice. This is just a snapshot of the available choices. The attention of students is there, but many are turned away. In 2008, 49,948 qualified applicants were turned away from baccalaureate and graduate programs due to insufficient numbers of faculty, clinical sites, classroom space, clinical preceptors, and budget constraints.[15] The shortage of faculty is of epidemic proportions. Preceptorship arrangements and service/education joint appointments are some of the arrangements that have been proposed to offset the need for instructional staff. How much can we dilute the academic tradition without risking return to an apprenticeship education? Today's faculty require the sensitivity to retain what is good of the past, yet anticipate the future their students will face. Nurses in community practice are increasing, and hospital practice is exceedingly complex. This introduces some serious thought about the most appropriate clinical placements for entry-level students.

Albeit much of what worked in the past has been retained, there is a need for more creative solutions better matched to today's needs, such as

1. Legislation providing capitation grants for nursing schools to increase their number of faculty and students
2. Use of technology to unburden the RN from much paperwork and improve the workplace
3. Redesign of the workplace to accommodate the aging worker
4. Restore practice autonomy to the RN
5. Governmental or professional policies that guarantee staffing in adequate numbers and of an appropriate skill level to be therapeutic
6. Maximize self-care through the nurse-patient relationship

■ HOSPITAL NURSING

As shown in Exhibit 11–1, most nurses work in hospitals. Hospitals differ in size, location, ownership, and kinds of patients. A hospital may be private or public, voluntary or public, general or specialized, for profit or nonprofit. The one element all hospitals have in common is that they are in existence primarily to take care of patients.

There are a variety of other characteristics that are important in predicting the quality of a hospital as a workplace. The organization that attracts and retains nurses values the service they bring to patients and expects them to be responsible for their own practice. This sentiment can be detected by the presence of a peer-review system and the fact that peer appraisals are taken seriously in promotion and retention decisions. In some situations this respect results in the decentralization of managerial functions to the unit level. Simply put, autonomy and intrapreneurship are not only tolerated but also encouraged. Staff nurses are treated as professionals, responsible for both their practice and the environment in which they practice. A salaried model of compensation rather than an hourly wage is more compatible with these expectations, but there is a need to be alert to abuses that become usual. Nurses find respect for the individuals in hospitals who provide the mechanisms for career advancement: career ladders, opportunity for internal promotion, financial assistance for both formal and informal education, and flexible work scheduling for personal needs, including the pursuit of educational goals. Salary and benefits are important, particularly flexibility within the limits of a total amount—a cafeteria approach. Beyond a fair compensation and benefit package, the greatest satisfiers to staff nurses are quality of care issues: support personnel to relieve RNs of non-nursing duties and participation in decisions about staffing and patient care policies. Nurses see themselves as part of a health care team and expect to be treated with the respect accorded to other provider professionals. They see their own status determined to a large extent by the status and respect accorded to the chief nurse executive (CNE). In other words, they value strong central leadership with optimum individual practice autonomy.

Nurses want to participate in decisions about the environment in which care is given, systems of nursing care, and one's personal practice.[16] How each of these relates to the other two and the nature of governance and control is of special interest and will differ from setting to setting. Terms such as *participative management* and *shared governance* characterize some models that are unique in the degree to which staff nurses assume responsibility and authority. The terminology may differ, but the process is familiar. In one model, called *collaborative governance*, day-to-day decisions take place at the unit level. Success required reeducation of the head nurse, retitled the *clinical coordinator*, in budgeting, team building, performance evaluation, counseling, and so on. In other examples of participatory management, all decision making is centralized; staff nurses and managers come together to develop policy and decide on aspects of operations, each holding an equal amount of authority (put simply, perhaps too simply).[17] Although not all hospitals require participation of this intensity or share authority to this extent, nurses weighing employment options need to consider the environment in which they would be most comfortable practicing. Some people prefer a more traditional relationship and structure.

The sections that follow provide a general description of the different levels and types of nursing positions. Many of these positions could be placed as readily in home care or LTC as hospital practice. To understand the intricate tapestry that is nursing, students will have to read carefully and make quantum leaps in their thinking from time to time.

General Duty or Staff Nurse

The first-level position for professional nurses is that of *general duty* or *staff nurse* and is open to graduates of diploma, AD, and BSN or other RN programs in nursing education. Individual assignments within this category will depend on the hospital's needs and policies as well as the nurse's preferences and ability.

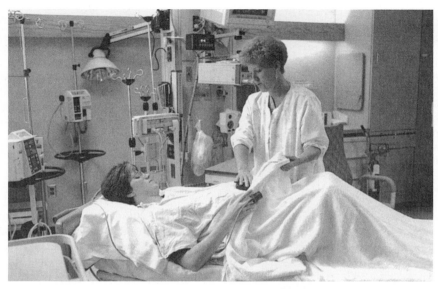

Today's labor and delivery nurses find themselves caring for more and more women with serious medical problems. (Courtesy of Magee-Women's Hospital, Pittsburgh)

Staff nursing includes planning, implementing, and evaluating nursing care through assessment of patient needs; organizing, directing, supervising, teaching, and evaluating other nursing personnel; and coordinating patient care activities, often in the role of team leader. It involves working closely with the health care team to accomplish the major goal of nursing—to give the best possible care to all patients.

To help attain this goal, in 2010 the ANA revised *Nursing: Scope and Standards of Practice.*[18] These are general standards; they apply to all RNs engaged in clinical practice, regardless of specialty, practice setting, or educational preparation, and serve as the framework for specialty standards. These standards consist of *Standards of Care* (patient centered) and *Standards of Professional Performance* (provider centered). Each standard is accompanied by measurement criteria to allow a determination on competence. *Assessment* is the first standard and is included here as applied in cardiovascular nursing. Exhibit 15–1 presents a list of ANA specialty practice standards and the year each was published.

Standard I: Assessment
The cardiovascular RN collects comprehensive data pertinent to the patient's health or the situation.

Measurement Criteria

1. Collects data in a systematic and ongoing process
2. Involves the patient, family, other health care providers, and environment as appropriate in holistic data collection, as well as the client, significant others, and health care providers when appropriate
3. Is involved in the assessment of patients of all ages across the continuum of care from acute to community care
4. Prioritizes data collection activities based on the patient's immediate condition or anticipated needs of the patient or situation
5. Uses developmentally appropriate evidence-based assessment techniques and instruments in collecting pertinent data
6. Uses analytic models and problem-solving tools
7. Synthesizes available data, information, and knowledge relevant to the situation to identify patterns and variances
8. Documents relevant data in a retrievable format[19]

Standards should remain stable over time. Criteria must reflect current practice, and so will change with advances in knowledge, practice, and technology.

■ **EXHIBIT 15–1. ANA Scope and Standards of Practice and Year Published**

Nursing Practice (1973, 2010)
Psychiatric–Mental Health Nursing (1973, 2000, 2009)
Medical Surgical Nursing (1974)
Orthopedic Nursing (1975)
Neurological and Neurosurgical Nursing (1977)
Urological Nursing (1977)
Pediatric Oncology Nursing (1978)
Cancer Nursing (1979)
Cardiovascular Nursing (1981, 2008)
Perioperative Nursing (1981)
Organized Nursing Services (1982)
Rheumatology Nursing (1983)
Maternal–Child Nursing (1983)
Professional Nursing Education (1984)
Perinatal Nurse Specialist (1985)
Child and Adolescent Psychiatric–Mental Health Nursing (1985)
Practice in Correctional Facilities (1985)
Rehabilitation Nursing (1986)
College Nursing (1986)
Community Health Nursing (1986)
Home Health Nursing (1986)
Hospice Nursing (1987)
Oncology Nursing (1987)
Primary Health Care Nurse Practitioner (1987)
Addictions Nursing (1987)
Organized Nursing Services (Revised) (1988)
Nursing Professional Development: Continuing Education and Staff Development (1994)
Nursing Informatics (1994, 2001, 2009)
Respiratory Nursing (1994)
Otorhinolaryngology Clinical Nursing (1994)
Gerontological Nursing (1995, 2001)
Acute Care Nurse Practitioner (1995)
Practice in Correctional Facilities (1995)
Pediatric (Clinical) Nursing (1996, 2009)
Oncology Nursing (1996)
Nurse Administrators (1996, 2009)
Advanced Practice Registered Nursing (1996)
College Health Nursing (1997)
Forensic Nursing (1997, 2009)
Clinical Nursing Practice, 2nd edition (1998)
Diabetes Nursing (1998)
Parish Nursing/Faith Community Nursing (1998, 2005)
Genetics Clinical Nursing (1998)

Developmental Disabilities and/or Mental Retardation Nursing (1998)
Home Health Nursing Practice (1999)
Public Health Nursing Practice (1999)
Nursing Professional Development (2000)
Pediatric Oncology Nursing (2000)
School Nursing Practice (2001)
Transplant Nursing (2009)

Literally hundreds of specific nursing tasks are involved in meeting these standards, some of which can be carried out by less-prepared workers. It is the degree of nursing judgment needed, as well as knowledge and technical expertise, that determines who can best help any patient.

Because the goals of the various kinds of nursing education programs differ, theoretically the responsibilities of each type of nurse should also differ in the staff nurse position. Unfortunately, this is not usual and the qualities that distinguish nurse from nurse based on education are not always respected. This is so common that there is even an inclination to praise as innovative those nursing services that do delineate nursing roles and responsibilities at the staff nurse level according to educational background (*differentiated practice*).

Three basic methods of assignment for delivering day-to-day care to patients in the hospital (and perhaps nursing homes and other inpatient facilities) are functional, team, and case. In *functional nursing*, the emphasis is on the task; jobs are grouped for expediency and supposedly to save time. For instance, one nurse might give all medications, another all treatments; aides might give all the baths. Obviously, the care of the patient is fragmented and the nurse soon loses any sense of "real" nursing; patients cannot be treated as individuals or given comprehensive care. Nevertheless, this approach is used in many hospitals, especially on shifts that are understaffed. The work gets done, but there is generally little nurse or patient satisfaction.

Team nursing presumes a group of nursing personnel, usually RNs, LPNs, and aides, working together to meet patient needs. For team leader, a BSN has been suggested by the Surgeon General's Consultant Group on Nursing as early as 1963, but there are still not enough baccalaureate graduates to fill these positions. Other team members are under the direction of the team leader, who assigns them to certain duties or patients according to their knowledge or skill. The team leader has the major responsibility for planning care and coordinating all activities, acting as a resource person to the team (although not always prepared to do so). In addition, if there are few or no other RNs on the team, the team leader may perform nursing procedures requiring RN qualifications. Often, the team leader is the only nurse directly relating to the physician, and too often, actual patient contact is infrequent or sporadic. The original concept of the team has been diluted. Planning and evaluation are seldom a team effort; conferences to discuss patient needs are irregular; and too frequently, the team leader carries out mostly functional nursing, performing treatments and giving medications in an endless cycle. Nevertheless, the professional nurse should expect to be part of a nursing team or, more likely, leader of this team, because most hospitals utilize some version of team nursing, at least to the extent that the RN supervises and directs other nursing personnel in patient care.

Primary nursing was instituted in the 1970s and is a somewhat confusing designation for the *case method*, in which total care of the patient is assigned to one nurse. A major difference between primary nursing and other methods of assignment is the accountability of the nurse. The patient has a primary nurse, just as she or he has a primary physician. A nurse is a *primary nurse* when responsible for the care of certain patients throughout their stay and an *associate nurse* when caring for patients while the primary nurse is off duty. Ideally, the primary nurse is responsible for a group of patients 24 hours a day, even though an associate nurse takes over on other shifts. The primary nurse is in direct contact with the patient, family or significant others, and members of the health team and plans cooperatively with them for total care and continuity. The head nurse then is chiefly in an administrative role. Almost always the primary nurse is an RN, often with a BSN. Sometimes the nursing team involved in primary nursing consists of all RNs, with the exception of aides who are generally limited to hotel service, dietary tasks, and transportation. There is almost unanimous agreement that the primary nursing model is the most satisfying to patients, families, physicians, and nurses and that high-quality care is provided. It is interesting to compare the role of the primary nurse with the clinical nurse leader (see Chapter 13).

Each method of assignment has its strong points and liabilities. Functional assignment may be the most administratively efficient because of its division of labor according to specific tasks, but almost no one says that either patient or nurse finds it preferable to others. Team nursing, when done according to the original concept, may be satisfying to the team who can give their attention to a small group of patients and also develop an esprit de corps that compensates for the time expended in conference and work coordination. It is often considered expensive because of the need for this additional time spent. Primary nursing, often considered the most professional of assignments, also has its detractors; additional stress, role overload, and role ambiguity are often mentioned.

Functional, team, and case methods are distinguished from one another by the extent to which they allow continuity of the provider of care, the use of assistants to the RN and the roles these assistants assume, the degree to which activities as compared with the complexity of the clinical situation drive decisions on the assignment of personnel, and the autonomy or decentralization of authority and accountability. Given these basic categories, there are endless variations on each theme.

In April 2008, a research project, Innovative Care Models, provided detailed profiles of 24 successful care delivery models, drawn from a field of over 100 original applicants. This project was conducted by Health Workforce Solutions LLC and was funded by the Robert Wood Johnson Foundation. Twenty-four successful delivery models were analyzed, and though they were very different, eight common themes were found among them, which included

1. Elevating the role of nurses and transitioning from caregivers to "care integrators." In 23 of the 24 models, the organization created at least one new role for nurses and often elevated the RN role to one of integrating care for the patient.
2. Taking a team approach to interdisciplinary care.
3. Bridging the continuum of care outside of the primary care facility.
4. Defining the home as a setting of care. (Six of the models rely on a patient's home as the primary location for care delivery.)
5. Targeting high users of health care, especially older adults.
6. Sharpening focus on the patient, including an active engagement of the patient and her or his family in care planning and delivery, and a greater responsiveness to patient wants and needs.

7. Leveraging technology.
8. Improving satisfaction, quality, and cost.

All of the models were developed in response to specific problems or concerns about patient quality, patient and provider satisfaction, or unsustainable costs and utilization.[20]

More information on each of these models can be obtained from the project's website at http://www. innovativecaremodels.com. The models can be categorized into three uniquely different systems: Acute Care, Bridge Continuum, and Comprehensive Care. New graduates should be aware of some of these variable models and of their own comfort zone in practice.

Another reality of nursing is the significant presence of assistive personnel, both those who provide environmental support and others who have some role in patient care. The work of environmental support personnel may include finding supplies and equipment, transporting patients and equipment, cleaning equipment, checking the work of other departments, and moving furniture. It is necessary that these people be carefully trained and that staff be oriented to their responsibilities. In the best of situations, they are accountable to the head nurse and are under the organizational control of the nursing department.

Environmental support staff must be distinguished from UAP who are trained to assist the RN in providing care, and are often referred to as *nurse extenders.* Delegation is essential to the RN–UAP relationship. In delegating, RNs transfer the responsibility for task performance from themselves to another person, but the accountability both for the process and the outcome of the task remains with the delegator. A further distinction is made between *direct delegation*, where there is verbal direction concerning a specific situation, and *indirect delegation*, which involves an approved list of activities or allowable tasks that are sanctioned by the organization. Although indirect delegation may offer some consistency, it can never substitute for or supersede the independent judgment of the RN. It is rare for RNs to be responsible solely for themselves, and in fact most professionals accomplish a lot of their work through others. Students should be prepared for this reality within their educational program. The ANA cautions that risk exists[21]

1. When the RN knowingly delegates a nursing care task to a UAP that only a licensed nurse can perform or when the delegation is contrary to law or involves a substantial risk of harm to a person or client

2. When the RN fails to exercise adequate supervision of the UAPs to whom patient care tasks have been delegated

3. When the RN knowingly delegates a patient care task to a UAP who has not had the appropriate training or orientation

The issue of UAPs and the RN is honeycombed with legal and ethical dilemmas. Can the RN plead ignorance of the extent of the UAP's preparation when a mistake is made and the patient is harmed? How adequate is the degree of supervision provided to UAPs in nursing homes? Will the certification of home health aides and nursing home assistants legitimize their work to the extent that they will eventually become independent of RN supervision? Because these two categories of nurse extenders have very little direct supervision and care for the most compromised of our public, how is safety to be assured?

The basic requirement for a staff position is graduation from an approved school of nursing and nursing licensure or eligibility for licensure. The new graduate may be designated as a graduate nurse (GN) and must take and pass the licensure examinations within a specific period of time. Sometimes a lesser salary is offered until the RN is acquired, and the new graduate may be limited to a general nursing unit, that is, not the coronary care unit or another that requires an investment of intensive additional education, albeit not necessarily formal education. Nevertheless, in the hospital, the variety of experiences is endless. Larger hospitals and those in medical centers may offer a greater variety of specialties, exotic clinical situations, and rare treatments, and the advantage of being in the center of medical and nursing research. Smaller hospitals may be less impersonal, are often in the nurse's own community, and provide the opportunity to be a generalist on smaller patient units (which does not necessarily mean a smaller patient load). There may be relatively little separation of specialties with the exception of obstetrics, pediatrics, and psychiatric care. When there is a declining census, hospitals are beginning to cooperate by consolidating specialties or using beds for a variety of patients regardless of clinical diagnosis. And the smaller nonteaching hospital may also offer many more opportunities in skills, whereas in a teaching center those hands-on experiences are often reserved for medical students. A nurse is usually hired for a particular specialty unit (except in very small hospitals), but it is not uncommon to be asked to *float*—replace a nurse on any unit. Floating should not extend to units that require special knowledge and skill unless the nurse is cross-trained. There should be clarity on the floating issue before you accept a position. In some hospitals, there are *float pools* or resource teams—highly skilled nurses who never have a regular unit.

In some cases, hospital nurses will be required to rotate shifts and work on holidays. For this reason, it is possible to work part time in most hospitals. Usually there are salary differentials for working evenings and nights. In recent years, flexible hours and shifts have become popular. Fringe benefits may include health plans, retirement plans, arrangements for CE, holidays, sick time, and vacation time. The amount of practice autonomy varies considerably.

Opportunities for promotion may be through clinical advancement or movement into managerial roles. Options may be incorporated into a career ladder. There are many variations of a career ladder. Most organizations use a committee composed of the CNE, other representatives of management, and staff nurses to develop and implement a career ladder plan, but other approaches are also used. Criteria are set, usually including educational levels, experience, clinical competencies, certification, continuing education, peer and supervisory evaluation, and seniority. Positions are categorized as I, II, III, and so on, based on these criteria. It is important that moving up the ladder not be a form of tokenism and that there be added rights and responsibilities as one progresses. In some settings added expectations are in areas such as patient and family education, leadership and coordination, and research. In others, the role status of the primary nurse may be linked to a specific rung on the ladder, and the nurse may choose not to progress any further. Both lateral and vertical mobility should be possible, allowing one to progress yet stay at the bedside or move into a managerial role. Where only clinical advancement is provided, this is more properly called a *clinical career ladder*. A ladder should allow for a change in patient population and in job pressures and expectations. In other words, a nurse may move to another type of nursing if qualified. Some nurses may choose realignment (downward mobility), perhaps as they choose to go to school. The guiding principle is for nurses to plan and develop their own careers. Through self-assessment—the first step—nurses identify their knowledge, skills, values, and interests in the context of the practice setting and additionally the rewards that are important to them. Salary increases are given with each change in level.

In preparing for the review that determines one's readiness to progress, the nurse usually prepares a portfolio that contains information demonstrating the ability to meet the performance criteria of a particular level of nursing practice. Information may include a case study, a patient teaching tool, a discharge plan, a nursing database, or other evidence of the nurse's abilities, as well as evidence of educational advancement (formal coursework or continuing education). The review process should be objective and involve both peers and superiors. If it is determined that the nurse does not meet the criteria, she or he should have a clear idea of what areas of behavior or practice need to be strengthened. Because both increased salary and prestige are at stake, career ladders must be carefully developed, managed, and explained.

Not everyone likes the career ladder. Some nurses find it time-consuming to develop a portfolio, even with help; some do not want peer evaluation. Others think it really does not measure a good nurse. Still others simply do not care and want to stay where they are. However, if their salaries top out, nurses may prefer to ladder instead of level. It should be mentioned that organizations seem more highly invested in career ladders during periods of workforce shortage. The career ladder conveys a sense of professionalism and career direction.

An employment option is to be placed in a position through a supplemental staffing agency sometimes called a temporary nursing service (TNS). Nurses who most commonly use TNSs are some new graduates, nurses enrolled in advanced educational programs, nurses with small children who cannot work full time or all shifts, or nurses who simply prefer the flexibility. The TNS pays them a salary for the hours worked, with the usual legal deductions, after billing the institution, patient, or client using the worker's services. There are some TNSs that treat the nurse as an independent contractor as opposed to an employee. The distinction is important; you are responsible for your own social security and tax payments as an independent contractor. You also forfeit the protections that are legally guaranteed to employees. There are local and national agencies, and selecting a reputable one is extremely important. Job assignments may be made an hour or a week ahead, but the nurse is not obligated to take it; however, no agency is interested in a no-show. In addition to a great deal of flexibility and variety, there are also disadvantages, even with a good TNS: there is no job security, sometimes only the minimum rate is paid by the area hospitals with no increases, and, of course, the constant reorientation to new nursing units and patients, even to new hospitals, although some nurses limit themselves to one particular hospital. The fact that *agency nurses* are sometimes looked down on by regular staff as incompetent (although they may simply be unfamiliar with that hospital's procedure) also creates problems for these nurses.

A variation of temporary nursing is the *travel* or *flying* nurse, who accepts short-term contracts directly with a hospital anywhere in the country and sometimes abroad. Arrangements are made through an agency. The hospital usually gives only the benefits required by law, but pays for the nurse's travel and sometimes arranges for or provides housing. The nurse must be licensed in each state where employed. Although the variety is exciting for many nurses, the place of work is seldom ideal, as there usually is a problem—strikes, extreme short staffing, or other poor practice conditions.

Because TNSs are widely used during a nursing shortage, some states are putting regulations in effect, both setting standards and limiting what can be charged. Nursing homes that use TNSs have been particularly concerned by what they consider outrageous costs.

■ NURSING SERVICE ADMINISTRATION

The administrative hierarchy in hospital nursing usually consists of a head nurse, supervisor, assistant or associate director of nursing, and director of nursing. The titles vary with the times and the philosophy of the hospital concerning nursing service administration. Some variation of this system is used in every health care organization—nursing home, home care, and so on.

A clear distinction is maintained between the executive and managerial levels of administration. Managers' strategic planning should be principally focused on the current operations of their program. The executive must have expanded vision and be able to weigh current decisions in terms of long-term consequences. Much of that sensitivity comes from a positioning that is very much in contact with events outside of the organization. The essential role of the nurse executive should never be minimized. In some organizations where nursing is seen as secondary, there may be no nurse executive, only nurse managers. This is an important indication of philosophy and values, regardless of lip service.

The nurse executive is complemented by the chief operating officer in nursing (director), middle manager (supervisor), and frontline manager (head nurse). The middle and frontline managers are the major securers of resources, facilitators of practice, and bridges for communication to the executive level. They control the environment within which care is given, whereas the professional at the bedside controls the care.

Realistically, in smaller hospitals there may be a less complex administrative hierarchy. The director of nursing may be the CNE. The important observation is to look for parity with other organizational units within the hospital and be assured that the executive functions are addressed on behalf of the nursing department.

Head Nurse

Head nurses are first-line managers and are in charge of the clinical nursing units of a hospital, including the operating room, outpatient department, and emergency room. Today, head nurses may hold a variety of titles, including *nursing* or *patient care coordinator*. They are sometimes also the charge nurse, although more sophisticated systems have a nurse designated as "charge" in addition. This may or may not be the assistant head nurse. In any event, the nurse designated "charge" manages the operations of the patient care area for the shift. Responsibilities may include staffing, admissions and discharge, and generally coordinating activities in the patient care area.

The deciding factor is who holds managerial authority. In a hospital functioning as a line and staff organization (as most are), head nurses are responsible to the next higher person in the organizational structure, usually the supervisor, or, in a smaller hospital, the assistant director or director of nursing. The head nurse position is the first administrative position most nurses achieve (or perhaps that of assistant head nurse, who may share some of the head nurse functions and substitute for the head nurse in his or her absence).

It is the head nurse's function to manage the nursing care and ensure its quality in a relatively small area of the hospital. How this is done, again, depends on the philosophy of nursing service and often on the individual's personality. If a democratic philosophy of administration prevails, the staff actively participates in decision making. Then the head nurse uses leadership skills in helping the group to make decisions as well as coordinating overall activities.

As the complexity of patient care increased, head nurses found themselves inundated with paperwork, which limited their major role in managing nursing care. Hospital administrators began to realize that it was less expensive and more efficient to employ clerical personnel to answer phones and questions, complete and route forms, order and check supplies and drugs, and perform the myriad other necessary clerical tasks that have kept the head nurse away from administration of patient care. *Ward clerks, ward managers, floor managers, unit managers,* and *service assistants* (or whatever the local term is) have a wide variety of responsibilities, with some ward clerks even taught carefully to transcribe doctors' orders. Hospitals utilizing computers have been able not only to cut down on every nurse's paperwork, but also to add greater assurance of accurate, rapid communication interdepartmentally. With decentralized decision making, the head nurse is more of an administrator and seen less as a clinical manager. Roles will differ dramatically from setting to setting.

Regardless of the staffing pattern, *staff evaluation* is a major responsibility of head nurses. They control the quality of care more than anyone else and often know best how to eliminate waste, improve utilization of personnel and dollars, keep communication systems open, and provide direct leadership.

Qualifications for head nurses are usually evidence of successful nursing experience and preferably a BSN degree. Many employers require a master's, but there are also many head nurses with no degree. The successful head nurse should have, besides nursing expertise, administrative ability. Unfortunately, in many hospitals, moving into administrative positions is still the only mode of advancement for RNs. Because a good clinician may not be interested or able in nursing administration, such promotions are not always successful. Employers may offer managerial courses to aid the transition. To some extent, the assistant head nurse position offers this training opportunity, but additional training and education are considered vital for most nurses assuming this position.

Head nurses usually earn more per year than staff nurses; other benefits may vary. Benefits acquired by staff through collective bargaining may or may not apply to the head nurse position. The head nurse is usually considered management and therefore unable to be part of a collective bargaining unit, although benefits awarded to staff are often passed on to managers. In most instances, the head nurse works only the day shift, but may alternate on weekends and holidays with the assistant head nurse.

Supervisor

It has been said that the role of the *nursing supervisor*, called a *middle manager*, is the most ill defined in the hospital hierarchy. Because basic management principles for span of control usually specify that no more than six to eight people should report to an administrator, the supervisor is usually needed for middle management. Some hospitals have

eliminated the supervisor, at least on the day tour of duty, placing responsibility directly on the head nurse. In general, however, the supervisor is responsible for several clinical units, delineated by either location or specialty. In a small hospital, the supervisor might be responsible for all the clinical units, and in any hospital the evening and night supervisors usually have larger areas to supervise. In many hospitals, these supervisors are the only administrative personnel available for any department after 5 PM. Therefore, they find themselves acting as temporary hospital administrators, devoting more time to overall hospital problems than to their main responsibility of nursing care. At times they dispense drugs because no pharmacist is present, thus violating the Pharmacy Practice Act in most states. Some of the larger or more progressive hospitals have now arranged for an assistant administrator to be available for general administration responsibilities, but this is still more likely to be the exception than the rule. Even when limited to nursing, the role of the supervisor often encompasses an enormous amount of responsibility and diversity: many aspects of personnel management, which may include hiring and firing; evaluation and improvement of patient care; and staffing and coordination of nursing systems (policies, procedures, and resources).

Generally, supervisors have been employed after showing evidence of ability in a head nurse or other administrative position. Clinical expertise may or may not have been a factor, but an advanced degree is probably a distinct advantage (even if not in administration). Increased emphasis is being put on the combination of clinical expertise, administrative skills, and at least BSN degrees. In larger hospitals, master's degrees are stressed, preferably with experience or a nursing administration major in the educational program.

Salaries may vary according to education and experience. Some fringe benefits, such as vacation time, may be greater than that of head nurses. Supervisors tend to remain on one specific shift, although they may also work weekends and holidays. Even more than that of the head nurse, employers consider the supervisor position administrative. This has made it difficult or impossible for these individuals to be included in collective bargaining with other nurses.

Assistant or Associate Director of Nursing

Assistant or *associate directors of nursing* work with the chief CNE in any or, occasionally, all aspects of the director's responsibility. Specific areas of responsibility may be assigned, particularly if the institution is large. The assistant or associate is generally expected to have at least some of the qualifications of the CNE or be in the process of acquiring them. As a rule, this individual is hired by the director and thus is expected to share a harmonious philosophical approach and be compatible in the work relationship with the director. Salary is often negotiable on the same basis as that of the director, although it is, of course, usually lower. Probably a great majority of the nurses assuming assistant or associate positions do so for the experience and as a step toward becoming a top nurse administrator. They do get that experience, but in a large hospital, many of their day-to-day activities are more likely to be in a direct relationship with staff and somewhat less involved in top-level hospital planning. There are opportunities to represent nursing service on hospital committees and to chair key nursing committees. A good CNE will relate to the associates as peers who participate in the determination of overall nursing service policies and strategies. It is a highly varied position, with no set routine, but extended hours.

Nurse Executive

The CNE position is the highest in the nursing service hierarchy. (Some CNEs are also formally responsible for other departments in the hospital.) The title may be *director of nursing, director of nursing service, director of patient care services, chief nurse, nurse administrator,* or, if this individual is considered part of the top echelon of hospital administration, *assistant or associate administrator for nursing, vice president for nursing,* or a variation of whatever title the administrator of the hospital carries. For years, nurses and others, including ANA and the American Hospital Association (AHA), have endorsed such a title with the concomitant responsibilities. Nursing service is generally the largest individual department in the hospital, often employing more than half the total number of employees. It affects and is affected by the functions of all other departments.

Actually, as a matter of two extremes, nurse administrators in very small hospitals and in large medical center hospitals have few similarities in areas of responsibilities. A director of a small hospital may be a jack-of-all-trades and have no associates or assistants and few managers. Because small hospitals are also usually in rural areas or small towns, management takes on a personalized dimension. On the other hand, in some medical centers, CNEs are also assistant or associate deans or deans of collegiate nursing programs and do little direct management. In larger, more complex systems, you may find layers of hierarchy. As described earlier in this section, the important observation is whether the CNE is on a par with other major department heads.

A survey of nurse executives and chief executive officers in hospitals revealed the following among the most valuable characteristics of the successful nurse executive:

1. Team player
2. A strong value system that is modeled through their behavior, and the expectation that subordinates emulate them
3. Humanistic and respectful of people
4. A vision that surpasses what is shared with staff (does not overwhelm staff)
5. Surrounds themselves with the best staff
6. Visible
7. Well educated, eclectic, and polished
8. Acts, looks, and speaks the part
9. Holds a higher standard for self than for others
10. No tolerance for detail
11. Constantly communicating
12. Well-developed business skills
13. Risk taker, and will sometimes operate on intuition
14. Charismatic
15. People skills are without a doubt their forte[22]

Minimum educational qualifications for administrators of nursing services should include completion of a BSN program that has prepared them for professional nursing practice and completion of a master's degree program with a focus both on clinical nursing and administration of organized nursing services. Completing dual master's degrees, one in nursing and another in business, is also popular. To assume this position in a health science center, academic medical center, or similarly sophisticated and complex setting, the doctorate has become essential. Professional experience should have contributed and enhanced the development of role competencies.

There is agreement in the field that the nurse administrator must be clinically knowledgeable, if not proficient, and that it is essential to have knowledge and skills in newer management techniques, including labor relations, personnel management, financial theories and skills, systems theory, and organizational theory, as well as knowledge of systems of health care delivery. There is also common agreement that education for this role should be based in schools of nursing.

Salaries for nurse executives are usually negotiated, but vary a great deal depending on location, size of hospital, responsibilities, and qualifications. This is a difficult, complex position with major responsibilities, frequently great pressure, and no routine 40-hour week in either time or activities. The director is often expected to be active in community, professional, and other activities, which extend beyond working hours. In some cases, dismissal can be instant and with no reason given (particularly if there is no contract) if the director has not pleased the administration or the hospital board of directors. On the other hand, leadership of a capable and farsighted director of nursing can create dramatic changes in the quality of nursing care and delivery of health services, and bring immense personal satisfaction and reward.

Staff Development

Although staff development still has a major responsibility for orientation and development of new staff, it is no longer a matter of a few lectures and demonstrations of new equipment. In most hospitals it is an organized, evaluated series of learning experiences based on nurses' needs and is sometimes done on the basis of self-paced learning activities. *Staff development* refers to those learning activities designed to facilitate the nurses' job-related performance. The three dimensions of staff development are orientation, in-service education, and continuing education (CE). Occurring at the start of each new employment or position, *orientation* introduces new nursing staff members to organizational culture and philosophy, goals, policies, role exceptions, and other factors necessary to function in a specific work setting. *In-service education* helps nurses to acquire, maintain, and/or increase their competence in fulfilling their assigned responsibilities. This may include how to use new equipment or changes in policies and procedures as well as various programs mandated by states or accrediting organizations. Mandatory programs may include subjects such as fire and safety, infection control, and universal precautions. *CE* includes learning based not just on the administration's concept of the learners' needs, but also on input from the learners.

Some of the current changes in staff development are enlargement of in-service staff for around-the-clock teaching sessions; better-qualified teachers; knowledgeable outside speakers; the utilization of more sophisticated teaching media; planned teaching on the clinical unit; and self-paced learning packages.

The responsibilities of the director include the organization, planning, evaluation, and often implementation of orientation, CE, and training programs for the nursing service department, and, increasingly, for other hospital departments. (For instance, all interested hospital personnel might be taught the fundamentals of emergency resuscitation and external cardiac massage.) The staff development educator must be aware of other resources available for the teaching program, but is personally responsible for the overall development of courses and programs. If there is a large staff development department, one or more instructors may share responsibility for the programs with the director.

Despite the fact that most staff development departments are still within nursing, a trend to be noted is the move toward hospital-wide training and education departments, which may include CE programs for all health professionals and support staff, and patient education. Nurses who have master's or doctorate degrees direct these departments, but may report to the VP of Patient Care Services, the Director of Professional Development, or the Human Resources Department.

Although some staff development directors or instructors have no degree, it is desirable that they have at least a master's degree with some knowledge of teaching principles and techniques (particularly in relation to the adult learner) as well as clinical expertise. They should also be able to work through and with others, with enough self-confidence to assume a staff role with little inherent authority.

Because of the cost of in-service education, there is also a need to develop both strong evaluation tools and programs that meet the goals of the institutions as well as the learner. Salary may depend on the qualifications and the kinds of responsibilities assumed; usually, salary and benefits are at the level of supervisors for the director and are lower for instructors. Of necessity, there will be some evening and night responsibilities, but the majority of activities are usually scheduled during the workday. This position is particularly attractive to nurses who are stimulated by teaching all levels of nursing personnel and who enjoy remaining in the hospital setting.

Other Positions for Nurses in Systems of Care

There are a number of other employment opportunities for nurses in hospitals, although they may have only a tangential relationship to nursing and are often in a department other than nursing service. Nurses on the *intravenous* (IV) *team* are specially trained, and are responsible for all the IV infusions given to patients (usually outside of the operating and delivery rooms). On the basis of a predetermined protocol, they may bring the appropriate IV solution to the bedside or obtain it on the unit, add ordered drugs, and start or restart the infusion. In some institutions they also start blood transfusions.

The *nurse-epidemiologist* or *infection control nurse* focuses on surveillance, education, and research. The surveillance aspect is designed for the reporting of infections and the establishment, over a period of time, of acceptable infection rates. Patients with infections are checked, and it is determined whether the infection was acquired after admission. Reports are used for epidemiologic research, and staff is educated in the prevention of infection.

A challenging role is that of *ombudsman* or *patient advocate*, in which a nurse (or a non-nurse) acts as an intermediary between the patient and the hospital in an attempt to alleviate or prevent problems related to the hospital or hospitalization. Nurses are also being employed in *utilization review*. This role is an outgrowth of the requirement for external monitoring of hospitals by a Professional Review Organization to ensure that Medicare recipients are admitted and discharged appropriately and that resources are used properly during the hospitalization. To avoid problems, hospitals have established Utilization Review Departments as internal compliance monitors of their utilization practices. Improper practices jeopardize reimbursement. It is not unusual to have certain procedures or hospital days decertified. (The government or other third-party payer refuses to pay for the service, because it was beyond the limits of the policy or program.) A selected nurse or nurses periodically check patients and their records to gather data for the Utilization Review Committee. The aim is to maximize the use of resources and avoid decertification. These positions do not require a nurse, but experience has proven that nurses are the best suited to this work.

Another position not requiring a nurse, but ideally suited to nurses is the *director* or *coordinator of quality assurance* (QA), with a variety of titles. Most are nurses because of their clinical background and advanced knowledge of systems. The primary function of these QA practitioners is to monitor and evaluate indicators of outcomes of care. The position arose partially in response to the Joint Commission's requirements for continuous quality monitoring as well as similar demands for accountability from the government, payers, and consumers.

■ ADVANCED PRACTICE NURSING

Advanced practice nursing is synonymous with specialization and specialization is the hallmark of a mature discipline. The advanced practice nurse (APN) is an umbrella term used for nurses who have specialized education and experiential requirements beyond their basic nursing program. In the past, those requirements were often satisfied within educational programs that awarded a certificate, and there were no admission criteria other than the RN. Many of these nurses continue to practice and they represent the vanguard of the advanced practice movement. Today, advanced practice nursing requires the knowledge, skills, and supervised practice that can only be obtained through graduate study in nursing (master's or doctorate). The APN includes the roles of the *clinical nurse specialist* (CNS), *nurse practitioner* (NP), certified *nurse-midwife* (CNM), and certified registered *nurse anesthetist* (CRNA).

The roles of the CNS and the NP are in a state of transition, and these roles are the major focus of this section. Nurse anesthetists (CRNAs) and certified nurse-midwives (CNMs) are discussed more completely later in this chapter. The CNS and NP roles evolved concurrently; the former legitimized expert clinical practice at the graduate level and the latter pioneered practice autonomy in those border areas of practice that intersect with medicine. NPs were more commonly involved in primary care, and CNSs were mostly secondary and tertiary providers (specialty and subspecialty services with patient access chiefly through referral). The two roles began to overlap to respond to the changing needs of the public, as should be the case. There was a growing need for primary care for many populations with chronic, complex health problems. Further, decreasing dollars for graduate medical education made it very useful for the CNS in acute, critical, and even LTC to assume a more active role in health assessment and the management of illness. The differences were additionally blurred as preparation for both roles moved decisively into graduate education, undergraduate students were expected to develop the skills of physical examination and history taking, and nurse faculty replaced medical preceptors who were once needed to teach physical assessment and the clinical management of illness to NP students.

In 1992, the ANA Councils of NPs and CNSs merged into a single Council of Nurses in Advanced Practice. This was not a step to be taken lightly and followed intense debate, testimony from practicing nurses, and a study of the educational programs that prepared one for the role. The education for these roles in 1992 was generally comparable. In reality, APNs seemed to view the roles interchangeably and saw the compartmentalization in education as an obstacle to their career options. It should be noted that the ANA had already linked the CNS and the NP in its legislative and regulatory strategy for reimbursement. NPs had become a very consumer-friendly provider, and legislators understood their role and the benefits they brought to the public. No doubt this was because of their primary care focus and ability to substitute for physicians. Linking the less commonly understood CNS with the NP in public policy hastened progress. A convergence of these circumstances allowed for more flexibility and a future that was certain, but had to be developed. The momentum for consolidation grew as several prominent colleges and universities merged what had been distinct NP and CNS graduate programs. Being more alike than different, crossover from one role to the other is possible. In selecting a graduate program, an individual should make sure that the faculty are consciously addressing the knowledge and skills to compete in a job market that is sensitive to the subtle distinctions between NPs and CNSs. Assessment skills should be highly developed, and pharmacology and pathophysiology should be major areas of study for both (see Chapter 13). For the purposes of this presentation, the roles will be presented separately.

The Clinical Nurse Specialist

The CNS, who may also be called a *nurse specialist*, *nurse clinician*, or *clinical specialist*, has become an increasingly important part of the nursing practice scene since the early 1960s. A clinical specialist is an expert practitioner within a specialized field of nursing or even a subspecialty. There are clinical specialists in all the major clinical areas, but also some concentrating on cancer, rehabilitation, and perinatal nursing, tuberculosis, care of patients with ostomies, neurologic problems, respiratory conditions, epilepsy, and many other subspecialties.

Expert practice is the sine qua non of the CNS. Ongoing experience with patients and their support systems directs participation in a range of subroles including direct care, research, teaching, consultation, and management. The CNS spends a great amount of time in mediated roles, in other words, working through other people rather than personally laying on of hands. The CNS is also a master of systems. CNSs in institutional practice may be either unit- or population-based and invest significant effort in the things that have to be done to maintain a quality system on behalf of their patients, such as quality assurance, policy development, and peer review. The basic element in CNS practice is continuing patient involvement, with practice more appropriately being within a nursing/social model as opposed to a medical model.

Originally, the intent was to position the CNS powerfully and award staff authority, that is, reporting directly to the chief nurse administrator and acting in an advisory or consultative capacity to the nursing staff and middle managers. However, a line position (superior–subordinate relationship) gives authority and there can be problems when a CNS makes patient care recommendations as a staff member and nurses and managers choose to ignore them. It is becoming more common for the CNS to also assume positional authority focused on nursing care.

The ANA has emphasized the importance of flexibility for CNSs in their work settings. Job descriptions and details of functions should not be standardized. Instead, rights, responsibilities, organizational placement, and role relationships should be negotiated between the CNS and the employer. The goal is the most strategic placement and involvement for maximum use of their abilities. The same standard applies in joint practice and partnership arrangements.

CNSs are expected to have a master's degree in nursing with emphasis on the specialty area and a functional role in advanced practice. Education for this role is in transition to the DNP (see Chapter 13). Advanced practice certification is not only preferred, but is also mandatory in most states to assume the role. According to the 2008 Sample Survey, there has been a decline in the number of nurses prepared as clinical nurse specialists since the 2004 Survey. In 2008, there were an estimated 59,242 clinical nurse specialists in the United States, compared with 72,521 in 2004, a drop of 22.4 percent.[23]

Frequently, there is a great deal of flexibility in the CNS's time. They may work no specific shift but care for patients selected according to the patients' and staff's needs, which may mean being available evenings or nights or, by choice, even available on call if a problem arises. (Telephone consultations with patients who develop problems or need support at home are not uncommon.) There should be time available for library research and home visits. A CNS usually has office space, preferably near the clinical units.

More than any APN, the CNS is the victim of misunderstanding and ignorance on the part of the health care industry and the general public and is often the recipient of double messages. There was a flurry of hiring CNSs in the early days of diagnostic related groups (DRGs) when every sector of health care was caught off guard by rising acuities and the movement of sicker patients into home and community care. Those CNSs who had the data to prove their contribution to the fiscal integrity of the organization flourished; others were eventually sacrificed to the need for economy. CNSs hold the answer to decreasing length of stay, increasing functional ability and self-sufficiency, avoiding complications, optimizing reimbursement, and gaining cooperation from nursing staff to pursue an ambitious clinical agenda. With a new flexibility on the part of both the profession and the industry, CNSs are sought for a variety of role configurations while maintaining a patient-centered focus and continuing their involvement in practice. CNSs can now be found in small as well as large hospitals and medical centers, nursing homes, ambulatory care, and virtually every service setting, including private practice. The prescriptive authority, reimbursement, and clinical privileging gains of recent years in many situations apply to the CNS and NP equally. This will be discussed later in this chapter. The presence of a CNS often indicates the seriousness with which an institution views nursing.

The Nurse Practitioner

The NP is no longer a new role. Chapter 9 should have adequately established the expectation that professions change with the times, and the NP is a good example. Many nurses would claim that there is nothing new at all, just legal recognition and broader consumer awareness of services NPs have always provided. Lillian Wald, a pioneer in public health nursing (PHN), made house calls, prescribed and dispensed medications and treatments, and counseled her client families as needed. In more recent times, the Frontier Nursing Service of Wendover, Kentucky, which was noted for its nursing on horseback midwifery services, has expanded its practice to overall family services.

However one views the role, it has proliferated. Nurse practitioners comprise 63 percent of nurses in advanced specialties in 2008, accounting for 158,348 nurses. In 2004, 141,209 nurses were prepared as nurse practitioners; the number of nurse practitioners thus grew 12.1 percent over 4 years. Of nurse practitioners in 2008, 19,134 were prepared as both a nurse practitioner and either a clinical nurse specialist or a nurse midwife.[24]

The NP movement had logical formal beginnings. The 1960s brought change, reform, Medicare, Medicaid, medical specialization at an accelerated pace, a larger market for primary health care services, and a shortage of primary care physicians. Nursing moved forward to fill the gap. In 1965, the first NP program was established by Ford and Silver at the University of Colorado. It is generally agreed that NPs have acquired additional knowledge and skills, some of which were previously considered the exclusive domain of medicine. Combining these new areas of service with the nursing role creates a comprehensive practice, requiring collaboration and consultation with a range of other provider professionals, including physicians. The NP is prepared to assume a primary care role. Although this means many things to many people, the essential definition includes the capacity to serve as the first and continuing contact for the client within the delivery system. Further, the primary provider is concerned with a broad range of services, including health promotion, disease prevention, the diagnosis and treatment of minor acute illness, and the monitoring and management of chronic conditions. The NP focuses on broad divisions of practice as compared with CNS practice, which often takes the form of more highly circumscribed specialties and subspecialties. NPs are prepared for practice in pediatrics, family practice, adult and women's health, geriatrics, and school and college health practice, to name a few. Their clients are commonly the well, even if that wellness is a new trajectory of normal with the constant of chronic disease. In comparison, CNS practice areas may be cardiovascular, orthopedics, oncology, geropsychiatry, medical-surgical, neurologic nursing, or others. As mentioned, the distinction has become largely artificial because once-differentiating knowledge and skills have become common to both.

NPs practice in a wide range of settings, such as public or private clinics, health maintenance organizations (HMOs), private offices, schools, and occupational health settings, as well as prisons and military facilities. They also provide care in home health care, LTC, and acute care settings; many are in private practices of their own. NPs provide health care to many diverse and underserved populations, such as the homeless, migrant families, Native Americans, and other ethnic minorities. The NP was a sensitive response to a very real consumer need. The role will continue to evolve in response to a changing health care environment.

A major trend in the education of NPs over the past 45 years has been the shift from certificate programs to the master's degree, and now the impending transition to the DNP (see Chapter 13). Much of this has resulted from positions taken by nursing organizations. For example, in 1984 the ANA House of Delegates adopted a resolution establishing 1990 as the target date by which all programs preparing NPs should be at the graduate level. Additionally, federal funding has been preferential to graduate as opposed to certificate educational programs. Now the DNP has been introduced by the AACN and specialty nursing organizations as the terminal degree for advanced practice, ideally by 2015.

No group has been more scrutinized and studied than the NP, probably because of the threat that they pose to the medical establishment and the fact that their success opens the door to a variety of other providers who may be better options than traditional providers. In 1986, a summary of existing studies on the effectiveness of NPs and CNMs was presented in a congressionally mandated Office of Technology Assessment Report. In 1993, the ANA funded a subsequent meta-analysis of research on nurses in primary care roles as they compared with physicians. NPs provide more health promotion activities, order more economical tests, recommend fewer prescription drugs, achieve higher scores on patient satisfaction and patient compliance surveys, and are more successful in maintaining or upgrading the functional status of their clients than physicians. They spent more time with their patients and complete an equal number of visits or encounters, yet the nurse's visit costs 40 percent less than the physician's, their educational preparation costs four to five times less, and it can be completed 4 years sooner. Research further shows that NPs can independently diagnose and resolve 80 percent of the primary care complaints of the American public; provide continuity of care where it has been fragmented; are accepted by consumers; save physician time; and are profitable to employers.[25]

Despite the positive aspects of collaboration, competition between MDs and NPs persists on many levels. Although some competition can be considered healthy, it is not so when it depletes time and energy that could be devoted to clinical practice. It becomes counterproductive given the large numbers of people who lack access to primary care and are in need of both NP and physician services. With the challenges of cutbacks in public health programs and the high cost of health care, collaboration between MDs and NPs can only be in the best interest of the public.

In 2010, NPs nationally earned an average salary of $90,000 to $109,000, depending on the geographic area.[26] NPs are frequently found in the private practices of physicians, not usually as partners but as employees. Careful negotiation of an employment contract in the latter situation is crucial.

Nurse-Midwife

Master's or post-master's educational preparation has become the standard, and certification is required for legal recognition and prescriptive authority in most states. CNMs are categorized as one of the advanced practice roles and have existed for some time. The

Maternity Center Association started the first school of nurse midwifery in 1931 in New York City. According to the American College of Nurse-Midwives (ACNM):

> Today, over 7000 certified nurse-midwives practice in all 50 states and many developing countries, according to birth control data. In 2005, CNMs attended over 306,000 deliveries, mostly in hospitals. This number accounts for almost 8 percent of all U.S. births. Furthermore, certified nurse-midwives continue to be highly regarded in the health care community. Two reports by the Institute of Medicine and the National Commission to Prevent Infant Mortality praise their contributions in reducing the incidence of low birthweight infants and call for their increased utilization.[27]

In 2010, a midwife in practice in the United States earned an average salary of $100,000.[28] They practice in a variety of settings where maternity and gynecological care are given—clinics, private offices, hospitals, birthing centers, or in the woman's home. Their practice may be interdependent within a health care delivery system, for example, a hospital obstetric service largely staffed by CNMs, where a physician might provide consultation or high-risk obstetrical care as needed. They might also have a formal written alliance with an obstetrician or another physician or group of physicians who have a formal consultative arrangement with an obstetrician-gynecologist. ACNM standards for practice require that CNMs base their care on knowledge, skills, and judgments that are reflected in written policies and practice guidelines. The fact that many mothers now seem to prefer a normal and natural birthing process when there are no potential complications has brought a resurgence of interest in nurse-midwifery.

CNMs receive much support from public and private agencies because of their documented effectiveness in managing the care of pregnant women and their infants. Specifically, studies have demonstrated that the care rendered by CNMs resulted in reductions in the rates of premature and low-birth-weight babies. A number of national studies on prenatal care have mentioned the value of CNMs and called for their increased utilization.

CNMs' clinical competence and nursing emphasis has contributed to their acceptance by consumers and professionals. Across the country, CNMs are gaining in recognition and popularity. For example, the number of hospital births attended by CNMs has increased nearly sevenfold, from 19,686 to more than 158,000 within a 15-year period. This growth is startling when one considers that only about 30 years ago, few states permitted CNMs to practice. New interest and political determination on behalf of CNMs has brought about legal changes that permit the nurse-midwife to practice, with a nursing license and ACC certification or whatever else is required under new midwifery laws. However, despite these trends, CNMs still face political battles in the clinical and policy arenas similar to those of NPs.

In the mid-1980s, CNMs faced a crisis in not being able to obtain affordable professional liability insurance. The situation threatened the viability of nurse-midwifery practice across the country and forced many CNMs to give up their practices. Since 1986, insurance has been available to CNMs through a consortium of companies. In addition, many employers offer coverage for the CNMs on their staff. ACNM provides information on insurance and sees it as a key part of nurse-midwifery practice.

A graduate degree is required for entry into nurse midwifery practice since 2010. There additionally is strong support for the DNP.[21] All programs include theory and practice in prenatal care, care of a woman during labor and birth, attendance of births in hospitals, immediate care of the newborn, care of the postpartum patient, family planning, and well-woman health care. After completion of an ACNM-approved program, the nurse-midwife is eligible to take the certification examination. The ACNM, located in Washington, DC, is the best source of information on careers and issues in nurse-midwifery practice.

Nurse Anesthetist

Certified registered nurse anesthetists (CRNAs) are anesthesia specialists who administer more than 65 percent of the 26 million anesthetics given to patients each year in the United States. They have been rendering quality anesthesia services in this country for more than a century. CRNAs practice in a wide variety of settings in which anesthesia services are required, in both urban and rural environments. CRNAs are the sole anesthesia providers in 49 percent of the hospitals in this country, and in over 70 percent of rural hospitals, enabling these medical facilities to provide obstetrical, surgical, and trauma stabilization services.

CRNAs administer anesthesia and anesthesia-related care in four general categories: (1) pre-anesthetic preparation and evaluation; (2) anesthesia induction, maintenance, and emergence; (3) postanesthesia care; and (4) perianesthetic and clinical support functions, such as resuscitation services, acute and chronic pain management, respiratory care, and the establishment of arterial lines.

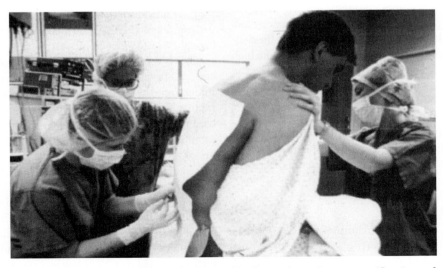

Nurse anesthetists are among the highest paid advanced practice nurses. (Courtesy of the American Association of Nurse Anesthetists [AANA])

CRNAs provide high-quality, cost-effective anesthesia care. In 1990, the US Department of Health and Human Services (DHHS) presented the results of a study of nurse anesthesia manpower needs conducted by the Center for Health Economics Research. This study concluded that a more efficient use of CRNAs to deliver anesthesia could save the nation $1 billion annually by 2010.[29]

CRNAs administer anesthesia for all types of surgical procedures, from the simplest to the most complex. CRNAs have the legal authority to practice anesthesia in all 50 states without anesthesiologist supervision. There is no study that shows that the anesthesia care an anesthesiologist provides is superior to that of a CRNA. In fact, the only studies that exist suggest that the quality of care is not significantly different.

The educational requirements to become a CRNA are as follows:

- Be a graduate of an accredited nurse anesthesia education program. Applicants to a program must have (1) a BSN or another appropriate baccalaureate degree; (2) a current license as an RN or (3) a minimum of 1 year's acute care nursing experience. There are currently 89 accredited nurse anesthesia educational programs in the United States; all offer a master's degree. Some programs offer DNP options for CRNAs.
- Graduates of nurse anesthesia educational programs must pass a national certification exam to become CRNAs.
- CRNAs are required to earn 40 continuing education credits every 2 years as one of the criteria for recertification.

Reflective of the high level of responsibility, CRNAs are one of the best-paid nursing specialties. In 2010, there were over 40,000 CRNAs in practice. CRNA's annual compensation in 2008 averaged $163,467, roughly 92 percent of the average $178,084 for 2007. While 54 percent of respondents were employer based, 42 percent had worked as an independent provider and 32 percent reported working on a contract basis exclusively. Nurse anesthetists in rural areas reported the highest salary average, as opposed to metropolitan and suburban areas. Twenty-five percent of CRNAs practice in rural areas; the rest were almost evenly split between major metro areas (38 percent) and suburban areas (37 percent).[30]

Depending on their employment situation, some CRNAs purchase their own professional liability insurance. St. Paul Fire and Marine Insurance Company, the underwriter for the American Association of Nurse Anesthetists (AANA) Professional Liability Insurance Program, has steadily reduced CRNA premiums owing to low claims losses.

Obstacles to Advanced Practice

The success of advanced practice has come only with much effort and tenacity. The goal has been direct access to patients without the intermediary participation of another provider, namely the physician. Direct access is critically dependent on *third-party reimbursement, adequate practice acts, prescriptive authority, practice privileges* in settings for service delivery, *professional liability insurance,* and *inclusion in managed care networks of providers.*

The history of CNMs and CRNAs predates that of NPs and CNSs, yet the barriers to patient access that frustrate their practices are the same. CNMs were faced with a major challenge in the 1980s. As the malpractice claims history of obstetricians skyrocketed, CNMs were seen as an equal risk by insurers. Their professional liability insurance premiums escalated to a point that could not be supported by their income. Interim coverage was provided through the carrier servicing the ANA. In time, a more permanent solution was found. This incident was a repercussion of the interdependent relationship that is required between CNMs and obstetricians. A similar effect is associated with CNSs and NPs as they enter into collaborative/joint protocol/supervisory relations with physicians to meet the requirements for prescriptive authority. In this case, it has been reported that physicians' malpractice premiums have increased in response to their supervisory role. The additional cost of practice is ultimately passed on to the consumer, frustrating the ability of these APNs to offer medical services at a price that is lower than traditional providers. CRNAs, NPs, and CNSs have had no difficulty obtaining coverage. Claims data show that they are an excellent risk, and consequently their premiums are very affordable, although more costly than the fee that would apply to a staff nurse. The insurance market has moved to the point where clear distinctions are made between advanced practice and staff nurses in policies.

The ANA linked the NP and CNS in public policy language in the early 1980s. In the early 1990s, the term *advanced practice nurse* was chosen to include the NP, CNS, CNM, and CRNA. Much of this public policy effort has been directed toward the third-party reimbursement agenda. All categories of APNs are reimbursable in the Federal Employee's Health Benefits Program (FEHB).

Similar provisions are included in TRICARE (formerly CHAMPUS), the program serving active-duty service members, National Guard and Reserve members, retirees, their families, survivors, and certain former spouses worldwide. The one TRICARE restriction is that only certified clinical specialists in psychiatric nursing are included under the CNS category. Medicaid includes mandatory reimbursement (at 70 to 100 percent of the physician rate) of pediatric and family NPs and CNMs, but defers to state discretion for CRNAs and CNSs. *Mandatory* in terms of federal legislation means that a provider must be reimbursed through Medicaid (or other federal programs as specified) for services within the provider's scope of practice as recognized within that state. None of the federal reimbursement laws supercede the states' responsibility for health and safety. Medicare has been the most resistant program, but was opened to direct reimbursement of APNs within the provisions of the Balanced Budget Act of 1997, although only at 85 percent of the fee received by physicians. Before the Balanced Budget Act, NPs and CNSs were limited to serving Medicare recipients in rural and medically underserved areas. This restriction has been removed. Nursing homes had been able to receive Medicare reimbursement for NPs who provided periodic medical monitoring, and recertification services, but the NP could not directly receive any fee. CNMs and CRNAs were already recognized in Medicare.

Indemnity and commercial insurances are governed by state statutes and recognize advanced practice to varying degrees. The picture is confusing and changes quickly. The situation is further confused by the reality that many APNs are reimbursed incident to the practice of physicians, and they like it that way. In that case, the fee is equal to whatever the physician would be paid. If the APN bills as an independent, the reimbursement is usually less than 100 percent of the physician's fee.

Some gains were recognized during the deliberations of the Physician's Payment Review Commission (PPRC), charged with proposing policy for Part B of Medicare. The PPRC, in an attempt to increase the attractiveness of general and primary care practice for physicians as compared with specialization, based its fee-setting techniques on the service provided as opposed to the nature of the provider. When it came to applying this same standard to APNs, they recanted and proposed that the extent of the educational investment for the role should be built into the reimbursement equation. The detail is tedious, and progress is slow and often illogical and unfair. The nursing community has been persistent and gains are obvious.

We are moving decisively and quickly toward managed care. Although everyone will never be enrolled in a managed care plan, managed care plans already dominate the health care industry. And whoever is recognized in fee-for-service models will have similar recognition and autonomy in managed care systems. Consequently, the struggle for recognition of nurses through reimbursement must continue. Chapter 19 includes more detail on legislation enabling reimbursement.

Prescriptive authority provides similar challenges. Studies of medical practice reaffirm the fact that most Americans expect to leave with a prescription when they visit a physician. Without prescriptive authority, APNs are unable to provide comprehensive services. Further, with either a joint practice arrangement or referral to a physician for prescription, the fee to the patient is equal to or greater than it would have been for the physician alone. In 2010, all states award NPs some variety of prescriptive authority, and in 23 states this authority was unassociated with physician supervision, collaboration, or oversight in prescribing, including controlled substances. Currently, 28 additional states are considering expanding the authority of nurse practitioners.[31] Prescriptive authority is addressed through state law. The regulations applying to NPs are sometimes applicable to CNSs as well. The current political strategy has been to secure whatever degree of autonomy is possible and remove restrictions at a later date. A good case in point is the success of New Hampshire nurses in the early 1990s. The requirement for physician supervision of prescriptive authority was carved out of an existing law through subsequent legislation. The AMA has been particularly adversarial over the prescriptive authority of APNs. Their attacks have focused on the inconsistent educational standard for APNs, and the tendency of the nursing profession to make exceptions by grandfathering current practitioners into a credentialed category as the requirements become more stringent. The economic threat to physicians is not frequently addressed, but it is obvious. An additional point of resistance to APNs having prescriptive authority has been the pharmacist. In some cases local pharmacists have refused to fill prescriptions when the order is from an APN. Most of these incidents have been successfully resolved. These occasions may be largely owing to incomplete information and inadequate communication or a reaction associated with pharmacy's own early struggle to achieve prescriptive rights.

APNs have also been hampered by confusion over the degree to which they should be recognized in legislation and governmental regulations. CNMs and CRNAs have been recognized as distinct providers for many years and their status is legally codified. In many states, this was accomplished through amendments to medical practice acts. In contrast, the original strategy had been to insist that CNSs and NPs need not be named because their practice is included in the scope of practice statements in nursing's licensing laws. This conviction was so strong that in the 1980s grant monies were provided from the ANA to roll back state laws that specifically referred to APNs. This strategy proved unwise; as reimbursement moved forward, states required that the advanced practice titles be explicitly included in public policy. An example is helpful here. Mandatory Medicaid reimbursement of pediatric and family NPs was denied in New Jersey based on the argument that there were no such providers in the state. Organized nursing in New Jersey had worked diligently to withhold the NP and CNS titles from public policy. To access reimbursement, these titles had to be codified in the law. The most current information on reimbursement, prescriptive authority, and licensing is available each year in the January or February issue of *Nurse Practitioner*.

Privileging—the right to admit patients to an institution and provide appropriate services (writing orders, consulting, treating, discharging) as part of a professional staff—is an area that has been given less attention. The ANA began to do the groundwork for privileging in working to reshape the definitions of professional staff included in public and private sector policy (the Centers for Medicare and Medicaid Services [CMS] and the Joint Commission). In these instances, professional staffs may include a broad range of providers. However, restrictions on membership may be imposed at the institutional level. It remains to be tested whether the withholding of privileges is an act of discrimination or restraint of trade. Regardless, privileges have become more common. The privileges themselves may be limited to admission, consultation, treatment (clinical), discharge, or some combination. It is common for NPs or CNSs who join a community-based physician practice to hold staff privileges and actively manage hospitalized patients. It is also common for these APNs to reject an offer of privileges, and the additional responsibilities and effort that they require. Another route to institutional access may be the recognition of independent APNs by the nursing staff organization in a facility (if one exists). Although admission privileges may not be possible through this route, clinical and consultation options may be.

But privileges are not the hottest issue. Rather, unencumbered prescriptive authority and membership in managed care provider networks seem to be greater areas of need. State laws in many instances have assured APNs the right of membership on managed care panels, but it is up to the consumer to demand our inclusion. We may be included, but we do not have to be.

■ FEDERAL HEALTH SERVICES

Professional nurses interested in a career with the federal government will find opportunities in both military and nonmilitary services. The military services include the Army, Navy, and Air Force. The Department of Veterans Affairs (VA) is not a military service, although it is closely allied. The other principal nonmilitary federal service employing nurses is the US Public Health Service (PHS).

US Public Health Service

Founded in 1798, the PHS is the principal health agency of the federal government. A component of the DHHS, the PHS is charged with improving and advancing the health of our nation's people. PHS programs are also designed to work with other nations and international agencies on global health problems.

The PHS is a vital force in advancing research in the health sciences, in developing public health programs, in providing therapeutic and preventive services, and in protecting the public health through the regulation of drugs, medical products, and foods. The PHS accomplishes its mission through 22 HHS and non-HHS offices and agencies, among them the Agency for Health Care Research and Quality (AHCRQ), Centers for Disease Control and Prevention (CDC), Food and Drug Administration (FDA), Health Resources Services Administration (HRSA), Indian Health Service (IHS), National Institutes of Health (NIH), and Substance Abuse and Mental Health Services Administration (SAMHSA). Refer to Exhibit 19–1 in Chapter 19.

There are opportunities in such fields as clinical care, nursing research, epidemiology, health services research, health promotion, regulatory science, community health, and environmental health. Most of the clinical positions are available in the IHS and the Clinical Center of the NIH. Commissioned Corps nurses may be detailed to the Federal Bureau of Prisons, US Coast Guard, Centers for Medicare and Medicaid Services (CMS), Immigration and Naturalization Service (INS), and the National Oceanic and Atmospheric Administration.

Nurses may enter the PHS by appointment to either the Federal Civil Service or the Commissioned Corps. AD, diploma, baccalaureate nurses, and nurses with graduate degrees may work in the civil service system. The BSN degree is the entry level for the Commissioned Corps. Other minimum requirements differ. To be considered for appointment into the PHS Commissioned Corps, a nurse must be a US citizen under 44 years of age, have earned a qualifying degree from an accredited program, and meet medical, security, and licensure requirements.

The *Commissioned Corps* is a personnel system composed entirely of health professionals; it is an all-officer corps. It is also one of the seven uniformed services of the United States, including the Air Force, Army, Navy, Marine Corps, Coast Guard, and the Commissioned Corps of the National Oceanic and Atmospheric Administration. In the event of a national emergency or war, the President may, by issuing an executive order, declare the PHS Commissioned Corps a military service. Pay, allowances, and other privileges are comparable with those of officers in the armed services. Rank appointments are made depending on the nurse's education and experience.

The PHS offers excellent opportunities for students in baccalaureate nursing programs for periods of 31 to 120 days throughout the academic year through the Commissioned Officer Student Training and Extern Program (COSTEP) and Senior COSTEP Program. Both programs are highly competitive and based on the needs of PHS agencies. COSTEP allows students to serve in assignments at any time during the year; however, the majority of students are hired for the summer months. On completion of their professional education, students may serve an extended active duty assignment with the PHS.

In Senior COSTEP, students are assisted financially during their final year of school in return for an agreement to work for the PHS after graduation. The student is appointed as an active-duty PHS officer during the senior year and receives monthly pay and allowances as an ensign (01) grade officer. Additional support, in the form of tuition and fees, may be paid by a supporting agency or program of the PHS. Following graduation, the student agrees to work for the agency or program that provided the financial support for twice the time supported.

As mentioned, most of the clinical positions are in the IHS and NIH Clinical Center. Almost half of the 5000 PHS nurses work for the IHS. The IHS is responsible for providing comprehensive care to over 1 million American Indians and Alaskan Natives in hospitals, health centers, and clinics across the United States. Most of the facilities are located west of the Mississippi. The NIH Clinical Center in Bethesda, Maryland, is a world-class facility for biomedical research. The center has experienced restructuring and downsizing comparable to other US hospitals. Approximately 550 nurses conduct research, help to design experimental treatments, monitor patient responses, analyze data, and educate patients and families. The NIH is composed of a number of institutes, including the National Institute for Nursing Research (NINR). The other PHS agencies employ nurses, although opportunities are more limited than with the IHS and NIH.

The National Health Service Corps (NHSC) is authorized to recruit health care personnel to urban and rural communities in the United States and its territories with critical health manpower shortages. The NHSC occasionally recruits, but most participants are expected to find their own placements that qualify as needy. In exchange for service or the promise of service, the NHSC offers educational loan repayment and scholarships.

Both COSTEP and NHSC federal financial assistance programs require participants to commit to 1 year of service in an underserved community for each year of financial support, and both require a minimum 2-year commitment.

Health professionals interested in NHSC opportunities are not federal employees; rather, they receive salary and benefits directly from the community-based system of care where they are employed. For additional information about the NHSC, call 1-800-221-9393.

Department of Veterans Affairs Nursing Service

The VA was established in 1930 (previously known as the Veterans Administration) as a civilian agency of the federal government. Its purpose is to administer national programs that provide benefits for veterans of the US armed forces. In 1989, the agency was elevated to cabinet status. The VA operates the nation's largest organized health care system. To accomplish its objective of providing high-quality health care, the VA has developed extensive programs in research and education. A majority of VA medical centers are affiliated with medical schools, schools of nursing, and other health-related schools in a network of health care facilities that cover the entire country. Individual hospitals range in size from approximately 110 to 1400 beds, most of which provide care for patients with medical and surgical diagnoses. A few hospitals are predominantly for the care of patients with psychiatric diagnoses. Many VA health care facilities have outpatient clinics and extended-care facilities, such as nursing home care units and domiciliaries.

To qualify for an appointment in the VA, a nurse must be a US citizen, a graduate of a state-approved school of professional nursing, currently registered to practice, and meet required physical standards. Graduates from a professional school of nursing may be appointed pending passing of state board examinations.

Nurses employed in the VA are covered by a locality pay system (LPS). The LPS is designed to ensure that VA nurses are paid competitive rates within local labor markets. As such, salary ranges vary according to facility location. There are several levels of salary grades for VA nurses.

Qualification standards relating to education, experience, and competencies are specified for appointment or promotion to each grade. The VA salary system recognizes excellence in clinical practice, administration, research, and education. Nurses, including those providing direct patient care, receive salaries commensurate with their qualifications and contributions. A Nurse Professional Standards Board reviews performance and recommends promotion or special salary advancement according to established criteria. A nurse appointed to one VA medical center may transfer to another with continuity of benefits and without loss of salary.

The VA has always been at the cutting edge of nursing practice. It is at the forefront of the Clinical Nurse Leader (CNL) movement (see Chapter 13). VA nurse leaders have actively participated in the development and implementation of this role. At VA, CNLs serve as the point person on patient care teams, and they are leaders in the health care delivery system across all settings in which health care is delivered. This revolutionary role is making a difference in patient care outcomes and professional role satisfaction for many staff nurses. Additionally, since 2005, the baccalaureate degree is the minimum preparation VA nurses must have for promotion beyond an entry-level position.

The VA Nursing Service emphasizes continued learning and advanced education. There is a Nursing Career Development Program to provide opportunities within the system. Nurse researchers are employed in some VA medical centers and in the national office. CNSs work in some VA health care settings. Also, NPs function in specific units, clinics, or satellite facilities. Applications and inquiries for full- or part-time employment should be directed to the Personnel Office at the VA Medical Center at the location of interest.

The Armed Services

Despite similarities, there are specific differences among the Army Nurse Corps, Navy Nurse Corps, and Air Force Nurse Corps. In recent years there have been a number of changes in qualifications and assignments to meet the changes in society and in the health care field. All the armed services have a reserve corps of nurses established by acts of Congress to provide the additional nurses that are needed to care for members of the services and their families in times of war or other national emergencies. Nurses may join the reserve without having joined the regular service; the requirements are similar. A certain amount of training (which is paid) is required, usually 1 weekend per month and 2 consecutive weeks a year, at local medical units related to that particular service. There are opportunities for promotion, CE, and fringe benefits such as low-cost insurance and retirement pay. More information is available from the reserve recruiter of the particular service. In all the services, nurses have the same economic, social, and health care benefits of all officers as well as the opportunity for personal travel. After discharge (or retirement, which is possible in 20 years), veterans' benefits are available.

Mergers are taking place in the military in the form of Military Treatment Facilities (MTFs). An MTF is a consolidation of personnel from two or three branches of the military into one site as downsizing and a greater use of community resources forces the closure of some of the military hospitals in an area. One example is in northern California, where Letterman Army Hospital and Oakland Naval have closed, leaving David Grant USAF Medical Center as the MTF for the entire region.

The Army Nurse Corps

Because it is the oldest of the federal nursing services, the Army Nurse Corps has had considerable influence on the development of nursing and the status of nurses in all of the armed services. When the Army Nurse Corps was established as part of the Army Medical Department in 1901, nurses were appointed in the Regular Army but did not have actual commissions. Their status was basically no status. Believing that they needed the authority of an officer to ensure accountability and responsibility for all nursing care delivered, the ANA, the New York Committee to Secure Rank for Army Nurses, and several other organizations tried to persuade Congress to legislate appropriate military rank and recognition. On June 4, 1920, the Army

Reorganization Act authorized relative rank for Army nurses, granting the ranks of Second Lieutenant to Major. This act also authorized the wearing of insignia but did not provide for equal pay or privileges such as retirement. During World War II, the federal government gave nurses serving in all branches of the armed services temporary commissions, but it was not until 1947 that female nurses achieved permanent commissioned status. Men in nursing had to wait until 1955 to be so recognized.

Basic qualifications for a commission in the Army Nurse Corps specify that an applicant must

1. Be a graduate of an educational program accredited by an agency recognized by the US Secretary of Education and acceptable to the Department of the Army. The educational program must prepare the individual for licensure as an RN.

   Applicants who enter active duty must possess a minimum of a BSN. Applicants who desire service in a reserve component must possess a minimum of a diploma in nursing, an AD in nursing, or a baccalaureate degree in nursing or nurse anesthesia.

2. Have successfully completed the National Council Licensure Examination for Registered Nurses (NCLEX-RN) and have a valid current license to practice as an RN in the United States, District of Columbia, Commonwealth of Puerto Rico, or a US territory.

3. Be engaged in practice as an RN for a minimum of 20 hours per week for a period of not less than 6 months in the 1-year period immediately preceding the date the application is received.

4. Be in the age range of 21 to 47$^1/_2$.

5. Be a citizen of the United States or lawfully admitted to the United States for permanent residence.

6. Be able to meet the physical standards prescribed for appointment.

7. Applicants can be married or single and have family members of any age.

An RN recently completing a basic nursing program will usually be commissioned as a second lieutenant. Applicants who have acquired noteworthy professional experience, received advanced nursing education, or served formerly as a commissioned officer may qualify for an initial appointment at a higher rank. Unless an applicant has previously served in the military, the service obligation is 8 years. For those applicants who enter active duty, at least 3 of the 8 years must be served on active duty. The remainder of the military service obligation may be served in either the active or the reserve components. Army Nurse Corps officers may advance to the rank of Brigadier General.

Army nurses may give direct patient care in any clinical specialty as staff nurses or head nurses and may serve as nursing consultants. They may serve as instructors for military or clinical courses in various hospitals or departments. They may become involved in administration in various clinical services or at Army headquarters. They may also function as nursing methods analysts, nurse researchers, health care recruiters, consultants to the Surgeon General, or advisers to military nurses of allied nations. Assignments may be in the United States or various parts of the world. Army Nurse Corps officers may also be selected to attend a college or university for advanced degrees with all or part of the costs paid.

Further information may be obtained from the local Army recruiting station (ask for the Army Health Care Recruiter), by calling the toll-free number (1-800-USA-Army) or by visiting their website at

http://www.goarmy.com

The Navy Nurse Corps

Although the Navy Nurse Corps was officially established by Congress in the twentieth century, Navy nurses were recommended by the first chief of the Bureau of Medicine and Surgery in 1811, and sisters of the Order of the Holy Cross served on the Navy ship *Red Rover* as volunteers in 1862. They were the first female nurses to serve aboard the first US Navy hospital ship. The first Navy nurses (called the *Sacred Twenty*) and a superintendent reported to Washington for duty in 1908. By 1910, nurses had expanded their activities to include the Far East, Hawaii, and the Caribbean. In World War I, female Navy nurses were assigned to hospitals in England, Ireland, Scotland, and France. Throughout World War II, Navy nurses brought nursing care to frontline casualties aboard 12 hospital ships and also to air evacuees. They served in foreign lands where American women had never been seen and some were prisoners of war. In 1944, the *USS Highbee* became the first combat ship to be named for a woman, the second superintendent of the Navy Nurse Corps.

During the Korean and Vietnam conflicts, Navy nurses served in station hospitals and aboard hospital ships caring for ill and wounded soldiers, sailors, and marines. Four Navy nurses received the Purple Heart for injuries received in Saigon, South Vietnam.

Today, Navy nurses provide care for patients; teach patients, corpsmen, and other health care team members; assume administrative positions; and serve as executive and commanding officers of medical facilities. They are assigned to hospitals, clinics, ships, headquarters staff, Officer Indoctrination School, Hospital Corps schools, and other duty stations in the United States and other parts of the world.

Initial appointments are made in grades of ensign to lieutenant, based on education and other professional qualifications. Nurses may advance to the rank of rear admiral. Basic qualifications for an officer commission state that the candidate must

1. Be a US citizen or a foreign citizen currently licensed to practice in the United States
2. Be a student or graduate in good standing of a US education program granting a bachelor of science degree and accredited by the appropriate state board of nursing or the National League for Nursing
3. Be licensed to practice in a US state, the District of Columbia, the Commonwealth of Puerto Rico, or a US territory (new graduates must obtain a license within 1 year of beginning Active Duty service)
4. Be willing to serve a minimum of 3 years of Active Duty
5. Be between the ages of 18 and 41
6. Be in good physical condition and pass a full medical examination

All Navy nurses are encouraged to continue their education through Navy in-service and CE courses, as well as courses leading to academic degrees. Qualified career officers may request assignment to full-time study for an advanced degree in nursing and related health care administration fields. Further information is available from the local Navy recruiting station or from the Director, Navy Nurse Corps, Bureau of Medicine and Surgery, Washington, DC.

The Air Force Nurse Corps

In 1947, with the passage of the National Security Act, the United States Air Force was established as a separate service. The United States Air Force Medical Service, including the nursing component, was established on July 1, 1949. Prior to that date, medical personnel in the Army Medical Service were assigned to duty with the United States Air Force.

The mission of the Medical Service is to provide the medical support necessary for maximum peacetime readiness and combat effectiveness of the Air Force. As an integral part of the mission, the Medical Service provides, to the greatest extent possible, a peacetime health care system for all eligible beneficiaries. The Air Force Nurse Corps, as one of the five components responsible for medical support of the Air Force, has a vital role in this mission.

Since its establishment, the Nurse Corps has undergone many changes, including increased authorization, increased rank, and new specialty codes. In 1955, male nurses were authorized to receive commissions and now approximately 25 percent are men. Over 50 percent of Air Force nurses are married and may have dependents of any age.

Air Force nurses provide quality nursing care in a variety of specialties and settings. They perform duties in one of 11 career fields, such as administration, mental health, operating room, anesthesia, clinical nursing, education, flight nursing, nurse practitioner, and midwifery. They are involved in clinical practice, patient teaching, supervision, and teaching of paraprofessional personnel, administration, education, and research.

The majority of the nurses are assigned to medical centers, hospitals, and clinics in the United States and overseas. Most medical treatment facilities are small community hospitals providing routine and emergency medical, surgical, pediatric, obstetric, and psychoneurological services for beneficiaries. One role unique to Air Force nursing is that of *flight nurse*. The Air Force has the Department of Defense responsibility for aeromedical evacuation in peacetime and during conflicts.

Nurses are assigned as flight nurses only after completing an intensive program at the School of Aerospace Medicine at Brooks Air Force Base, Texas. Since the first class graduated in February 1943, the course has been conducted continuously, with over 12,000 graduates. The course includes didactic and practical experiences in aerospace physiology, basic sciences, specialized techniques necessary for the safe and efficient transportation of patients by air, and survival and life support principles, procedures, and equipment. It provides students with the knowledge and skills required for management and nursing care of patients in flight.

Air Force nurses are given every opportunity to grow, both academically and professionally. Nurses are encouraged to continue their formal education at civilian colleges and universities located near Air Force medical treatment facilities. Under a tuition assistance program, the Air Force may pay up to 75 percent of their tuition costs for off-duty courses. Many Air Force nurses compete regularly for undergraduate and graduate study opportunities. A certain number are selected each year to pursue full-time graduate studies in civilian universities. Air Force–sponsored students receive their normal pay during the school terms, plus educational assistance covering tuition and required expenses. Accepting this educational assistance requires an additional active-duty obligation commensurate with the length of the education program.

Tuition assistance is available for generic nursing students via the Reserve Officer's Training Corps (ROTC) programs on most university campuses. Applications are accepted from BSN students who meet certain criteria during their senior year. This program offers an excellent opportunity for a wide variety of clinical experiences to new graduates. Applicants accepted for this program participate in a 5-month nurse internship program before reporting to their first assignment. Nurses in the intern program have the opportunity to apply basic nursing knowledge and skills and acquire new, specialized skills. Rotations through several clinical areas help prepare nurses for a variety of nursing duties.

Air Force nurses have two professions; they are professional officers and professional nurses. The ranks of Air Force nurses range from second lieutenant to brigadier general. Most applicants receive their commission as officers in the grade of second lieutenant. Nurses with additional professional experience and education may be appointed at a higher rank after review of records and in accordance with current policy.

To qualify for appointment, the applicant must

1. Hold at minimum a Bachelor of Science in Nursing degree from an accredited college or university
2. Have a current registration in any state or the District of Columbia
3. Meet physical and professional requirements
4. Be at least 18 years old
5. Be a citizen of the United States

Additional information may be obtained by contacting a local Air Force recruiter or by writing to HQ USAF Recruiting Service/RSHN, Randolph Air Force Base, TX 78150. In addition to a full-time career as an Air Force officer, commissions are also available via the Air Force Reserve and Air National Guard Programs. Information on Air Force Reserve Programs may be obtained by writing HQ Air Force Reserve/SG, Robins Air Force Base, GA 31098 or HQ ARPC/SG, Denver, CO 80280. Information on Air National Guard programs may be obtained by writing National Guard Bureau/SG, Room 2E369, The Pentagon, Washington, DC 20310 or ANGRC/DPR, 3500 Fetchet Ave, Andrews AFB, MD 20331-5157.

■ NURSING IN EXTENDED AND LONG-TERM CARE FACILITIES

The distinction between skilled and intermediate beds in nursing homes has been largely abandoned. All of today's nursing home residents are frail and seriously compromised in their self-care. Instead, the most important distinction is the payer source, mostly Medicare and Medicaid. *Medicare recipients* are confined for a limited period on the assumption that their conditions are transient and there will be positive progress. In contrast, *Medicaid* funds continuing LTC to the financially needy. The difference in reimbursement rates between the former and the latter are considerable. Residents of these facilities are not only the elderly, but include people of many ages and stages of disability, including those with neurologic problems, victims of trauma, those with multiple sclerosis, and so on. More RNs are working in nursing homes today, although the majority of caregivers are practical nurses and certified nursing assistants (CNAs).

Nurses may have positions in nursing homes similar to those in hospitals, with the additional role of *facility administrator* being assumed by some nurses. In this case, the nurse must be certified for the position, and although the individual's knowledge of nursing may be extremely helpful in understanding the need for quality care, being a nurse is not a requirement for certification.

The *director of nursing*, who has the same kinds of responsibilities as any other director of nursing, is sometimes expected to act as the administrator's assistant. In small nursing homes, the director might assume both roles. Because most facilities are for-profit, financial management is extremely important. The administrative nurse should be well prepared in managerial skills; unfortunately, that is rare.

In most nursing homes the pace is slower and the pressure less than in other settings for care. Nurses interested in nursing home care enjoy the opportunity to know the patient better in the relatively long-term stay and to help the patient maintain or attain the best possible health status. This is not the area of practice for someone impatient for quick results. Both rehabilitative and geriatric nursing require a greater amount of patience and understanding. In rehabilitation, nurses work closely as a team with related health disciplines—occupational therapy, physical therapy, speech therapy, and others. In geriatric nursing, the nurse works to a great extent with nonprofessional nursing personnel and acts as team leader, teacher, and supervisor. It may well be that there is only one licensed nurse in a nursing home per shift, with practical nurses as charge nurses and aides giving much of the day-to-day care.

Because the patients are relatively helpless and often have no family or friends who check on them, the nurse must, in a real sense, be a patient advocate. Physicians make infrequent visits, and in some cases, where there are limited or no rehabilitative services, the nurse is the only professional with patient contact.

For this reason, *geriatric nurse practitioners* (GNPs) are considered a tremendous asset in nursing homes. The GNP is responsible for assessing patients and evaluating their progress, performing certain diagnostic procedures, and interpreting the results. She or he diagnoses and treats minor acute illness, monitors and manages chronic conditions, promotes health, and prevents disease. Additional important functions are assessing personal and family relationships, patient and staff relationships, and life situations that may affect the patient's health status. In some nursing homes, the GNP is on 24-hour call.

Requirements for employment are similar to those in hospitals for like positions, although often the need for a degree is not emphasized. Conditions of employment and salaries have improved, but are not as good as those in hospitals. Because, under Medicare, orientation and subsequent in-service education are mandatory, the nurse has an excellent opportunity to learn about LTC and the concepts and techniques of geriatric nursing. Because the increase of older people is one of the trends in society, geriatric care is being given greater attention, and workshops, courses, and programs are available in the field. With an aging population, there are also likely to be good job opportunities for some time to come.

■ PUBLIC HEALTH/COMMUNITY HEALTH NURSING

PHN synthesizes the knowledge from the nursing and public health sciences to promote and preserve the health of individuals, families, and communities. This area of specialization is population focused, the community is the client, and the provision of personal health services is only important as they benefit the community as a whole. The goal is to improve the health of the community by identifying subgroups (aggregates) within the population that are high risk for illness, disability, or premature death; directing resources toward these groups; and monitoring the adequacy of the response to these efforts. *Home care* is also a part of the community health agenda, recognizing that outreach to the sick and vulnerable in their homes is a community responsibility. Home care is not just service to the acutely and chronically ill brought into the home as an option to the hospital. The setting creates new rights and responsibilities for both the nurse and the patient.

ANA has revised standards for community health, public health, and home health nursing practice. The standards for public health and community health nursing practice have been consolidated given their mutual focus on populations, and home health practice has been recognized as a distinctive area of personal care services.

From the very beginning of PHN in 1893, under the inspiration of Lillian Wald and the Henry Street Settlement on New York City's Lower East Side, nurses made visits to people in their homes, schools, or where people and neighbors gathered. Health teaching and care of the sick were intertwined with preventive services and linked with the social and political concerns of the times.

Today, public health nurses practice in many settings. Most are employed by agencies that may carry the title of public health, community health, home health, or visiting nurse. They may be official—governmental and tax supported (e.g., a city or county health department); nonofficial or voluntary—agencies supported to a great extent by community funds (e.g., visiting nurse or home health service); or proprietary—for profit. These agencies range in size and services from small, employing only one or two public health nurses, to very large, employing a sizable staff of professional nurses, other health professionals, practical nurses, and home health aides and homemakers.

PHN employment opportunities are not limited, however, to these agencies. Nurses may also be employed by hospitals to conduct home-care programs or to serve as liaison between the hospital and the community. They may work with other organizations, private and governmental, in need of the kinds of services the public health nurse is prepared to provide in schools, outpatient clinics, community health centers, walk-in clinics for drug addiction and sexually transmitted diseases (STDs), migrant labor camps, and rural areas.

As part of the official public health services, every state, every US territory, and many counties, large towns, and cities have a public health department. Health departments may be freestanding departments or combined with hospital and medical care regulatory agencies, environmental health agencies, or welfare and social service agencies. In some instances, these functions may be subcontracted to the private sector. Public health services focus on health promotion and disease prevention, community health protection, personal prevention, and assistance in gaining access to care. Examples of such programs and services follow.

Health Promotion and Disease Prevention

1. Education about risk factors for STD and human immunodeficiency virus (HIV) and acquired immunodeficiency syndrome (AIDS)
2. Promoting seatbelt use
3. Teaching school children about the health benefits of good nutrition and physical activity

Community Health Protection

1. Ensuring a safe environment through safe housing, workplaces, food, and water
2. Aiding households and communities exposed to hazardous waste sites or chemical spills
3. Reducing the occurrence and harmful effects of air pollution
4. Disaster response preparedness programs

Personal Prevention

1. Early and periodic screening for childhood diseases
2. Screening and treatment for infectious diseases such as tuberculosis (TB) and STDs
3. Behavior change counseling

Services to Improve Access to Care

1. Coordinating public and private responses to community health needs
2. Providing outreach services to individuals, families, and groups at risk for specific diseases
3. Public health nursing visits to the home for high-risk pregnant women

Public health offers extraordinary opportunities for the imaginative, competent, and resourceful person to originate and develop ideas that may greatly affect the health of the community. There is a need for collection of data, constant monitoring of trends, and epidemiologic surveillance of both communicable and chronic diseases. Public health

nurses are constantly collecting data, investigating adverse health conditions, monitoring the outcomes of medical care services in families and communities, and assisting with health policy development at the state or local level. Public health nurses may also work for various international agencies assisting with the development of public health programs in developing countries. There is growing recognition of the role public health nurses can play in combating serious world health challenges such as AIDS or childhood diseases that can be prevented with vaccination.

Nurses make up the largest group of professional public health personnel, and their influence is considerable. However, PHN positions are increasingly threatened as other nonclinical workers are employed in public health. Funding for public health nurses has been cut because of costs, yet no other worker has the vast repertoire of skills. This trend is a major concern and has captured the attention of the nursing community. Workers in the field of public health include physicians, social workers, sanitary engineers, nutritionists, dentists, physical therapists, speech therapists, and others. Members of these groups may work alone or as a team. All public health workers, therefore, need an overview of the entire program to understand their place in the organization and the scope of their own work. An effective public health program requires excellent working relationships with other agencies, both health and nonhealth, because public health activities reach every segment of the community. Although situations differ, nurses in official agencies may make home visits, but their responsibilities are primarily in community health clinics focused on the needs of that agency's population. Traditionally, these have been family planning, maternal-childcare, and communicable disease; in a number of communities these agency nurses are also the school nurses and, occasionally, are contracted to do some occupational health nursing.

The *visiting* or *home health nurses*, regardless of their place of employment, also carry out these functions and may, in addition, provide physical care and treatments. With the advent of earlier discharge from hospitals, patients are sicker when they go home and nurses are required to know how to provide home care for the acutely ill. If the nurse's assessment indicates that the patient's care does not require professional nurse services, home health aides and homemakers may be assigned to a patient or family, with nurse supervision and reassessment. Visiting nurses have also set up clinics that they visit periodically in senior citizen centers or apartments, as well as in the single-room occupancy (SRO) hotels commonly used for welfare clients and the homeless in large cities. There are multiple liaison roles with hospitals, HMOs, clinics, geriatric units, and various residences for the long-term disabled and mentally ill or retarded, primarily to assist in admission and discharge planning, as well as coordinating continuing patient care. Nurses in managerial positions in PHN agencies have responsibilities similar to those in hospitals in terms of general managerial skills.

Schools of professional nursing have long recognized that nurses who plan to enter the field of public health need special preparation for it. Most diploma and AD schools give students theoretical instruction in PHN, conduct orientation visits to community health agencies, provide several hours of experience in prenatal and well-baby clinics, and integrate public health aspects of nursing wherever possible in all clinical areas. One of the problems in giving experience to students in these schools is the lack of clinical facilities (agencies) for practice. What experience is available is usually reserved for BSN programs, because preparation for PHN is usually a major educational objective of these programs, and students have taken a considerable number of courses in preparation. However, their experiences should not be limited to official and nonofficial agencies, because public health and community health nursing practice deserve to be experienced in a broader context.

Besides state licensure, and for some agencies, prior nursing experience, one major qualification for PHN work is ideally graduation from a BSN program. Many graduates of these schools go on to earn a master's degree and are thus prepared educationally for a lifetime career in this field. Because of the shortage of nurses with the prescribed PHN preparation at the present time, however, graduates of diploma and AD programs can and do find positions in this field, working at the entry level and under supervision. In some areas they work only in clinics. Some employers encourage nurses to work toward a BSN by providing tuition or scholarship grants.

In 2008, 97,210 RNs worked in community or public health settings, including state or local health departments, community-based home health agencies, various types of community health centers, student health services, and occupational health services. In the past, public health nurses enjoyed standard daytime hours, with most working Monday through Friday. However, with the move toward more care in the community on a 24-hour basis, public health nurses are expected to rotate shifts and work weekends, much the same as nurses employed in institutions.

A unique and distinct aspect of PHN practice is the self-sufficiency and autonomy required when working in a setting without walls. You have to know a lot, be clinically versatile, a critical thinker, have a quick mind, and be willing to confront your own biases.

Nurses in community practice have to relinquish the implied authority of hospital practice. Control is in the hands of the patient who will decline or grant access to his home. Anticipating this, nurses should have the personality attributes that allow them to deal successfully with such situations. Even if the setting is a clinic, there is no force that can make a client come or return or, for that matter, follow any prescribed regimen.

Many studies have documented the need for public health nurses to use interventions with clients and families that are specific to ethnic, cultural, and social values. Families may reject health teaching if it is perceived to be judgmental or prejudiced on the part of the health care provider.

Professional nurses who select PHN as a career need an outstanding ability to adjust to many types of environments with a variety of living conditions, from the well-to-do in a high-rise apartment house to the most poverty-stricken in a ghetto or rural area, and to appreciate a wide range of interests, attitudes, educational backgrounds, and cultural differences. They must be able to accept these variations, understand the differences, communicate well so as to avoid misunderstandings and misinterpretations, and be able to give equally good nursing care in every situation. Public health nurses in any position must use excellent judgment and are expected to use their own initiative. They have the opportunity to work with persons in other disciplines and other social agencies to help provide needed services to the clients, services that may include financial counseling, legal aid, housing problems, family planning, marital counseling, and school difficulties. In some instances, public health nurses are not only case finders, but also case coordinators—patient advocates in every sense.

■ SCHOOL HEALTH NURSING

In 2008, there were 84,418 RNs employed in school health settings according to the Division of Nursing's sample survey of the *Registered Nurse Population*.[30] This includes nurses who are employed in public and private elementary and secondary schools, and college health services. These numbers include RNs with no advanced or specialty preparation, certified school nurses (requirement differs by the state), and school nurse practitioners (SNPs) who are APNs qualified to deliver a full range of primary care services. In some cases, school nurses are expected to have the same educational credentials as teachers. The salaries for these positions vary by region, but in the beginning are lower than for hospital employment. School nurses employed by large urban school districts eventually can earn and even exceed some hospital salaries. Salary growth is often associated with the same variables that apply to teachers, increasing the base salary for further formal education beyond the BSN and seniority. Formal coursework must often be in areas of education to qualify for tuition remission or salary gains; therefore, many school nurses have not been encouraged to pursue degrees in nursing, which puts them at a disadvantage in their own profession.

School nurses in elementary and secondary schools ideally work with and through school health councils to plan and execute their programs. School health councils consist of school and community health administrators, parents, students, senior citizens, teachers, nurses, business people, individuals working for the media, attorneys, and elected officials with an interest in school health. Consequently, community development and coalition-building skills (e.g., team building, negotiating, needs assessment abilities, and an awareness of how community governance works) are necessary abilities for someone entering the school health field.

Local school districts vary in size throughout the country. The majority (75 percent) has a total student enrollment of 2500 students or fewer. School nurses may work in more than one building. Here, nurses perform a wide range of services, including basic screenings for vision, hearing, growth measurements, and risk factors that would interfere with the development of healthy lifestyle habits. Case management services are also provided for students at high risk for health impairments and school failure. Unfortunately, school nurses are often spread too thin to work adequately and intensively with students who need it most. The National Association of School Nurses (NASN) suggests a ratio of 750 students to one certified school nurse in schools with mainstreamed populations (accommodating students with special needs in the regular classroom), and even lower ratios in schools that serve special populations.[31]

Almost every school nurse is responsible for activities in the areas of (1) health service, (2) health education, and (3) environmental health and safety. The programs they implement may range from very basic services for students as a whole, such as health risk appraisals, to one-on-one primary health care services provided in a school-based student health center. It depends on the wishes of the community, as often represented by its Board of Education, and the actions of the school health council, where one exists.

All nurses working in schools must be clinically prepared to work with students with special health needs. Since the passage of the Individuals with Disabilities Education Act (IDEA) in the 1970s, students with complex chronic diseases, emotional disorders, and developmental disabilities as well as those who are dependent on technology (e.g., ventilators) are entitled to a free and appropriate public education. This means nurses must be prepared to perform a number of clinical procedures (e.g., gastrostomy feedings, suctioning, dressing changes) to ensure that these students have ready access to education. Additional legislation has since expanded the age range of children with special health needs served by schools from the previous 5 to 18 years of age to birth through adulthood. Consequently, school nurses today must be prepared to work with students of all ages. Furthermore, school nurses in many districts also provide employee health services for school administrators, faculty, and staff, including the processing of workers' compensation claims.

School nurses function in accordance with the Standards of Professional School Nursing Practice as established by the NASN. These standards include clear expectations for both the services delivered to the client and behaviors of the school nurse as a member of a profession. Measurable outcome criteria for each standard further reinforce the school nurse's intent of being accountable to the public.

Because school nurses have ties to both the health and education fields, the following national health criteria related to *Healthy People 2010* further define their goals for children:

1. Increase participation in daily physical education activities at school.

2. Provide school lunch and breakfast programs with menus consistent with nutritional principles contained in the Dietary Guidelines for Americans.

3. Provide nutrition education from preschool through 12th grade.

4. Include tobacco use prevention in the curricula of all elementary, middle, and secondary schools.

5. Provide children in all primary and secondary schools with educational programs on alcohol and other drugs.

6. Increase the proportion of children and youth who have discussed human sexuality with their parents or received information from parentally endorsed sources such as schools.

7. Increase the proportion of elementary and secondary schools that teach nonviolent conflict-resolution skills.

8. Provide academic instruction on injury prevention and control.

9. Increase the proportion of schools that have age-appropriate HIV education curricula.

10. Include school instruction on preventing STDs.

Schools have become an important site for the delivery of primary health care to school-age children and youth. SNPs working as members of interdisciplinary teams are often primary health care providers. Other advanced practice school health nurses manage and coordinate school-based student health centers and other aspects of the school health program that are part of an integrated, comprehensive service package for students. Still other school nurse specialists provide mental health counseling within student assistant programs, serve as active members of the school team responsible for athletic programs, and design, implement, and evaluate health promotion programs for the entire student body.

How successful and satisfying is school nursing? As an example, an NP working in a middle school health clinic has made a tremendous difference in the lives of economically deprived children. The NP works in an inner-city school on the East Coast and provides primary health care to students who otherwise have very limited access to health services. Since the opening of the school-based clinic, this NP has been a vital member of a health team that has witnessed a significant drop in the teen pregnancy rate, a notable decrease in suicides, an increase in the attendance rate, and an increase in the number of mental health problems diagnosed and treated. The health team has been so successful that even the school principal and staff are crediting the NP and the school-based clinic facility with keeping the students healthy enough to learn.

It is important to recognize that the patterns for school nursing practice vary according to the needs perceived and the limits set by school boards. In one pattern, the nurse might assume responsibility for the total school health program assisted by an aide to do clerical work and to triage simple conditions. In a second pattern, a senior nurse or specialist may visit a number of schools, assessing and evaluating children and leaving the follow-up to the regular school nurse. Or one nurse may routinely circulate between a number of facilities in a district. In another situation, the practice might be limited to performing physical exams or evaluating children with learning difficulties. School-based clinics (SBCs) or school-linked health clinics with SNPs provide comprehensive health care service. In some, family planning services are included, which has generated controversy.

Colleges and universities also provide a setting for the nurse interested in student health, although obviously there is considerable adult health involved. Responsibilities vary according to the size of the institution and the types of services offered. College students often pay a health fee that entitles them to specific benefits. Services may include mental health counseling, family planning, and care for minor illnesses or injuries. SNPs and NPs with other related specialty areas are becoming the dominant providers in college health, and more commonly the directors of college health services are nurses, with physicians as members of the staff.

Many school districts hire their own nurses, but others contract with the local public health agency for school health coverage. School nurse positions are often considered particularly desirable because the time schedule is the same as for teachers, with weekends and summers off. Schools with SBCs may operate the health centers year-round so that health care services for children are not interrupted.

Several years ago, a large coalition of nursing organizations cited schools as a key facility for primary care under health care reform. It is likely that nurses who are creative and interested in primary care and prevention will find school nursing a rewarding career. A graduate degree will become essential for the complexity of the role in the years to come.

Opportunities for advancement are found primarily in the larger systems, and are still often linked to supervisory positions. The possibility of professional growth is limitless in systems where nurses are able to assume a full professional role and have an impact on the health of school-age populations. School nursing is an evolving field that offers dramatic practice opportunities.

■ OCCUPATIONAL HEALTH NURSING

Occupational health nursing (OHN), once called *industrial nursing*, reportedly began in 1888 with services provided by Betty Moulder to a group of coal miners in Drifton, Pennsylvania. In 1895, the Vermont Marble Company hired Ada Mayo Stewart to care for ill and injured workers and their families. She is generally credited with being the first industrial nurse; much has been reported about her activities.

Two department stores were the next to provide similar health services for their employees: the John Wanamaker Company of New York in 1897 and the Frederick Loeser Department Store in Brooklyn in 1899. Early in the 1900s, more and more industries on both the East and West Coasts recognized the economic value of keeping employees healthy and established similar health services. Adding impetus to the trend was the enactment of workers' compensation laws (beginning in 1911), which emphasize accident prevention to employees on the job and provide for disability compensation for work-related injured or ill workers and encourage immediate and expert attention to injuries received at work. This development brought more industrial nurses into the workplace. World Wars I and II were also strong influences in the growth of OHN because they created increased respect for the value of the worker.

For many years, nurses employed in these positions called themselves industrial nurses. In 1958, however, industrial nurses voted to call their field *occupational health nursing*, which reflected the broader and changing scope of practice within the specialty. A key factor in the change in terminology was the enactment in 1970 of the Occupational Safety and Health Act (see Chapters 6 and 19). This act created the National Institute for Occupational Safety and Health (NIOSH) to provide education to occupational health and safety professionals through the establishment of Educational Resource Centers (ERCs), to research occupational health problems, and to recommend health and safety standards. With the establishment of the ERCs, specialized education in OHN is now available to prepare NPs, nurse managers, and nurse specialists to assess workplace hazards, design intervention strategies to minimize risk, and promote worker health and healthy working conditions.

The Occupational Safety and Health Administration (OSHA) was also established to guarantee a safe and healthful workplace. OSHA inspects the nation's workplaces for health and safety hazards, but its effectiveness has been blunted by lack of funds and the resistance of some employers, who have sometimes sued and won to limit the access of OSHA's inspectors. Nevertheless, unions, environmentalists, and other interested citizens have pressed for more action.

The occupational health nurse may work in a multidisciplinary setting or multi-nurse unit; however, more than 60 percent of occupational health nurses work alone. Physicians are often employed on a contractual basis and provide medical services as needed, but in most cases the occupational health nurse is the manager of the unit.

Whether this nurse functions in a sophisticated manner in the delivery of health care depends on his or her education and experience, and the policies of the employer. As an NP, the nurse provides primary care and makes a clinical diagnosis. She or he assesses the worker's condition through health histories, observation, physical examination, and other selected diagnostic measures; reviews and interprets findings to differentiate the normal from the abnormal; selects and carries out the appropriate action and referral as necessary; counsels; and teaches. The practitioner must also be concerned with the physical and psychosocial phenomena of the workers and their families, their working environment, community, and even recreation.

When the nurse does not function in an expanded role, standing orders or directions, prepared and signed by the medical director, give the necessary authority to care for conditions that develop while the employee is on the job. In a more conservative environment, where a nurse does not have specialized preparation, activities may be limited. However, these usually include first aid or emergency treatment, assisting the physician, carrying out certain diagnostic tests, and keeping health records. The ability to take and recognize abnormalities in electrocardiograms and perform eye screenings, audiometric testing, and certain laboratory tests and x-rays is also important. In addition, the nurse must be vitally concerned with the safety of the employees and often conducts worksite tours with management and the safety engineer to help plan a practical safety program.

The scope of OHN practice has broadened considerably. More emphasis is being placed on health promotion activities to keep the worker well. There is an increased emphasis of concern on worker health problems that may or may not be directly caused by the job but affect worker performance—alcoholism, emotional problems, stress, drug addiction, and family relations. In many cases, the nurse may be involved in developing employee assistance programs and in counseling and therapy.

In addition, occupational health nurses are assuming the role of manager of the occupational health unit and administration of the overall program. There are a number of legal issues about which the nurse must be knowledgeable. These include the serious and not infrequent responsibility of giving immediate care to workers with serious injuries, often with no physician present, which may have major legal implications. Occupational health nurses should be familiar with the laws governing the practice of nursing, medicine, and pharmacy in their own states and discuss them with the physician and management to make sure that they all understand the legal scope of nursing functions. In addition, the nurse must be fully cognizant of laws that govern employee health. This requires the interpretation of regulations and the design and implementation of standards to protect worker health. The nurse should be involved in policy decisions affecting worker's health and safety.

Graduation from a state-approved school of professional nursing and current state registration are basic requirements for the occupational health nurse. More employers are requiring a college degree and many find a graduate degree desirable. A career occupational health nurse may seek certification by the American Board for Occupational Health Nurses, an independent nursing specialty board authorized to certify qualified occupational health nurses.

Salaries and fringe benefits vary according to the size of the industry or business and its location. The usual company benefits include vacations, sick leave, pensions, and insurance. Working hours are those of the workers; thus, in an industry with work shifts around the clock, nurses are usually there as well. Although some industries carry professional liability insurance that supposedly covers the occupational health nurse, it may not apply in all cases of possible litigation. It is advisable, therefore, for the nurses to carry their own professional liability insurance.

■ OFFICE NURSING

Office nurses are employed by physicians and ambulatory care multispecialty practices and usually see their patients in an office. Office nurses may provide the nursing care needed themselves or assign certain duties to other personnel who work under their direction and supervision. When working for several doctors in a group practice or in a larger multispecialty center employing numerous personnel, a supervising nurse may oversee a staff of RNs, LPNs, and medical assistants; clerical, billing, and insurance personnel; receptionists; and other technical personnel.

Nurses may work in a one-doctor (solo) practice with a generalist, internist, or family practitioner. This requires the nurse to have general skills and knowledge. Or nurses may be employed in a specialist's office, which necessitates skills in the specific specialty. For instance, a surgeon (ophthalmologist, plastic surgeon, orthopedist) may employ a nurse who can also act as a scrub nurse in surgery at the hospital or assist in office surgery. With a current emphasis on primary care, preventive care, and managed care, many physicians are establishing practice groups in which physicians of the same or different specialties provide comprehensive medical care for their patients. This means a greater dependence on the office nurse to coordinate the activities in the office and address new problems in the delivery of ambulatory office care. In the larger practice or clinic milieu, several nurses are usually employed as part of a larger staff. Nurses may be employed as part of a team with other technical and professional personnel providing services such as x-ray, laboratory, electrocardiograms, and other cardiac procedures, electroencephalograms, physical therapy, pharmacy, nutrition counseling, laser procedures, preventive maintenance, and wellness counseling.

Providing patient education, often of a preventive or rehabilitative nature, is one of the primary functions of office nurses. Office nurses must have excellent teaching and communication skills, exhibit organizational and leadership abilities, possess good assessment skills, be familiar with community resources, and have good insight to anticipate and interpret the needs of their patients. In today's competitive health care climate, they are also called on to assist the physician in marketing the medical practice, to be a public relations agent to promote the retention of existing patients, and to function as a patient advocate as the patient moves through the maze of support services.

Although more physicians and larger clinics are employing NPs to assume responsibility for patient care, smaller offices depend on the RN to assume these responsibilities along with accountability for running the office; scheduling patients; hiring, evaluating, and scheduling staff; and generally overseeing the smooth operation of the office. Today, office nurses are seeking continuing and collegiate education specific to office practice, office management, and organizational leadership.

All office nurses must be licensed to practice and be currently registered in the state in which they work. Although not usually required, education beyond the basic nursing program is desirable. In most cases, nurses have also had previous nursing experience.

Salaries and working conditions in this field, generally speaking, are varied, based on the needs of each specialty practice, the region of the country, and the employer. Salaries may be lower than those offered to acute care nursing counterparts, and benefits are also negotiable with the employer. Office nurses sometimes say that they are willing to make some financial sacrifices because there are other benefits: There are no shift rotations, they often do not work weekends, and they can negotiate their schedules to meet their current needs. There is, however, the possibility of evening or overtime hours based on practice needs.

Some of the most common fringe benefits include paid vacation and holidays, paid sick leave, year-end bonus, and free medical care for the nurse and family. A point of negotiation when seeking employment is medical-surgical or hospitalization insurance, malpractice insurance, pension or retirement plans, tuition reimbursement, and time off to attend CE courses and meetings. Although they may be named on the physician's malpractice insurance policy, nurses should carry their own malpractice liability insurance.

Those considering a career in office nursing should discuss all aspects of their work and employment conditions in detail with their prospective employer. It is important to make sure that the nurse will be free to function in a nursing capacity and that the employer is in accord with what the nurse expects the role to be. A written job description is critical to mutual understanding of the role and its responsibilities. A written contract setting forth the professional and personal agreements between the nurse and the employer can also be mutually beneficial.

■ NURSING EDUCATION

Nursing is not only in the midst of a general shortage, but a grave shortage of faculty is an obstacle to moving on with recruitment and enrollment in schools of nursing. Over one-third of baccalaureate programs have pointed to faculty shortages as the reason for not accepting all qualified applicants for 2010. Budget constraints in higher education, an aging workforce, and job competition from clinical sites have all contributed to this crisis.[32] Additionally, there has been substantial growth in part-time and adjunct faculty in all program types, but so has there been for higher education in general.

The qualifications of faculty beyond the basic academic credential are another issue. Faculty in baccalaureate and higher degree programs must compete on the basis of a scholarship standard that is on a par with other members of the academic community. For faculty in all programs there is the issue of clinical credibility and new practice patterns and settings that are foreign to their own background. Most teachers of nurses expect to teach in the area of their clinical expertise, but different programs may make additional demands. The teacher may be expected to teach a variety of nursing subjects in AD and practical nurse programs. This only further complicates the issue of clinical credibility (see Chapters 12 and 13), and there is the ongoing debate over educational credibility. Just because you can do it, can you teach it?

The philosophy, objectives, students, and conditions of employment vary in different kinds of nursing education programs. Nurses planning to teach should give thought to the kind of program with which they can identify philosophically and in which they can function effectively. The number and types of positions within each program depend on the size of the student body, the curriculum content, the faculty organization, and the school's philosophy, aims, and budget. There is a place in some schools for a nurse instructor of sciences; however, in most schools, students take courses in physical and social sciences taught by non-nurse instructors.

Certain aspects of a faculty position are the same regardless of the educational setting. Faculty have responsibilities to the total program, usually through committees. Some are development and updating of philosophy, objectives, conceptual framework, and selecting appropriate courses to meet those objectives; selection, evaluation, and promotion of students; assisting in developing educational and faculty standards, policies, and procedures; participating in promotion and tenure of faculty; developing special projects; and planning for the future. In a university or college setting, the teacher is expected to participate in campus-wide committees of the same nature. In relation to the student, a basic role is teaching in the classroom and on-line, laboratory, and clinical setting, individually or in groups, using appropriate and effective techniques with current knowledge and practice in the area of expertise. Advisement and personal and career counseling of students are also important; some teachers are class or student committee advisers and consultants as well. In the college and university settings, research and publication are major expectations; generally the teacher must seek outside funding for research. Almost equally important is service to the profession and the community, as officers of organizations, members of committees, consultants, or speakers.

Differences in teaching in the various programs relate to both the setting and the level. In universities, particularly medical centers, there is a trend toward joint appointments, with the teacher carrying a patient caseload and, occasionally, administrative responsibilities in the clinical setting. In some cases, teachers are reimbursed additionally for this duty. Some set up a group faculty practice arrangement in which their compensation benefits both themselves and the school.

Graduate faculty are expected to be scholarly and research oriented, because, as well as teaching, they direct graduate students' research. They are encouraged to work closely with graduate faculty in other disciplines. Working with graduate students on special projects and guiding or supervising their research may mean spending hours with a student in conference and committee presentations for the master's thesis or doctoral dissertation, including certain administrative details.

Faculty in college- or university-based programs have the advantage of being in an academic setting with broad interdisciplinary contacts and campus activities. They may have joint appointments in other departments or schools and other responsibilities there. They also have the benefits and problems of being in such a setting; the policies and regulations are less directly controllable.

Students in collegiate programs affiliate or rotate through a number of hospitals, agencies, or facilities. Unless the program is in a medical center or the teacher holds a joint appointment, students and teachers maintain something of a guest status and find it more difficult to effect care. If other students are also present, there is competition for good teaching patients.

On the other hand, in diploma programs, basic nursing education is significantly influenced by the hospital. Nursing classes and often clinical practice are given in that particular school and hospital, although students may go to other clinical settings. Because of geographic proximity and the fact that hospitals often think of the diploma students as their students and future employees, there may be a closer relationship between nurses in the clinical area and the faculty. Often the CNE has overall responsibility for both nursing service and nursing education, and there are opportunities for both service and education personnel to plan and work together on joint projects that hold mutual benefit to the school and hospital. Usually there is more national prestige in being affiliated with a university program, but other schools with strong community ties are highly respected locally.

The teaching opportunities in practical nurse programs offer another type of challenge to the nurse educator. The method of teaching and the philosophy of vocational education differ somewhat from those of professional education. The course of study usually is limited to 1 year. The setting may be in hospitals, public schools, or community colleges, among which both philosophy and environment vary considerably. It is important that the professional nurse teaching in these programs understands and respects the role of practical nurses in providing patient care and be able to teach accordingly.

Besides the educational requirements, teachers in all nursing programs are expected to have knowledge of nursing in general and continuously updated knowledge and clinical expertise in the subject area in which they expect to teach. They also need knowledge and skill in curriculum development, the teaching-learning process, and teaching methods and techniques. It is equally important for any prospective teacher to establish rapport with students and to be open-minded and secure enough to welcome differences in opinion. Evaluation of teacher effectiveness is an ongoing process in a progressive educational setting and includes self-evaluation and evaluation by students, peers, and administrators. The quality of teaching is considered in retention and promotion of faculty.

Tenure in colleges and universities means basically that the individual has a secure place in that institution and cannot be dismissed except under unusual circumstances. Usually there is a span of time (6 years) during which the person works toward tenure or leaves, unless they are placed in some special category outside the tenure track. The more prestigious the institution, the higher the standards for appointment, promotion, and tenure. If university teaching is to be a nurse's career, a doctoral degree is essential, and a postdoctoral research experience would be wise (see Chapter 12). The pursuit of tenure is very stressful, and collegiality among faculty can provide the support needed to succeed. Many of the major university schools of nursing have established a clinical appointment system that provides for the appointment, reappointment, and promotion of faculty who are exceptionally talented in their practice. Such a status does not usually allow progression toward tenure.

Salaries and fringe benefits vary, and in an institution of higher education they are supposed to be the same for individuals of the same rank regardless of discipline. A full professor at the last salary step may earn as much as or more than the administrator of that particular program. Salaries are reported frequently by the American Association of Colleges of Nursing (AACN), and there is a yearly salary study of academics conducted by the American Association of University Professors (AAUP) and published in *Academe*, their official publication.

Teaching positions in any educational program usually demand irregular working hours. Except for scheduled classes, the amount of time a teacher spends at work is unpredictable because there are so many influencing factors, such as class and clinical preparation time, student conferences, student evaluation, participation in school committees and meetings, library use, and participation in student activities and university social events.

Teachers are also involved in professional activities, updating their own clinical practice, and advancing their education. Depending on where they teach, they may be able to set their own hours as far as presence in the school is concerned (except for scheduled classes). It is estimated that the average university nurse faculty member spends about 56 hours a week on the job. However, faculty are usually freer than other nurses to attend educational and other meetings. Nurses selecting a career in this field will want to analyze the conditions of each employment opportunity to make sure that it offers them as much as possible of what they want most in both material and professional rewards as well as an atmosphere in which they can do their best work. For a teacher, often the greatest reward is the intellectual and personal stimulation of an educational environment, including interaction with students and peers.

Administration in Nursing Education

At the head of each education program in nursing is a professional nurse who is both administrator and teacher. Nursing education administrators need preparation in administration as well as teaching. Again, it is best, and sometimes required, that the director of the program takes graduate courses in educational administration.

Such courses are only rarely available in graduate nursing education programs, so those whose goal is education administration often acquire experience as assistants to a top administrator or in minor administrative positions and apply principles from non-nursing management courses. In some colleges and universities, department chairmen or deans are appointed administratively on recommendation of the faculty for limited terms, after which they return to nonadministrative faculty positions. This approach has advantages and disadvantages: It gives presumably competent faculty members an opportunity in the administrative role, but it may not be considered desirable by the individual whose primary interest is educational administration and who must then relocate to secure a top administrative position.

Qualifications for nursing administration positions in education usually include experience in nursing and nursing education and frequently in administration of some kind. This nurse should be able to relate well to others in the nursing program, the profession, the particular setting of the school, and the community. The need for leadership qualities is frequently cited. A minimum of a master's degree is usual, and the dean, director, or chairman of a collegiate or university program in nursing is expected to have a doctoral degree. It is also not uncommon to expect these candidates to have achieved national prominence in the nursing field, be a scholar, and have been published. Frequently, when a top administrative position is open, a search committee composed according to institutional criteria looks for, screens, interviews, and recommends an individual after a national search.

The top administrative post of any nursing education program usually requires both long hours of work on the job and active participation in professional activities. If in a college or university, the administrator is expected to be a leader in campus-wide committees and activities. There may be pressure from the faculty, students, administration, and community, all trying to achieve their own ends. Often there are financial problems for the school. There is little time for nurse administrators to keep abreast of their own clinical field because the demand to keep current on administrative, educational, and general nursing trends is immediate. This is not a position for someone who cannot learn and act quickly and who wilts under pressure. The rewards, however, can be great professionally, in the satisfaction of accomplishments of the nursing program, its faculty, and students, and in the opportunity to be in a leadership position in nursing and health care. Insights into some desirable attributes for this role may be found in the section on the nurse executive earlier in this chapter.

Salaries, fringe benefits, and sometimes rank and tenure tend to be negotiable and usually depend on a number of factors related to the position, the community, and the qualifications of the nurse.

■ NURSE RESEARCHER

Nurses in research may function in a variety of roles, depending on their educational preparation. If the nurse has not had doctoral preparation or research training, working on a research team as a research assistant or associate, collecting data, or doing some data analysis may be a start. Fully prepared nurse researchers are in great demand. They may find employment in universities and health institutions or may choose to freelance as consultants. The need is greater than either the supply of qualified nurses or the funds available for research. Many nurses with doctoral degrees have taken positions in universities and colleges, either as professors of nursing or as administrators, where they engage in both research and teaching. This is considered a compatible and necessary combination, because not only do these nurses increase their knowledge of nursing, but they also train other nurses in research and guide their studies as well as teach from the products of their own scientific investigations. The need to recruit nursing students early in their careers for graduate study and research is important.

A particularly encouraging trend is the employment of nurse researchers in practice settings, such as medical centers, home care, government, and more. In these positions, nurse researchers may have responsibility for studying patients' nursing needs; defining and evaluating patient care effectiveness; setting up testing situations for the development of new nursing techniques, equipment, or procedures; acting as advisers or consultants to nurses developing patient research projects; and planning with other disciplines for the improvement of patient care. Nurse researchers may also become research project directors, directors of research institutes, or full partners in an interdisciplinary research team.

Nurses engaged in research as described here are expected to have research training and ability that are verified both through their educational credentials, the doctorate, and their experience. Personally, they must have the ability both to do creative thinking and to carry through the orderly process of research, which, with human beings, is seldom static or orderly, and the writing skill to report their findings. Nurses holding university positions earn the same salaries and benefits as other nurse teachers in that setting. Although time may be allotted for research, the funding of this research is often the responsibility of the teacher-researchers, and they must become adept at grantsmanship. There are also nurses hired by universities to head or participate in specific research projects, without teaching responsibilities. These positions are often on a short-term basis. Most researchers find that they devote considerable time to their studies, and working hours are often not in a regular 40-hour-a-week framework. This is particularly true if the researcher also has teaching or administrative responsibilities.

If employed in a clinical setting, the nurse researcher's salary is probably negotiable, depending on her or his background. Although such positions may be budgeted, there may be very limited budgeting for other personnel and equipment needed for specific research projects. Again, funds must be sought from other sources, such as foundations, individuals, or, most frequently, governmental agencies. The availability of these funds has fluctuated, which has been a detriment to nursing research.

For nurse researchers, however, the satisfactions are great, in terms of both the personal satisfactions of research and the knowledge that they have made meaningful contributions to the nursing field. With all the opportunities available to nurses with doctoral degrees, it is certain that those engaged in research do so because it is their first preference.

■ CASE MANAGER

All nurses manage the care of their patients. The presence of case managers, case coordinators, or discharge planners does not eliminate that responsibility. The case manager as discussed here is a very intense and empowered role necessary for the most complex and costly of patients.[33] It is not the case method for organizing the daily care of patients that was discussed earlier in the chapter, although there is a shared philosophy of comprehensiveness. The case manager is best situated in an integrated system of services (or unrelated to the systems that serve the patient), although many case managers are hospital based and terminate their services with discharge and successful community or extended care placement. The benefit of moving with the patient across a continuum of services has resulted in a thriving market for independent case managers and employment by third-party payers or managed care programs.

The case manager strives to secure the services that are preferred by the patient within the constraint of available resources. The case manager fosters independence, advocates on the patient's behalf, and supports decisions that are outcome driven and fiscally sensitive. The case manager ideally can authorize the disbursement of resources, but does so cautiously in anticipation of the long-term needs of these patients, who are usually very resource intensive. Practice occurs within an interdisciplinary model, which requires that case managers be secure in their identity as a nurse and able to command respect from other disciplines.

Although social workers have performed aspects of case management for years, today's more complex patients need a holism and clinical sophistication that makes the nurse the most appropriate case manager. Eighty percent of case managers are nurses. A minimum of a baccalaureate is required, with a master's preferred. APNs with a specialty in the target population or community health experience are ideally suited as case managers.

■ ENTREPRENEURS AND INTRAPRENEURS

Nurses in private practice seem to be a growing phenomenon. It is estimated that some 20,000 nurses have their own businesses. An *entrepreneur* is defined as one who organizes and manages a business undertaking, assuming risk for the sake of profit. Most of the studies on the characteristics of entrepreneurs, not thought to be typical of women, have focused on white males. However, Aydelotte, in the first study of nurses in private practice, summarized the demographics and characteristics gleaned from a number of studies of female entrepreneurs. In general, these women are 35 to 45 years old, married with two to five children, have a father who was an entrepreneur, are firstborn children, and start their venture because of job frustration, interest, and recognition of an opportunity. They have a need for achievement, describe themselves as risk-takers, and score high on masculine-associated traits such as autonomy, aggression, independence, and leadership but not as high as female managers.[34]

Aydelotte went on to study nurse entrepreneurs themselves. The vast majority (96.7 percent) were women; most were between 30 and 50 years old, married, with one to three children. More than two-thirds had master's or doctoral degrees and 10 to 25 years' experience; they were certified in their specialty and belonged to one or more nursing professional organizations. Experience was a major factor; only about 9 percent had less than 10 years' experience. Their reasons for initiating the entrepreneurial venture included a wish for independence, the opportunity to do so, and a lack of control and decision making in the workplace. Unlike non-nurse entrepreneurs, they did not say they were frustrated. Slightly over half were sole proprietors of their business and worked full time. The services they offered are largely consultation, counseling, direct client and home care service, client education, and nursing CE, although a variety of other services were offered and more than one service was usual. Referrals came from clients, nurses, physicians, hospitals, clinics, and public health departments; these nurses also had contracts with agencies. Advertising was done through speaking engagements, flyers, newspapers, magazines, and newsletters (and today would likely include the Internet). A few used radio and television. A number worked in other positions, especially as educator, staff nurse, and manager, to supplement their income.[35]

Aydelotte also notes current patterns and future directions of entrepreneurial models, such as a preferred professional nurse provider organization and nursing service organization, all somewhat similar to the managed care arrangements described in Chapter 7. In these cases, a nurse group would contract their nursing services to an individual, hospital, or other agency.

For those who want to set up a private practice it is essential to understand that setting it up and running it must be a businesslike process. There are basic decisions to be made: What kind of organization should be created (corporation, partnership, for-profit, nonprofit); by whom (nurses and other professionals); for whom; at what fees; what kind and how many employees will be needed; how to get clients (marketing); types of advertising; how to relate to other health professions; where the services will be offered; at what hours; and policies about telephone counseling or home visits (house calls). Early expenses include lawyers' and accountants' fees, space, furniture, equipment, supplies, telephone, insurance, stationery, postage, advertising, and brochures. Repeated obstacles or problems to most are the normal process of business for the entrepreneur: employee contracts, salaries, benefits, tax deductions, fee preparation and collection, and the multitude of forms, records, and electronic systems that are essential. When federal or other contracts are involved, still more records are necessary.

Intrapreneur is a term coined to describe a person who takes hands-on responsibility for creating innovation of any kind within an organization. As opposed to entrepreneurs, who leave a place of employment to start their own business, intrapreneurs work within the system to create exciting new things.

The reader is referred to Pinchot's early work on intrapreneuring. In analyzing both the system and personal characteristics for the successful intrapreneur, he used the case study technique, interviewing pioneer intrapreneurs from a variety of backgrounds. He calls the intrapreneur the hedge against the "dead wood" syndrome in corporate America. Neither the entrepreneur nor the intrapreneur is taking the safer route; they are not better or worse, just different. The intrapreneur

1. Wants freedom, but access to resources (not willing to be totally self-reliant)
2. Recognizes an urgency to meet a timetable to some degree established by the system
3. Is cynical about the system, but confident of her or his ability to outwit it
4. Has an inside-outside orientation, regardless of position in the hierarchy
5. Likes risk, and is unafraid of being fired
6. Hides risky projects until comfortable about their eventual success
7. Mocks traditional status symbols, but plays the game flawlessly . . . is manipulative
8. Values the presence of accessible networks
9. Seeks friends in high places for protection[36]

Examples of successful intrapreneurial activities may be setting up a high-end substance abuse unit or a 24-hour outpatient center for patient education; supporting and gaining admitting privileges for APNs; supporting joint hiring of a strategic nurse subspecialist with another facility; and establishing a consultant group of APNs for "on call" access to clients, organizational or individual.

Depending on the arrangements made, the nurse may receive royalties, direct payments, profits shared with the institution, income for the nursing department to be used in a variety of ways, or nothing extra financially at all, just freedom and excitement. An interesting intrapreneureal/entrepreneureal idea is that of a self-managed group of nurses running a unit and being paid by the hospital.

■ INTERNATIONAL NURSING

The nurse with a taste for adventure and a desire to see the world may enjoy a position with one of the agencies concerned with nursing in areas outside the United States. Such positions are almost invariably challenging and a little off the beaten track. At the same time, the qualifications are usually high, including special preparation in the area in which the nurse will be working.

World Health Organization

One agency to which nurses have turned for international health employment is the World Health Organization (WHO) and its regional office, the Pan American Health Organization (PAHO). Their major concerns currently are in primary care, but related activities in terms of education may also have priority. Because of changing emphasis and varying needs, it is best to contact these agencies for information on the type of positions available, requirements, and conditions of employment. However, generally it is necessary to have advanced education, experience, and language capability. The WHO headquarters is in Geneva, but PAHO can be contacted at 525 23rd St NW, Washington, DC 20037.

Peace Corps

Since the Peace Corps began in 1961 it has employed nurses as both volunteers and paid staff. Nurses serve in many of the 60 Peace Corps countries in the preventive and curative program developed to care for the volunteer. Here, too, there are changing priorities and variable funding, depending to an extent on the politics of the moment. Whether interested in a paid or volunteer position, it is best to contact the Peace Corps, P-301, Washington, DC, 20526, for available opportunities and requirements. As a rule, it has been necessary for the nurse to be an RN, a US citizen, and to have appropriate language skills for the country assigned, good health, stamina, and, of course, the necessary nursing skills.

Project HOPE

The purpose of Project HOPE has traditionally been to bring the skills and techniques developed by the American health professions to other peoples of the world in their own environment, adapted specifically to their needs and their way of life. HOPE is now engaged in a number of projects in the United States, as well as continuing some of its international activities. It is best to get updated information from Project HOPE, Millwood, VA 22646.

Other International Nursing Opportunities

A number of agencies place nurses internationally. Almost every religious denomination supports some kind of missionary work in foreign countries. Nurses are usually welcomed in such activities because missionary work often includes some form of professional or semiprofessional health care activities. Nurses who select missionary nursing as their life's work must have a strong desire to nurse the sick and underprivileged, often in primitive surroundings; an ability to teach religious principles by example, and possibly in religious classes; and knowledge of the language of the people in the regions assigned. They will have many opportunities to teach citizens and health workers of other lands. *Missionary nurses* must expect to find their rewards principally in personal satisfaction because missionary nurses usually earn a low salary for long hours of hard work. Nurses can obtain specific information about missionary nursing from their own church. Some mission groups accept volunteers who are not of their own religious faith.

Another major possibility in international nursing is *occupational nursing* for major industries (the multinationals) with overseas branches. On occasion, the governments, universities, hospitals, or industries of foreign countries also seek American nurses with all types of educational preparation. In recent years, Mideastern countries particularly have used recruiters to fill staff and other positions in their hospitals. It is especially important to clarify the job role and functions, as well as personal living conditions, and to learn about the country because some female American nurses have found it very difficult to adjust in Moslem countries. Limited opportunities are found with the federal government in countries where federal personnel are stationed, but these positions are first filled by transferring career personnel already in the agency.

In all cases, there are usually advertisements in newspapers or professional journals for these positions. If not, the nurse should make inquiries to the private company concerned or the appropriate federal agency.

■ OTHER CAREER OPPORTUNITIES

It would be impossible, or at least extraordinarily lengthy, to give information about every career possibility available for nurses. A list of specific positions, directly related to nursing, not even including specialization or

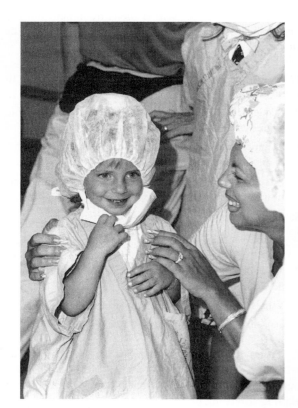

EXHIBIT 15–2. There are many novel practice opportunities such as this nurse who is conducting a hospital preadmission orientation for a child. (Courtesy of the Valley Hospital, Ridgewood, New Jersey)

subspecialization, runs into the hundreds when the diverse settings in which nursing is practiced are considered. Overall, these are clinical nursing, administration, education, or research (or a combination of all), but the specific setting brings its own particular challenges. These positions may require knowledge of another culture and the physical or psychosocial needs of these groups, such as nursing on an Indian reservation, or a new orientation to practice, such as working in an HMO, juvenile court, the prison system, or a methadone maintenance clinic.

In some cases, specialization or subspecialization, usually requiring additional education and training (because most generic education programs present only a brief exposure), becomes a new career path. There are a number of these, and as each becomes recognized as a distinct subspecialty, involved nurses tend to form a new organization and develop standards of practice.

Specialization and subspecialization are not really new; operating room nurses have been practicing since the beginning of American nursing, and coronary care nurses or enterostomal therapists are into their fourth decade. More recently, there is an emphasis on educational programs in such areas as women's health care, family planning, thanatology, and sex education, all of which have an interdisciplinary context that brings additional dimensions to the practice.

When nurses assume positions such as editors of nursing journals or nursing editors in publishing companies, they draw not only on their nursing background, but must learn about the publishing field and acquire the necessary skills. Editing is not the same as writing, and the responsibility for putting out a journal or other publication has financial, administrative, legal, philosophical, and policy-making components.

In the same vein, nurses employed as lobbyists, labor relations specialists, executive directors or staff of nursing associations, nurse consultants for drug or supply companies, and staff for legislators or governmental committees all use aspects of their nursing knowledge, but must learn from other disciplines not related to nursing and develop new role behaviors. If they choose to remain close to nursing, the association will enrich the profession.

As health care and nursing expand, some nurses will develop new positions themselves and the need and the qualifications cannot now be determined. It seems safe to say, however, that opportunities and challenges in nursing today are practically unlimited.

KEY POINTS

1. Nursing has been plagued by cyclical shortages and surpluses.
2. Because of the social and economic factors that can create rapid and unexpected demands in health care, it is difficult to predict the number of nurses that would provide a balance of supply and demand.
3. Our most recent shortage is one of supply: low enrollments in basic educational programs, an aging workforce, low workforce participation by current RNs, and a patient population with a need for clinical sophistication.
4. The hospital is still the largest employer of RNs.
5. Staff nurses want control over their practice and to receive respect for the work that they do.
6. Nursing positions are available or can be developed in every setting where health care is provided.
7. There continues to be disagreement as to whether differentiated practice should be built on competence or education.
8. Standards of practice describe a competent level of nursing care and a competent level of behavior in the professional role.
9. Three basic models for delivery of patient care exist: functional, team, and case, with endless variations.
10. It has become rare for nurses to be only responsible for themselves; they accomplish much of their work through others.
11. There is no consensus as to whether the case management role is reserved for the advanced practice nurse.
12. School health and occupational health nursing are ideally suited to primary health care.

REFERENCES

1. Aiken L. Charting the future of hospital nursing. In Lee P, Estes C (eds): *The Nation's Health*, 4th ed. Boston: Jones and Bartlett, 1994, pp 177–197.

2. Aiken L. The hospital nursing shortage. A paradox of increasing supply and increasing vacancy rates. In Harrington C, Estes C (eds): *Health Policy and Nursing*. Boston: Jones and Bartlett, 1994, pp 300–312.

3. Secretary's Commission on Nursing. *Final Report*, volume I. Washington, DC: US Government Printing Office, 1988.

4. McKibbon R, Boston C. An overview: Characteristic impact and solutions, Monograph I. In *The Nursing Shortage: Opportunities and Solutions*. Chicago: The American Hospital Association and the American Nurses Association, 1990.

5. Buerhaus P. Is another shortage looming? *Nurs Outlook* 46:102–108, May–June 1998.

6. Pay levels rise to record highs at NYC hospitals. *Am J Nurs* 93:71, July 1993.

7. Commission on the National Nursing Shortage. *Final Report*. Washington, DC: US Government Printing Office, 1991.

8. Shindul-Rothschild J, Berry D, Long-Middleton E. Where have all the nurses gone? *Am J Nurs* 96:25–39, November 1996.

9. Decision Data Collection. *Report of Survey Results: The 1994 ANA Layoffs Survey*. Submitted to the ANA, November 7, 1994 (unpublished paper).

10. Aiken L, Salmon M. Health care workforce priorities: What nursing should do now. In Harrington C, Estes C (eds): *Health Policy and Nursing,* 2nd ed. Sudbury, MA: Jones and Bartlett, 1997, p 174.

11. Buerhaus P. May–June 1998, loc cit.

12. Nally T. Nurse faculty shortage: The case for action. *J Emerg Nurs* 34(3):243–245, June 2008.

13. Aiken LH, Clarke SP, Sloane DM, Lake ET, Cheney T. Effects of hospital care environment on patient mortality and nurse outcomes. *J Nurs Adm* 39(7–8 Suppl): S45–51, July–August 2009.

14. Buerhaus P, Auerbach D, Staiger D. The recent surge in nurse employment: Causes and implications. *Health Affairs* 28(4):657–668, June 2009.

15. AACN. Nursing Shortage. May 2010. http://www.aacn.nche.edu/media/FactSheets/NursingShortage.htm. Retrieved May 4, 2010.

16. Bretschneider J, Eckhardt I, Glenn-West R, Green-Smolenski J, Richardson C. Strengthening the voice of the clinical nurse: The design and implementation of a shared governance model. *Nurs Adm Q* 34(1):41–48, January–March 2010.

17. Dietrich SL, Kornet TM, Lawson DR, Major K, May L, Rich VL, Riley-Wasserman E. Collaboration to partnerships. *Nurs Adm Q* 34(1):49–55, January–March 2010.

18. ANA. *Nursing: Scope and Standards of Practice*, 2nd ed. Silver Springs, MD: The Association, 2010.

19. ANA. *Cardiovascular Nursing: Scope and Standards of Practice*. Silver Springs, MD: The Association, 2008.

20. AMN Healthcare. New Health Care Delivery Models Are Redefining the Role of Nurses. 2009. http://www.nursezone.com/Nursing-News-Events/more-features/New-Health-Care-Delivery-Models-are-Redefining-the-Role-of-Nurses_29442.aspx. Retrieved May 5, 2010.

21. American College of Nurse Midwives. Midwifery Education Programs. 2010. http://www.acnm.org/map.cfm. Retrieved May 9, 2010.

22. Anderson BJ, Manno M, O'Connor P, Gallagher E. Listening to nursing leaders: Using national database of nursing quality indicators data to study excellence in nursing leadership. *J Nurs Adm* 40(4):182–187, April 2010.

23. National Sample Survey of Registered Nurses. 2008. http://bhpr.hrsa.gov/healthworkforce/rnsurvey/initialfindings2008.pdf. Retrieved May 8, 2010.

24. Ibid.

25. AACN. Nurse Practitioners: The Growing Solution in Health Care Delivery. April 1998. http://www.aacn.nche.edu/. Retrieved May 9, 2010.

26. PayScale. Salary Snapshot for Advanced Registered Nurse Practitioner (ARNP). http://www.payscale.com/research/US/Job=Advanced_Registered_Nurse_Practitioner_(ARNP)/Salary. Retrieved May 9, 2010.

27. American College of Nurse Midwives. A Brief History of Nurse-Midwifery in the US. http://www.mymidwife.org/history.cfm. Retrieved May 9, 2010.

28. My Salary. Certified Nurse Midwife. May 2010. http://swz.salary.com/salarywizard/layoutscripts/swzl_salaryresults. Retrieved May 9, 2010.

29. Study of Nurse Anesthetist Manpower Needs. Washington, DC: DHHS, USPHS, National Center for Nursing Research, February 1990.

30. *CRNA Jobs*: http://www.crnajobs.com/crna-careers/main.aspx. Retrieved May 5, 2010.

31. Healy B: *The newdoctors in the house*. April 15, 2010. http://www.usnews.com/education/best-medical-schools/articles/2010/04/15/the-new-doctors-in-the-house.html. Retrieved May 3, 2010.

32. USDHHS, HRSA: The Health Professions. *2008 National Sample Survey of Registered Nurses*. http://bhpr.hrsa.gov/healthworkforce/rnsurvey/2008/nssrn2008.pdf. Retrieved October 20, 2010.

33. Interview. President, National Association of School Nurses, May 10, 2010.

34. AACN. New AACN Data Show the Impact of the Economy on the Nurse Faculty Shortage. September 18, 2009. http://www.businesswire.com/portal/site/home/permalink/?ndmViewId=news_view&newsId=20090918005431&newsLang=en. Retrieved May 3, 2010.

35. Thomas P. Case management delivery models: The impact of indirect care givers on organizational outcomes. *J Nurs Adm* 39(1):30–37, January 2009.

36. Aydelotte M. *Nurses in Private Practice*. Kansas City, MO: ANA, 1988.

37. Ibid.

38. Pinchot G. *Intrapreneuring*. New York: Harper & Row, 1985.

Updates can be found at **www.kellysnursing.com**

Leadership for an Era of Change

Autonomy, leadership, power, and change are presented together in this chapter because of their interdependence. Each is described and the dynamics of each are discussed. They are applied to nursing situations to provide a flavor of reality, and so become more personally meaningful to the reader. These are not abstract concepts, but qualities that distinguish nurses in all their dealings with the public. Professions are expected to change with the times, and nowhere is change more guaranteed and dramatic than in health care. Although human nature may tempt us to drag our feet, nursing will have to change to accommodate the world around it.

Previous chapters presented a challenging future with discussions of hospital downsizing, a shift of services into community settings, emergent markets for nursing services, an industry-wide movement into managed care, a focus on disease prevention and health promotion, new consumer rights, and the prominence of advanced practice nurses (APNs). If this were not enough, we are confronted with a variety of models for restructuring the way day-to-day services are provided to our patients and the manner in which nurses are governed or directed in their work. It is necessary for nurses to know when change occurs for the sake of change and when it is in the best interest of the public. The magnitude of the decisions and the instability of the practice environment can work to our advantage, given that we understand the meaning of autonomy and are clear on what we see as a preferred future for nurses and the American public.

■ AUTONOMY

The public allows professionals a generous amount of freedom as they conduct their affairs. This freedom, better called *autonomy*, is based on the assumption that professionals are the stewards, not the owners, of their areas of service. Because of the complexity of their work, professionals have superior judgment on the internal affairs of their field. However, whatever they do, they do on behalf of the public, and any violation of that contract can result in restrictions on self-governance.

Sociologists have identified autonomy as the most strategic (and cherished) distinction between a profession and an occupation or semi-profession. We show our continuing appreciation for that autonomy through maintenance of our systems of licensure and certification, control of our educational systems, and adherence to a code of ethics. There is a distinction between *job content autonomy*, the freedom to determine the methods and procedures to be used to deal with a given problem, and *job context autonomy*, the freedom to name and define the boundaries of the problem and role relationships with other providers. The keys to autonomy as applied to nursing are that no other profession or administrative force can control nursing practice and that the nurse has latitude in making judgments in patient care within the scope of nursing practice as defined by the profession and the state Board of Nursing. Ideally, the definition of *scope* is one and the same for both.

There are a number of reasons why nursing does not have full autonomy. Early nursing in America did not assume an autonomous stance. In part, this was because most nurses were women, and female status was low at the time. Nurses, usually female, were constantly admonished to obey the physician, usually male, and to abide by his judgment about the patient's condition. Even though nurses were trained to observe, the next step was to report and wait for further direction. For nurses to act on their own judgment of what to do for the patient was a very risky area. Added to this was the nurse's position in the male-dominated hierarchy of the hospital (which, as it became larger, developed into a male-dominated bureaucracy).

As Ashley reported in her now-classic work, nurses have been expected to be mother figures, giving freely (in the financial as well as the social sense) of their time and efforts to meet the needs of all members of the hospital family, from patients to physicians. She attributed nurses' lack of progress and accompanying low status to the fact that they are mostly women and their work has been virtually ignored and trivialized in comparison to that of physicians. "Nursing's problems, rooted in the tradition of economic exploitation, inadequate education, and long-standing social discrimination, have plagued the profession for the greater part of its history."[1]

The fact that there were some early nurses who struggled free and were able to practice independently, primarily in public health settings, is evidence. From the beginning there was health care practice that was uniquely nursing. It is possible that we may have enjoyed more freedom in the past than in modern-day practice. Current restrictions on autonomy are both experienced in one's personal practice and by the discipline as a whole. The common practice for government to consult with the American Medical Association (AMA) on health care legislation has often been presented as proof of the autonomy of American medicine. We can debate whether the interpretation is correct, but given that it is, American nursing has moved closer to that standard through the American Nurses Association's (ANA's) prominence on Capitol Hill.

Ashley's theory that economic exploitation is one factor that has retarded the development of autonomy in nursing is well taken. By the 1990s, nurses had realized some significant salary gains. Additionally, as is common in the rest of the population, many households were then and still are headed by a woman. This unique set of circumstances allows many women to make autonomous decisions about the use of their money. The success of fundraising by the ANA Political Action Committee (ANA-PAC) reflects these changing times.

There are other indicators of progress toward autonomy for nurses. Shared governance models that bring staff nurses and nursing service managers together to problem solve, peer review as a mechanism in retention and promotion, nursing staff organizations, the growing number of APNs with professional staff privileges in hospitals and other facilities, nurses as primary care providers in managed care systems, the growth in the number of community nursing centers, and significant gains in reimbursement and prescriptive authority are all benchmarks in the progress toward full autonomy. However, the term *full autonomy* may be misleading given the necessity for interdisciplinary management of care.

Most nurses do not identify with the issues of autonomy as they are played out on the state or national level. They are more concerned with their personal practice. Yet, nurses have gravitated toward roles that hold the promise of autonomy, although they may not call it that. In advanced practice this has usually been the APN, and for the staff nurse it has been primary nursing, or some variation of what we call primary nursing. Both of these roles are highly focused on the essential relationship between the client and the provider, yet both remain externally controlled. Autonomy for the NP hinges on reimbursement, prescriptive authority, clinical staff privileges, and recognition in managed care networks. Primary nursing's autonomy is contingent on how these qualities are played out given the presence of an administrative hierarchy.

Issues of professional autonomy may be particularly frustrating when the professional is an employee. The nature of these conflicts surfaced in a US Supreme Court decision in May 1994 (see Chapter 25). The decision places in question the distinction between those actions that an employed professional initiates as part of their autonomous practice in contrast to those that are initiated on behalf of the employer. The distinction is important and will be questioned more as professionals less frequently become entrepreneurs.

■ A LEADER AMONG LEADERS

Leadership is "every nurse's domain." In a contrary tone, Marriner reverts to the defeatist interpretation that nurses are overwhelmingly drawn from individuals low on self-esteem and initiative and higher on submissiveness and the need for structure than people in other occupations.[2] Malone observes that nursing is captivated by the allure of leadership and engages in a constant search for leaders, but is afraid of the essential relationship between leadership and power. It is this ambivalence about power that disempowers us.[3] Although this might have been true of past generations, current recruitment patterns offer hope of a better future. Nursing has become the preferred choice for more mature learners, often coming from an earlier work life that held a variety of leadership successes, and who feel secure in their abilities and comfortable with power. They expect state-of-the-art preparation for a challenging future that they are anxious to meet head on. Although this older, more experienced cohort of students contributes to the aging of nursing, they also have real potential for expanding our leadership corps.

In the ordinary course of events, leadership is often confused with management. In today's prevailing bureaucracy we are most usually over-managed and under-led. The dichotomy between nurse-executives and nurse-managers is a good point of reference (see Chapter 15). In many ways, the executive in that comparison was the leader, although a leader does not always have positional status. Managers focus on specific organizational goals and the tasks to accomplish those goals. The manager is assigned to a role. The leader has the interpersonal ability to cause people to respond because they want to (and sometimes at considerable personal cost and inconvenience). In the best of worlds, managers have leadership ability, but it is not guaranteed. Neither are leaders always managers.

Theories of leadership are numerous. Traditional theories emphasize control, competition, power wielding, and rationality, and imply a hierarchy. Most were developed using the scientific method, aiming to describe, understand, predict, and prescribe that elusive quality known as leadership. The comments on leadership theory presented here are very condensed and aim to whet the appetite for further reading about the topic.

Leadership is both a process and a property. As a process it is the strategic use of power to move others toward a shared vision. As a property it is a cluster of qualities that allow one person to successfully achieve with and through others. Followers are essential ingredients; without followers there are no leaders.[4] The formula for success requires a good fit between the people who will make things happen, the leader, and the circumstances that have brought them together (see Exhibit 16–1). There is considerable difference of opinion between traditionalists and contemporary theorists in how they see leadership. Once aspiring leaders were encouraged to select an approach most suitable to themselves and the situation at hand. Finding no clear direction for a suitable match, the option was to create an eclectic style, borrowing from a variety of orientations. If only it were that simple.

Leadership theories focus on who leaders are, what they do, and how they adapt to changing situations. Trait,

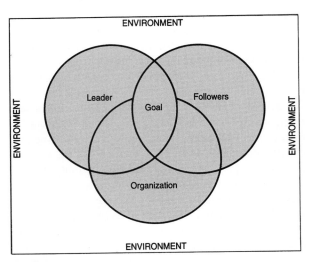

EXHIBIT 16–1. The Interplay of Forces in Leadership

behavioral, and contingency theories provide the general framework for the conventional knowledge about leadership, and variations on these themes provide additional perspectives.

- *The great man theory*: As old as Aristotle, this tells us that some are born to lead and others are born to be led. Confusion exists here over which traits are necessary to acquire leadership and which are needed to maintain it. Personality is not viewed as an integrated whole, and the impact of environmental and situational factors, including followers, is ignored. A better interpretation would be that one may be born to a position, but that does not guarantee that it could have ever been achieved or will be maintained.

- *Charismatic theory*: The ability to lead is dependent on an emotional commitment from followers. Followers feel secure in the presence of the leader, which is particularly helpful when sacrifices that could only be expected based on personal loyalties are asked of followers. Many of our most successful revolutionary leaders have been described as charismatic. Note that the allegiance is to a specific person. Removal of that person can often result in loss of progress, unless there has been a planned strategy to transfer leadership to a new personality.

- *Trait theory*: Personality studies abound. The traits of successful leaders closely approximate those observed in successful executives (see Chapter 15). They are described as endowed with vision, motivating followers to buy into that vision, sharing just enough of their vision to motivate people without overwhelming them, and distinguishing their relationships with humanism. They live with human respect and expect no less from their followers. Other traits associated with leadership include intelligence, emotional maturity, creativity and the ability to see novel solutions for problems, initiative, careful listening skills, the ability to derive meaning from even clouded communications, persuasiveness, good people judgment skills, and social adaptability.

- *Behaviorists*: Leaders have their styles, which place them on a continuum from bureaucratic to autocratic to participatory to consultative to democratic and finally laissez-faire. The distinguishing qualities are whether followers need to be motivated by internal or external forces and how much of a role followers actually have in decision making. The ultimate external locus of control is the bureaucrat who follows neither self nor followers, but defers to organizational policies. Laissez-faire does not assume that the followers are directionless, but that they need to be left alone to decide how to complete their own work.

- *Contingency theory*: This school of thought is situational and prescriptive. It involves a three-dimensional model that aims to create the best fit between leader–follower relations, the task at hand, and the resources or support that can be accessed by the leader owing to her or his position or status.

- *Path-goal theory*: The leader structures work for subordinates and removes obstacles so that they can be successful. Caring and consideration are added to the leadership prescription based on the needs of the group, one variation of contingency theory.

- *Life cycle theory*: The most appropriate leadership style is based on the maturity of the followers. With growing maturity there is less need for structure and a greater need for followers to assume an active role in the work at hand. The leader must be able to adjust to periods of regression if they should occur.

- *Dual factor theory*: A motivational theory that presents satisfaction and dissatisfaction not as direct opposites, but as separate entities. An increase in satisfaction is brought about by attention to humanistic aspects of leadership and results in greater cooperation and productivity. The removal of the dissatisfying elements does not necessarily result in satisfaction. These principles

have been widely applied to nursing during periods of shortage.

- *Transactional leadership*: Built on the principles of social exchange theory, where social interactions are expected to be a give and take of social, political, and psychological rewards. The leader defines the expectations, and interaction rarely moves to the point of shared values. The meaningfulness of the rewards keeps the exchange going and the process could break down if the leader misreads the followers. The goal is maintaining equilibrium or a steady state. There is a division of labor and competitiveness within the group. Control is centralized and a hierarchy develops.

Contemporary theories of leadership build on these traditional perspectives, but evolve into something new and different that better fits the tempo and values of life as it is at this point in time. The leader and followers are fused into a whole that is greater than the sum of its parts. The process is to break down old hierarchies and build commitment around a shared vision. The leader may facilitate and support, but only lead at the pleasure of the followers. Disequilibrium is not something to avoid but inevitable, and is sometimes the stimulus for action. Networking outside of the group is seen positively. Stability comes from human relationships. This represents the converse of earlier models, where the presumed instability was in the human relationships. A body of knowledge has begun to take shape around the dynamics of this *transformational leadership*. Earlier work, which was largely transactional, assumed that differences between leader and follower were sure to be an obstacle and demanded attention in planning and execution. In a transformational context, these concerns are not primary; rather, the goal is for the leader and the followers to evolve toward a shared agenda. All parties grow and develop through the process. History does not repeat itself, but patterns recur as cyclical events that challenge any leader to be self-sufficient. A comparison between transactional and transformational leadership qualities is found in Exhibit 16–2.

These transformational leadership qualities are applied in Senge's discussion of strategies that will allow organizations to survive and even thrive in our age of turbulence:

- *The whole is greater than the sum of its parts*: You cannot think of your work in isolation. Whereas earlier studies of leadership expected only the designated leader to be sensitive to external events, newer thinking expects that

■ **EXHIBIT 16–2.** Qualities of Transactional and Transformational Leadership

Quality	Transactional	Transformational
General orientation	Technical	Philosophical
Assumptions	Instability in human relations; stability in the environment and organization	Instability in the environment; stability in human relations and relative stability in the organization
Response to goal	Reactive	Proactive, visionary
Plan for action	Predetermined by the vision of the leader	Creation of shared vision
Prevailing focus	Content	Process
Roles	Division of labors	Group unified by goal; roles emerge over time and in response to work plan
Group dynamics	Competitive	Collaborative, catalytic
Emotions	Work to distance feelings	Accept and recognize feelings and work them through
Cognition	Rational, objective, strive to decrease complexity and ambiguity	Acknowledge complexity and ambiguity; value intuition
Decision making	Directive	Participative
Governance	Managerial	Self-governance
Human relations	Work to ensure stability	Assume and exploit stability
Leadership style	Command/control	Facilitate/protect/empower
Leadership goal	Team building	Integrate assets of the group
Distribution of power	Centralized	Decentralized
Structure	Hierarchy	Networking

all participants will have this broadened view. A good example is that hospitals presumably operate within a budget, and if nurses achieve significant salary increases, will it mean layoffs for other departments (and ultimately more work for nurses), cutbacks in supplies, or a bigger budget?

- *Look internally for solutions to problems:* It is more comfortable to blame our misfortunes on external circumstances or personalities. They are often beyond our control, so failure is less personal. From a position of strength, the first step in problem solving should be to straighten any of your own thinking or behavior that contributes to the problem. This whole scenario is actually a by-product of the tunnel vision described in the first characteristic. As we become too preoccupied with ourselves, we cease to appreciate that what we do has consequences beyond the boundaries of our system and will come back to haunt us. As we are exposed to this boomerang effect, it becomes uncomfortable to admit how we participated in our own problems.

- The voguish strategy is to become proactive or to *rise to address difficult issues* before we are faced with crisis management and forced into a reactive mode. All too often, we are still reacting, although at an earlier stage in the development of the issue. In other words, the illusion of taking charge is just that—an illusion. The best advice is to set aside labels and just plan to avoid a crisis; invest in early intervention.

- We are hampered by our preoccupation with events and short-term planning. Survival in today's environment of rapid change demands a *search for themes and the identification of patterns over time.* Dig under events for the real themes. Diagnostic related groups (DRGs), final directive requirements, and Peer Review Organizations (PROs) are each events that drew strong reactions from the health care community. Managing those issues diverted our attention from the more basic concerns: the need for cost reduction in acute care, the struggle of consumers to regain control of their choices in the health care system, and public suspicion of the industry and provider professionals.

- *We tend to adjust to a bad situation* and learn to live with it, focusing on the reality of the moment. The deep penetration of the Japanese into the US car market occurred over a period of many years. Seeing threats for what they are requires us to slow down, compare situations across time, and attempt to forecast.
- Given the rapid pace of change, it is *difficult or impossible today to learn from your mistakes*. Decisions made at one time and place will impact people and events in a distant time and place, often generations away. Consequences of many of our actions will be forever hidden from our eyes. The best hedge against doing harm is to ensure that leadership for the far-reaching issues is a blend of people from many perspectives. Examples of the application of this strategy can be seen in the Robert Wood Johnson Teaching Nursing Home Program of the 1980s and the later Pew Charitable Trust's project to strengthen hospital nursing.[5,6] In each of these instances, the active participation of the entire executive team from each funded site was required.
- The traditional concept of the *team is useless for today's problems*. Over time most teams invest more effort in maintaining their image of cohesiveness than participating in the process of change. Better suited to the times is a model where everyone has something to contribute and no proposal is dismissed. This is a decidedly transformational style. The role of the leader evolves into one of developing people, actually instigating openness and honesty, while removing the threat of reprisals. The leader often assumes the position of consultant on process and facilitator, as opposed to expert and controller. This is a very difficult role transition for those socialized into a traditional mode of leadership.[7]

Transformational leadership focuses on creating the social architecture to sustain a vision and the attitudes and behaviors that allow progress in these uncertain times. This brand of leadership builds on organizational trust first, because of the organization's likelihood of greater permanence, and then on leaders with positive self-regard and a capacity for humanism.

The trick is to bridge the gap between transactional and transformational leadership. The insights generated by the transactional school of thinking are not to be dismissed, but should be enhanced by new assumptions and ways of operating. The autocratic, democratic, and laissez-faire styles of management (often equated with leadership) are naive. Rather, as an intermediate step in the transition, the literature supports directive, collaborative, and collegial leadership patterns, each selected to suit the mix of individuals and the challenge at hand. Nurses will be expected to lead as they manage their practice and the care of each patient. Broader leadership challenges will find nurses as leaders among leaders. The collegial style is proposed as the natural complement for leadership among peers, such as peer review, shared governance, self-directed work teams, and co-leadership choices. In this context, leadership is relative and functional only once it is legitimized by the group. In other words, the claim to leadership must be achieved. Collegial leaders are catalytic, not merely consultative. They do not build teams but integrate the assets of the group. Although the buck does stop somewhere, leadership is shared, as is the responsibility and recognition for success. Communication is authentic and multidimensional, with emphasis on the content and the manner in which it is received rather than the form. Supervision and motivational techniques are nonexistent because these qualities reside in the individual. Shared vision, responsibility, and accountability are more than rhetoric and prompted the federal government to design a pay-for-performance merit system that would properly recognize contributions of individuals working as a group, it being impossible to distinguish the efforts of any one person from another.

Despite any transformations or miracles, the leader still stands out and fulfills some useful role. One such role admittedly smacking of paternalism, but real and valued by followers, is that of buffer or protector. Leaders may advocate for their followers, protecting them from external forces, the organization, other members of the group, fellow employees, medical staff, top administration, and even one another. Buffering may take the form of more closely coordinating work and being clearer on the unity of command (orders come from one person and only one person unless specifically instructed otherwise). Other situations may require conflict resolution, confrontation, or negotiation.

During the late 1970s and 1980s, there were a series of studies of leadership in nursing that used an inductive or case study approach. In chronological order the investigators or authors were Safier, Vance, Kinsey, and Schorr and Zimmerman.[8,9] Each of the influentials studied demonstrated their leadership acumen. In their self-evaluation, they ranked the following qualities as most important to their success (in the order presented):

- Communication skills
- Intellectual ability

- Willingness to take risks
- Interpersonal skills
- Creativity
- Ability to mobilize people
- Recognition in the profession
- Charisma

An unremarkable and highly predictable list. However, there is one remarkable observation that comes from these biographers. In other professions, leaders are as likely to be drawn from the ranks of practitioners (those who directly do the work of the field) as from individuals who maintain a career identification but do not practice their profession directly (positional leaders), such as teachers, researchers, and administrators. This was not true for nursing in these studies, where most influentials were positional leaders, as opposed to clinicians.

Much is written, in these studies and elsewhere, about the price of leadership: the loneliness at the top, for instance. It has been said that a good leader must get over the need to be loved and learn to function without the need for the approval of others. No leader can please all of his or her constituents all the time. To lead inevitably requires commitment; at times the leader must sacrifice personal desires, interests, and time. The rewards, of course, are to meet goals that one believes in and to know that this might not have happened without your leadership.

■ ASPECTS OF POWER

Autonomy and opportunities for leadership do not come to the spineless, powerless, indifferent, or downtrodden, or those who think they are. As members of a profession who are obliged not only to participate in change, but also to provide the leadership to make things happen, an understanding of the dynamics of power is essential.

Power is the ability to influence the behavior of others to produce certain intended effects. Power can be actual or potential (indicating power as latent or undeveloped, but still a force to be reckoned with). Power can be directly applied to the point where effect is desired, or indirect so that the nature or source of the power is more discreet or even undetected. Power can be a means to an end, or even an end in itself (the existence of latent power can sometimes achieve the desired results). Power varies in quantity, scope, legitimacy, its degree of humanism (benevolent versus destructive), and whether it is situationally unilateral or bilateral.

Power is usually seen as a social relationship. It is given, maintained, or lost within those relationships. Individuals

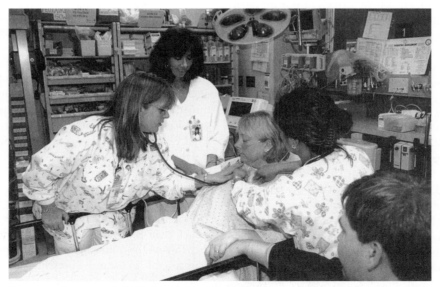

The power for nurses is in their practice, which allows them to make a rich contribution to interdisciplinary patient care. (Courtesy of Hackensack University Medical Center, Hackensack, New Jersey)

derive power from certain sources or bases and then use that power according to their personal power orientation. This orientation indicates how an individual perceives or values power. Is power an essential part of one's identity, even if it is never used constructively? "He could do so much good if he only wanted to." Is power interpreted as an exclusive possession, something that is not shared? "You never quite feel that she is telling you everything."

A typology of power bases (where your power comes from) deriving from the work of many authors follows:

- *Coercive power*: Real or perceived fear of one person by another
- *Reward power*: Perception of the potential for rewards or favors by honoring the wishes of a powerful person
- *Legitimate power*: Power that derives from an organizational position rather than personal qualities (authority)
- *Expert power*: Knowledge, special talents, or skills held by a person
- *Referent power*: Power flowing from admiration, or charisma, usually rooted in similar backgrounds or some other mutual identification
- *Information power*: Exclusive access to information needed by others
- *Connection power*: Privileged connections with powerful individuals or organizations
- *Collective power*: The ability to mobilize a critical mass or a system on your behalf

It is well to emphasize that power is given. Further, we often infer that people who claim to have power actually do, but when studied more carefully, they have no claim or legitimacy. Additionally, power invariably fills any vacuum. People generally want peace and order. In situations of stress or chaos, someone will come forward and be given or take the power to restore order.

Observing the power base of individuals in combination with their power orientation allows a prediction on how they will function and can even provide you with a model to identify your own capacity and style. Power orientations (how you use your power) can be exclusive to one of the following or in a combination of several:

- *Good*: Power as natural and desirable and used in an open and honest manner; would probably build on expert, reward, and legitimate power bases
- *Resource dependent*: Power depending on possession of things, including information, property, and wealth; associated with withholding patterns in the information power base; greatly diminished in a computer age and the growing presence of transformational leadership
- *Instinctive drive*: Power as a personality attribute, usually associated with referent power
- *Charismatic*: Influence over people through personal magnetism; power often given to people who are ill prepared or even destructive, and could stifle the growth of those who do the giving
- *Political*: Drawing heavily on referent, connection, and collective bases, power is linked to an ability to negotiate the system
- *Control and autonomy*: The power broker always calls the shots operating from a base of coercion, information, and connection

Power and *influence* are sometimes equated, because both affect or change the behavior of others; however, when they are separated, it is on the theory that power is the potential that must be tapped and converted to the dynamic thrust of influence. Almost all authorities agree that a person or group must be valued on some level to have either power or influence, again reinforcing the interpersonal dimension of the concept.

Maraldo claims that "power to influence others requires a high level of skill in the strategic manipulation of impressions toward others. . . . Seekers of power who are skilled at cajoling, flattering, comforting, hedging, exhorting, exploiting, and exciting colleagues and higher-ups alike have an emporium of all the instruments they need to influence others."[10] She adds that manipulation is not always bad and gives an example of how a lobbyist successfully manipulated someone who would not listen to her by having a number of people that person respected and liked (because of their power, position, or other characteristics) show support for the worthwhile project the lobbyist was promoting. Maraldo also noted that powerful persons have some of the same pain over failure and rejection, the same fears and inadequacies as others, but never let it show. They always appear to be in command of the situation, even when they are quivering inside.[11]

Does nursing have power? Considering the things we have discussed, it is clear that nursing has the potential for power with its overwhelming numbers, its special knowledge and skill, and its place in public trust and has, in fact, already exercised that power successfully. Nursing leaders also have power of various kinds, including positional power in high government policy-making positions. But what of nurses as individuals? They are still complaining of lack of power on the job—the lack of autonomy and involvement in budget setting and in policy making. Yet nurses do not seem to reach out to fill any vacuum, mobilize their constituency, or capitalize on their position at the center of health care information networks. Is it a historical pattern of obedience to authority, which has been transmitted by education and practice? Is it their social, cultural, or economic background? Is it because, according to personality tests, nurses have a low power motive? Is it that they think they do not have what it takes to be powerful and influential—for whatever reason? Groups or individuals choose to remain uninvolved for a number of reasons: habit, fear of sanctions, moral obligation, self-interest, psychological identification with someone in charge, indifference, and lack of self-confidence. No doubt there are nurses who fall into one or more of these categories.

However, those who maintain that lack of self-confidence is the root cause for nurses' apparent lack of interest in gaining power should remember that "both the powerful and the powerless tend to take existing social systems for granted and rarely recognize that it is not talent, but rather laws, customs, policies, and institutions that, in reality, keep the powerless . . . powerless."

■ PARTICIPATING IN CHANGE

Early in the chapter we established the expectation that professionals have a responsibility to change with the times as stewards to the public. Their practice must change, as must the organizational systems that support their practice. Further, in the process of caring, patients must be helped to adjust to change or change so that they can adjust. The magnitude of change is often measured by the size of the system involved. Whether it is changing the health care practices of the newly diagnosed diabetic, or the body image of the traumatic amputee, a transition from team to primary nursing, or the decentralization of all management decisions to the unit level, the theoretical constructs and strategies are much the same.

Change is any significant departure from the status quo. Change may be planned or accidental. *Planned change* is a deliberate, conscious effort intended to improve a situation and facilitate acceptance of that improvement by the parties involved. In comparison, *accidental change* is that minor shift that occurs to maintain balance between a system and its environment. In his classic work on change, Watzlawick and associates describe *first- and second-order change*. In first-order change, change occurs but the original system remains unaltered; in second-order change, the system itself changes. The difference here is one of accommodation versus assimilation.[12] An example might be a project to increase nurse–physician collaboration, established with all the components of joint practice, integrated patient records, comprehensive critical paths, and multidisciplinary patient conferences, yet nurse–physician relations remain unchanged. If the supportive systems are held in place long enough, will assimilation or second-order change occur?

Lewin's theory of change is probably the basis for the adaptations of most other theorists. He identifies three basic stages: *unfreezing*, in which the motivation to create change occurs; *moving* (the actual changing) when new responses are developed based on collected information; and *refreezing*, in which the new changes are integrated and stabilized. Hence, Lewin's model illustrates the effects of forces that either promote or inhibit change. Specifically, driving forces promote change while restraining forces oppose change. Change will occur when the combined strength of one force is greater than the combined strength of the opposing set of forces. A further notion is that in all changes there are driving forces that facilitate action and restraining forces that impede it. Each must be identified—the first so that they can be capitalized on, and the second so that they can be avoided or modified.

Lippitt, Watson, and Westley extend Lewin's Three-Step Change Theory. Lippitt, Watson, and Westley created a seven-step theory that focuses more on the role and responsibility of the change agent than on the evolution of the change itself. Information is continuously exchanged throughout the process. The seven steps are as follows:

1. Diagnose the problem.
2. Assess the motivation and capacity for change.
3. Assess the resources and motivation of the change agent. This includes the change agent's commitment to change, power, and stamina.
4. Define progressive stages of change.
5. Ensure that the roles and responsibilities of change agents are clear and understood. Examples of roles include the motivator, facilitator, and subject matter expert.

6. Maintain the change through communication, feedback, and group coordination.

7. Gradually remove the change agents from relationship, as the change becomes part of the organizational culture.[13]

The change agent should gradually withdraw from her or his role over time. This will occur when the change becomes part of the organizational culture or the client's self-care system. Lippitt, Watson, and Westley point out that changes are more likely to be stable if they spread to neighboring systems or to subparts of the system immediately affected.[14]

Changes are better rooted. Three examples are the individual meets other problems in a similar way, several organizational units adopt the same innovation, or the problem is encountered in the care of several patients. The more widespread imitation becomes, the more the behavior is regarded as a permanent solution. Lippitt's theory includes seven phases within Lewin's stages—a delineation that is useful in thinking through action follows.

Unfreezing

- Identification of the problem
- Assessment of the motivation and capacity for change
- Assessment of the change agent's motivation and resources

Moving

- Development of progressive change objectives
- Identification of appropriate role for the change agent

Refreezing

- Maintenance of the change once it has been started
- Termination of a helping relationship

A useful nursing-oriented approach based on Lewin/Lippitt's model is summarized as follows:

1. Identification of a need for and verification of the desire for the change
2. Development of a change relationship between the agent and the client system
3. Clarification of the client's problem, need, or objective
4. Examination of alternative routes and tentative goals and intentions of actions

5. Transformation of intentions into actual change behavior
6. Stabilization
7. Termination of the relationship between the change agent and the client system

The Lewin and Lippitt models paint a very simplistic picture of the change process. On the contrary, even the most adventuresome participants have trepidation because human nature fears the unknown. The test will be in the day-to-day arduous implementation process. A review of the numerous change strategies and tactics reported in the literature urges the following conditions to make change more acceptable:

- Ensure that the need for change is justified, even if there is not agreement. This requires total honesty, exquisite communication, and sensitivity to the cues that you have heard. Change for the sake of change is never justified.
- Try to safeguard the future security of those who are involved in change.
- Diffuse anxiety by having those involved create the vision for change.
- It is helpful to work from a previously established set of impersonal principles.
- Change is best received when it follows other successes rather than failures.
- It is better to space events so that prior change is assimilated before the system is asked to accommodate another.
- People new to the organization react more comfortably to change than people with longevity in the system targeted for change (vested interest).
- Try to guarantee that there will be personal benefits to those who participate. Things should be better, not worse, after the change.
- Establish a venturesome environment by making change and improvement a priority.
- Choose the change agent with psychological sensitivity to serve as a bridge to other participants.
- Focus attention on the future, not the past.
- Allow for failure, treating it as a growth experience. Nothing is forever; be open to more change if there is justification. Be ready to compromise during planning and development once everyone is clear on the bottom line.
- Provide assurance of administrative support and freedom to act without the constant need for approvals.

- Encourage open expression of concerns.
- Never withhold information; be sure people see the big picture and know what they are doing.

Conflict of some kind is probably inevitable. It is important that the change agent develop effective methods of dealing with conflict. Action, rather than reaction, is the better course, but it should be recognized that the emotions associated with change must be dealt with. If not all participants are won over, the decision must be made to stop or go ahead, trying to anticipate the negative aspects of what may become covert resistance if the resister is outvoted. Just how a nurse handles resistance may be a matter of individual style and the particular situation.

Because of their central position in systems of care, and their large numbers, nurses often find themselves in the role of change agent. The *change agent* guides the change project. The extent to which the change agent is the architect of the process is determined by the strategic approach to change. The manner in which the change agent participates can also vary, but the concept of the role is to provide a catalyst that will disengage from the project after change is complete and transfer continuing aspects of the role to individuals internal to the changed system. Ignoring this need for transition may cause the loss of much that has been accomplished.

The skills necessary to participate in change and even initiate change projects are an integral part of the curriculum for entry into professional practice. The role of change agent is more demanding. Although it may require more highly developed skills or experience, it is a role that can be legitimately and effectively assumed by a nurse at an early stage of career development.

Whether working as an insider or outsider (each of which has advantages and disadvantages), knowing the process of change, planning carefully and thoroughly, and acting strategically and with an appropriate sense of timing are essential. Because a change agent is a leader in that instance, the leadership role must be assumed and the individual usually must start out by selling her- or himself first before the idea for change is seen as acceptable for consideration.

■ RELATED STRATEGIES AND RELATIONSHIPS

Nursing does have influence and power. This is particularly evident in areas of politics and public policy. It is also evident in the increased status of nursing and in the expansion of nursing practice to every conceivable setting. Hand-wringing is not in order. It is probably a healthy sign that so many nurses are saying, "But compared to what we can do and should do, it is not enough," and they are right. The major problems within nursing have been caused by the lack of cohesiveness; the lack of agreement on professional goals; the lack of planned leadership development; the heterogeneity of nurses in background, education, and position; the lack of internal support systems; and the divisiveness of nursing subcultures, all coping with a rapidly changing society. If nursing is to have the full autonomy of a profession, there must be unification of purpose and action on major issues. Leadership is vital, but it must be a transformational leadership, focusing on shared power directed at accomplishing the profession's goals. Those goals must be agreed on jointly. Although nurse leaders may indeed influence them, the feedback from the grass roots must be a part of the final decision, or achievement of the goals will continue to be an uphill struggle. Therefore, the strategies and relationships that are discussed in the following section are the responsibility not just of nursing leaders, but also of all nurses.

Mentors, Networks, Collegiality: The Great Potential

The term *mentoring* is usually defined as a formal or informal relationship between an established older person and a younger one, wherein the older guides, counsels, and critiques the younger, teaching him or her (the *protégé*) survival and advancement in a particular field. Mentoring is part of a patron system, a continuum of advisory support relationships that facilitate access to positions of leadership, authority, or power. When individuals function literally as patrons, they assume the roles of protector, benefactor, sponsor, champion, advocate, supporter, and/or adviser.

At the far end of the continuum is the *mentor*, the most powerful, most influential individual, and the relationship with the protégé is the most intense (and perhaps the most stressful). Next is the *sponsor*—a strong patron, but less powerful than a mentor in shaping or promoting the protégé's career. The *guide* is next, less able than either of the other two to serve as benefactor or champion, but capable of providing invaluable intelligence and explaining the system, the shortcuts, and the pitfalls.

At the beginning of the continuum are the *peer pals*, peers who help each other to succeed and progress. This first step is highly important, more like the concept of people helping people, more egalitarian, less intense and exclusionary, and therefore more democratic, by allowing access to a large number of young professionals. It is the mentor relationship, restrictive though it might be, that gives the biggest career boost, whereas the peer-pal relationship is often a bootstrap operation. However, mentorships are not democratic. Selection may be very idiosyncratic, as described later, and there are always strings attached—if nothing else, the demand to succeed.

Peer pals can create their own new order networks. There is a male corollary (not exclusively male, but the example makes sense)—the good-old-boy networks that, through an informal system of relationships, provide advice, information, guidance, contact, protection, and any other support that helps a member of the group, an insider, to achieve his goals, goals obviously not in conflict with those of the group. The "good old boys" frequently share the same educational, cultural, or geographic background, but whatever the basis of their commonalities, mutual support is the name of the game. It could be group pressure; it could be a word to the right person at the right time; it could be simply multifaceted information sources, but it exists. You can count on it; you can take risks; you will not be alone. (You do not necessarily have to like each other or agree on everything.) Could this work for nurses? It already does among those who share certain common backgrounds. It would be a good project to identify some of these networks and search for evidence to either verify or disprove their usefulness.

Suppose more systems of support could be established in nursing. Not a good-old-nurse network—no need to duplicate the nearsightedness of the men in their narrow system that so frequently excludes women—but a good-nurse network that promotes the support of nurses for nurses, men or women. A network provides backup for the risk takers until all can become risk takers for a purpose. A network that shows unified strength on issues that can be generally agreed on, so that the profession as well as the individual practitioner can put into practice the principles of care to which both voice commitment. A network that avoids destructive self-competition and instead develops new leaders at all levels through peer pals, mentors, and role models. A network that encourages differences of opinion, but provides an atmosphere for reasonable compromise. In essence, a network that develops and utilizes the essential abilities of nurses to share, to trust, and to depend on one another.

Because networking is "in" and is sometimes seen as a quick fix for moving up, and because it is also new to many, it is being abused by some. Networkers are advised to observe both common and uncommon courtesies: do not make excessive requests; be appreciative; be sensitive to your contacts' situation; and be helpful to others.

Of the nurse networks already in operation, many have been initiated by a nursing organization or subgroup made up of nurses with common interests, clinical or otherwise. The participants help each other to make contacts when they relocate, or they supply needed information or suggest someone else who would know. They alert each other to job opportunities and suggest their colleagues for appointments, presentations, or awards. They give visibility to nurses, boost each other, and praise each other, instead of being unnecessarily critical. But they also critique supportively for professional growth.

Could this also be called collegiality? In a sense. A *colleague* is usually defined as an associate, particularly in a profession. Yet, beyond this basic phrase, the term is rich in meaning. In a thesaurus, we also find ally, aide, collaborator, helper, partner, peer, friend, cooperator, coworker, cohelper, fellow worker, teammate, or even right-hand man (or woman) and buddy. The implications are even richer. Colleagues may be called on confidently for advice and assistance, and will give it. Colleagues share knowledge with each other, together rounding out the necessary information to enhance patient care. Colleagues challenge each other to think in new ways and try new ideas. Colleagues encourage risk taking when the situation requires daring. Colleagues provide a support system when the risk taker needs it. Colleagues are equal, yet different—that is, they may have varying educational preparation, experience, and positions, perhaps even belong to another profession, but when they work together for a particular purpose, that work is bettered by their cooperation. To take it a step further, a collegium may be formed—a group in which each member has approximately equal power. Clearly, nurse colleagues are part of a nurse network. But developing that spirit of collegiality requires trust, and the trust must be mutually deserved. Then it can also extend beyond the borders of nursing to include other health professionals.

Returning to the patron system, neither the guide nor the sponsor has been given much attention in the literature, perhaps because of semantics. *Sponsor* is often used interchangeably with *mentor*, and both terms often refer to a relationship that is more at the guide level. For instance, reference is often made to neophytes who are being mentored, when actually those individuals are simply assigned to more experienced people for guidance.

Mentors are never assigned; they choose. In most situations, the level of participation is more at the guide level, perhaps progressing to sponsor if a suitable relationship is established. However, most of these senior persons are never mentors; they simply are not powerful enough, and in the time given and considering the number of "protégés" involved, they probably do not have the interest or commitment to be mentors. Nevertheless, there are mentors who participate in a very intense and deliberate relationship and who have a great impact on their protégés' careers.

Mentorship demands a high degree of involvement between a novice in a discipline and a person knowledgeable and wise in that area. On a cognitive level, the mentor is involved with the novice as a whole person. The mentor–protégé relationship is a "serious, mutual, non-sexual, loving relationship" voluntary on the part of both. The lack of a protégé is a developmental handicap. Mentoring is part of what Erickson calls *generativity*, in which the primary concern is establishing and guiding the next generation. A mentor acts as

- *Teacher* to enhance the young person's skills and intellectual development
- *Sponsor* to ease the neophyte's entry and advancement into the workaday world
- *Host and guide* to welcome the initiate into a new occupational and social world with its unique values, customs, resources, and cast of characters
- *Exemplar* to serve as a personal example of virtues, achievements, and ways of life
- *Counselor* to provide advice and moral support
- Most important, the mentor is given the opportunity to leave a legacy in the form of his or her protégé

A mentor supports a younger adult's dreams and helps him or her make them a reality, and is a protector and supporter who provides the extra confidence needed to take on new responsibilities, new tests of competence, and new positions. (Emphasis on competence is of paramount importance; the mentor teaches, supports, advises, and criticizes.) Sometimes the mentor is equated with a role model, preceptor, or the master in a master–apprentice situation, but it is more than that. In other words, the protégé must show that she or he is someone worth investing in, someone who will show a measure of return by success in the field. And the obligation of the protégé goes further

than that. The protégé often becomes the one to catch the mentor as his or her own days of power and status decline.

Mentors may be or have been role models or preceptors, but role models and preceptors are not necessarily mentors. A *role model* can be just that—someone to emulate and admire, even with minimal contact. It is really a passive process. Some preceptorships are carried out with almost total impersonality; *preceptors* may overtly carry out their responsibilities to their students and yet withhold a vital element of role development. Role models, too, have been known to have a negative impact on new graduates, as when they socialize them into a bureaucratic orientation.

Because of the time and effort mentors put forth for their protégés (usually for one at a time), protégés are carefully selected. And they are selected. True, someone who wants another for a mentor can bring him- or herself to that person's attention, but the protégé must be seen as worthy. One group of executives cited certain qualities that they looked for in potential protégés: has depth, integrity, a curious mind, good interpersonal skills; wants to impress; has an extra dose of commitment; has a capacity to care; can communicate; understands ideas; can identify problems and help find solutions; is ambitious, hard working, and willing to do things beyond the call of duty; someone looking for new avenues and new challenges; someone dedicated to a purpose; and always someone who would be a good representative of the profession. Usually the individual is also expected to be well groomed and appropriately dressed. Of utmost importance, the chemistry has to be right between the mentor and the protégé.

There is no question that, although protégés get plenty of help, they are expected to produce, to be worth the mentor's time, and to make him or her proud. The mentor's rewards are many—seeing someone's potential fulfilled, acquiring a following, and preparing leaders for the profession. There are dangers to both. The mentor can be overwhelming and try to mold the protégé in his or her image or the protégé can become too dependent. On the other hand, the protégé can take over the mentor's position; this is one reason that the relationship often ends on a bad note, usually in business. Protégés do outgrow mentors and may move on to another mentor or become mentors themselves. It also happens that a person may be mentor to one person and also give attention to another, although not as intensely.

There is now much literature on mentoring, particularly in business and education and in research studies. Although almost everyone says that being mentored is a key to success, others disagree. After all, there are not enough true mentors for every ambitious person, and yet many succeed with no mentor at all. There is not yet enough research on mentoring to answer all the questions raised. However, almost everyone had help from someone along the way, and everyone can find someone to be helped by and later someone to help, somewhere along the continuum of the patron system.

Interest in mentoring in nursing has been rising in terms of preparation for scholarliness, development of minority nurses, and leadership in general. In relation to the last item, it is particularly important to note several pieces of extensive research, all of which point to the importance of mentors in the development of today's nursing leaders.

In Vance's study, 83 percent of the leaders reported having had mentors and 93 percent were mentors to others.[15] In Kinsey's replication, the percentages were about the same. In both studies, the mentors were primarily female nurse educators (teachers) or teacher colleagues, advisers, and educational administrators. They, in turn, tended to mentor students and professional colleagues. All cited the importance of mentoring in their success. A more extensive nursing study of 500 female graduates of doctoral programs also showed the effect of mentoring.[16] Those mentored attributed much of their development to their mentors, and those not mentored often cited the deprivation. Those mentored were slightly more productive and satisfied with their work and with nursing as a career than the others. Many other details on mentoring are given in this in-depth study. One interesting point is that with the exception of a very few, the mentors and protégés parted amicably and are now friends.

It is generally agreed that mentoring can help develop nurses who can rise to the future's challenges. The commitment of today's nursing leaders to be those mentors is essential.

Risk Taking and Role Breaking

Nurses have had to bear up under the constant insult that they are deferential, retiring, prone to suffer in silence, and so on. Their seeming lack of progress toward autonomy has been blamed on internal discord over basic issues. In fact, solidarity has not been so rare. Those who wish to condemn nurses often do so for their own purposes. The speed with which the nursing community can mobilize its critical mass has become evident in a host of recent attacks chronicled elsewhere in this text (unlicensed assistant personnel, shortage, wage and salary issues, workplace safety). The fact that only 12 to 15 percent of registered nurses (RNs) belong to a state constituent of ANA is regrettable, but networks have been put in place to reach almost 75 percent of the RNs in the United States through the state nurses' associations and specialty nursing organizations. These networks penetrate to the grass roots and have put petty differences aside in favor of winning for the profession and its future generations.

The risk takers and role breakers are there for nursing. It is no wonder, given nursing's courageous past. The profession has its roots in the early, uncharted territory of community health and in the holism of the social welfare movement. That pioneering spirit was temporarily chilled as cure, hospitals, high-tech, and their association with medicine began to dominate. Nurses did not lose their vision but were distracted until leaders and issues surfaced to remind them of the reason they chose nursing.

Nurses have everything it takes for successful risk taking: the issues, the consumer appeal, and the strategic position. When considering risks, incorporate a healthy dose of foresight:

- Carefully observe patterns over time.
- Be cautious not to waste effort responding to isolated situations.
- Realize that your actions may affect many others unrelated to your target group.
- Try to anticipate the eventual consequences of your actions, even though they may be beyond your time and place; you have some responsibility.
- You deserve no credit for adjusting to an intolerable situation.
- First try to identify how you contribute to your own problems; it is easier to readjust your own behavior than someone else's.
- Allow all those potentially affected to participate in problem solving; once you begin to think you have an edge on wisdom, you are doomed.
- Educate your constituency (or yourself) that today's changes are only interim steps toward a grander vision, and that today's wins may have to be purposely undone later.

Nurses have been criticized because many RNs seem to have a tenuous commitment to a field that demands professional intensity. Nursing is no different from other disciplines.

Regardless of the rigor of preparation, each field has those who see the work as an interlude in their lives, draw firm lines between work time and private time, and care very little about the politics of the discipline. In fact, most RNs continue to nurse for a lifetime, moving in and out of full- and part-time status. Conversely, all RNs may not be professionals in the classic sense of the term, setting aside the educational distinctions that have fueled internal warfare for generations. Chapter 9 alerted us to the changing nature of professionalism. There is no doubt about the basically decent and proud work we do as nurses; we believe it and so does the public. Proceed with caution in risk taking and role breaking. The times will take care of some of the reshuffling.

Political Action

Politics may be defined as the art or science of influencing policy. There is a legitimate tendency to think of politics in the context of government, but affecting policy and operations at the institutional level is often just as important in the work life of a nurse. The term *in-house law* has been used to describe the power nurses can have if they can participate in establishing policies and procedures that affect daily practice.

It is vital that nurses participate actively in the agencies or community groups where decisions are being made, such as local or state planning agencies. The strategy used to gain input may vary. A basic principle is applicable: Before, during, and after gaining entrée, nurses must show that they are knowledgeable, have something to offer, and can put it all together into an action package. There are many places to start, because most community groups are looking for members who work and are willing to hold office (e.g., church groups, societies, and parent–teacher associations). These activities may be seen as (1) a way of gaining experience on boards, using parliamentary procedure to advantage, politicking, and gaining some sophistication in participating and guiding decisions and (2) being visible to other groups and the public. Many community groups interlock, and, by being active in some, nurses come in contact with others. It also helps to gain support of women and men other than nurses. But participating nurses must be capable; there is nothing worse than having an incompetent as the first nurse on a major board or committee. At this stage of nurses' reach for influence, it could do the profession more damage than having a non-nurse; it appears that newcomers still have to be better than those already in power to gain initial respect.

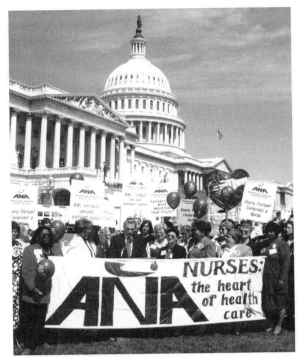

Nurses are exceptionally effective political reformers. Here nurses demonstrate for patient safety on the grounds of the U.S. Capitol. (Courtesy of the American Nurses Association, MATTOX Commercial Photography)

Another aspect to consider and use is the potential economic power of nurses. A nurse executive who controls a multimillion-dollar budget can wield power in how that money is spent. Nurses who have major responsibility for patient care but no budget control can transform their pivotal role in consumer satisfaction into economic power. But this transformation takes effort and motivation.

Community nurses are particularly good resources, because most make strong community contacts. Today, the participation of the consumer in health care decisions is increasing. An activated consumer who supports nursing can impact local decision making as well as on state and national legislation. A legislator is more inclined to hear the consumer who presumably is a neutral participant, as opposed to an obvious interest group. But nursing must sell that consumer the profession's point of view and balance consumer needs and nursing goals.

Although it is often through the influence of consumer groups and the community's traditional power figures that nurses get on decision-making committees, boards, and similar groups, after that they are on their own and must be prepared, perceptive, articulate, and under control. In meetings and at coffee breaks, the politicking and the formation of coalitions may well determine which way a decision goes. Nurses who have not learned to play that game had better take lessons and use role-play, assertiveness training, group therapy, group process, or speech lessons—whatever is necessary.

On the level of governmental politics, nurses can influence and have influenced not only such issues as Social Security, quality assurance, patient rights, care of the long-term patient, and Medicare, but have a vital interest in such issues as reimbursement for nursing services, nurse licensure, use of technology, children's services, funds for nursing education, and workplace safety. The specifics of the legislative process and guidelines for action are described in Chapter 18. Nurses should be encouraged to run for public office. They are intelligent, well educated, and know a lot about human relations. Those holding state offices are not only effective, but also often offer extraordinary insight into health issues. Some have been responsible for major legislative breakthroughs for nursing and health care. This is equally true of the dynamic group in regulatory agencies and congressional offices. These influentials always point out the importance of nurse involvement in health policy formation.

Regardless of the setting, there are some basic guidelines for effective political action. The first guideline is to know the social and technical aspects of professional practice; second, to know the current professional issues and the implications for various alternative actions; third, to be aware of emerging social and political issues and trends that will affect health care and nursing; fourth, to learn others' points of view (those of potential supporters or opponents) and come to terms with what policy changes are possible as well as desirable; and fifth, to seek allies who can espouse or at least see the desirability of a particular course of action.

Feminism and Sexist Stereotyping

When it is asked why nurses, with so much potential influence, do not seem to be able or willing to use it, the point is often made that nursing is still overwhelmingly a woman's profession, and, even with changing legislation and attitudes, women as a whole are still subject to discrimination and harassment and still are often victims of female socialization (see Chapter 6).

For many years, most female nurses looked at nursing as a useful way to earn a living until they were married and a job to which they could return if circumstances required. Most nurses did marry and most married nurses did drop out to raise families, working only part time, if at all. Unmarried female and male nurses were more inclined to stay in nursing; however, women, unlike men, frequently did not plot an orderly path to positions of authority and influence. This is similar to the career patterns of other women. In business, most women have traditionally been in their 30s or 40s before they realized that they either wanted to or would be forced to continue working, and by then they were often frozen in dead-end, low-prestige (however productive) jobs. When they decided to compete for power positions in management, they were up against an old-boy network that prevented or deterred their progress. Moreover, they had to overcome their own reluctance to be aggressive and reject traditional female social goals. This is changing, but progress is slow and tedious and limited to the few, rather than characteristic of the many.

Nurses have tended to move into the administrative hierarchy more through default than intent, perhaps gathering credentials on the way. But until the last few decades, relatively few had attained power outside nursing, either as recognized expert practitioners within a practice setting or as representatives of nursing in health policy determination.

Has the women's movement had an impact on this situation? As noted in Chapter 6, despite many obstacles still in the path of women on the way up (and even of those who are not interested in this path) the women's movement has had a tremendous influence in improving many aspects of women's lives. Yet, nurses have had an uneasy relationship with feminists as a group, in part because many feminists have incorrect knowledge about nursing and were more interested early on in encouraging women to move into the powerful male bastions of law, medicine, and business. On the other hand, many of the issues concerning nurses, such as comparable worth and child care, are also feminist issues.

Feminism can be defined as a world view that values women and confronts systematic injustices based on gender. There are a number of feminist theories and ideologies, but none are anti-male; they are simply opposed to the male-defined systems and ideologies that oppress women. Feminists point out that, even now, women believe that they must choose between the male-defined feminine role and the more interesting male role. Overall, they feel that nursing, with its largely female component, follows oppressed group behavior and also tries to emulate what they see as powerful, that is, male.

Nursing tends to identify with the oppressor (administration? medicine?) and is sometimes self-aggressive. An example of this self-aggression is given in relation to the long-standing entry-into-practice battle. Debate is largely taking place on the professional organization level, to which most nurses do not belong, ignoring the fears of those without a baccalaureate and the means or motivation to get one. The fact that nurses blame themselves and each other for failure to solve the complex dilemmas of the profession is seen as another form of antifeminist self-aggression.

One danger in feminism is the temptation to adopt an anti-male attitude, for which some feminists are judged guilty. Although men in nursing may not suffer gender discrimination as such from other men, they do from some female nurses. In certain instances they may even suffer wage discrimination. There are reports that the salaries of some male nurse executives, for instance, are not comparable to those of other men with equal status and responsibilities in the same institution. Being a nurse counts for less than being a male. If nursing is to become stronger, both men and women in the field need to work together toward that common cause.

The winds of change blow constantly. As we enter the new century, there is a decided change in the feminist perspective. Feminists today choose a more low-key and gentler approach to their issues. They emphasize the differences between men and women as opposed to their similarities. This shift in ideology comes on the scene as nursing is more influenced to define its own uniqueness as caring. The works of Watson and Benner have already been noted. The emergent *soft feminism* is comfortable and persuasive to nursing. You could well see these constituencies converge on the issue of women's health.

Physician–Nurse Relationships

Physician–nurse relationships are a large, if not major, factor in nurse autonomy and deserve special consideration. (A variety of issues and incidents on this topic are included elsewhere in the text.) There is necessarily a fine line between overstating and understating the problems, or, as some would have it, between paranoia and servility. Physicians' recognition of nurses as coprofessionals and colleagues has been present almost since the beginning of nursing, but a hard core of physicians who see and prefer a nurse hand-maiden role, although less common than even a decade ago, still exists. Some individual physicians and, to some extent, a part of organized medicine seem to have limited, stereotypic images of nurses and resist nurse autonomy—either because they honestly doubt nurses' ability to cope with certain problems (bolstered, unfortunately, by the behavior of some nurses they work with) or because they are threatened by the expansion of nursing roles. More serious is the periodic action of certain medical societies and boards to restrict expanded nursing practice by opposing reimbursement for nursing services unless there is physician supervision, or using their power to limit nursing practice in a particular community or health care settings.

The reasons for problems in nurse–physician relationships have been examined repeatedly. One reason given is that physician education tends to impress on the medical student a captain-of-the-ship mentality and a need for both omniscience and omnipotence (Aesculapian authority), whereas nursing education often has not developed nurses as independent and fearless thinkers. This is also seen as one cause of the doctor–nurse game, in which the nurse must communicate information and advice to the physician without seeming to do so, and the physician acts on it without acknowledging the source. This game has an inhibitory, stifling, and anti-intellectual effect on open dialogue.

Other reasons include the different socioeconomic and educational status of doctors and nurses; the doctors' lack of accurate knowledge about nursing education and practice, and vice versa, which enables nurses and doctors to work side by side without really understanding each other or communicating adequately (prompting some authors to compare their behavior to the parallel play of toddlers); different orientations to practice, including physician disapproval of the nursing emphasis on the psychosocial aspects of patient care; the difference in attitudes about their professions as a long-term career commitment; nurses' lack of control over their practice, particularly in hospitals; physician exploitation of nurses; and general male misogyny (although some find that female physicians may not act much differently).

With nurses looking toward expanded practice, the fact that many physicians do not seem comfortable in having nurses carry out responsibilities that were traditionally medical has caused considerable misunderstanding. This is particularly true when nurses feel that they must prove themselves to be accepted in new roles and that there is a role challenge thrown out by physicians. Again, apparently interrelated is the male–female role, the dominance–deference pattern that has had such strong historical roots that as someone stated, the nurse/woman (primarily women) must feel like a girl, act like a lady, think like a man, and work like a dog.

On the other hand, an increasing number of physicians encourage and promote nurse–physician collegial relationships and see them as inevitable and necessary for good health care. Joint practice and other collaboration, both at the unit level and in various manifestations of physician–APN practice, are evidence of this cooperation. The secret seems to be to establish mutual respect one on one. Large-scale initiatives have been less than successful.

That doctors and nurses are willing to work together, that is, to collaborate, has a more serious meaning than symbolism. Over the years, an impressive amount of data have been gathered to show that nurse–physician collaboration has significant implications for patient well-being. Collaboration had positive results by improving the conditions of geriatric patients in several settings, including lowering mortality, lowering costs, increasing patient satisfaction, improving professional nurse–physician relationships, and decreasing the patient's length of hospital stay. A study team headed by a physician reported the most dramatic instance of the importance of collaboration. Thirteen hospitals were ranked according to their ratio of actual to predicted deaths of 5030 patients in intensive care units. The differences, considering all factors, were clearly owing to physician–nurse relationships. In the best hospital, excellent communication between physicians and nursing staff was ongoing to ensure that all patient needs were met. The charge nurse could cancel major elective surgery if not enough nursing staff were available. A similar degree of respect extended to other physician–nurse interactions. In the worst hospital there was an atmosphere of distrust between doctors and nurses and poor communication. The pattern matching collaboration with good results and vice versa was consistent throughout the study.

Stein, who named the *doctor–nurse game* and restudied this phenomenon after 20 years, notes major changes. He admits that in some places the game still functions as described 20 years ago, but he predicts that the changes visible elsewhere will spread. One factor is that "the image of nurses as handmaidens is giving way to that of specialty-trained and certified advanced practitioners with independent duties and responsibilities to their patients."[19] Many physicians have come to depend on this special expertise. Stein adds that the many other influential roles nurses take in utilization review and quality assurance may threaten doctors' authority in clinical decision making. In explaining how and why the physician–nurse interaction has changed, he stresses the nurses' goal of becoming autonomous practitioners; changes such as the civil rights and women's movements and the nursing shortages; nurses' education, in terms of both content and socialization of nursing students to relate to physicians differently than in the past; and the improved environment of some hospitals. The effect on those physicians who still see the RN as primarily carrying out their orders is bewilderment; they often turn to LPNs who cheerfully do what they are told. Although Stein reiterates the positive aspects of a collegial relationship, he also suggests that both participants might be a little uncomfortable with the new roles. Yet, "When a subordinate becomes liberated, there is potential for the dominant one to become liberated, too."[17] Is Stein too optimistic? Given his caveats that the doctor–nurse game still exists and realizing that everything takes time, probably not. In recent years, there have been many more reports of health care settings where the new, interdependent mode prevails. Resolving this overall issue is a part of the challenge that both medicine and nursing must face.

KEY POINTS

1. To lead others to personally meaningful change will be a constant requirement of your practice.
2. Without followers, there are no leaders.
3. The most logical view of leadership for today assumes general instability and requires that the leader and followers fuse their strengths and move toward mutual goals.
4. Power is the by-product of social relationships and is given, or it does not exist.
5. Nursing has the potential for power in its overwhelming numbers, its special knowledge and skills, and its place in the public trust.
6. Planned change allows us a degree of control.
7. Because of their central position in systems of care, nurses often find themselves in the role of change agent.

KEY POINTS

8. Nurses who are women must overcome some of the stereotypes about what women can and cannot do.

9. The most influential mentors to hospital staff nurses are peers and nurse managers.

10. Physician–nurse relationships can be problems or assets, depending on how the two professions understand each other and whether each sees the other as rival or colleague.

11. Networking is an effective way to broaden professional opportunities.

12. Nurses can have a strong impact on health policy making by their effective participation in community groups.

13. Nurses who have pride in nursing themselves and one another can move nursing forward toward a preferred future.

REFERENCES

1. Ashley J. *Hospitals, Paternalism and the Role of the Nurse.* New York: Teachers College Press, 1976.

2. Marriner A. Theories of leadership. In Hein E, Nicholson M (eds): *Contemporary Leadership Behavior,* 5th ed. Philadelphia: Lippincott, 1999, pp 55–61.

3. Malone B. Nurses in nonnursing leadership positions. In McCloskey J, Grace H (eds): *Current Issues in Nursing,* 6th ed. St. Louis: Mosby, 2001, pp 293–298.

4. Joel L. The leader–follower connection. *Am J Nurs* 97:7, July 1997.

5. Small N, Walsh M. *The Teaching Nursing Homes: The Nursing Perspective.* Baltimore: National Health Publishing, 1988.

6. The Pew Charitable Trusts, The Robert Wood Johnson Foundation. *Strengthening Hospital Nursing: A Progress Report.* St. Petersburg, FL: The Authors, 1992.

7. Senge P. *The Fifth Discipline.* New York: Doubleday, 1990, pp 17–26.

8. Safier G. *Contemporary American Leaders in Nursing: An Oral History.* New York: McGraw-Hill, 1977.

9. Schorr T, Zimmerman A. *Making Choices, Taking Chances.* St. Louis, MO: Mosby, 1988.

10. Maraldo P. The illusion of power. In Wieczorek R (ed): *Power Politics and Policy in Nursing.* New York: Springer, 1985, pp 64–70.

11. Ibid.

12. Watzlawick P, Weakland J, Fisch R. *Change.* New York: Norton, 1974.

13. Lippitt R, Watson J, Westley B. *The Dynamics of Planned Change.* New York: Harcourt, Brace and World, 1958.

14. Project Management. Lippitt's Phases of Change Theory. September 24, 2008. http://en.wordpress.com/tag/change-management/. Retrieved May 3, 2010.

15. Vance C. Mentorship. *Annu Rev Nurs Res* 9:175–200, 1991.

16. Spengler C. Mentor-Protégé Relationships: A Study of Career Development Among Female Nurse Doctorates. Unpublished PhD dissertation. University of Missouri-Columbia, 1982.

17. Stein L, Watts D, Howell T. The doctor–nurse game revisited. *N Engl J Med* 322:546–549, February 22, 1990.

HELPFUL WEBSITES FOR PART II, SECTION FOUR

American Academy of Nurse Practitioners: http://www.aanp.org

American Association of Colleges of Nursing: http://nche.aacn.edu

American Association of Nurse Anesthetists: http://www.aana.org

American Association of Occupational Health Nurses: http://www.aaohn.org

American Association of Office Nurses: http://www.aaon.org

American Association of Retired Persons: http://www.aarp.org

American College of Nurse Midwives: http://www.acnm.org

American College of Nurse Practitioners: http://www.nurse.org/acnp

American Hospital Association: http://www.aha.org

American Medical Association: http://www.ama-assn.org

American Nurses Association: http://www.nursingworld.org

Case Management Society of America: http://www.cmsa.org

Center for Health Care Strategies: http://www.chcs.org

Change Management: http://en.wordpress.com/tag/change-management

International Council of Nurses: http://icn.ch

National Center for Continuing Education: http://nursece.com

National Council of State Boards of Nursing: http://www.ncsbn.org

National Institute of Nursing Research: http://www.nih.gov/ninr

National League for Nursing: http://www.nln.org

National Student Nurses Association: http://www.nsna.org

Nurses Organization of Veteran's Affairs: http://vanurse.org

The Nurse Practitioner (Journal): http://www.springnet.com/np

Legal Rights and Responsibilities

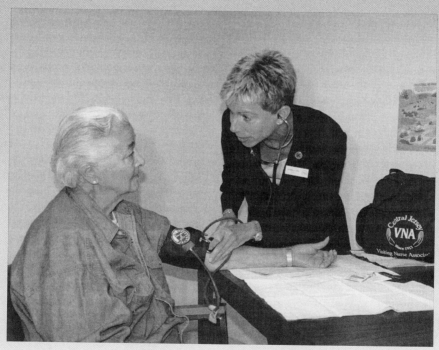

Community-based health promotion programs for the elderly are part of the role of the public health nurse.
(Courtesy of the Visiting Nurse Association of Central Jersey, Red Bank, New Jersey)

An Introduction to the Law

Law has been defined as the sum total of rules and regulations by which society is governed, designed to assist people to order their society, organize their affairs, and settle their problems. It is man-made and regulates social conduct in a formal and binding way. It reflects society's needs, attitudes, and mores.[1] The more complex the society is, the more complicated the legal system that governs it, and also the more likely that the law will be in a state of change. Everyone dealing with law knows that there may be no final or absolute answer—something that is quite frustrating for those who want to know exactly what they can or cannot do. Yet, there are certain principles that serve as guidelines and as a basis for understanding American law.

■ ORIGINS OF MODERN LAW

The leaders of primitive peoples who found they could not live successfully in groups without rules or codes to govern them probably introduced the first *laws*. Prevailing customs and traditions were often set down as the basic law of the land. One of the early tasks was to distinguish between sensible laws and those that were merely taboos or superstitions.

The most illustrious lawgiver of ancient history was Hammurabi, king of Babylon (2067–2025 BC), who developed a detailed code of laws to be used by the courts throughout the empire. Known as the *Code of Hammurabi*, the text was inscribed on stone columns, the ruins of which are now in the Louvre in Paris.

The laws governing Greece remained unwritten until about 621 BC, when Draco, an Athenian statesman and lawgiver, codified them. Although the code was a marked advance toward equal justice under the law for all people, it was so stern (demanding the death penalty for nearly all crimes) that the word *Draconian* is still used to describe an unduly cruel person or action. Draco's Code was replaced by a milder one prepared under the direction of Solon (circa 638–558 BC). Plato (circa 428–348 BC) later revised the code.

In Rome, Emperor Justinian I (AD 483–565) appointed a commission of legal experts to prepare a revision—actually a consolidation—of Rome's various laws, which had developed over a period of approximately 1000 years.

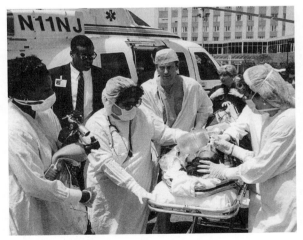

Complex high-tech care has created new issues in the areas of ethics and patient's rights. (Courtesy of Saint Barnabas Hospital, West Orange, New Jersey)

This revision, the *Corpus Juris Civilis*, which was issued in four parts, serves as a basis for civil law in most European countries and England. Later, it had considerable influence on the structure of laws in the United States. The third part of the document, the *Digest* (AD 533), was intended for use by judges and practitioners of the law. It contained the law in concrete form and was by far the most important section, influencing jurists and scholars for many years, possibly even to this day.

Another famous code of laws, parts of which are still in effect in France, was prepared under the leadership of Emperor Napoleon of France (1769–1821). The legal system of the state of Louisiana, once a French colony, was originally based on the *Napoleonic Code*; all other colonies based their laws on the English system of common law.

In England, centuries ago, the king reigned supreme, but because of great distances and limited capacity for communication, the king found it necessary to enlist the help of lords and barons in settling disputes in their geographic areas. He, however, retained the privilege of overriding or vetoing their decisions if he deemed it to the crown's or the kingdom's advantage to do so.

The lords and barons, in turn, passed on authority for settling certain disputes to persons of lesser standing, retaining the power of veto over their decisions. To achieve a degree of order and uniformity, the same persons traveled from place to place in the manner of circuit judges to hear arguments pro and con and serve as mediators in settling controversies. It was quite natural for these *judges* to make similar decisions when cases presented similar sets of circumstances.

As so often happens, the administrative official (in this case, the king of England) became concerned lest some of his power be stripped from him, and he took steps to regain and centralize control over the dispensation of justice throughout his land. The king accomplished this by assuming responsibility for the appointment of judges to preside over hearings to be held in designated places called the king's courts. To facilitate their work and serve as guides for future deliberations, the judges often kept written records of their decisions for their personal use. Later, the keeping of such records became mandatory. These records and the principles found therein were the foundation of common law.

With the introduction of written decisions, one of the most important principles known in the law was born, the principle of *stare decisis*, which is Latin for "to stand by things decided." *Stare decisis* is essentially the doctrine of precedent. Courts cite to *stare decisis* when an issue has been previously brought to the court and a ruling already issued. Generally, courts will adhere to the previous ruling, though this is not universally true.

> When a previous case involving similar facts has been decided in the jurisdiction, the court will be strongly inclined to follow the principles of law laid down in that prior adjudication. Unless precedents are carefully regarded and adhered to, uncertainty would be both perplexing and prejudicial to the public. However, when the precedent is out of date or inapplicable to the case before the court, the principle of stare decisis will not be followed and the court will announce a new rule.[2]

Courts of law presided over by competent lawyers quickly gained the confidence and respect of the English people. As a result, common law achieved extraordinary power, perhaps even greater than that of the reigning monarch, whose arbitrary despotism remained almost unquestioned until the barons forced King John to sign the Magna Carta in 1215 at Runnymede. The following excerpts from the Magna Carta are applicable to some of the current issues in our society.

> No freeman shall be taken, or imprisoned, or outlawed, or exiled, or in any way harmed, nor will we go upon or send upon him, save by the lawful judgment of his peers or by the law of the land. [Article 39]
> To none will we sell, to none deny or delay, right or justice. [Article 40][3]

These clauses were the antecedents of due process of law and the guarantee of trial by jury. The Magna Carta also provided for a committee of 25 barons to enforce it. This was the beginning in England of a government that provided a system of checks and balances that would keep the monarchy strong but prevent its perversion by a tyrannical or inept monarch. Although severely tested at times, government in England from then on meant more than the despotic rule of one person; custom and law stood even above the king.

The British Parliament, the supreme national legislative body, was established in 1295 and is actually an outgrowth of the Magna Carta. It marks the beginning of self-government in England. It took its name from the French *parlement* (derived from *parler*, "to speak"), which in France was originally used to describe any meeting for discussion or debate. The English form of parliament was initially used to designate a debate and later a formal conference.

The laws enacted by this body or parliament were termed *statutory law,* as contrasted to common law. The rules and regulations developed to guide the deliberations of Parliament, and now widely used in other countries, are often called *parliamentary law.* They are not laws, however, and are more correctly termed *parliamentary procedure.*

■ THE UNITED STATES LEGAL SYSTEM

As the American colonies were founded one by one, the manner in which they would be governed was a vital and primary consideration. The edicts of the governments in the homelands of the settlers were a persuasive force. In addition, the colonists were influenced greatly by their own previous experience and knowledge. From the beginning, self-government became their goal, a goal that seemed more attainable in the English colonies than in those originally settled by the Spanish or French.

One of the early problems was to establish methods of dealing with disputes over property and personal injuries. To handle such disputes, the Pilgrim Fathers adopted a system similar to that of the common law then in effect in England. Judges were appointed and courts established, but because life and customs were so different in America from those in England, it often proved impractical and unfair to apply decisions that had been made in the mother country. Furthermore, the problems and experiences within the colonies varied so widely that a judge's decision regarding a dispute in one colony was not necessarily applied by a judge to a similar set of circumstances in another colony. Each colony, therefore, developed its own procedures and laws, both common and statutory, based on its peculiar needs.

From this evolved the concept of *states' rights,* which has played an important role in the history of the United States. For many years, any infringement of these rights either from the federal government or from other states was vigorously opposed. There has been less resistance over the years to the initiation of federal programs that assume or share responsibilities that were formerly carried by the individual states. Nevertheless, the concept of states' rights has been increasingly invoked with regard to major federal legislation such as welfare reform and health care, when the state government felt that specific pending legislation was not in the state's best interest.

It is not unusual, of course, for several states to adopt in their separate legislatures an identical law, such as a law governing the age at which people may vote if they meet other qualifications. The fact remains, however, that a state that enacts its own laws can retain, revise, or repeal them without interference from other states or the federal government. Relinquishment of this right is a serious matter in a democracy, because doing so sets a precedent that may be difficult to overcome. On the other hand, variance in state laws also gives rise to a great deal of confusion, misunderstanding, and red tape. The fact is that sovereign states each set their own rules.

The founders of the United States did not depend on common law alone to govern the colonies; nor did they give unlimited power to the governors and councils appointed by the governments of their homelands. To establish and maintain a degree of control, each of the original 13 colonies early in their history established legislative bodies elected by the voters. The first was the House of Burgesses, which met in Jamestown, Virginia, in 1619 and was attended by two burgesses (citizens) from each of 27 plantations.

Such localized government was considered adequate as well as advisable until 1774, when the colonies felt the need to unite to voice their collective grievances against England's colonial policies. In that year, the First Continental Congress, attended by representatives of all colonies except Georgia, met in Philadelphia from September 5 to October 26. The Congress did more than express grievances; it also created an association to impose extensive boycotts against British trade, thus firmly establishing the tradition of pooling strengths and resources in time of national stress and emergency.

By 1775, war had begun and the Second Continental Congress, meeting in session from May 10, 1775, until December 12, 1776, created a Continental Army under the direction of George Washington to oppose the British. With the Declaration of Independence, formalized on July 4, 1776, the colonies were launched on a course of liberty from which they—and the states that were later formed—never retreated, although discussions, disagreements, financial difficulties, jealousies, and friction hampered progress time after time.

The Continental Congress continued to meet annually for varying periods of time in several different cities. With limited funds and little experience in affairs of state, the representatives maintained the will and courage to advance toward full independence. In 1778, the Congress submitted the Articles of Confederation to the legislatures of the states for ratification. Ratification finally occurred in 1781. The states considered themselves practically as separate countries, delegating to the central government only those powers that they could not handle individually, such as the authority to wage war, establishing a uniform currency, and making treaties with other nations. The Articles of Confederation made no provision for an executive head of the central government.

The Articles of Confederation proved to be too weak to hold the colonies together, giving rise to fears that foreign powers might reconquer part or all of the country. Under the leadership of farsighted patriots such as George Washington and Alexander Hamilton, a movement toward nationalization took place. As a result, in 1787 a Constitutional Convention met in Philadelphia to draw up the Constitution of the United States, a concept that had originated in English and earlier colonial history. Ratification of the Constitution by a majority of the 13 colonies established the permanent structure of the Congress of the United States, which held its first meeting in New York on March 4, 1789. The first meeting in our present capital, Washington, DC, was held in 1800. The Constitution also directed that a president, elected by the people, should be at the head of the government.

Since colonial times, the volume and complexity of problems facing the Congress have increased tremendously. Numerous departments and councils have been set up to assist in the work of making laws. The principles guiding their work are embodied in the Constitution of the United States—the law of the land—which, although amended 27 times (the last in 1992), could scarcely be improved on were it rewritten from the start today. Its basic principles are as relevant today as they were in 1789.

Constitutional Amendments

Shortly after the adoption of the Constitution, it became apparent that the government's police power, that is, the power to provide for the health, safety, and welfare of the people, needed to be limited by spelling out the rights of the states and the individual citizen.[4] Congress therefore submitted to the states 12 amendments to the Constitution intended to clarify these rights, 10 of which were ratified by the states in 1791 and became known as the *Bill of Rights*. Social and political developments in recent years have placed renewed emphasis on these rights. It may be well, therefore, to review these amendments to form a basis for later discussion of the legal rights and responsibilities of citizens, and particularly nurses.

The *First Amendment* guarantees US citizens freedom of religion, speech, press, and the right "peaceably to assemble and to petition the Government for a redress of grievances." This amendment is often the center of controversy in disputes related to the freedoms guaranteed therein. In the last few years, it has been invoked and upheld, even when related to situations most Americans abhor, such as the marches of neo-Nazis, or about which there is public disagreement, such as the picketing of abortion clinics.

The *Second Amendment* gives the people the right to keep and bear arms, because a well-regulated militia is necessary to the security of a free state. Even with recent federal and state restrictions on what kind of arms and the procedures for obtaining them, this amendment, too, is firmly defended, particularly by some groups and certain states, although others argue about its interpretation for modern times where crime is an important concern. The *Third Amendment* refers to the quartering of soldiers in a private home in times of peace or war.

The last seven amendments included in the Bill of Rights have direct or indirect bearing on crimes, trials, and other legal matters in which nurses might become involved. They give protection against search and guarantee the right to due process of law: clarity on accusations, the role of the grand jury and a jury of one's peers, representation by counsel, and protection against excessive punishment. The *Tenth Amendment* establishes and clarifies the nature of states' rights. The reader is referred to earlier editions of *Dimensions of Professional Nursing* for a fuller presentation of the Bill of Rights.

Later Amendments

The *Eleventh Amendment* (1798) is concerned with judicial powers; the *Twelfth* (1804) with the method of electing a president and vice president; and the *Thirteenth* (1865) abolished slavery. The *Fourteenth Amendment*, added in 1868 during the Reconstruction period following the Civil War, guarantees equal protection under the law to any citizen faced with state action that threatens loss of rights. The *Fifteenth Amendment*, ratified in 1870, provided former slaves the right to vote. The *Sixteenth Amendment* (1913) authorized Congress to levy and collect income taxes; the *Seventeenth* (1913) refers to the election of US senators; the *Eighteenth*, adopted in 1920 and repealed in 1933, prohibited the manufacture, sale, or transport of intoxicating liquors or beverages within the United States and all territories subject to its jurisdiction. The *Nineteenth Amendment*, known as the Women's Suffrage Amendment, went into effect on August 26, 1920. The *Twentieth Amendment*

(1933) specifies the dates on which the terms of the president, vice president, senators, and representatives shall assume office. The *Twenty-first Amendment* (1933) repealed the Eighteenth Amendment; the *Twenty-second* (1951) limited the presidential terms of office to two; the *Twenty-third* (1961) gave citizens of the District of Columbia the right to vote for presidential and vice presidential candidates.

The *Twenty-fourth Amendment* (1964), which was enacted because of laws passed by certain states to make it impossible, or at least very difficult, for black citizens to vote, outlaws making the right to vote contingent on a poll tax or any tax. The *Twenty-fifth Amendment* (1965) deals with the disability of a president or a vacancy in the office of vice president and stipulates how the offices shall be filled in the event of an emergency. The *Twenty-sixth Amendment* (1971) lowered the voting age to 18.

For a while, there was great hope that the *Twenty-seventh Amendment* would be passed, barring legal discrimination against women based on sex. The bill, passed by Congress (1971–1972) and sent to the states for ratification, read: "Equality of rights under the law shall not be denied or abridged by the United States or any State on account of sex." To be adopted, two-thirds of the states (38) needed to ratify the amendment by a specific time. When it was apparent that this goal would not be reached by the legal deadline of March 22, 1979 (three votes were still needed by mid-1978), both the House and the Senate voted to extend the deadline to June 30, 1982. At the same time, a proposal to allow states that had already ratified the amendment to rescind their decisions was defeated, but the final decision on whether rescinding was possible remained open. Most of the states in which the Equal Rights Amendment (ERA) was defeated were in the South (Alabama, Arkansas, Florida, Georgia, Louisiana, Mississippi, North Carolina, Oklahoma, South Carolina, and Virginia), but the legislators of Arizona, Illinois, Missouri, Nevada, and Utah also voted not to ratify. The required number of states was never won, so the bill was defeated in 1982 by lack of ratification. What is rather amazing is that more than a decade later, no new bill has been passed in Congress. Finally a *Twenty-seventh Amendment* (1992) was passed that limited Congressional pay increases.

The Constitution and its amendments encompass some of the basic provisions that ensure the rights of individuals to protection under the law and to fair and just practices in the application of laws at any political level. Protection against usurpation of the privileges and authority of individuals, as well as state and local authorities, is also provided. Beyond this, it is up to the states, counties, townships, and municipalities to develop laws and legal procedures to protect their citizens. It is the individual's responsibility to be well informed about the laws governing his or her geographic area and especially those that are applicable to his or her status and vocation. This will help avoid legal problems and provide some protection as individuals insist on their rights.

■ LEGAL STRUCTURE OF THE UNITED STATES

Under the US system of government, the law is carried out at a number of levels. The Constitution is the highest law of the land. Whatever the Constitution and the federal laws established under its authority do not spell out, the states retain the power to legislate for themselves (Tenth Amendment). Because states can create political subdivisions, units of local government—counties, cities, towns, townships, boroughs, and villages—all have certain delegated legal powers within their geographic boundaries. On all levels, but most obviously on the federal and state levels, there is a separation of power: legislative, executive, and judicial. The legislative branch makes the laws, the executive branch carries them out, and the judicial branch reviews the laws, a system that the founders of the United States believed would create a balance of power.

Besides constitutional law, there are three basic sources of law: statutory law; executive, administrative, or regulatory law; and judicial, or common law.

Statutory law refers to laws that are enacted (codified) by legislative bodies, declaring, commanding, or prohibiting something. Statutes are always written, and can be altered only by amendment or repeal. The federal government's explicit powers come from the Constitution, but the states have broader inherent power. Both have broad powers to legislate for the general welfare, for instance, health and safety. The Nurse Education Act that, over the years, has provided funding for nursing education is one example of a federal law. A law requiring professional nurses to be licensed before they can legally practice nursing is an example of a state law. In the federal system, the laws are published in the United States Code; state laws are published in that particular state's code. (The legislative process is described in Chapter 18.)

Executive, administrative, or *regulatory law* refers to the rules, regulations, and decisions of administrative bodies, to which the statutes have delegated authority. For example, the Department of Health and Human Services (DHHS) Division of Nursing develops the regulations that determine the requirements for the various programs in the Nurse Education Act; the State Board of Nursing spells out the requirements for a nursing school; a city health code may adopt a patient's bill of rights as a requirement for hospitals in the city. All have the effect of law. The state's police power to provide for and protect the public health, a basic, inherent power of the government, is also delegated to lower levels of government (county, municipal, etc.). This includes promulgation of health and sanitary codes, rules and regulations for hospitals and nursing homes, housing, plumbing, as well as for health services such as municipal hospital systems and school health services.

Judicial law, also called *decisional*, *case*, or *common law*, as distinguished from law created by legislatures, comprises a body of legal principles and rules of action that derive their authority from usage and custom or from judgments and decrees of courts based on these usages and customs. Courts are agencies established by the government to decide disputes. (The term *court* is also sometimes used to refer to the person or persons hearing a case.) There is usually only one judge for a trial (with or without a jury) and two or more to hear the appeals (with no jury). The particular court in which a case is brought depends on the offense or complaint.

There are also various classifications of law. *Criminal* or *penal law* deals with actions harmful to the public and the individual and designates punishment for offenders. Three gradations of criminal acts are recognized by the law: (1) offenses, such as traffic violations or disorderly conduct; (2) misdemeanors, such as small thefts, forgeries, conspiracies, and assaults without the use of weapons; and (3) felonies, such as major robberies, assault with a dangerous weapon, arson, rape, and murder. The state or local government prosecutes criminal actions.

Civil law involves the rights of individuals and stipulates methods of maintaining or regaining such rights. The word *civil* means "citizen"; civil laws, therefore, pertain to the individual citizen. Many acts of negligence, libel and slander, and commercial disputes are examples of cases that are subject to the application of civil law. A civil wrong is a tort. Civil law is distinct from criminal law. An aggrieved plaintiff prosecutes civil suits.

There are many subdivisions of civil law. One of particular interest to nurses is *contract law*. Contract law governs all legal actions related to the making, keeping, or breaking of legal contracts of any type—for example, employment contracts, marriage contracts, and contracts for the sale of property. Contract law also deals with fraudulent contracts. No fraudulent contract is binding against an innocent person unless that person elects to make it so.

Laws are additionally classified by subject matter, such as labor laws, maritime laws, mercantile laws, tax laws, motor vehicle laws, and others. Two other categories of law are martial and military law.

Martial law involves the suspension of civil law in times of emergency and the enforcement of military law on the civilian population.

Military law is a branch of national (or state) law that governs the conduct of national (or state) military organizations in peace or war. The rules or laws are enacted by the legislative body and administered in *court martial*—a court consisting of military officers where personnel are tried for breaches of military law or discipline. Nurses enrolled in the armed forces as commissioned officers are subject to military law, which applies to all branches of the military services.

Enforcement of Laws

Besides generally adhering to the principle of *stare decisis*, courts also abide by another basic legal principle—that the court must have jurisdiction over the person or property involved, that is, that the proceeding must be initiated in a court where the defendant resides or does business, where the action occurred, or where the property in dispute is located. An exception occurs when, because of extraordinary publicity or emotionalism, the defendant claims that she or he cannot expect a fair trial in a particular jurisdiction and requests a change of venue—to be tried in some other jurisdiction.

The US Constitution provides for the enforcement of federal laws by establishing a system of courts (sometimes called constitutional courts because they hear cases involving matters mentioned in the Constitution), headed by the Supreme Court, the only court specifically mentioned in the Constitution. Other federal courts—courts of appeal, district courts, and others—have been established for all states and territories. Staffed by judges, lawyers, and other personnel employed by the federal government, these courts try all cases arising under the Constitution and laws of the United States except those over which the Supreme Court has original jurisdiction. For example, cases involving violations of federal income tax laws, civil rights, and the passing of counterfeit money are tried in federal courts. In addition to jurisdiction over federal questions, the federal courts also have *diversity jurisdiction*, when the action is between citizens of different states and the amount in controversy exceeds $75,000.

Most citizens are not involved in legal action handled by a federal court. Misdemeanors are usually dealt with on a local level, often by a justice of the peace court, common in rural areas and small towns, or, in urban areas, by a magistrate's court, sometimes called a *municipal* or *police court*. A district court, often called a *county court*, may hear cases in one county or in several. Matters related to estates and wills often are handled at the county level in surrogate courts (sometimes called *probate courts*) under the direction of surrogate or probate judges.

At the state level, no two states have court systems that are precisely identical. They may differ in the names of the courts, their methods of selecting and removing judges, the number of jurors needed to convict the defendant in criminal cases, and in other ways. They do not differ widely, however, on fundamental principles or in their conduct of judicial affairs.

State courts have jurisdiction over all cases arising under common law and statutory laws in their respective states, except in Louisiana, which still operates partially under the Code of Napoleon, which makes other provisions. All states have a high court for the trial of cases, and appellate courts that ensure that the trial courts correctly interpret the law and that the litigant's rights were observed in the trial courts.

To meet changing times and new challenges in the field of law, reform of the courts at all levels is almost constantly under consideration by the state legislatures. It is a slow process, however, because it involves a change in the law and possibly the enactment of new laws. In some states a constitutional amendment is necessary.

Juries

A *petit jury* is a group of citizens, usually 12, but now often 6, sworn to listen to the evidence at a trial and pronounce a verdict. The right to trial by jury is guaranteed by the Constitution of the United States and by the constitutions of the individual states.

A juror must have the qualifications specified by the statute that applies in a particular situation and be free from any bias because of personal relationships or interests. A person cannot serve as a juror on a criminal case if she or he has formed an opinion beforehand on the guilt or innocence of the accused (which is, of course, difficult to determine and may be based on what the prospective juror states when being placed on the jury).

Jurors are supposed to be selected impartially. Jury duty is one of the privileges of a citizen in a democratic society, and many persons find it challenging, educational, and rewarding. It may also be boring. Some jurors are excused from a trial panel because they are not the type of individual desired by one or the other of the opposing lawyers, who have a certain number of peremptory challenges, requiring no explanation. Prospective jurors may spend their entire time of service in a jury room waiting to be empanelled. There is a definite technique to jury selection, intended to produce a panel most favorable to a lawyer's client. For instance, in malpractice or accident cases, nurses are sometimes not selected to serve because they know too much and may be unsympathetic, according to some lawyers. To lessen the effect of jury selection, jurors are questioned by the judge rather than the lawyers in some courts.

Blacks and women have been particularly affected by the use of peremptory challenges. It was common for prosecutors, assuming that black jurors would be sympathetic to black defendants, to use their challenges to create an all-white or nearly all-white jury. In a 1986 landmark decision (*Batson v. Kentucky*), the Supreme Court barred prosecutors from using their peremptory challenges to remove black jurors from criminal cases involving blacks, ruling that the Constitution's equal protection guarantee did not permit assumptions about group behavior to determine a person's ability to serve on a jury. In subsequent rulings, the court expanded that ruling to civil trials and to private litigants as well as government prosecutors.

Over the years, a woman was often excused from jury duty if she had home and family responsibilities that would suffer because of her absence, or if she was pregnant. In some states, nurses, or women in general, were not called or were quickly excused. Because this violates the woman's right to serve if she so chooses and is able, women's rights groups have fought those restrictive laws. In 1975, the Supreme Court ruled that it is constitutionally unacceptable for states to deny women equal opportunity to serve on juries. The decision was based on the Sixth Amendment guarantee of a jury trial by a cross-sectional representation of the community. Women comprise over 50 percent of the population; therefore, systematically excluding them would deny those rights. In 1994, the high court barred sex as a standard for picking jurors.

Harry Blackmun, who retired later that year, said, "Discrimination in jury selection, whether based on race or on gender, causes harm to the litigants, the community, and the individual jurors who are wrongfully excluded from participation in the judicial process." A warning note was sounded by Justice Sandra Day O'Connor, however, although she concurred with the majority. She wrote, "We know that like race, gender matters," citing research that showed that in rape cases, female jurors are more likely to convict than male jurors. She added, "Moreover, though there have been no similarly definitive studies regarding, for example, sexual harassment, child custody or spousal or child abuse, one need not be sexist to share the intuition that in certain cases, a person's gender and resulting life experience will be relevant to his or her view of the case. . . . Individuals are not expected to ignore as jurors what they know as men or women. Today's decision severely limits a litigant's ability to act on this intuition."

A person must have a very good reason to be excused from jury duty, although those with pressing duties, such as doctors, lawyers, members of a fire or police department, and the armed forces, may be exempted. Various reasons for requesting release from a call to jury duty are accepted in all states, although these people may be called later, and the trend is to narrow exemptions and acceptable excuses. A juror receives a modest daily fee. Many employers keep an employee on full salary while he or she is on jury duty. Jury service is usually for a relatively short period of time, unless one is assigned to a long trial. The length of increasing numbers of trials today, extending into months, is creating new problems for jurors and employers, especially when the jurors are sequestered. For the self-employed, jury duty is often a financial hardship.

A *grand jury* is a group of persons, usually numbering from 12 to 23, whose principal function is to examine the accusations against someone charged with a crime and to determine whether or not she or he should be indicted, that is, brought to trial before a petit jury. The grand jury system is based on the English system dating from the thirteenth century, which was intended to prevent a citizen from being imposed on by a despotic government and charged with a crime based on insufficient evidence. Some states rarely use a grand jury, although indictment by grand jury is provided for in all states. Members of the grand jury are selected even more carefully than members of a petit jury. They usually serve at intervals over a longer period of time, and are paid somewhat more for their services.

■ LEGAL STATUS OF YOUNG PEOPLE

US citizens of any age are endowed with the rights of freedom of religion, speech, press, petition, and other rights as set forth in the Bill of Rights. Furthermore, most people agree that all are entitled morally (at least until they forfeit the privilege through their own actions) to respect, tolerance, and understanding from their fellow man. Children born into citizenship in the United States have certain civil rights and responsibilities, some of which are in effect all of their lives; others they relinquish when they become adults and take on new rights. Traditionally, parents' duties to their children include support, protection, education, and control, the last duty allowing parents to make rules by which their children will live. The children's duties are to obey (reasonable orders and rules), render reasonable services (chores), and live with parents until majority.

In the last few years the threshold of legal adulthood or majority has been in a state of flux, but even more so has been the question of the rights of young people in the nebulous state between minority and the age of majority. Legislation has begun to deal with the rights of children in relation to privacy, informed consent, and many health-related matters. Some of the major legal decisions concerning health care and youth are discussed in Chapter 22, but a few basic facts on the legal status of young people should provide useful background.

Infant, minor, child, and *juvenile* are terms, often used interchangeably, for someone who has not yet attained majority. The *age of majority* is the age designated by state law at which a citizen of the United States becomes an adult for legal purposes and is entitled, therefore, to assume full civil rights and responsibilities. This status, sometimes abbreviated to majority, is synonymous with full or legal age. Each state adopts its own law setting the age of majority. With the exception of Alabama, Delaware, Mississippi, and Nebraska, the age of majority is 18 since the passage of the Twenty-sixth Amendment, which established the voting age of 18. On attaining legal age, individuals are permitted by statutory state law to perform certain acts with or without the consent of parents or guardians. Nevertheless, even within a particular state, the law may vary with respect to the activities or purposes involved. The state has the right to set the age of qualification for such activities as serving on a jury; marrying without parental consent; buying, possessing, and drinking alcoholic beverages; buying tobacco products; making a contract; drawing a will; inheriting money; working for wages;

obtaining a license to drive a motor vehicle; attending school; receiving juvenile court treatment for illegal or criminal conduct; using the courts to sue another person or one's parents; and receiving medical care without parental consent. Most laws have a bias toward parental authority.

Emancipation describes the condition whereby children are released from some or all of the restrictions of childhood and receive the rights and duties of adulthood before the age of majority. Emancipation may be partial or complete. Theoretically, only the court or a specific state law can determine emancipation except under certain classic circumstances such as the young person's marriage or membership in the armed services. Parents can petition the court for a declaration of emancipation, which releases them from their legal obligation to the child—the duty to support, maintain, protect, and educate. They give up the custody and control of their child and the right to receive services and earnings. On the other hand, when young people leave home or earn an independent living, and are otherwise free from the authority and control of parents, this may be grounds for de facto emancipation. Usually the petition for emancipation requires the consent of both the parents and the child, but the reality is that unless there is a serious problem, an individual in such independent circumstances is considered emancipated for all general purposes. Minors can also be emancipated with the express consent of their parents, even without formal permission.

In cases involving consent for medical treatment, the term *mature minor* may be used, indicating that the child is sufficiently intelligent to understand the nature and consequences of treatment.

Right of Sustenance and Shelter

Besides the constitutional rights cited earlier, minors have additional legal rights. From the moment of birth until legal age, children are entitled by state law to such food, shelter, medical care, and clothing (legally termed *necessities*) as the parents can reasonably afford. State laws are changing from the traditional focus on father to include the mother, because both parents are recognized as having obligations to their children.

Wherever minors may be—in school, recreation camp, hospital—they always have the right to food, clothing, and shelter provided by their parents, either directly or through a written or unwritten contract with the agency or individual under whose care any children have been placed

temporarily. Failure to provide for a child in this way (including medical care) is termed *child neglect.*

In cases of extreme parental neglect or abandonment, the state is obligated to intervene and either see that the parents assume their responsibility for the child's care or the state will remove the child from them, temporarily or permanently, and place the child in the custody of a guardian, foster family, or institution. The state must also assume financial responsibility for the child until or unless other means of support are available. The concept that the state has an interest in the welfare of children is expressed in the doctrine of *parens patriae* or the state as guardian.[4]

Although many young people are earning money—sometimes enough to live on—before they are 18 or 21, they theoretically are entitled by law to continue receiving sustenance and shelter provided by their parents or a legally appointed guardian. Also, theoretically, the parents are entitled to that minor's earnings. It is unlikely that a court would require a parent to support a wage-earning child under circumstances of hardship without requiring the child to contribute at least part of his or her earnings. Neither is it likely for the court to require the child to turn over a full paycheck to the parent. When a person reaches legal age, parents no longer are liable for child support, nor are they permitted to confiscate the child's earnings.

Right of Protection

The law requires parents to protect their children from danger and harmful exposures of all kinds. Failure to do so constitutes *negligence.* A parent who in a fit of rage or as a means of inflicting punishment seriously injures a child is guilty of battery, which is unlawful beating or other physical violence inflicted on a person without his or her consent. On the other hand, if physical punishment is permissible for the purpose of punishment, it must be reasonable and never excessive, not resulting in great physical injury or mental distress. Differentiating between what is *reasonable* and what is *abuse* is not always easy, and the determination may end up in the courts, where decisions are often inconsistent.[5]

Child abuse is reportable in every state, although it is defined differently. Hospitals, all health professionals (including nurses), and sometimes schoolteachers are required to report reasonable suspicions of child abuse. Failure to do so may expose the individual and the employer to civil and perhaps criminal charges. In most states, those reporting in good faith are insulated from civil liability (lawsuits) for having made the report.

Nurses should ask three questions about a child's injury. Has the child suffered injury or harm? Does the injury appear nonaccidental or inconsistent with the history given? Did the parent or caretaker cause the injury or fail to prevent it? If yes, the nurse should report a case of suspected child abuse and carefully gather and report specific information.

Sexual abuse is usually part of the statutory definitions of child abuse even if no physical injury has occurred. Among the specific forms of sexual assault identified are rape, incest, sodomy, lewd or lascivious acts on a child under 14, oral copulation, penetration of a genital or anal opening by a foreign object, and child molestation. Much attention has been directed recently to adults who make overtures to minors through Internet chat rooms.

The entire issue of identification and reporting has become particularly sensitive because the sexual abuse of children has become more visible and children have died. The question has been raised as to whether it is always in the best interest of the child and family to report the situation if changes are being made. On the other hand, health professionals, teachers, and social agencies have been sued for not reporting or following through on these cases. The minor's right of protection extends to her or his school where, in most states, the law stipulates what punishment a teacher can employ to maintain discipline in a classroom or school. Private schools are not always subject to the same legal restrictions on discipline as public schools.

The law requires the administrative officers of schools, hospitals, places of amusement, all public buildings and vehicles, transportation systems, health and beauty salons, and others to observe specific rules of safety for the protection of all citizens, minors and adults alike. Such establishments must have and enforce regulations intended specifically to protect the young child or risk legal difficulties of various degrees of seriousness. Furthermore, they must employ persons capable of providing the services offered safely and competently.

Right to Give Consent

Under the law, consent means that a person gives permission in writing or orally for the performance of a certain act. In many cases, minors have not been able to consent to health care, but many changes are occurring (see Chapter 22).

Female minors are protected against sex crimes to a certain extent by penal laws that state at what age a girl can legally consent to sexual intercourse. The age varies in different states—from 10 to 18. A person who violates the law is guilty of *statutory rape* and is subject to the punishment prescribed by law regardless of whether the minor consented. The law is frequently inadequate in its handling of sex offenses against both young boys and girls, but the issue is gaining increased attention legally and socially in terms of child abuse legislation.

Right to an Education

Children are legally entitled to a free education until they complete elementary school or reach a certain age. This right makes it mandatory for parents or legal guardians to see that their children or wards attend school regularly. Children cannot legally be deprived of their rights to an education, even if they are needed at home, without special permission from school authorities. Neither can children be excluded because of disability or illness, unless contagious.

Rights of Marriage and Parenthood

Every state has its own statutory laws governing the right of a couple to marry with or without the consent of their parents, guardian, or a superior court, and with or without reputable witnesses. The majority of states permit a couple to marry without the consent of their parents or anyone else at age 18. State laws also stipulate the ages at which a couple can marry with the consent of their parents or other responsible person. They are usually lower than the ages required for marriage without consent. Minors who marry declare their independence by so doing and therefore assume the same legal responsibilities as adults who marry. Minors in general have the right of custody over their children, but whether or not the mother can consent to the adoption of her child without parental consent or notifying the father varies from state to state. This inconsistency has caused problems for adopting parents in recent years. Children born when their parents are not married have the same legal rights as children born in wedlock. Within the last few years, courts and legislatures have overturned or deleted old statutes discriminating against these individuals.

Right to Make Contracts and Wills, Inherit Property, and Sue

Most states do not consider a contract binding if one of the parties is a minor. This does not mean that the contract cannot be carried out, but that the child may disaffirm it. Therefore, many adults do not enter into contracts with minors unless there is a parental signature; the parent, as an adult, cannot repudiate a legal contractual obligation. Contracts that cannot be voided by minors are those for necessities (food, clothing, shelter, and medical care), marriage, enlistment in the armed forces, and, in some states, educational loans and automobile and motorcycle insurance.

A contractual agreement to work, written or unwritten, can be legal, subject to the laws of the state that delineate the kinds of jobs that children can hold, at what age, and under what circumstances (hours, hazards, and so on). Most states require work permits, which, in turn, require parental consent and proof of age. Acquisition of a Social Security card is also necessary. Generally, salaries and fringe benefits should be the same for adult and child workers, male and female. Exceptions may be in the areas of babysitting, housework, and agricultural work.

In most states, the law does not recognize a will made by a minor as a legal document. Exceptions are sometimes made, particularly if a minor is married. A minor may inherit money or property, but usually does not have control over it until a specific age or the age of majority, based on the assumption that the minor cannot manage an estate. Therefore, the court or an adult designated in the will may act as a guardian of the minor. The guardian or trustee has the legal responsibility for safeguarding the estate.

Sometimes the disbursement of money inherited by an infant is subject to the discretion of an orphans' court, which might release money to pay for the minor's education, medical expenses, or other purposes.

There appears to be no hard-and-fast rule that states at exactly what age a person may witness a will or other legal document, serve as a witness in legal action, or serve as a legal witness at marriages and other ceremonies. The courts have permitted testimony of children as young as 7 years old. It is not so much a question of age as of intelligence and understanding. Some children have more ability and demonstrate better judgment than persons of considerably older age. A witness must be mentally capable of knowing what he or she is doing. This obviously excludes the mentally deficient witness and the child who is too young to realize the import of his or her acts. The issue of children testifying in cases of sexual abuse is quite controversial. Questions have arisen as to whether the children had been coached by the prosecution or might be intimidated by the perpetrator. Some courts have allowed videotaped testimony; others have not. More decisions are pending.

A minor can sue or be sued to enforce any civil right or obligation. Before any action against the child can be taken, however, if there is no parent or legal guardian, a court of law must be asked to appoint a guardian to institute the action on behalf of the minor or to act for the minor. This person is generally referred to as a *guardian ad litem*, that is, the capacity as guardian ceases when the action or claim is settled.

If a child is suing, an adult, such as a parent, guardian, or "friend," must bring the suit for him or her. In a few states, a child may bring suit against parents or other family members for negligent or deliberate injurious harm; other states have an *intrafamily tort immunity* law. Even in the latter circumstances, a child can often sue for damages to personal property or willful personal injury.

The law involving the arrest, detention, trial, and punishment of juveniles has been in a constant state of change in recent years, both in terms of protecting the minor and protecting the public from the minor. Horrendous crimes committed by some juveniles have focused attention on the need to protect the public.

■ THE LEGAL RIGHTS OF WOMEN

There was a time when adult women were considerably restricted by the law, simply because they were females (see Chapters 3, 4, and 16). Married women were even more limited than single women, because husbands were entitled to their wives' worldly goods and usually represented them in the execution of all legal procedures. Even if the woman was not married, she was usually under the control of a male family member. The history of women's struggle for equal rights precedes the Constitution, at which time Abigail Adams warned her husband, the future president, that if the new legal codes did not give attention to women, their absence would eventually ignite a rebellion. Over 200 years later, women are still at a legal disadvantage.

The women's suffrage amendment drafted by Susan B. Anthony was introduced into the Senate in 1875, but ratification was not certified until 1920. Efforts toward an ERA have been under way for more than 50 years with no success as yet.

Between 1920 and 1963, little legislation was passed that was useful in securing equal rights for women. However, because of the civil rights, black power, and women's rights movements that gained strength in the 1960s, new energies seemed to be released. Dumas cites and describes 43 pieces of legislation related to women's rights or of special interest to women that were enacted into law between 1963 and 1978 alone.[5]

Most of the laws that Dumas cites specifically prohibit sex discrimination in employment, military service, or education. However, even with legal protection, women are not necessarily granted equal work opportunities and equal pay for equal work, even in state and federal agencies.

This is evident in the number of court cases won (and lost) since these laws were passed, as well as the thousands of complaints of sex discrimination filed under the 1964 Civil Rights Act. As discussed in Chapter 19, the erosion of that law by Supreme Court decisions resulted in the introduction of new civil rights legislation to restore those rights. Over 300 cases, many involving women, have been dismissed because of those decisions. A few Supreme Court decisions have supported affirmative action for women. One was considered particularly important because it ruled that an employer could take sex and race into account when making employment decisions. Another, which found that sex stereotyping had been a major factor in denying a woman partnership in a large firm (the employer thought she did not dress or act feminine enough), was seen as applicable to other settings, such as in higher education where covert sexism and racism affects employment and promotion decisions. Another action (1988) backed a New York law ending sex bias in large private clubs that play an important role in business and professional life. Nevertheless, much discrimination is still evident, overtly or covertly.

Comparable Worth

Comparable worth (equal pay for different jobs that require similar levels of training, education, and responsibility) is an issue in which nursing is particularly involved because, in many situations, nurses are still paid less than men in jobs requiring much less training, education, and responsibility. In 1984, when the state of Washington was ordered to pay its female workers up to $1 billion in back wages because of pay inequities, women thought that they had moved a giant step. However, the US Court of Appeals for the Ninth Circuit overturned that lower court decision in 1985. Earlier that year, the Federal Civil Rights Commission chairman contended that comparable worth amounted to "middle-class white women's reparations" and referred to the concept as "the looniest idea since *Looney Tunes.*" The comparable-worth concept was officially rejected. However, the Washington State legislature mandated that a comparable-worth system be put in place by 1993, and in 1986 it signed a $482 million accord with its largest employee union, increasing the salary of workers, mostly women. The state also agreed to measure the worth of different jobs in terms of skill, effort, training, education, responsibility, and working conditions.[6] Although many court decisions still rule against comparable worth and others are dismissed, the National Committee on Pay Equity, a nonprofit coalition in Washington, DC, notes that there appears to be a grass-roots movement to recognize and act on such inequities. Some 20 states, led by Minnesota in 1982, began to reassess the public workforce, a move that is filtering down to municipalities. Not surprisingly, it has been found that women, and often minorities, start and stay at lower pay levels. In 1986, when Minnesota instituted pay equity for state employees, clerical workers and health care workers, almost all women, reportedly accounted for 90 percent of the employees who received raises. However, the battle is not over. In 1990, Washington state officials reported that men were shunning government jobs for private industry because the salaries were not high enough.

In 1998, a woman was earning 80 cents compared to each dollar earned by a man. Since then ground has been lost. In 2003, the ratio descended to 75.5 cents on the dollar; in 2006, 75 cents to the dollar; and in 2009, the ratio was 71 cents to a dollar earned by a man in a comparable job with similar experiential and educational background.[7]

Clearly, there is still much ground to be covered. Besides legislation, legal suits, and union action, all of which have their ups and downs, job evaluation and focused research activities will also be useful in resolving the comparable-worth issue.

Sexual Harassment

The problem of sexual harassment of women by their employers or superiors has also had some visibility, despite limited positive legislation, but with some judicial response and Equal Employment Opportunities Commission (EEOC) action. In 1980, the EEOC ruled that sexual harassment was a violation of the 1964 Civil Rights Act. Then, in 1986, the US Supreme Court affirmed that sexual harassment is a violation of Title VII of the Civil Rights Act (*Meritor Savings Bank v. Vinson*). The court recognized two forms of actionable harassment: quid pro quo and hostile environment. In each instance, the underlying premise is that Title VII proscribes unwelcome sexual conduct. *Quid pro quo* sexual harassment is the more blatant and explicit form—the demand for sexual favors for favorable job benefits or continuation of employment. These are actually the minority of complaints made or cases filed, perhaps because the plaintiff must be able to prove that the advances were unwelcome and that job benefits or retention actually depended on submission to these demands. Because such situations usually occur in places and at times in which only the two parties are present, a case may be hard to prove. Some also contend that even though such a threat may not have occurred, a woman who was not capable in her job might use a sexual harassment complaint as a way to retain her job or receive promotion, without concern for the reputation of the supervisor. The *hostile environment* allegations are much more common, but also more difficult to quantify. The complainant must show "that the harassment was based on his or her gender; that he or she was subjected to unwelcome sexual conduct; that the harassment either affected a term or condition of employment; or the conduct was so serious or pervasive as to have created a hostile or offensive working environment (*Meritor Savings Bank v. Vinson*)." In its 1993–1994 term, the US Supreme Court also ruled unanimously that if the environment "would reasonably be perceived, and is perceived, as hostile or abusive," Title VII was violated and the plaintiff need not show that the harassment had caused them "severe psychological injury," which lower courts had required (*Harris v. Forklift Systems*). This ruling makes it easier for employees or ex-employees to bring suits against their employer.

Why all the attention to sexual harassment issues now, when most women, even if they have themselves not been victims, acknowledge that sexual harassment in the workplace has been going on for a long time, perhaps as long as women have been employed in male-controlled environments? One reason is the visibility that the subject has received in recent years. This includes the accusations leveled against a Supreme Court nominee and a well-known senator and the sexual harassment by Naval officers at the infamous 1991 Tailhook Convention, which was followed by a cover-up and limited punishment. The resignation by a noted female physician from a distinguished university medical school because she was tired of the sexual harassment by some of her male colleagues was followed by an AMA survey in which 41 percent of female physicians indicated that they had been sexually harassed in their practice, primarily by management staff or a colleague. (Another survey revealed that 75 percent had been sexually harassed by patients.) These and other incidents are receiving considerable media attention. As a result of case law and EEOC rulings, an employer is potentially liable for the acts of independent contractors as well as those of management and employees.[8] Such interpretations have served as a catalyst for establishing prevention and training programs to hedge against costly litigation. Many employers are now making greater efforts to sensitize employees to the kinds of behavior that might be seen as hostile environment sexual harassment. Although some harassing behavior, whether verbal or physical, would seem to be clearly identified as such, in reality it may be subject to dispute. What some might find offensive and unwelcome, others would not. It is important that both male and female executives be trained to recognize behavior that might prompt a complaint and that they communicate that such behavior is unacceptable. Complaints should be promptly investigated and resolved, with the offender being educated, counseled, and disciplined appropriately.

Sexual harassment is certainly present in the nurse's workplace, and both male and female nurses are victims. For instance, in an environment that is dominated by women, some male nurses have been on the receiving end of sexual jokes that, if the role were reversed, women would find offensive. In this case, a female executive who is not sensitive to the situation may regard the incident as only good-natured fun.

In 1998, the US Supreme Court clarified the law on sexual harassment in two important decisions (*Burlington Industries v. Ellerth* and *Faragher v. City of Boca Raton*) holding that an employee who resists a supervisor's advances need not suffer a tangible job detriment, such as loss of promotion or dismissal to maintain a lawsuit. The suit, however, cannot succeed if the employer has an anti-harassment policy with an effective complaint procedure and the employee fails to use it.[6]

Other Areas of Discrimination

Once retirement plans were reluctant to give women the same retirement benefits as men. The argument was that women lived longer than men and therefore should not receive as much as men. However, a series of Supreme Court rulings now ban employers from offering retirement plans with unequal benefits for men and women.

Women's rights initiatives that have resulted in legislation include preventing testimony on a rape victim's sexual history and victim's rights in general. However, in the very important area of abortion rights and family planning, the judicial and legislative action changes with the political climate (see Chapter 22).

The fact that action on women's rights has been so fragmented, frequently contradictory, and not always implemented is a major reason that the ERA is still considered so important. The misunderstanding about what it will or will not do has been widespread, particularly in relation to the support and protection of women. (It is important to remember that the ERA prohibits discrimination against either sex.) Some of the projections of what ratification of the ERA would mean in relation to some controversial issues are

1. Decisions about the support obligation of each spouse and about alimony after divorce would be based on individual circumstances and resources, instead of on gender. It is unclear what would happen in the distribution and control of marital property, but presumably property would be equitably distributed, as is presently the law in many states.

2. Women would be permitted to volunteer for military service, or be drafted, if necessary, with appropriate exemption. They would be assigned to duty compatible with their physical and other qualifications and service needs.

3. In school, enrollment in certain kinds of courses could not be limited to a particular sex; only legitimate, activity-related physical qualifications could be used to set restrictions.

4. Labor laws that provide real protection for women would probably remain and be extended to men also, but those barring women from certain occupations would be invalidated.

5. The constitutional right to privacy is expected to permit continued segregation of public toilets and sleeping quarters in dormitories, prisons, and so on.

6. Homosexual marriages would not automatically be permitted or prevented; this issue is generally a state matter.

7. Private or business relationships between men and women would not be affected in any legal sense.

Because some of these changes are already occurring as a result of the action of individual states or courts, or a lack of objection, some will say that enactment of the ERA is not necessary, and that the trend toward equality between women and men is so strong that lack of a constitutional amendment will not stop it. Nevertheless, because trends do not take care of the problems of here-and-now and equal rights decisions, as noted in Chapter 6, and because laws are often inconsistent, grossly unjust treatment for thousands has resulted.

KEY POINTS

1. Laws are man-made, unique to the mores and attitudes of a people, and intended to bring order and justice to their society.

2. The US Constitution is as relevant today as the day it was written.

3. The first 10 amendments to the Constitution are known as the Bill of Rights.

4. The twenty-seventh proposed amendment to the Constitution, the Equal Rights Amendment, was never passed, but many of the changes it hoped to evoke have come to pass anyway.

5. There are three major sources of law: statutory, administrative, and judicial.

6. A system of federal, state, and local courts enforce laws.

7. The right to a trial by jury is guaranteed by the Constitution. The petit jury listens to the evidence and pronounces a verdict. The grand jury determines whether or not a person should be brought to trial before a petit jury.

8. Parents are generally responsible for the support, protection, education, and control of their children.

9. Many changes are occurring in the rights of children to consent to health care.

10. An adult making sexual overtures to children through Internet chat rooms is a new spin on sexual offenses.

11. Sexual harassment may be either quid pro quo (explicit) or by the creation of a hostile environment (implicit).

12. Rulings of the Supreme Court ban the offering of retirement plans with unequal benefits for men and women.

REFERENCES

1. Creasia J, Parker B. *The Bridge to Professional Nursing Practice*, 4th ed. St. Louis, MO: Mosby, 2007, p 256.

2. Creighton H. *Law Every Nurse Should Know*, 5th ed. Philadelphia: Saunders, p 7.

3. National Archives and Documents Administration. The Magna Carta. http://www.archives.gov/exhibits/featured_documents/magna_carta. Retrieved May 10, 2010.

4. The United States Constitution. http://www.usconstitution.net/const.html. Retrieved May 3, 2010.

5. Dumas R. Women and power: Historical perspective. In *Nursing's Influence in Health Policy for the Eighties*. Kansas City, MO: American Academy of Nursing, 1979, pp 68–73.

6. US Department of Labor. Establishing an Effective Anti-harassment Policy. www.dol.gov/oasam/programs/crc/DraftHarassmentPolicy.ppt. Retrieved May 3, 2010.

7. American Association of University Women. Pay Equity Statistics. http://www.aauw.org/act/laf/library/payequity_stats.cfm. Retrieved May 3, 2010.

8. Equal Rights Advocates. Know Your Rights: Sexual Harassment at Work. http://www.equalrights.org/publications/kyr/shwork.asp. Retrieved May 3, 2010.

The Legislative Process

CHAPTER 18

■ IMPORTANCE OF ACTION

The successful functioning of a democracy depends on the willingness of its citizens to participate in their government. Perhaps the most important activity involved in a successful democracy is exercising the right to vote, with understanding of the issues concerned and the potential impact of election of the candidates. Further involvement might include participating actively in campaigns or in organizations that promote or oppose certain legislative issues; contacting legislators about issues; giving testimony at hearings; and even helping to originate and encourage the enactment of specific legislation.

Nurses, particularly, need to take on these responsibilities of citizenship, not only on general principles, but because so much of their professional lives are, and will continue to be, affected by legislation. The nursing practice act of each state controls nursing education and practice and can be eliminated, amended, or totally rewritten in the legislative process. Laws authorizing expanded nursing practice and reimbursement for nursing services can only be enacted if nurses excel in the political arena.

Furthermore, any law involving health care, general education, or almost any other social issue might well have an impact on nursing. For example, at the end of one session of a state legislature, there were 149 bills of interest to nurses in some way. Included were bills for changes in the practice acts of professional nurses, practical nurses, physicians, physical therapists, pharmacists, dentists, and chiropractors; practice of other paramedical workers; treatment of drug addiction; funds for nursing education; funds for scholarships; funds for health facilities; staffing standards; abortion; birth control; malpractice; and matters related to consumer protection. On the national level, existing or pending legislation for Medicare, Medicaid, Social Security, health programs, funding for nursing education, standards for health maintenance organizations (HMOs), nursing research, mental health grants, public health services, workplace protections, labor relations, and more all have an impact on nursing practice.

There has been an increasing recognition that nurses must become involved or find that someone else has made the legislative decisions regarding health care and workplace issues that affect nurses' practice, economic security, and patients. Serving in state legislatures has been an effective training ground for many of these nurses who have gone on to serve in elected and appointed positions nationally. An interesting development is that a number of nurses have successfully run for office. In fact, over half of the states report nurses holding political office on a local or state level; and in 2010, three nurses held seats in the US Congress.

Many students with political know-how are taking a part in influencing legislation at all levels. Nursing students, in their heterogeneous groups of the young and the not-so-young, with their variety of backgrounds, have become increasingly active and their impact has been felt. In one state they were a powerful influence in the enactment of child abuse legislation. Their influence has also been felt at the national level. Although they initially began giving testimony on federal funding for nursing education, along with their licensed nurse colleagues, they have expanded into other public policy issues.

As a group, nurses have become more sophisticated in the legislative process and political action. They have achieved significant steps in developing influence as individuals, and as members of a profession. In part this results from knowledge of the process itself, the ways in which they can make their power felt, and the best time to take action. This chapter presents a pragmatic view of the legislative process, strategies for enhancing nurses' political savvy, and actions to ensure nurses' full participation.

■ BECOMING KNOWLEDGEABLE IN THE LEGISLATIVE PROCESS

There are a number of ways in which nurses can become more knowledgeable in the legislative arena. To begin with, the American Nurses Association (ANA) and its state and local constituent groups take an active part in shaping legislation. Because ANA represents the profession, it may take part in developing a bill, testifying, and lobbying on behalf of its members, and has the responsibility to do so.

The major legislative activities of the nursing organizations are discussed in the chapters on these organizations and in Chapter 19. Pertinent at this point is the means by which members are kept informed about legislation. All major nursing journals, particularly the *American Journal of Nursing*, report key legislative movements on the national level and, if particularly significant, those on the state level. *Capitol Update* is published 10 times a year by ANA and presents legislative, regulatory, and political news on issues that impact nurses. It is available in electronic format at http://www.nursingworld.org/.

Capitol Update is an informative summary of current policy-related issues that ANA is actively pursuing, and it is an excellent resource for nurses, covering a wide range of social policy issues. ANA also uses unscheduled newsletters for action alerts, urging nurses to contact their legislators, the administration, or regulators about a particular issue. State nurses' associations publish legislative newsletters or have legislative sections that describe legislation on national, state, or local levels in their journals, electronically, and through other means of communicating with members. Directors of nursing or heads of nursing education programs often post these legislative newsletters so that all nursing personnel have access to them. (And if not, they can certainly be requested to do so.)

Some institutions have special legislative groups who keep abreast of pertinent legislation and see that the other nurses are informed. Students may be involved in these groups on their own. The National Student Nurses' Association (NSNA), with its various communications, is also a means of gaining current information about legislation important to nursing. The National League for Nursing's (NLN's) newsletters and legislative reports in its journal are excellent, and many specialty organization publications feature legislative updates on topics relevant to their area of practice.

The kind of legislative information available in the newspapers depends on their editorial policies. Feature articles, news stories, and editorials on particular legislation are usually published, and many of them are relevant to nurses and their patients. Some newspapers list the major bills in the state legislature or in Congress and report action taken and current status. They may also report the vote of the legislators of that particular region on major bills. This enables readers not only to follow the action of a particular bill, but also to see how their own legislators vote in general. The League of Women Voters and various political action groups often publish some sort of legislative roundup for varying subscription prices. Legislators may also send newsletters to voters.

There are several ways for individuals to find out the names of their legislators, the numbers of their legislative districts, and where they are supposed to vote. Calling the local Board of Elections is the most reliable way to obtain this information. A local or state League of Women Voters branch will also usually give this information and for a minimal fee will often send pamphlets or more detailed and useful information, such as the committees on which the legislators serve. Similar detailed information might be available from the district and state nurses' association. Another possible source is local political clubs. Probably the best source of information today is the Internet. For your senator, their e-mail address, location in Washington, and phone number go to http://www.senate.gov/general/contact_information/senators_cfm.cfm. Similarly, find your member of the US House of Representatives at http://www.house.gov/house/MemberWWW_by_State.shtml.

It might be educational to see whether family, friends, or neighbors know the names of their legislators. In addition to knowing the national legislators, it is essential to become acquainted with state and local legislators, because of the number of health-related issues that are the responsibility of state and local government.

■ THE LEGISLATIVE SETTING

It is not possible to influence legislation unless there is a clear understanding of how a bill becomes a law and the setting in which this happens. Presumably, legislators, whether state or national, are elected on platforms of their own or their party's that set their goals, and on certain promises for action that they make to their constituents. Fulfillment of these goals and promises, of course, means successful passage of appropriate legislation, but also voting on other, perhaps unforeseen, legislation to the general satisfaction of the folks back home. It is important to remember that most legislators want to be reelected at the same or a higher level, and many of their actions reflect this desire. It is equally important to know that it is not unusual to have hundreds or even thousands of bills introduced in a state assembly (or house) and senate. On the national level, over 25,000 bills may be introduced in the 2-year course of a congressional session. Legislators must have pertinent information on at least those that are likely to be of importance to their areas of interest and constituents. For this, legislators have staffs of varying size, depending on seniority and other factors. The staff total for both houses is well over 19,000 people and rising. Some perform secretarial and other similar duties, but others act as aides, assistants, or researchers. These are individuals who gather, sort out, and sum up background material on key bills and brief the legislator on specific issues and on his or her constituents' feedback. The legislator generally uses this information to decide how to vote. Staff in the legislator's office share the power, if not the glory. Committee staff do the preparatory work that comes before committees and subcommittees, drafting bills, writing amendments to bills, arranging and preparing for public hearings, consulting with people in the areas about which the committee is concerned, providing information, and frequently writing speeches for the legislator.

Because these staff members get information from numerous sources, representatives of organizations, individuals, and lobbyists find it wise to become acquainted with them, maintain good relations, educate them, and provide accurate, pertinent information about the issues with which that particular legislator must deal and about his constituents. When representatives of nursing have not done so, they have found that the information about nursing that a legislator gets may be inaccurate, incomplete, out of date, or simply skewed in the direction favored by another informant.

A measure of the influence a legislator has is placement on committees, where most of the preliminary action on bills occurs. Appointments are influenced or made by party leaders in the House or Senate. It is customary that the chairmanships of committees, extremely powerful positions, are awarded to members of the majority party, usually senior members of the House or Senate, although this is changing as more aggressive younger members have begun to demand a chance to compete for these positions. Some committee assignments are more prestigious than others and are eagerly sought. There are cases in which the chairpersons of some of these committees, particularly on the national level, have remained for years, but the makeup of a committee may change with each new session. The legislator's performance on assigned committees may be a means of gaining attention and prestige with colleagues and constituents, particularly if major issues arise and there is attendant news media coverage. It is, however, not unknown for her or him to lose a favorable position because of clashes with party heads. It is vital to know on which committee your legislators sit, because the action of committees affects the future of a bill. It is also important to know who chairs the major congressional committees with jurisdiction over health care and whether your legislator sits on any of those committees. See Exhibit 18–1 for a listing of congressional committees for health issues. The websites designated earlier also contain information on national committee chairs and membership. Comparable websites are available for each state.

Other useful people to know are the party *whip* at both the state and national levels. They are selected by their party or delegation and have the job of whipping in the vote, seeing that all party members are present for a particular vote or persuading the recalcitrant to vote a certain way. In times of stress, the whips can offer all kinds of political favors. If they fail, the party leaders take over. The function of the whip goes back to 1769, when the British parliamentarian Edmund Burke, in a historic debate in the House of Commons, used the term to describe the members of parliament who had sent for the colleagues of their own party as "whipping them in"—derived from the term *whipper-in*, the man who keeps the hounds from leaving the pack during a hunt.

Influencing the Legislative Process

There are many elements to be considered before a legislative body or even individual legislators make a final decision on how to vote on a piece of legislation. Some are undoubtedly personal—how the legislator feels about an issue. Some are internally political—support of the party leadership or a favor owed to a colleague. But likely to be most influential is the voice of the legislator's *constituency*—the folks back home.

■ **EXHIBIT 18-1.** Key Congressional Committees and Subcommittees with Health Legislation Responsibilities

Committee or Subcommittee	Select Areas of Health Involvement
House of Representatives	
Committee on Energy and Commerce Subcommittee on Health and Environment	Most health programs in DHHS, including Medicaid and Medicare Part B
Committee on Ways and Means Subcommittee on Health	Taxes, Social Security, Medicare Part A
Committee on Appropriations Subcommittee on Labor, Health and Human Services, and Education	Allocation of tax funds in the budget for DHHS health programs, except for Medicare and Medicaid
Committee on Budget (no health subcommittee)	Budget resolutions: Overall priority setting
Committee on Veterans Affairs Subcommittee on Hospitals and Health Care	All veteran's benefits and affairs, oversight of veteran's treatment facilities
Senate	
Committee on Health, Education, Labor and Pension (no health subcommittee)	Most health legislation, jurisdiction over the Public Health Service Act (most programs in DHHS)
Committee on Finance Subcommittee on Health	Taxes, Social Security, Medicare, Medicaid
Committee on Appropriations Subcommittee on Labor, Health, Human Services, and Education	Allocation of tax funds in the budget for DHHS health programs, except Medicare and Medicaid
Committee on Budget (no health subcommittee)	Budget resolutions: Overall priority setting
Committee on Veterans Affairs (no health subcommittee)	All veteran's benefits and affairs, oversight of veteran's treatment facilities

In other words, if the constituents do not see that legislator, whether national or local, voting as they wish, the intractable or insensitive legislator is replaced. Of course, what is important to them may not be the great national or international issues, but those that affect their own lives and livelihood. But just who are these powerful constituents—the ordinary householder or a power conglomerate? Actually they are both, as interested individuals or interest groups.

The purpose of interest groups is basically to represent and promote the policy preferences of their constituents and use the power of the group to influence public decisions that affect them. Interest groups have been categorized as economically motivated, such as business and labor; professionally motivated, with emphasis on service rather than economic gain, such as ANA and the American Medical Association (AMA); and public interest groups that claim to speak for the public or a segment of the public (even if they do not always seem to express popular views), such as the American Civil Liberties Union, Citizen's Coalition for Nursing Home Reform. The reality is that such categorization does not hold in the rough-and-tumble of politics and in today's environment of overlapping interests.

Professional groups may be at odds with each other as they lobby for the interests of their constituents. ANA has been steadfast in the fight to ensure that labor protections apply to nurses. The American Hospital Association (AHA) has vehemently opposed this. The AMA's attempt to exempt physicians from the Federal Trade Commission's authority is unacceptable to ANA where ensuring marketplace competition for the advanced practice nurse is a priority. However, because success in influencing legislation is so often a matter of power through numbers, there is a tendency for a variety of interest groups to form coalitions to support or oppose an issue, sometimes on a very short-term basis. This process of building intricate networks is correctly described as *pluralism*. These coalitions penetrate every socioeconomic stratum and include a variety of strange bedfellows who come together around a mutually important issue. Nursing has been creative and successful in network building, with success in financing research, education, and the prevention of human immunodeficiency virus (HIV) transmission, civil rights, pay equity, pension reform, women's health, nursing home reform, and so on. ANA has long been the convener of women's groups in Washington, a seemingly disparate but powerful coalition of liberals and conservatives, one-issue and broad-based interest groups.

One method used to influence legislation is to support a legislator, either for election or for reelection. In the 1970s, changes in federal election laws limited the amounts that individual donors can give to a political campaign. This created a window of opportunity for political action committees (PACs), or more correctly the political action fund of membership organizations. The PAC became the vehicle for small donors to pool their dollars and support candidates who were sympathetic to the issues of their parent organization. PACs do no direct lobbying. Their only function is to provide financial and other support for political campaigns; they raise and disperse funds. These dollars donated to political campaigns gain access to elected officials who share a political philosophy. The PAC offices may be located in the same space as its parent organization, but funds are not commingled, and budgetary and policy decisions are the responsibility of a separate board of directors.

ANA-PAC can boast of a "war chest" in excess of $1 million for every election cycle (2-year periods) since 1994 (see Chapter 25). ANA-PAC is the fourth largest health care PAC in Washington, only outsized by AMA ($8 million), American Dental Association (ADA) ($6 million), and AHA ($1.5 million). The support of nurses is an even greater asset than dollars; where nurses believe in the candidate, they usually provide a functional grassroots network with a rich spirit of volunteerism. In the most recent election cycle the ANA-PAC endorsed 103 candidates for public office, with an 89 percent success rate.[1] Currently the ANA-PAC is reconsidering its strategy. Will nursing achieve more legislative support if fewer candidates are endorsed and more funds and volunteerism are provided for a select few?

PACs are criticized for the dollars they give and the influence they wield. Periodically, a consumer group will publish a legislator's voting record, matching it to the source of campaign contributions—and they do match more often than not. Although the public may be poised to demand some type of financing reform, the cost of political campaigns has spiraled well into the millions, and reform efforts have been frustrating and largely unsuccessful.

In 1993, ANA established a grassroots network, Nurses Strategic Action Team (N-STAT). N-STAT consists of a leadership corps of nurses who are highly invested in political action and are members of their state nurses' association. These volunteers participate in a rapid response network to exert pressure on behalf of nursing's issues. Additionally, ANA's Government Affairs Department recently established the Nurse Political Action Leaders (N-PAL) program. This program, in conjunction with N-STAT, is the heart of ANA's efforts to ensure that members of Congress hear the voice of nursing. N-PAL and N-STAT both promote grassroots action. ANA members who are chosen as Nurse Political Action Leaders will be ANA's liaisons to legislators and their staff in assigned legislative districts. ANA and its state association collaborate to appoint an N-PAL volunteer for each Congressional District and for each senator.[2] Members with a personal connection to their legislator are particularly sought. Individually, they build liaisons with specific federal legislators. They supply these legislators and their staff with information on health care issues, educate them to nursing's positions, recommend to the PAC Board of Trustees regarding candidate endorsement for reelection, and participate in campaign activities if this legislator proves to be an advocate for nursing. ANA-PAC endorsements of candidates for the US Congress are always reviewed by the state.

Another important component of lawmaking is lobbying. *Lobbying* is generally defined as an attempt to influence a decision of a legislature or other governmental body. Because it is a type of petition for redress of grievances, lobbying is constitutionally guaranteed. Lobbying exists at several levels, from a single individual who contacts a legislator about a particular issue of personal importance to the interest groups that carefully (and often expensively) organize systems for monitoring legislation, initiating action, or blocking action on matters that concern them. Lobbying is a subtle dance, often two steps forward and one back. The important thing is to be clear on the bottom line of your lobbying efforts.[3] What are the principles that are nonnegotiable? An example may help here. The nursing home reforms of 1987 were to assure the significant presence of registered nurses (RNs) in long-term care (LTC) facilities. During the staging and refinement of this legislation, the word *registered* was replaced by *licensed*. ANA felt that it was better to accept some gain and work toward a higher standard in subsequent legislation. Others felt that a principle had been sacrificed and the legislation should have been stopped from proceeding.

Professional lobbyists must be registered with the Clerk of the House and the Secretary of the Senate. They spend all or part of their time representing the interests of a particular group or groups. A good lobbyist makes it his or her business to know everyone and to cultivate such friendships. There are numerous ways in which lobbyists attempt to influence legislators; much lobbying is done on a personal level, sometimes in the semisocial setting of a lunch, dinner, cocktail party, golf date, or other such activity. Lobbyists provide information to legislators and their staff (not necessarily objectively) and introduce resource people to them. Lobbyists are knowledgeable in the ways of legislation and are often familiar with legislators' personalities and idiosyncrasies. They are invaluable in keeping their interest group informed about any pertinent legislation and the problems involved, and in aiding the group in taking effective action. It has been said that the skill with which a lobbyist monitors, analyzes, and participates in the political process is a major influence on success, but one should never minimize the ability of an interest group with its passion over an issue and its unique blend of resources to sway opinion among those who are neutral and opposed, as well as to hold the allegiance of allies.

A skilled lobbyist can have great influence on lawmakers, and many times this is all to the good. When done properly and controlled, lobbying is a desirable and accepted way of bringing important information and sound arguments to the attention of legislators. In this sense, lobbyists act as ombudsmen. Unfortunately, some lobbyists present biased information to influence opinions and decisions in a group's favor. Lobbying may lead to bribery, which has already created state and national scandals and caused great public concern, as mentioned earlier in this chapter. Legal measures have been taken to curb dishonest lobbying, rarely with complete success. The Congressional Reform Act of 1946 requires federal lobbyists to register and file statements of expenses incurred to influence legislation.

This organized approach to lobbying exists at both the federal and state levels. Effective though it is, it should not overshadow the efforts of the individual who, in effect, lobbies when she or he contacts the appropriate legislator about an issue. Groups such as nurses, who do not necessarily have millions of dollars to spend, have proven to be very effective in lobbying by coordinating the efforts of individuals for unified action on an issue important to nursing. Therefore, how well and how much the individual citizen lobbies can be crucial in political action.

The most effective influence comes from the constituency of a legislator. Commonly called *grassroots lobbying*, it may take the form of telephone calls, telegrams, and letter-writing campaigns, as well as letters to the editor, press conferences, and various other media activities. It is often most effective if it includes not only the group most involved, but also other influential people.

Influencing the legislative process requires first of all, information, and second, lobbying strategies. Later in the chapter, some sources of information are listed, as well as effective techniques for grassroots lobbying.

■ HOW A BILL BECOMES A LAW

Anyone can initiate a bill. Legislation is basically a citizen's demand for action because of discontentment with an existing situation or because of an emerging need. A vocal group is more likely to get action than one that is silent. A citizen who takes his or her complaints to a legislator is more likely to get a response than one who just complains. And the larger and more politically active the complainer group, the better the chance of being heard. There have been instances of legislation based on the concerns of one individual, but most commonly groups, which may or may not be organized, suggest ideas for a bill. Some common originators of bills are organizations representing various interest groups; a governmental administrator, agency, or department; a delegation of citizens in a legislator's district; a legislative committee; or the legislator him- or herself. A prolific source of legislation is the executive communication—a letter from the President, a member of his Cabinet, or the head of an independent agency transmitting a draft of a proposed bill to the Speaker of the House and the President of the Senate. This communication is then referred to the standing committee that has jurisdiction over that particular subject matter. The chairman of that committee usually introduces the bill promptly, either in the form received or with changes he or she considers necessary or desirable.

In general, the enactment of a law follows the same procedure in all states and the federal government (Exhibit 18–2). The differences are slight and do not have an effect on the citizen's participation in the legislative process.

Basically, there are two types of bills: authorizations and appropriations. An *authorization* bill is a legislative prerequisite for an appropriations bill. Congress passes authorizing legislation to initiate or continue a federal agency or program, establish program policies, and put a ceiling on monies that can be used to finance programs. Once an authorization bill is passed, the appropriations process determines the actual amount of funds that will be available for that particular piece of legislation.

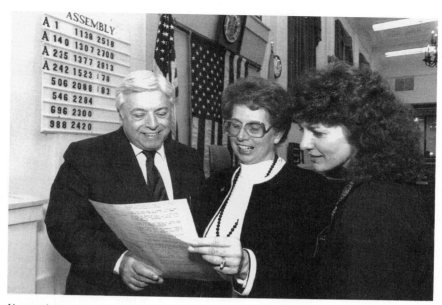

Nurses have a natural talent as legislators. Here Assemblywoman Barbara Wright (R—NJ) discusses a bill with colleagues. (Courtesy of the New Jersey State Nurses Association)

To keep the explanation of the process as simple as possible, introduction of a bill in the House of Representatives will be used as an illustration. Only the major steps are given, but the details, which can be quite complex, are both useful and interesting and can be found in a variety of basic books on the legislative process.

A bill may be sponsored or introduced by one or more legislators. The legislator whose name appears first on the bill is often known as the author and has the responsibility for the procedural handling of the bill. Although a legislator may be requested to sponsor a bill simply because he or she is from an interested citizen's district, sophisticates in legislation choose more carefully. The more senior, more prestigious a legislator is, the better the chance for a bill's enactment. Bipartisan sponsorship is desirable, but on occasion a key member of the majority party alone can be just as effective. To have one or more sponsors who are members of the committees to which the bill will be sent is also a highly strategic factor. Junior members of Congress often seek senior cosponsors to enhance the opportunity for their bills to succeed.

Before a bill can be introduced, it must be put into legal language. Although an organization may have its own knowledgeable attorney to do this, the bill is always put in its final form by a government legislative counsel. The drafting of statutes is an art requiring considerable skill and experience.

After introduction in the House (which is commonly called putting the bill in the hopper), the bill is assigned a number by the Speaker. (The *Speaker of the House* is a member selected by the House membership to preside and is usually of the majority party.) Numbers are given consecutively as bills are introduced in each session; if the bill is reintroduced in the next session, it is unlikely to have the same number. The number is preceded by an HR in the House (an A or AB for Assembly in some states) or an S in the Senate. When the bill is read in the House by its number only, that is known as the first reading. (In the Senate the sponsor introduces the bill more fully.) The Speaker then refers the bill to an appropriate committee or subcommittee (health, education, judiciary, etc.) and the bill is released for printing. Usually the printed bill includes the branch of Congress, the legislative session, bill number, by whom introduced, date, committee referral, and amendment to particular law (if pertinent). Consecutive numbers precede each line of the bill for easy reference. Definitions of key words may be given. Amendments to existing laws may be shown by having deleted words or phrases crossed out or put in parentheses and having new words or phrases put in italics or underlined.

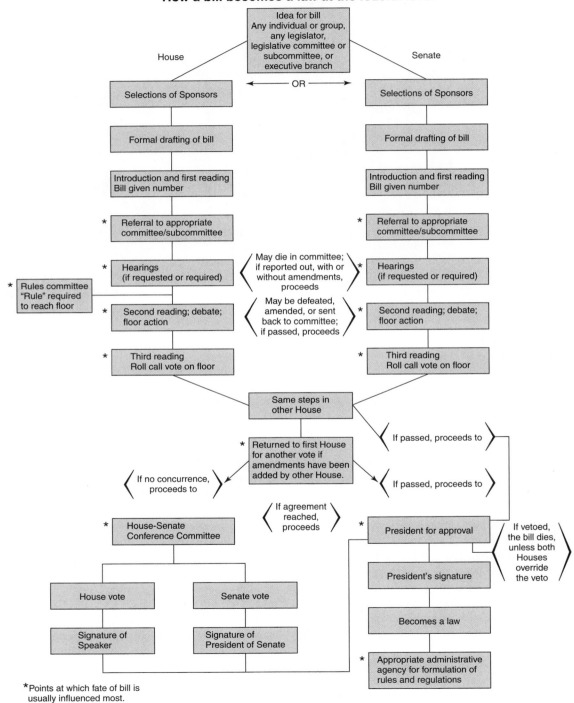

THE LEGISLATIVE PROCESS
How a bill becomes a law at the federal level

*Points at which fate of bill is usually influenced most.

EXHIBIT 18–2. The legislative process.

Copies of bills may be obtained from the sponsor or from one's own senator or representative. Better yet, in the spirit of Thomas Jefferson, legislative information including the text, summaries, and status of federal bills can be obtained electronically from the Library of Congress at http://Thomas.Loc.gov.

A great deal of a legislator's time is spent in committee. Some committees may go on simultaneously with the House session, and when the bell rings to indicate a roll call, members quickly go to vote, presumably having made their decisions previously. The committee to which the bill is referred is the first place where its fate can be influenced. If the bill is never put on the committee agenda or is not approved, it will generally proceed no further. The chairman has the power to keep the bill off the agenda or, conversely, to introduce it early or at a favorable time.

Open or public hearings may be held, at which any interested person may present testimony. The date and time of public hearings are published. The committee then considers the bill—sometimes in executive (closed) session, if it is so agreed by open roll-call vote—and either kills it or approves it (reports it out) with or without amendments, or drafts a new bill. This activity is called *mark-up*.

Committee action is determined by a voice vote or roll call, but no record is kept of individual votes. (For this reason, there is some pressure toward having open committee meetings and voting.) For favorable action, the majority of the total committee must vote affirmatively. To get the desired vote, interested persons begin their legislative action at the committee level. Letters, phone calls, telegrams, faxes, and personal contact are used in reaching the chairman and other committee members. This is usually most effective if done by the legislator's own constituents, by whom he or she is understandably more influenced. Here, also, written testimony or oral statements can be given. ANA and other nursing groups regularly testify at congressional hearings. Their expert witnesses have helped win passage of key pieces of legislation.

In Congress, the Director of the Congressional Budget Office submits a financial estimate of the cost of the measure if enacted. This is included in the report written by a member of the committee. If the bill is recommended for passage, it is listed on the calendar and is sent to the Rules Committee (House only). In the House, the Rules Committee, with more majority than minority members, is most powerful; it can block the bill or clear it for debate. Presumably, the purpose is to provide some degree of selectivity in the consideration of measures by the House. The Rules Committee may also limit debate on the bill at the second reading. If a bill is blocked (no rule obtained), a discharge petition signed by a certain percentage of the House members can obtain its release from the Committee and access it to the floor, but this seldom occurs.

A bill that survives all committee action is then scheduled for action *on the floor*, meaning the total membership of the House. When the bill and number are read, that becomes the second reading. Amendments may be proposed at this stage and are approved or rejected by the majority.

Moving the previous question cuts off debate. If it is carried, the Speaker asks, "Shall the bill be engrossed and read a third time?" If approved, first the amendments and then the bill are voted on; if the required number of objections exist, action may be postponed. If a group whose bill of interest seems to be in danger of defeat (or the reverse, if the aim is defeat) can influence at least the minimum number of congressmen to object, they can buy time to try some other approach to achieve their goals. Delay may also be desired if the amendments appended in committee or in the House are undesirable to concerned individuals. Locking on amendments to a bill that seems sure to pass is a technique for putting through some action that might not succeed on its own and that may be only remotely or not at all connected to the content of the original bill. For instance, in one year in which the administration wanted to authorize only $12.2 million for the Nurse Training Act, the congressionally approved appropriation of $52.5 million was tagged on to another appropriations bill that the President could not veto for political reasons. Nursing also achieved many successes through amendments to the Omnibus Budget Reconciliation Acts (OBRA), traditionally one of the last bills to be brought to the Congress at the close of a session, with a positive vote necessary to comply with budget requirements. Nursing was successful in nursing home reform, creating community nursing organizations, and a variety of reimbursement options for nurses. On the other hand, amendments that are totally unacceptable to the bill's sponsors may be added as a mechanism to force withdrawal or defeat of the bill. In general, amendments are introduced to strengthen, broaden, or curtail the intent of the original bill or law. If passed, they may change its character considerably. When debate is closed, the vote is taken by roll call and recorded. Passage requires a majority vote of the total House or a two-thirds vote for certain types of legislation. (Some legislators who, for some reason, do not wish to commit themselves to a vote find it convenient to be absent at the roll call.)

If the bill is passed, it goes to the Senate for a complete repetition of the process it went through in the House, and with the same opportunities to influence its passage. A bill introduced in the Senate follows the same general route with certain procedural differences. Also, the president of the Senate is the vice president of the United States.

A major difference between the House and the Senate is that bills that are not objected to are taken up in their order and debated. There is no Rules Committee. *Filibustering* is also a unique senatorial process—a motion to consider a bill that has been objected to is debatable, and senators opposed to it may speak to it as long as they please, thus preventing or defeating action by long delays. It takes a three-fifths vote to invoke cloture (closing debate and taking an immediate vote). This is quite difficult to achieve for political reasons of senatorial courtesy.

At times, the same or a similar bill is introduced in both houses on certain important issues. The introduction of bills for nursing funding is an example. If these bills are not the same when passed by each house, or if another single bill has been amended by the second house after passing the first and the first does not concur on the amendments, the bill is sent to a conference committee consisting of an equal number of members of each house. The conference committee tries to work out a compromise that will be accepted by both houses. Sometimes the two houses are not able to arrive at a compromise and the bill dies, but usually an agreement is reached and the compromise version of the bill is returned to each house for approval.

After passing both houses and being signed by each presider, the bill goes to the President, who may obtain opinions from federal agencies, the Cabinet, and other sources. If he signs it or fails to take action within 10 days, the bill becomes law. The President may choose the latter route if he does not approve of the bill, but for political reasons, such as a big margin of votes, cannot afford to veto it. He may also veto the bill and return it to the house of origin with his objections. A two-thirds affirmative vote in both houses for repassage is necessary to override the veto. Because voting on a veto is often along party lines, overriding a veto in both houses is difficult. The National Center for Nursing Research was established in 1985 through a veto override of a National Institutes of Health authorization bill, demonstrating the political strength of nurses and others who lobbied for the bill. If the Congress adjourns before the 10 days in which the President should sign the bill, it does not become law. This is known as a *pocket veto*. All bills that become law are assigned numbers, not the same as their original number, are printed, and are attached to the proper volume of statutes.

Another type of legislation is a resolution. *Joint resolutions* originating in either house are, for all practical purposes, treated as a bill but have the whereas-resolved format. Concurrent resolutions usually relate to matters affecting both houses. They are not considered law, but are used to express facts, principles, opinions, and purposes of the two houses. They do not require the President's signature if passed. These are identified as *H. Con. Res.* or *S. Con. Res.* and a number. Simple resolutions concern the operation of one house alone and are considered only by the body in which they are introduced. They are designated as *H. Res.* or *S. Res.* and a number. State legislatures use similar procedures.

One of the criticisms of the legislative process is that action is slow at the beginning of a session and relatively few bills are introduced, debated, and voted on. Many bills may be introduced near the end of a session and receive inadequate attention. It is not unusual for a tremendous number of bills to be acted on in the last weeks of a session (often passed), with some question as to whether they have been studied carefully. A technique used by some state legislatures is *stopping the clock*; the clock is figuratively stopped before midnight of the last day of the session (which has been predetermined) and all-night legislative action goes on until the necessary bills, frequently budgetary in nature, are acted on.

With so many checks and balances provided by due process of law in this democratic government, often accompanied by extreme political pressure from within the government and the influence of lobbyists, one can readily understand why it is so difficult and time-consuming to translate an idea for legislation into statutory law, urgent though the need may seem to those who originated and promoted it. Some policy makers contend that this type of deliberating safeguards Congress against acting in an impulsive manner.

A particularly good illustration of the time-consuming nature of policy making is the federal budget process (Exhibit 18–3). It is important to keep in mind that the federal government's fiscal year is designated by the calendar year in which it ends. Thus, the period from October 1, 2010, to September 30, 2011, is fiscal year 2011. Also, the budget process originates in the Executive Branch, wherein each agency submits its budget requests 2 years in advance of the intended fiscal year.

The President (Executive Branch) submits his budget to Congress for the next fiscal year in approximately January or February. The Congressional Budget Office (CBO) completes its analysis and forwards the budget to the House and Senate Budget Committees where hearings are held and a congressional budget plan is drafted for each respective legislative chamber. By May, a budget resolution is developed, which is a compromise between the two houses. While this process is occurring, appropriations committees in the Congress are considering the dollar amounts that should be allocated to new and continuing programs. These amounts are then incorporated into the budget as proposed. Subsequently, the Office of Management and Budget (Executive Branch) and CBO independently estimate the final amount of the budget (balanced, deficit, or surplus). Once their analysis of the budget has been reconciled, final action is taken on the appropriation bills. In most states the governor has the prerogative to make line-item vetoes, therefore carving out parts of a bill (authorization or appropriation) without vetoing its entirety, often for the sake of economy. This right does not exist at the federal level, seeing it as vesting too much power in the executive branch (president) of government. This is a very debatable point of law, and the scholar should seek to inquire more about it. The line-item veto has been found unconstitutional by the Supreme Court. The Court sees a Constitutional amendment as necessary to its enactment.[4]

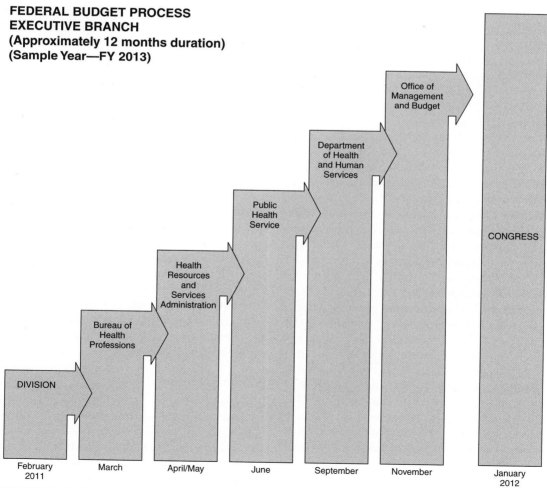

FEDERAL BUDGET PROCESS
EXECUTIVE BRANCH
(Approximately 12 months duration)
(Sample Year—FY 2013)

Office of Management and Budget

Department of Health and Human Services

Public Health Service

Health Resources and Services Administration

Bureau of Health Professions

DIVISION

CONGRESS

February 2011   March   April/May   June   September   November   January 2012

EXHIBIT 18–3. The federal budget process (Adapted from DHHS, FMB, BHPr.)

If final action has not occurred by the beginning of the new fiscal year, Congress passes a continuing resolution, which provides access to money to run the government until final approval of a complete budget. The reader is also alerted that each bill, as it is presented, includes a financial analysis. In passing legislation, Congress authorizes a set amount of dollars for the programs in the legislation. In effect, this authorization sets a ceiling on the amount. Program amounts are then considered again during the budget process, and specific amounts are appropriated. In other words, a piece of legislation with a 3-year program commitment cannot be included in the budget until an appropriation amount is determined, and this is not always the amount authorized. Exhibit 18–3 depicts the budget process, from its beginning in the Division of Nursing to presentation to Congress, where it takes yet another 9 months for completion.

However, action on a law does not end with its enactment. Laws are usually general; too much specificity makes them obsolete too rapidly and requires another trip through the legislative process to add amendments. Therefore, through the process of rule making, the governmental agency or department within whose purview the law falls develops rules and regulations. For instance, rule making to allow enforcement of the Nursing Practice Act is the responsibility of the department under which the state board of nurse examiners falls. On the national level, health legislation is sent to DHHS. Advisory committees of citizens are usually appointed, as spelled out by the law or the department. There is public notice of hearings for the proposed rules so that interested individuals may respond. These are published in the *Federal Register*. (States have comparable publications.) Regulations have the force of law. ANA and other nursing organizations are affected by regulations that DHHS promulgates such as standards for nursing home care, Medicare, or family planning. It is possible to influence the interpretation of legislation at this point and to strengthen or weaken the intent of the law. For example, rules and regulations that delineate a particular piece of legislation, such as nursing home reform, may be flexible, rigid, or extremely loose, and a facility must adhere to them to become and remain approved. The opportunity to contribute to the development of regulations is available to interested organizations, which may make recommendations for individual appointments on advisory committees or offer informal participation and cooperation. They may also testify at the hearings on regulations. Regulations have been changed after hearings because of major protests by interested groups, the presentation of well-thought-out alternative regulations, or letters written in response to proposed rules. The role of the public is to provide information, education, and interpretation to the regulatory agency. It is illegal to lobby at this point in process.

■ NURSES AND POLITICAL ACTION

As noted in Chapter 16, nurses, both as individuals and as a group, are becoming more politically active for a variety of reasons. On the political scene, momentum has been building for a number of years, and organizations such as the ANA, NLN, AACN, and American Organization of Nurse Executives (AONE) have taken leadership roles in mobilizing nurses in grassroots lobbying efforts. Among the approaches are educational programs and political consciousness-raising sessions both to teach nurses techniques and strategies and to make them aware of issues. ANA and other nursing organizations have set up networks, where the lobbyist or a monitoring group in the state or national capital alerts the organization about the status of a bill at a crucial time and an action plan begins. Usually not all members are mobilized, only select volunteers. The network is activated through a state legislative committee and a telephone tree that passes on the "act now" directive, or simply by mailgram, first-class mail, e-mail, or fax. If, as often true, mass action is not needed, the difficult part is to select the nurses who are best suited for the situation. For instance, if the legislator is particularly sensitive to a constituency such as the elderly, an influential citizen, or a particular part of the legislator's district, the member(s) fitting that category are called on to act. Another type of categorization is by expertise. It is essential for any serious political group to develop a coded database that classifies each volunteer according to select characteristics that fit most political situations. Using but not overusing the network is also essential to success, as is follow through to determine what worked and what did not.

Personal Contact

It is sensible for nurses to become acquainted with their legislators before a legislative crisis occurs. This gives them the advantage of having made personal contact and shown general interest, and gives the legislator or staff member the advantage of a reference point. In small communities, legislators often know many of their constituents on a first-name basis through frequent contacts. This personal

interested in the legislators' positions, attitudes, and problems. Nurses who generally agree with their legislator's approach will find that it is also politically astute to contribute to a reelection campaign or offer their services in the campaign. These might include house-to-house canvassing to check voter registration or to register voters; supplying transportation to the polls; making telephone calls to stimulate registration and voting; acting as a registration clerk, poll challenger, block leader, or precinct captain; raising funds; preparing mailing pieces; planning publicity; writing and distributing news releases; making speeches; answering telephones and staffing information booths; planning campaign events; or having coffees to meet the candidate. Groups or organizations can become more extensively involved if they are able to do so legally and financially. Most nurses who have participated in political action have found it stimulating and educational.

Testifying at Hearings

Committee hearings are intended to get the opinions of citizens on particular bills or issues. Student nurses and nurses can be effective speakers for health care but, if poorly prepared, can cause just as negative an impact.

Attending public hearings of the committee to which health issues are referred is both an educational experience and a good preliminary before testifying yourself. It provides an opportunity to become more familiar with the atmosphere and setting of hearings, as well as the attitudes and personalities of the committee members, and to become acquainted with them individually.

It may be disconcerting for someone testifying to find only the chairman present at a hearing or, on the other hand, to find a full committee and hundreds in the audience. A nurse or organization may or may not be specifically invited to give testimony. Either way, it is a courtesy (and may be mandatory) to notify the committee of the intent to appear or to request placement on the agenda and provide a copy of the testimony if possible. Prior presentation of testimony does not exclude the possibility of adding appropriate remarks verbally or in answer to committee questions.

It can have a negative effect to request the opportunity to present testimony if the bill is of marginal interest or if a statement inserted in the record would serve as well. Testimony should be prepared well in advance, or as much as possible, because hearings may be called on short notice and sloppy testimony is worse than none. The ground rules applicable to the hearing (time limitations, length of testimony, number of copies to be submitted, and deadline

for submitting advance copies) should be requested from the committee staff and be followed.

Legislators, lobbyists, and others interested in legislative action have suggested some guidelines for giving testimony before legislative bodies.

1. Be prepared to adjust your schedule so that you can participate as the committee schedule permits. Hearings may start late, be cut short, run late into the night, be recessed and reconvened later, or otherwise changed.

2. Learn about your audience in advance, with accurate names and titles. Pronounce names correctly.

3. Although you have the right to disagree with your professional organization, totally independent action confuses the issues for legislators. It is better to work within the organization, ironing out differences. A collective voice usually carries more weight than isolated testimony.

4. Pay attention to protocol; be sure to thank the committee for the opportunity to address it.

5. Introduce yourself with a very brief biographical sketch; state the issue on which you are testifying, and note whether you represent a group or only yourself.

6. If the testimony is in writing and has been given to the committee, they may prefer that the information be briefly recapitulated rather than read completely. Be prepared with both a long and a short text.

7. Be brief and concise (about 10 to 15 minutes); discuss only the specific bill or issue concerned, refrain from irrelevant comments, and speak plainly and without professional jargon. Relate your arguments to people, not abstractions.

8. Be secure in your knowledge of the facts, totally honest, and comfortable in speaking to a group. Have additional data available to help in answering questions accurately. It is disastrous to present false information or a dishonest interpretation. If possible, know the data on which your testimony is based and do not simply read a statement prepared by someone else.

9. When being questioned, it helps to be able to think under pressure, remain cool, not become angry, and have a sense of humor. (Some legislators use committee hearings as stages; some may not be friendly to the nurse's cause; others have predetermined ideas and prefer to keep them.) Never try to bluff; if you do not know the answer, it is best to say so and perhaps volunteer to provide the answer to the committee before the vote or have it placed in the record.

10. As in any other situation, appearance is important. Be appropriately dressed; a uniform is not appropriate except in unusual circumstances.

11. Be aware that appearing at a hearing is often all that is necessary. Testifying may not be the best action for various reasons and should not be forced. The appearance of a large number of nurses and students at a hearing indicates that it is of major concern to them. Behavior should be courteous. This is also no time for intraprofessional quarreling.

12. Be aware that everyone appearing before a committee represents a special interest group; legislators weigh conflicting views to make their own decision.

13. Do not be alarmed or disillusioned if the vote goes against you at the hearing. Votes may have been promised to colleagues at this initial stage, even before the hearing, but may be reversed on the floor. If the bill is filed, a new version may be introduced, with changes made to minimize the opposition.

14. Always be courteous, whether in the audience or testifying. Catcalls, boos, or similar noises from the audience are not taken well. Even certain kinds of body language can have a negative effect. In one televised hearing, a senator on the side of those testifying chastised them for rolling their eyes and making other gestures at the words of another committee member.

Politics is often a matter of compromise. Adherents of a bill must be prepared to yield on some issues as necessary, meanwhile holding firm on the most vital issues and allowing opponents to compromise on these points. Most of all, it is essential that nurses continue to be involved in political action, becoming ever more knowledgeable, sophisticated, and effective.

4. A program may be approved in legislation, but there are no dollars for operation until success in the appropriation process.

5. PACs are criticized for the dollars they give and the influence they wield.

6. The most effective influence comes from the local constituency of a legislator and is known as *grassroots lobbying*.

7. A bill becomes a law through a long, tortuous process filled with checks and balances.

REFERENCES

1. Capitol Update. The ANA-PAC's Political Endorsement Process. March 5, 2010. http://www.capitolupdate.org/index.php/tag/ana-pac/. Retrieved May 3, 2010.

2. ANA. Wanted: Nurse Political Action Leaders. www.nursingworld.org/mainmenucategories/ANApoliticalpower/federal. Retrieved May 12, 2010.

3. Joel LA. Policy Development in nursing. In Dickson G, Flynn L (Eds): *Policy—A Nursing Phenomenon.* New York: Del Mar, 2008, pp 319–328.

4. Wikipedia. Line-Item Veto. http://en.wikipedia.org/wiki/Line-item_veto#Line_Item_Veto_Re-enactment_Activity_of_2009. Retrieved May 12, 2010.

KEY POINTS

1. The success of a democracy depends on the willingness of its citizens to participate in the process of government.

2. The Internet provides endless networks for the retrieval of information related to governmental affairs.

3. A measure of the influence of a legislator is his or her committee assignment.

CHAPTER 19

Major Legislation Affecting Nursing

Federal and state laws have a major impact on nursing practice and education. At the state level, nurses need to know about their own nursing practice acts, and they should be acquainted with the licensure laws of other health practitioners. These are discussed in Chapter 20. Other state legislation affecting the health and welfare of nurses may be equally important, and nurses should keep abreast of both proposed and enacted legislation. One of the best ways to keep informed is to be an active member of a nursing association. Such organizations provide leadership and information that is invaluable for nurses who want to have input into health care policy.

This chapter focuses on federal legislation that affects the practice of nursing and the rights of nurses. State laws will be discussed only as they pertain to federal issues. Obviously, there are a plethora of health bills and laws that are relevant to nursing, but only those that have particular significance will be highlighted here.

■ OVERVIEW OF FEDERAL AGENCIES

The federal agencies with responsibility for health care are primarily within the Department of Health and Human Services (DHHS), although other departments administer certain health-related programs. An example is the Food Stamps Program, which the Department of Agriculture administers. Within DHHS, there are 11 major agencies. Those most central to our discussion here are the Centers for Medicare and Medicaid Services (CMS), the Agency for Healthcare Research and Quality (AHRQ), National

Institutes of Health (NIH), Centers for Disease Control and Prevention (CDC), Health Resources and Services Administration (HRSA), the Substance Abuse and Mental Health Services Administration (SAMHSA), and the Food and Drug Administration (FDA). In 1994, Congress passed legislation that authorized a separate Social Security Administration, effective March 31, 1995. Until then, the Social Security Administration was an agency within DHHS, but legislators presumed that making it a separate entity might help increase its visibility, accountability, and administrative efficiency.

The Centers for Medicare and Medicaid Services (CMS), formerly HCFA, administer the Medicare and Medicaid programs. The Division of Nursing within the HRSA and the National Institute of Nursing Research (NINR) at the NIH are focal points for nursing initiatives at the federal level and are discussed later in this chapter. However, nurses are involved in every agency listed, and the activities of each agency have an impact on nursing practice. It behooves nursing students and faculty to be knowledgeable about them and provide input whenever possible. It is also important to note that the organization of federal programs for health and social services often undergoes revisions, especially at the beginning of a new presidential administration. Thus, the structures depicted in Exhibit 19–1 are subject to change at any point.

Follow-up of federal legislation requires close attention. In addition to the law itself, regulations implementing the law are also important. On one hand, some legislators have charged that regulations circumvent or exceed the intent of

356

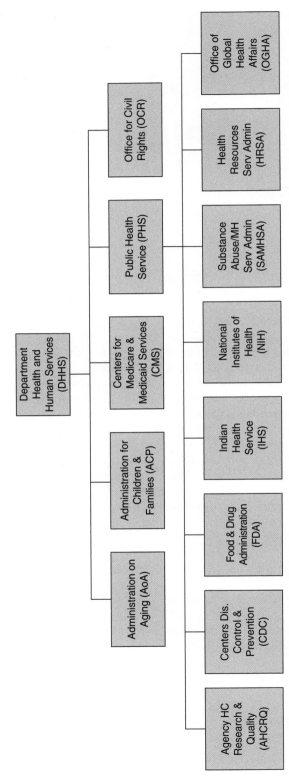

EXHIBIT 19–1. US Department of Health and Human Services: Operating Divisions of Particular Importance to Nursing

the law. On the other hand, especially with controversial issues, lawmakers have been known to omit details in legislation and leave them to the regulatory agency to finalize. Federal agencies—such as the FDA and Federal Trade Commission (FTC)—are created by law and responsible for particular issues. Agency decisions can affect nursing practice, as illustrated by various examples throughout this chapter.

■ SOCIAL POLICY AS A CONTEXT FOR HEALTH CARE

Health care is one facet of America's complex social policy scheme. Compared with other industrialized nations, the United States has been reluctant to establish a government-sponsored social policy system. The Patient Protection and Affordable Care Act of 2010 aims to provide health care services for every American through a combination of personal responsibility and government-sponsored initiatives. Though there will essentially be universal coverage once all of the provisions of the bill are developed, its good is accomplished by a union of public and private sector resources. This is a far cry from the government-provided social welfare programs that are common in many other countries. Government-sponsored health care has been alien to the traditional American belief that individuals should be self-sufficient and the strong emphasis that Americans have traditionally placed on individualism and market economics. Subsequently, over the course of the twentieth century, political trends and factors have produced a patchwork of social welfare programs in the United States.

One of the earliest social insurance programs developed in the United States was for what is known as *Social Security*. The origin, funding, authorization, and development of Social Security are relevant to those of other social and health programs.

Social Security

Beginning in the mid-1920s there was a growing sense that federal and state governments should play a larger role in helping to meet people's unmet needs, and that certain risks of a growing industrialized nation could best be met through the development of social insurance programs. By the late 1920s, almost every state had enacted some type of workers' compensation program. But these programs could hardly meet the growing needs of individuals and families in an industrialized state. The economic depression of the

1930s intensified the urgency for some type of government intervention in social policies and culminated in the Social Security Act of 1935. The lawmakers who produced the original act based it on the conviction that a program of economic security must have as its primary aim the assurance of an adequate income to each human being in childhood, youth, middle age, or old age—in sickness or in health—and that it must provide safeguards against all of the hazards leading to destitution and dependency.[1]

The Social Security Act (SSA) is the origin of most health and social welfare in this country. Each *title* (or component) covers a specific social program. The act is far broader than the Social Security program. Its later amendments provide many benefits: federal Old-Age and Survivors Insurance (OASI); unemployment compensation; federal grants-in-aid to states to promote special health and welfare services for children; and matching funds to help finance state-administered relief programs for dependent children and other needy persons who are aged, blind, or permanently disabled. *Disability* insurance programs were enacted in 1956. Since 1965, the *Medicare program* (Title XVIII of the SSA) has financed a large share of the medical and hospital costs of persons over 65. Title XIX, *Medicaid*, passed at the same time, was a hasty compromise on the part of Congress and can probably be best described as a cooperative federal-state medical assistance program for the poor or near-poor. Medicare and Medicaid are discussed in detail later in this chapter.

Old-Age and Survivors Insurance

The average citizen who talks about Social Security is typically referring to the federal Old-Age, Survivors, and Disability Insurance (OASDI) program. OASDI provides a monthly payment from the federal government to replace, in part, the income that is lost to a worker and his or her family when the wage earner retires, becomes disabled, or dies. OASDI has two components: Social Security and disability. Although the funding mechanisms are similar, the administration of the two programs is somewhat different.

Contributions to OASDI are made under the Federal Insurance Contributions Act (FICA) of the Internal Revenue Code through a dedicated payroll tax. In most cases, coverage is universal and compulsory for all employees. Approximately 95 percent of all jobs in this country are covered through contributions made by employees, even if self-employed, and matching taxes paid by employers. Employee contributions are withheld from wage and salary payments. They are based on wages and earnings up to an annual maximum taxable wage base and appear on employees' paycheck stubs under FICA. In 2010, employers and employees each paid 6.2 percent of wages up to the taxable maximum of $106,800, while the self-employed paid 12.4 percent up to that same wage base. In 2010, 87 percent of total OASI and DI income came from payroll. The remainder, or 11 percent, came from interest earnings, and 2 percent came from the taxation of OASDI benefits. The payroll tax rates are set by law for OASI and DI. This wage/earnings base rises as average wages increase.[2] As discussed later in this chapter, a similar but separate mechanism exists for financing Medicare.

Monthly cash benefits under Social Security were paid to almost 53 million individuals in 2010. These included retired workers and their dependents (37.8 million) and their eligible survivors (6.4 million), and qualified disabled individuals and their dependents (9.8 million). Benefits awarded through the Social Security program amounted to $7.7 trillion in 2010. Further, the dependency ratio was 49 percent. That means that for every 10 working adults, there are 4.9 people that are either too young or too old to work, compared to the number of people within working age. A lower dependency ratio is better for economic growth.[3] Not only does it mean that more people in the workforce are contributing to national productivity, but also that more resources can be directed toward investments in growth initiatives.

Retirement age is officially 62 for both men and women. If an individual prefers, however, she or he may wait until 65 or 70 to start drawing benefits; if so, monthly checks will be higher than if begun at 62. Neither is there any penalty to individuals 65 years of age or older who wish to work in addition to receiving Social Security benefits; they are merely taxed on the entire amount of their income. Before 2000, a beneficiary under 69 could only earn $14,500 before benefits would be reduced $1 for each additional $3 of earnings. Beginning with 2001, the retirement age was gradually increased until it reached 66 in 2009 and it will be 67 in 2027.[4]

The look of post-retirement income has changed dramatically since 1962 when the first data were collected on this program. Even after adjustment for inflation, since 1962 the median income for both married couples and non-married persons has increased dramatically, 88 and 93 percent, respectively. In 2008, almost two-thirds of the retired population claimed some personal asset income, 35.2 percent had a pension, 89.9 percent were covered by Social Security, and 20.7 percent worked post-retirement.[5] For a worker retiring at age 66 in 2010, the monthly Social Security benefit amount is $2,346. This figure is based on earnings at the maximum taxable amount for every year after age 21.[6]

The Social Security Advisory Council, a group of prominent private citizens established by the law, has periodically made suggestions (with no guarantee of acceptance) to Congress and the President. One of the council's recommendations was that all Social Security credits and benefits be shared equally by husbands and wives, and that every retired person have minimal Social Security benefits at age 65 plus whatever benefits may be earned as workers. Based on the reports of the Advisory Council, as well as pressure from interest groups representing the elderly, Congress has periodically made changes in the Social Security program. For example, since 1984, all federal employees and those in nonprofit organizations must be covered by Social Security. Also, under the *Omnibus Budget Reconciliation Act (OBRA) of 1986*, Social Security is exempt from automatic spending cuts required to reduce the federal budget deficit. (See Chapter 18 for a discussion of the federal budget process.) In 1990, Congress enacted legislation requiring the SSA, on request, to provide individuals with statements of their contributions and estimates of their future benefits. In 2000, Congress removed any penalty to retirees over 65 for earnings in addition to Social Security benefits.

To a great extent, Social Security was originally and still is slanted toward the male wage earner, with the assumption that most couples remain married, that the husband is the main breadwinner, and that the wife stays home. These trends have been offset by the longer life span of most women compared with men and the rising labor force participation rates of women of all ages, even those with young children. Thus, the Social Security system has not fully kept pace with the changing roles of men and women. For example, women's wages remain lower than men's, resulting in lower benefits paid to women when they retire. Furthermore, women are still likely to spend less time in the workforce than men because they also carry the major responsibilities for home and children. Future changes in Social Security might include adjustments to correct these imbalances.

Disability Insurance

Contributions to the Disability Insurance Trust Fund from employers and employees are made in the same manner as those for Social Security. However, unlike Social Security, which is solely under the jurisdiction of the federal government, disability insurance is administered through both federal Social Security offices and state disability determination services. As mentioned, about 9.8 million individuals were receiving disability benefits in 2010, and the numbers have been increasing each year.

An insured worker of any age, male or female, who becomes totally disabled can begin receiving benefits after a 5-month waiting period. Benefits are also paid to dependent spouses, widows (or widowers), and dependent children of those who are disabled. To be eligible for these benefits, the worker must (1) have been covered by Social Security for a specified number of years (5 to 10); (2) have a physical or mental disability of indefinite duration; and (3) be so badly disabled that she or he cannot work at gainful employment.

In recent years, payments and benefits for disability have expanded and shifted in several notable ways. For example, there has been an increase in the proportion of women receiving disability benefits, reflecting the surge of women in the paid labor force. In addition, the percentage of disabled who have mental, psychiatric, or personality disorders has grown, whereas the percentage of those with circulatory conditions has decreased.

In sum, Congress periodically revises OASDI policies based on shifts in the target population and lobbying efforts on behalf of those involved with the programs. The over 53 million Social Security and disability beneficiaries comprise a formidable interest group for politicians. The size and success of the Social Security system in protecting many elderly and disabled against poverty means that it will continue to hold a prominent place on the legislative agenda for years to come.

Unemployment Insurance

Another major provision of the Social Security Act of 1935 is a system of unemployment insurance to protect workers who are without work through no fault of their own. State governments administer unemployment insurance. Federal law specifies a maximum and minimum benefit, and the states must remain within these limits. Each state has its own law governing the amount of weekly benefits allowed to the unemployed person and the number of weeks for which it will be continued. This is because the cost of living and employment conditions vary so widely in different sections of the country. Thus, unemployment policies are very much dependent on state laws.

Changes in federal and state unemployment laws usually parallel trends in the economy, in particular, unemployment

rates. For example, during the economic recession of the early 1990s, Congress enacted several Emergency Unemployment Compensation laws to assist the long-term unemployed. These laws supplement standing unemployment policies to assist those who have been out of work for an extended period of time. At certain points, the laws allowed for an additional 26 weeks of unemployment payments.

Information pertaining to state eligibility requirements and administration of benefits is available from local unemployment offices. To collect unemployment insurance, a person must have been out of work for at least 1 week; must be able to work and be willing to take a job in his or her line of work at the prevailing rate; and must not have left the previous job without good cause or not have been asked to resign because of misconduct. In some states, marriage, pregnancy, and further education do not qualify one to claim unemployment insurance, and a mother cannot collect unemployment benefits for a certain period after childbirth.

Supplemental Security Income

Known as Title XVI or SSI, this program was passed in 1972 and provides direct cash benefits to the aged and disabled whose income and resources fall below a certain level. SSI is for US citizens with few exceptions and is totally federally funded, and the amount of benefit paid is based on need, not prior contributions to the Social Security Fund. This income supplement has allowed many persons to reside in their own homes rather than with relatives or state institutions. SSI is often associated with the migration of the chronically mentally ill into board-and-care homes and other group living arrangements. In this case, Social Security or SSI provides for room and board, and Medicare or Medicaid covers medical costs.

Medicare Benefits and Coverage

Since enacted into law in 1965, Medicare (Title XVIII of the Social Security Act) has provided Hospital Insurance (*HI* or *Part A*) for those (and their spouses) who have worked in Medicare-covered employment for at least 10 years, are 65 years old, and are citizens or permanent residents of the United States. Younger persons with a disability or with end-stage renal disease (ESRD; permanent kidney failure requiring dialysis or transplant) might also qualify for coverage. Individuals who qualify for Medicare Part A can purchase Supplemental Medical Insurance (*SMI* or *Part B*) for payment of a monthly premium. In

2010, that monthly fee is $96.40, and most individuals enrolled in Part A also participated in Part B of Medicare. Medicare, when originally proposed, was extremely controversial, with some citizens and legislators not completely committed to the idea and the AMA rigorously and uncompromisingly opposed to it. ANA, however, supported it. Passed in 1965, Medicare went into effect on July 1, 1966. Medicare is the largest single payer of health care services in the United States, and benefit outlays are expected to total $504 billion in 2010—15 percent of the federal budget.

Medicare was expanded in 1972 to include people under age 65 with permanent disabilities. People under age 65 who receive Social Security Disability Insurance (SSDI) generally become eligible for Medicare after a 2-year waiting period, while those with ESRD and amyotrophic lateral sclerosis (ALS or Lou Gehrig's disease) become eligible for Medicare when they begin receiving SSDI payments.[7]

Most Americans, on turning 65, are automatically enrolled in Part A, which consists of HI. Those over age 65 who do not qualify for Part A can pay a premium to enroll; that premium is currently anywhere from $254 to $461 a month depending on the individual's Medicare-related work experience. Part A is financed out of payroll taxes collected under the Social Security system in a manner similar to the funding for OASDI. That is, employees and employers each contribute 1.45 percent on an employee's total earnings to the HI Trust Fund. All HI benefits and administrative costs are paid out of this trust fund.

In 2008, almost 45 million aged and disabled were covered under Part A. Almost all of those entitled to Part A of Medicare also choose to enroll in Part B. Given trends of increased longevity and the aging baby boom generation, the number of beneficiaries covered under Medicare will inevitably increase.

Part A includes inpatient hospital, skilled nursing facility and home care, and the option of hospice for the terminally ill. The recipient of hospital and skilled nursing facility services is responsible for a deductible or copayment, which has been increasing. In 2010, the hospital deductible for each benefit period of 1 to 60 days was $1,100. The concept of a *benefit period* is important. The period starts when the beneficiary first enters a hospital and ends when there has been a break of at least 60 days since inpatient hospital or skilled nursing care was provided. A copayment of $275 per day is required for each hospital day after 60 days in a benefit period up to 90 days. The copayment provisions are complex and both penalize the affluent beneficiary and discourage the use of expensive hospital services. Medicare will pay some nursing home costs for Medicare beneficiaries who require skilled nursing or rehabilitation services. To be covered, you must receive the services from a Medicare-certified skilled nursing facility after a qualifying hospital stay. A qualifying hospital stay is the amount of time spent in a hospital just prior to entering a nursing home. This must be at least 3 days. Care in a skilled nursing facility also requires a copayment of $137.50 after the first 20 days, and Medicare assumes no responsibility for skilled care that exceeds 100 days in a benefit period. Hospice care for those with a life expectancy of 6 months or less is covered for 210 days. There are no copayments or deductibles for home care, but the beneficiary must be referred to a Medicare-certified agency and be homebound.[8]

After an annual deductible of $155, Medicare Part B pays for 80 percent of the allowable charges for physicians' services.[9] The *allowable charges* are a constant source of controversy between the medical community and the government. Additional specific services covered under Part B are laboratory and other diagnostic tests; outpatient services at a hospital; therapeutic equipment such as braces and artificial limbs; home health services for those services not covered under Part A; mammography; and respite care consisting of in-home personal services that allow the homebound enrollees' usual caretakers to take respite. These details are presented to acquaint the reader with the general flavor of these programs, and the most current benefits and payment liabilities can be found through the Medicare Internet site included in the references for this chapter.

The *Balanced Budget Act of 1997 (BBA97)*, P.L. 105-33, created other unconventional options for the elderly. The government's agenda continues to be to cut costs, provide choice, and expand benefits including preventive services. *Medicare + Choice or Part C* of Medicare allows the beneficiary to derive services from a variety of risk-adjusted plans, most notably,

1. *Coordinated care plans*, including HMOs, PPOs, and a variety of other plans as yet undefined that will meet approved standards

2. *Private, unrestricted fee-for-service plans* in which providers agree to the plan's payment terms and conditions and in exchange minimize their own risk associated with volume and rates

3. The *Medical Savings Account* (MSA) option, which allows beneficiaries to select a high deductible and

deposit the difference between the Medicare capitated rate and their premium into an MSA, with the dollars to be used at the discretion of the beneficiary

The latest addition to the Medicare program is *Part D*, Prescription Drug Coverage. The benefit package focuses on the needs of those beneficiaries who are the heaviest users of prescription drugs. The Medicare Prescription Drug, Improvement, and Modernization Act of 2003 created this benefit, which was added to Medicare in January 2006. Medicare recipients will be able to join a drug plan, which is run by private companies. These plans offer a variety of choices for prescription drug coverage with an estimated monthly premium of $35. Once the $250 annual deductible is met, Medicare pays 75 percent of prescription drug costs for the next $2,000. The individual is responsible for a 25 percent copayment. A beneficiary who has used $2,250 in covered prescription costs is responsible for paying 100 percent of the next $2,850 of expenses. This is referred to as the "donut hole." After a beneficiary reaches $5,100, Medicare will pay for 95 percent of any remaining covered costs for the rest of the year. This is another step in progress, but competes with state-based programs, some of which offer much more generous benefits.[10]

The financial liabilities incurred by Medicare beneficiaries (copayments, deductibles, and uncovered services) may be paid by the recipients themselves, a third party such as private Medigap insurance purchased by the beneficiary, or Medicaid if the person is eligible. Given the gaps in Medicare coverage, many private insurance companies sell *Medigap policies* to absorb the personal financial liabilities under Medicare. In 1990, Congress enacted legislation that established standards for Medigap.

The Medicare program is the responsibility of the CMS within DHHS. However, much of the daily operational work of Medicare is under the auspices of intermediaries, who handle claims from hospitals, home health agencies, and skilled nursing facilities. CMS contract with intermediaries regionally, and their responsibilities include conducting reviews and audits, determining costs and reimbursement amounts, and monitoring for fraud and abuse.

Similarly, CMS contract with carriers—typically Blue Cross/Blue Shield plans and commercial insurance companies—to handle claims from doctors and other suppliers of services under Part B. The use of intermediaries and carriers is considered by some to not only add another layer of bureaucracy, but also to increase costs. However,

the administrative costs of Medicare are approximately 5.7 to 6.4 percent of total outlays, whereas comparable services for private plans are 11.4 to 13.2 percent.[11]

Long-term care (LTC) is an area to which Congress and health policy experts are devoting more attention. There is deliberate movement to expand the nature of services to the aged and create options that challenge our traditional models. LTC is moving out into the community, and skilled nursing facilities are only one, and perhaps not the most preferred, choice for those who are seriously disabled.

BBA97 included a provision called Programs of All-inclusive Care for the Elderly (PACE). PACE consolidates Medicare and Medicaid resources and offers those 55 and over who qualify the choice of an alternative to institutionalization for a nursing facility level of care. The program is administered by the state within broad federal guidelines. For those choosing PACE, services may be delivered in day care centers, the home, hospitals, or nursing homes, and all services (health, medical, and social) are provided by the PACE team. The priorities are dignity, independence, and quality of life for the individual. PACE uses a capitated rate and there is no copayment. All services guaranteed by either Medicare or Medicaid must be available to the recipient, regardless of cost. PACE may be the first step in eliminating the sometimes artificial barrier between episodic care and LTC, and delegating responsibility for these health care entitlement programs to the state. As of 2010, PACE is operating in collaboration with Medicare Part D.[12]

Expanding Medicare benefits in any way would require placing a greater financial burden on beneficiaries, lowering provider reimbursement rates, or raising taxes on employers and employees (or some combination of these alternatives). The political stakes involved in any of these options create fierce competition and turmoil in the legislative arena. Regardless of what route federal lawmakers take to pursue health care reform, Medicare will endure, given its large constituency. However, this does not make it immune from changes in reimbursement, benefits, payments, and other policies.

Medicaid Benefits and Coverage

Medicaid was authorized in 1965 as Title XIX of the Social Security Act to pay for medical services on behalf of certain groups of low-income persons. It is a federal-state means-tested entitlement program under the aegis of the CMS, but administered by the state. By law, the federal contribution to the state cannot be less than 50 percent of the total cost of the program, nor more than 83 percent. On the average, the federal government pays 56 percent of the benefit costs and states pay the rest. Wealthier states have a smaller portion of the cost of their program absorbed by the federal government. The amount of federal outlay for the program has no set limit under the law. Certain groups of people (i.e., the aged, the blind, the disabled, members of families with dependent children, and certain other children and pregnant women) qualify for coverage if their incomes and resources are sufficiently low. Each state designs its own Medicaid program, setting eligibility and coverage standards within broad federal guidelines. As a result, substantial variation exists among the states in terms of persons covered, types and scope of benefits offered, and amount of payments for services. In 2010, there were approximately 60 million, or one in five Americans, enrolled in state Medicaid programs. Seventy percent of these beneficiaries were enrolled in managed care plans. The rapid rise in Medicaid costs is of concern to state and federal lawmakers. Total Medicaid outlays increased from $90.5 billion in 1991 to $194.6 billion in 2000, and to almost $290 billion in 2010.[13]

Until 1986, Medicaid eligibility was tied to welfare. In that year, Medicaid was extended to include certain women with low incomes and their children who were not covered by the Aid to Families with Dependent Children (AFDC) program. This change was important because state poverty levels are considerably lower than the federal poverty level, and when the state poverty level was used to determine AFDC eligibility, many poor women and children were excluded from receiving necessary health care. The BBA97 categorically eliminated AFDC and established Temporary Assistance to Needy Families (TANF), which is discussed later under block grants.

It is important to note that Medicaid does not cover all poor people. In addition to income, assets and resources are considered in determining eligibility on a state-by-state basis. Furthermore, besides the poor, other medically needy individuals can be eligible, based on federal and state criteria.

The Medicaid program also provides services to a diverse elderly population, mostly in terms of nursing home care. Medicaid remains the nation's major program of financial support for persons needing nursing home care. Approximately two-thirds of the bill for freestanding (as compared with hospital-based skilled nursing facilities) nursing home costs is paid by Medicare. Despite the burgeoning number of older Americans, national trends in nursing home occupancy are declining. This may be due to several factors. First, today's elderly are healthier, therefore delaying the need for skilled nursing services. The vastly increased availability of independent and assisted living and other community-based support, such as day care and home care, are also delaying or eliminating the need for institutional care.

The American Association for Retired People is waging a campaign for "money to follow the people" in LTC, as opposed to "people following the money." Many of the frail elderly and disabled are forced into nursing homes because other choices are not funded. But in fact, nationally, nursing home care averages about $75,190 per patient each year. In contrast, care in the home, through such services as meals-on-wheels and daily visits by a health aide, averages $18,000. Momentum is slowly growing for this program, but by 2009, 31 states were participating and almost 38,000 individuals had been returned to community living.[14] It is often difficult for nursing home residents to reenter the community, and so the real chance for change lies with those who have never been introduced to institutional living.

Another notable aspect of Medicaid is that the proportion of beneficiaries in a particular category does not necessarily correspond to the percentage of funds that are allocated to that group. For example, in 1999, children under age 21 comprised approximately 45.5 percent of Medicaid recipients, but received less than 13 percent of resources.[15] The historically low proportion of payments going to families with children, especially given the number of children and pregnant women lacking adequate health care, spurred Congress to enact a number of laws expanding Medicaid coverage and eligibility for children and pregnant women. These laws are discussed in later sections.

Major Amendments Affecting Medicare and Medicaid

In the years following enactment, much criticism was directed toward Medicare and Medicaid. As a result, frequent amendments were enacted, with the intent of controlling soaring costs and eliminating fraud and abuse of funds. There are now rigid regulations about the length of institutional stay that will be reimbursed, level of care requirements for skilled nursing home services, payment for specific services, and coverage of particular groups. A growing concern over quality of care has resulted in legislative amendments. Although any institutions participating in Medicare must be certified by DHHS and those participating in Medicaid must abide by standards set by each state, the quality of care that beneficiaries receive has often been criticized.

One legislative initiative aimed at improving the quality of care under Medicare was the *Professional Standards Review Organization* (PSRO) amendment in 1972, which mandated the establishment of PSROs within all states to improve the quality of health care and make it more cost-effective. The intent was to involve local practicing physicians in the ongoing reviews and evaluation of health care service rendered under Medicare and Medicaid. PSROs were primarily the responsibility of and under the control of physicians.

Despite the activities that PSROs generated in quality assurance and utilization review, they still presented several problems: lack of adequate funding, lack of uniformity among PSROs, difficulty in changing physician practice behavior, and lack of agreed-on measures of success. In 1982, P.L. 97-248 changed PSROs to Peer Review Organizations (PROs) and permitted quality assurance by private entities in a competitive market. PROs review only Medicare services. Medicaid and other reviews are left entirely to the states. There is only one PRO per state, with some subcontracting with regional units in larger states. The PRO monitors the appropriateness of admission and discharge and the use of resources during the period a beneficiary is hospitalized. PROs have had much more input from nurses and consumers than PSROs, some of which has been required by law. In 2001, the PROs were renamed Quality Improvement Organizations (QIOs). They have been recontracted by CMS in 3-year cycles, the latest being 2008, retaining the same mission and reporting relationships, but incorporating the additional theme of "transformational change" to be achieved through accelerating the rate of quality improvement, raising the bar for performance, and facilitating profound cultural change by incorporating Health Information Technologies.[16]

In 1986, as part of another effort to improve quality under Medicare, Congress enacted the *Health Care Quality Improvement Act* (P.L. 99-660). Among its provisions was the establishment of a National Practitioner Data Bank (NPDB) to help in identifying and disciplining practitioners who engage in unprofessional conduct and to restrict the ability of incompetent practitioners to move from state to state without discovery. The NPDB pertains to physicians, nurses, and other practitioners. The Medicare and Medicaid Patient and Program Protection Act of 1987 clarified the responsibilities of the NPDB and of registered nurses

(RNs) in relation to the NPDB. In short, nurses may be reported to the board for adverse licensure actions or adverse professional actions. They may also be reported for medical malpractice claims paid with certain stipulations. The NPDB has generated concern among many physicians and nurses that the federal government is monitoring their practice too closely and infringing on their rights. However, the potential for the NPDB to safeguard the public from the dangers of unqualified health professionals seems to outweigh its drawbacks, as long as professional organizations such as ANA continue to work to protect the rights of the practitioners with regard to NPDB activities.

In addition to concerns about quality, the problem of funding Medicare reached panic proportions by the 1980s. The system's trustees reported that even under the most optimistic conditions, either disbursements would have to be reduced by 30 percent or financing would have to be increased by 43 percent to prevent exhaustion of the Hospital Insurance Trust Fund by 1996. Two ongoing problems were the escalating growth of the over-65 population and the shrinking tax base. Workers in the United States and their employers each paid into the Trust Fund, but this was dwarfed by the rising cost of hospital care.

At the same time, the newly elected Reagan administration clearly stated that it was not interested in large-scale federal subsidies of health care. Costs had escalated tremendously but had been grudgingly absorbed in each new funding year. Medicare was a political hot potato, especially with an active "graying America" lobbying force (and after all, most everyone will someday grow old and may be threatened by serious illness). Medicaid had always stirred controversy among federal and state politicians. Thus, cuts were inevitable—in fact, they had been creeping up since the end of Johnson's Great Society. Legislation affecting the Medicare–Medicaid program came in various guises, some directly aimed at resolving its problems, some as part of other laws. Some actually increased benefits.

The Omnibus Budget Reconciliation Act of 1981 (P.L. 97-35) (OBRA 81) held major legislative reforms with far-reaching results. About $1 billion of cuts in health care spending for fiscal year (FY) 1982 were from Medicaid. Federal payments were cut progressively for each year through 1984. Medicare funding was also cut, and all but one public health hospital were closed.

Even more dramatic were the provisions of the *Tax Equity and Fiscal Responsibility Act of 1982* (TEFRA) (P.L. 97-248). It required the development of Medicare prospective payment systems (PPS) for hospitals, skilled nursing facilities, and, to the extent feasible, other providers. Additional cost-cutting mechanisms affecting health care facilities and providers were also included.

The work on the prospective payment mechanisms resulted in the enactment of P.L. 98-21, variously called the *Social Security Amendments of 1983*, the *Social Security Rescue Plan*, or simply the *DRG law*. This legislation established a PPS based on a case mix of 467 Diagnosis Related Groups (DRGs) that allowed pretreatment assignment of patients to billing categories. This system was put into place for almost all US hospitals reimbursed by Medicare. Separate payment rates applied to urban and rural areas. Psychiatric, LTC, children's, and rehabilitation hospitals continued to be reimbursed under the cost-based system. However, over time, the feasibility of PPS for these types of facilities (as well as home care and nursing homes) was also explored and implemented, with various degrees of success. The DRG category to which a patient is assigned is determined by his or her principal diagnosis (reason for entering the delivery system), age, the presence or absence of surgery or a major procedure, and complications or secondary diagnosis (comorbidity).

The DRG system was phased in over 3 years. What DRGs mean to a hospital is that if a patient is kept more than the number of days designated by the patient's DRG category or treatment is more costly than expected, the extra costs must be absorbed by the institution. If the patient goes home early, a portion of the amount designated for the scheduled days is the hospital's clear profit. Some predicted that hospitals would encourage doctors to admit more patients who were not potential problems or those who were self-paying or self-insured.

Needless to say, the DRG system had a direct impact on nursing. In some cases, hospitals, desperate to cut costs, chose to retain lower-paid nursing personnel rather than RNs. Others chose to turn to all-RN staffs that could actually save money by teaching patients or by anticipating potential complications, so that the patient would be discharged in a shorter period than the DRG anticipated length of stay.

Since the enactment of prospective payment in 1983, there have been a series of revisions in Medicare through legislation and regulation. Many of the new laws deal with prospective payment rates, based on recommendations of the Medicare Payment Assessment Commission (MedPAC, formerly the Prospective Payment Assessment Commission or ProPAC) and the Physician Payment Review Commission

(PPRC). These Commissions deal with rates and financial issues associated with hospital and physician payment under Medicare.

One of the most fascinating episodes in Medicare history was the enactment and 1 year later the repeal of the *Medicare Catastrophic Coverage Act of 1988*. The legislation was to provide a new Part B drug program to cover prescription drugs; extend coverage for skilled nursing facility, hospice, and respite care; and cover other services, such as mammography. In 1989, in response to protests from beneficiaries over the rising costs they were forced to incur, Congress repealed the act, eliminating all of these Medicare benefits. (Some components of the bill were maintained.)

Many policy makers thought that the repeal of catastrophic coverage would hit states the most, because state Medicaid programs would have to pick up much of the burden of health care for the elderly. Once the mood in Congress subsided after the stormy sessions over the catastrophic repeal, some legislators expressed interest in restoring a few of the benefits the act had provided (and adding some new ones). Congress in the *Omnibus Budget Reconciliation Act of 1990* reinstated biennial mammography screening and elimination of a limit on hospice care.

It is difficult to ascertain what the exact effect of PPS has been on quality of care, primarily because no study has uncovered a systematic pattern of diminished quality as a result of DRGs. Nonetheless, certain trends were discernible early in the history of PPS. Average hospital stays dropped 18 percent (1.8 days) between 1981 and 1990. Hospital patients were more acutely ill, requiring more nursing resources. Nursing home admissions increased nearly threefold over approximately the same period. Medicare and other patients were discharged in more clinically unstable conditions than in previous years, placing greater demands on family members, community resources, and providers.

As we move further into the new millennium, there are more recent observations that begin to contradict those made earlier. We now have empty nursing home beds, the average hospital length of stay has leveled off, and managed care will decrease the overall acuity of hospital patients (by stressing prevention and early intervention). The movement toward community services continues and health care resources are being moved in that direction.

Medicare policies have also expanded and occasionally reduced reimbursement opportunities for advanced practice nurses (APNs). *The Omnibus Budget Reconciliation Act of 1987* (OBRA 87) included a provision for Medicare payment to certified nurse-midwives (CNMs) working in HMOs, and to nursing homes for the services of gerontological nurse practitioners. OBRA 89 authorized nurse practitioners (NPs) and clinical nurse specialists (CNSs) working in collaboration with a physician to certify and recertify the need for skilled nursing facility care under Medicare. Finally, provisions of the *BBA97* guaranteed direct Medicare reimbursement to NPs, CNSs, and physician's assistants for services allowable under state law, regardless of their geographic location or practice setting, although at 85 percent of the physician rate for the same services. See Chapter 15 for more details.

In 1989, certified registered nurse anesthetists (CRNAs) succeeded in obtaining direct reimbursement under Medicare Part B for anesthesia services that they are legally authorized to perform in a state. In previous years, CRNAs lobbied successfully to ensure that the cost of their services was not included (bundled) in hospitals' DRG rates, but would be passed through on the basis of reasonable cost. On a more negative note, in November 2001, CMS reversed a rule passed in the last few hours of the Clinton administration that would have allowed CRNAs to administer anesthesia without physician supervision, and as a by-product bill Medicare independently for their services. Exemptions to this rule are possible on a state-by-state basis, only if the governor follows a cumbersome internal process of consultation and consents. Thirty states do not have a "physician supervision requirement" in nursing or medical board regulations or in the state's laws. The "opt out" option could therefore be activated by the governors of those 30 states and any others if their state laws were changed.[17] Thus, the controversy moves from Washington to the state level.

Nurses also improved their reimbursement under Medicaid, reaching an important milestone in 1989 when Congress enacted legislation providing for coverage of family and pediatric NPs (FNP, PNP) services under Medicaid (as long as they are practicing within the scope of state law). This was important in improving access to care for many pregnant women and children. Payment rates are determined by individual states and vary considerably.

OBRA 89 (P.L. 99-509) included major revisions in reimbursement to physicians under Medicare Part B, prompted by the dramatically rising costs of services under that program. The bill revamped the system of paying doctors on the basis of customary, prevailing, and reasonable fees, and replaced it with a Medicare fee schedule (MFS) that based payments on the resource costs involved in providing care. The resource costs included the nature of the service provided, practice expense, and cost of malpractice insurance. The new system, which went into effect in January 1992, is called the Resource-Based Relative Value Scale (RBRVS) and compensates based on the service rendered as opposed to the person rendering the service. This could be viewed as a strategy to reduce the number of physicians attracted to specialty practice on a monetary motive. The reimbursement of a general practitioner was comparable to that of a specialist performing the same procedure.

These changes in physician reimbursement under Medicare provided incentives for further review of nonphysician and noninstitutional reimbursement. OBRA 89 mandated a PPRC study of nonphysician providers, to be submitted to Congress by July 1, 1991. Nurses had input into the call for this study through their representatives on the PPRC and the lobbying efforts of ANA and other nursing organizations. In 1992, the PPRC made recommendations to Congress based on this study. The PPRC found a tremendous amount of variation in how nurses were paid for their services under Medicare, especially with regard to services incident to those of physicians. (Services *incident to* a physician's are those provided by nonphysicians that are an integral, although incidental, part of the visit and necessary for diagnosing or treating an injury or illness.) The PPRC recommended that all services provided by nonphysicians should be identified as such on the claims forms. In 1993, the HCFA issued rules allowing nonphysician providers to be eligible for incident to compensation at the full physician reimbursement rate, under physician supervision, even if a physician did not provide care to the patient at the time of the visit. These provisions increased the financial advantage APNs brought to a medical practice, but did little to establish their autonomy.

The PPRC also recommended that nonphysician providers (including NPs, CNMs, and CRNAs) be reimbursed at rates less than those for physicians to reflect differences in educational investment. This was in direct contrast to the position of nursing organizations, such as ANA and the National Alliance of Nurse Practitioners, who argued that the services NPs provide should be reimbursed at the same rate as comparable services provided by physicians. By 1994, payment of APNs under Medicare varied, depending on the location of the service and the setting. For example, NPs in rural areas were eligible for direct payment for their services, although at a percentage of the physician rate if not "incident to."

Medicaid reforms for the elderly have focused largely on quality of care in LTC facilities. The *Nursing Home Reform Act of 1987* (P.L. 100-203) included requirements for a minimum data set for resident assessment, new nurse staffing requirements of one RN 8 hours a day and 24-hour licensed nurse coverage, guidelines for nursing assistant training, and rigorous standards for the use of chemical or physical restraints. Much of this legislation was in response to the findings of a 1986 Institute of Medicine (IOM) report, *Improving the Quality of Care in Nursing Homes* (see Chapter 7).

The BBA of 1997 mandated the implementation of a PPS for Medicare reimbursement to nursing homes. A Minimum Data Set (MDS) consisting of over 300 indicators of functional ability, health, mental status, and treatment places each resident into a classification category (Resource Utilization Groups, RUGs) that distinguishes residents by their resource use and establishes an all-inclusive, capped rate of payment per day.[18] The BBA also legislated Medicare + Choice and the PACE Program as discussed earlier in this chapter. Although the BBA initiated many new programs, its primary purpose was to cut costs. It was overzealous in this mission and gained Congressional support based on incorrect information. Since then, the Balanced Budget Refinement Act (BBRA) of 1999, and the

Medicare, Medicaid, and SCHIP Benefits Improvement and Protection Act (BIPA) of 2000 have been designed to reinstate some of the funding cut under the BBA. These bills restored $51 billion over a 6-year period and refined many other aspects of the BBA.

Other very significant changes in Medicaid were enacted throughout the 1980s. When President Reagan came into office, he and his staff were intent on removing many of the working poor from the Medicaid program, as well as reducing AFDC eligibility levels. Decreases in funding and eligibility criteria for Medicaid ensued. Between 1981 and 1984, Medicaid's average annual growth rate slowed to 7.5 percent, down from an average of 15 percent between 1975 and 1981. In response to lobbying from many maternal and child health interest groups, most notably the Children's Defense Fund, the end of the 1980s brought expansion of Medicaid eligibility criteria and renewed interest in maternal and child health initiatives in Congress and the Reagan and Bush administrations. Three factors were mostly responsible for the prompt legislative action in these areas: (1) the high rate of poverty among children (approximately 25 percent); (2) the large proportion of the uninsured who are individuals under 18 (approximately 66 percent); and (3) the nation's embarrassingly high infant mortality rate and large number of unimmunized preschool children.

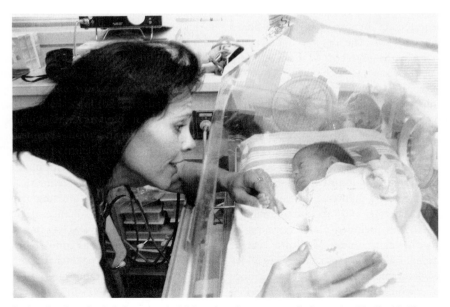

Caring for America's infants and children has become a priority under Medicaid. (Courtesy of the Valley Hospital, Ridgewood, New Jersey)

The expansion of Medicaid in recent years has occurred incrementally, with intense deliberations at state and federal levels of government. The discussions focused on what states were required and had the option to provide under Medicaid. The changes have had a significant impact on access to and the financing of health care for America's women and children.

Most significantly, the *Sixth Omnibus Reconciliation Act* (SOBRA) of 1986 gave states the option of extending automatic Medicaid coverage to pregnant women and children younger than 5 years of age with family incomes below the federal poverty level but above state AFDC eligibility levels. This option represented a major shift toward ending the dependency between AFDC and Medicaid programs.

Through federal legislation enacted in the late 1980s and early 1990s, Medicaid is required to cover all pregnant women and children under age 6 who are eligible for AFDC in a particular state or whose family income is at or below 133 percent of the federal poverty level. In addition, Medicaid must cover all children born after September 30, 1993, in families with incomes at or below the federal poverty level. This phased-in coverage is an attempt to ensure that all children under age 19 from poor families have health care benefits.

Making children's health a priority was the theme of the *Children's Health Insurance Program* (CHIP) created through provisions of the BBA97. There are 5 to 10 million uninsured children in this country, 3 million of whom are eligible for Medicaid, making it wise to move ahead with case finding and outreach. The CHIP program targets children who are from working families that are making too much to qualify for Medicaid, but not enough to sustain the cost of private insurance. These dollars take the form of a grant to states, and there is the expectation that CHIP is coordinated with the state Medicaid program. CHIP is directed by CMS, jointly financed by the federal and state governments on a matching basis, and is administered by the states. Within broad federal guidelines, each state determines the design of its program, eligibility groups, benefit packages, payment levels for coverage, and administrative and operating procedures. Children began receiving benefits through CHIP in 1997, and the program helped states expand services to over 5 million of the nation's uninsured children. The program was reauthorized on February 4, 2009, when the President signed into law the Children's Health Insurance Program Reauthorization Act of 2009 (CHIPRA). CHIPRA finances CHIP through FY 2013.[19] It will preserve coverage for the millions of children who currently rely on CHIP and provides the resources for states to reach millions of additional uninsured children. Some of the following Medicaid changes are expected: presumption of eligibility until proven ineligible, targeted enrollment of low-income children, and acceleration of the phase-in of low-income groups for children up to age 19.

■ PUBLIC HEALTH PROGRAMS RELEVANT TO NURSING PRACTICE

Block Grants

In addition to Medicare and Medicaid, there are several important public health initiatives relevant to nursing practice. *Block grants* have been in existence for many years, but they became increasingly popular under President Reagan, who favored block grants over categorical funding for separate programs. Block grants, funded through federal- and state-matched funds, shift much of the political and administrative accountability to the states without subsequent increases in state funding. The result is often inequities among states in terms of populations covered by the programs and competition among the various programs funded under a block grant in a particular state. The major advantage to block grants is the streamlining they provide at the federal level by consolidating programs into clusters for legislative and programmatic purposes.

In 1981, several health block grants were formed: maternal and child health, preventive services, and mental health (including alcohol and drug abuse). Congress originally designated a primary care block grant that consisted of community and migrant health center programs, but it was never officially made a block grant, and today these remain categorical programs.

In 1992, under P.L. 102-321, which reorganized the administration of mental health treatment and research services at the federal level and created the new SAMHSA, the mental health block grant was divided into two components. First, the Substance Abuse Prevention and Treatment Block Grant was formed in recognition of the scope and costs of substance abuse and of the fact that more attention was needed in that area. It became the largest specialized form of support for substance abuse. Each state must spend at least 35 percent of this block grant for the prevention and treatment of alcohol addiction and at least another 35 percent for drug abuse and treatment services. The second mental health block grant is the Community Mental Health and Services Block Grant, which provided support to states to develop community mental health services, emphasizing networks of families, providers, and other community resources.

By the mid-1990s, Congress addressed the Maternal and Child Health Block Grant. This includes programs for children with special health care needs, immunizations, school health, prenatal care, and other child health services. The Prevention Block Grant was funded by the mid-1990s and covers activities as diverse as health education, rape crisis intervention, fluoridation, hypertension prevention, and funding for tuberculosis and immunizations. Since the late 1980s, federal funding for the public health block grants has increased, albeit very incrementally. They still lack the support needed to reach members of the populations they are intended to serve, and their future depends on budget resources and the extent to which their advocates can successfully compete for political support.

The *Personal Responsibility and Work Opportunity Reconciliation Act of 1996* (Welfare Reform Bill) has initiated a not-so-quiet revolution in the nation's welfare programs, and there will be a direct impact on both health care and nursing. States receive a block grant for a fixed percentage of the money they spend on public assistance pre–welfare reform. The bill includes a host of initiatives that were once separately funded, such as SSI, nutrition programs, food stamps, Medicaid, and TANF. The TANF block grant replaces AFDC, which matched state funds designated for the program. State flexibility in TANF is broad, but there are some compulsory requirements to qualify: Public assistance is limited to a total of 60 months; adults in families receiving assistance must work after 2 years; if not, community service must begin within 2 months of receiving benefits; unmarried minor parents must reside within an adult supervised relationship; eligibility of aliens and naturalized immigrants for federal benefits is dramatically reduced; a parent receiving benefits must cooperate in paternity determination; and deadbeat parents will be pursued across state lines and then some to expedite child support.[20] A lot of pain and disenfranchisement of children has been predicted; others see success and a strategy similar to Roosevelt's Works Progress Administration (WPA) of the Depression. The judge is still out and the data too fraught with inconsistencies. However, able-bodied welfare beneficiaries must accept occupational training and jobs in more than 20 states, and the number is growing.[20]

Health Planning Legislation

One of the early health services laws that provided funds (on a matching grant basis) for constructing and expanding health care facilities was the *Hospital Survey and Construction Act of 1946*, popularly known as the *Hill-Burton Act*. It was highly successful, providing funds for more than 30 percent of the hospital beds in this country in its first 20 years, and funding was renewed several times.

Under Hill-Burton, states received money for developing a planning program, supposedly based on need. As might be expected, however, politics was a more important factor than any rational basis for planning. This resulted in a substantial oversupply of hospital beds and contributed to the inflation of health care costs as it became imperative to keep those beds filled.

After the enactment of several unsuccessful health planning laws in the 1960s, Congress passed the *National Health Planning and Resources Development Act of 1974*. It was designed to set up a new system of state and local health planning agencies and to integrate into those agencies a program for the support of certain kinds of health facility construction. Under the act, each state was required to establish a state health planning and development agency (SHPDA) and a state health coordinating council (SHCC) to advise the agency. Health Systems Agencies (HSAs) were responsible for collecting and analyzing data concerning the health care status of the residents in their designated health service area, the state of the area's health care delivery system, and its utilization, among other things. Most HSAs were private, nonprofit organizations with governing boards of 10 to 30 persons, the majority being consumers. Nurses served on a number of these boards. Their power lay in their ability to review and approve or disapprove the use of certain federal funds in their areas. HSAs were always accused of playing politics. Moreover, there was often poor communication and coordination among HSAs and state and national agencies.

In 1979, the *Health Planning and Resources Development Amendments* were signed into law. Agreement on the amendments was delayed for 3 years because of the various conflicts about the effectiveness of the law. Too much provider influence was one accusation. Another was related to the *certificate of need* (CON) power of the HSAs, without which existing health facilities cannot buy certain expensive equipment or expand.

Health planning provisions squeaked through under the *Budget Reconciliation Act of 1981* but lost authorization in 1986. This was in part because they failed to do enough to keep costs down (even though the original intent of health planning was not cost control). In addition, the political and administrative burdens they imposed often outweighed any type of planning effectiveness. Since then, most states continue health-planning efforts on their own without a federal mandate. They continue to operate CON programs, even if they have liberalized requirements, exempt certain types of projects, or expand the CON purview.

Although no longer mandated under federal law, HSAs left a legacy on the health planning landscape that is not easily erased. In particular, they demonstrated how even the best-laid plans for consumer and provider collaboration can fall prey to political maneuvers, and they left many government and health professionals leery of trying such a structured, bureaucratic route for regulating health care. In the wake of health care reform, states have developed new options for health planning. Many have initiated studies or commissions to determine the state's health needs or to focus on particular populations. These projects are often coordinated with public health initiatives while making the most efficient use of state dollars and resources.

Human Immunodeficiency Virus/Acquired Immune Deficiency Syndrome

During the 1980s, federal funding for AIDS became a hot topic. Federal policies for AIDS remain extremely fragmented, lacking well-coordinated programs in health care or education. Nonetheless, the government supports a wide range of programs, which many AIDS advocates believe is still insufficient given the need for research, community-based alternatives, and support for health professionals.

The AIDS Commission appointed by President Reagan urged broad and comprehensive plans to fight the epidemic. One of the most controversial issues pertaining to AIDS is whether the federal government should be allowed to limit immigration to this country of people who are infected with human immunodeficiency virus (HIV). AIDS activists and many members of the AIDS Commission are against such measures, arguing that it violates human rights. Other more conservative players and government officials have taken a different stand. They claim that AIDS is a public health threat, that neither the federal government nor the American taxpayer can afford to care for these individuals and that lenient immigration policies with regard to AIDS increase the public's risk of HIV/AIDS transmission. This policy was enacted into law under the 1993 NIH reauthorization bill (P.L. 103-43). However, the US Attorney General has the right to grant waivers from the exclusion. Nurses, public health professionals, and

other civil rights groups continue to challenge this exclusionary policy because HIV is not spread by casual contact and the policy restricts the freedom of many individuals—in particular, refugees seeking political asylum here. Under the same 1993 NIH law, the federal government created an Office of AIDS Research within NIH, the director of which would be the leading federal official responsible for AIDS research. This was an important move for centralizing AIDS research and planning and advancing AIDS research at NIH.

President Clinton, attempting to improve policies for AIDS, appointed a National AIDS Policy Coordinator, known colloquially as the AIDS Czar. The first person to fill the position was a nurse, Kristine Gebbie, RN, MPH. She resigned in August 1994, criticizing Congress and the Clinton administration for lack of sufficient funding to implement important AIDS programs, especially in the area of HIV prevention. Thus, although the federal government had allocated millions of dollars for research to prevent and treat AIDS, given the challenges that AIDS presents to health care providers and practitioners, the consensus among those in the field is that services for people with AIDS remain under-funded. AIDS-related policies continue to be hampered by lack of steady leadership and coordination, and reluctance on the part of the federal government to fund many AIDS initiatives. Nurses have been at the forefront of efforts to reverse these trends.

One of the ongoing concerns of AIDS activists has been the lack of funding for the Ryan White Comprehensive AIDS Resource Emergency (CARE) Act, enacted in 1990 and reauthorized four times as amended. The CARE Act is the largest single source (next to the Medicare and Medicaid programs) of federal funding for HIV/AIDS care for low-income, and uninsured and underinsured individuals. As such, the Ryan White HIV/AIDS Program fills gaps in care not covered by other funding sources. The Ryan White legislation has been adjusted with each reauthorization to accommodate new and emerging needs, such as an increased emphasis on funding of core medical services and changes in funding formulas.[21]

Agency for Health Care Research and Quality

In the late 1980s, one of Congress' attempts to combine concerns about the costs and quality of health care was the establishment of the AHCRQ (originally called the Agency for Health Care Policy and Research) within the PHS. The agency was authorized under OBRA 89 (P.L. 101-239), replacing what had been the National Center for Health

Services Research and Health Care Technology Assessment. The mission of the AHCRQ includes conducting research on the quality and effectiveness of health care services, developing practice guidelines, and assessing technology. The agency has the primary responsibility for implementing the Medical Treatment Effectiveness Program (MEDTEP) within the DHHS. The purpose of the medical effectiveness initiative is to improve the effectiveness and appropriateness of health care services through better understanding of the effects of health care practices—including nursing—on patient outcomes. The effectiveness initiatives are of particular importance because many policy makers look to effectiveness research as a way of controlling health care costs and streamlining medical practice. The AHCRQ convened a Nursing Advisory Panel on Guideline Development to provide input to effectiveness research as it pertains to nursing. It is important for nurses to understand and contribute to the agency's programs as much as possible, because its recommendations will affect nursing practice.

In many ways, MEDTEP is a backdoor approach to stemming the litigious environment by empowering consumers. Providers have been directed to reach consensus around the preferred treatment for select disease conditions that are highly variable in their treatment despite a substantial body of scientific evidence on clinical management. This consensus process yields guidelines for consumer use. The guidelines are not meant to drive reimbursement, nor do they limit the provider's ability to propose alternate treatment. It does place the burden on providers to justify their alternate recommendations. In seeking legal opinion on MEDTEP, the ANA has determined that these guidelines potentially have the force of law and establish the standard for clinical management in these specific situations.

In 1992, AHCRQ released its first clinical consensus-driven, evidence-based practice guidelines. They were for postoperative pain management, urinary incontinence in adults, and the prevention of decubiti. Since then, AHCRQ has issued many other guidelines including areas of otitis media in children, depression, strokes, managing patients with unstable angina, and much more. Many nurses have high-level positions at the AHCRQ and have provided input and leadership to the committees on clinical practice guidelines, as well as directing several of the AHCRQ research activities. Three of the consensus panels were chaired or co-chaired by nurses. The publications, resources, and information that AHCRQ provides are useful for nurses

engaged in many aspects of research and are relevant to advancing health care policy. AHCRQ has been very proliferative in guideline development, and you can find the archives of its work at http://www.guideline.gov, Immunizations.

One domestic priority has been to improve the immunization status of the nation's children. By the early 1990s, approximately 40 percent of American children between the ages of 1 and 4 years were behind in their immunizations, with higher rates for certain minority groups. To remedy this situation, Congress enacted a new childhood immunization entitlement program to assist states in bringing more children up to date with their vaccines. The program was to augment existing funds for immunizations that had been in existence for many years. The new law was enacted in 1993, as part of the fiscal 1994 budget reconciliation bill. It requires states to provide free vaccines to all children under age 19 who lack health insurance, are not covered by Medicaid, or are Native American. It would also assist children with health insurance who are unvaccinated and provide their immunizations at community or migrant health centers. Under the new law, DHHS negotiates a discounted price for the vaccines from the manufacturers, sets up a government vaccine warehouse, and then arranges with states to administer them to eligible children. States are responsible for the administrative costs of the program, and neither states nor providers are allowed to charge the family for the costs of the vaccines, although they can charge a limited fee for the administration of the vaccine. Implementation of the immunization program was delayed because of concerns that the law provided discounted and subsidized vaccinations for children who had health insurance or whose families could ostensibly afford to obtain vaccines without federal assistance. The conflicts depict how even a basic preventive program, such as childhood immunizations, can fall prey to political conflicts over eligibility, financing, and the allocating of responsibility for health care between public and private sectors.

■ NURSING PRACTICE, EDUCATION, AND RESEARCH

To understand the dynamics of current legislation for nursing, it is useful to establish a historical perspective. Except for the Bolton Act during World War II, it was not until Congress enacted the *Health Amendments Act of 1956* that members of the health professions received any substantial government funding. This act, now a section of the Public Health Service Law, provided dollars (called traineeships) to nurses to prepare for clinical, teaching, administrative, and other aspects of public health work. The traineeship program set the stage for years of subsequent federal funding for nursing. The government agencies that focus solely on nursing and those resources designated for the use of nurses are the Division of Nursing and the NINR. Each deserves to be presented separately.

The Division of Nursing

The Division of Nursing is an agency of the PHS. In turn, the PHS has been a component of DHHS since it was created in 1953 (originally named the Department of Health, Education, and Welfare). The PHS is an exceedingly important federal agency as far as health is concerned. Established in 1798 as a hospital service for sick and disabled seamen, the PHS has steadily expanded its scope and activities over the years and is now the federal agency charged with overall responsibility for the promotion and protection of the nation's health.

The Division of Nursing is exclusively concerned with nursing education and practice. It is within the Division of Nursing that the PHS focuses on the nation's nursing situation. However, nursing's roots go far back into the history of the PHS. In 1933, the first public health nursing unit was created within the PHS, primarily to implement the health provisions of the Social Security Act and to conduct the first national census of nurses in public health work. In 1941, the PHS established a unit on nursing education to administer federal programs, among them the United States Cadet Nurse Corps, which produced nurses during the emergency caused by World War II. In 1946, the Division of Nursing was established within the Office of the Surgeon General. Formally, the Division of Nursing was known as the Division of Nurse Education. During 1949, the PHS was reorganized to better coordinate its activities. The Division of Nursing in the Surgeon General's Office was abolished and its functions were taken over by the Division of Nursing Resources of the Bureau of Medical Services. In 1960, a restructuring of the PHS again occurred, uniting the Division of Nursing Resources and the Division of Public Health Nursing into the present-day Division of Nursing.

The Division's overall purpose is to work toward the achievement of high-quality nursing care for the nation's growing population and to approach this goal through aid to nursing education and consultation; the analysis and evaluation of nursing personnel; and the preparation of nurses for expanded roles in the primary care and teaching of patients. The Division identifies what exists in nursing, what is needed, and how improvements can be made. The Division is a catalyst for progress.

The Division supports programs related to the development, financing, and use of educational resources for the improvement of nurse training; conducts and supports a national program to improve the quality of nursing practice and health care, including innovative demonstration practice models; conducts studies and evaluations of nursing personnel supply, requirements, utilization, and distribution; and provides support to develop or maintain graduate nursing education programs and to prepare RNs for expanded roles in primary health care in various health care settings. It formerly funded research projects to expand the scientific base of nursing practice and education. However, its research functions and responsibilities were transferred to the National Center for Nursing Research, now the NINR, at the NIH when the Center was established in 1986.

The Division (and its predecessor units) has exerted significant influence and leadership within the nursing profession. Over the years, the Division has developed many significant publications as well as significant reports of special committees, such as that on the extended role of the nurse, which helped launch federal financing for NPs (see Chapter 5). Consultation services in many nursing areas are available through the Division. For example, schools wishing to expand the enrollment of professional nursing students, or those interested in developing or expanding nursing practice arrangements in noninstitutional settings to demonstrate methods for improving access to primary health care in medically underserved communities may receive help from the Division. The Division also conducts data collection on a continuing basis to determine the current and projected supply and distribution requirements for nurses within the United States and each state. The National Sample Survey of Registered Nurses, initiated in 1975, is the profession's major source of comprehensive personal and professional data on RNs, whether or not they are employed in nursing.

DHHS has 10 regional offices throughout the United States, each headed by a Regional Health Administrator. PHS has always recognized the importance of nursing in the total scheme of providing health services, and there is scarcely a PHS program that does not have a nurse involved in some way. At one time, there was a regional nursing program director in each region, but in the cut-back of the 1970s that position was abolished. Further information may be obtained online at http://bhpr.hrsa.gov/nursing.

The Division will only be as successful and prominent as funding allows. With the advent of Medicare and Medicaid and the expansion of facilities, health personnel became an urgent issue to Washington. At the same time, nurses were becoming more vocal, their organizations stronger, and their politics more sophisticated. Nurses had a self-assured and convincing presence as they appeared before legislative committees and met with their representatives. As a result, several new laws were enacted in the early 1960s that are noteworthy. Most significant among these was the Nurse Training Act of 1964 (Title VIII of the Public Health Service Act). The purpose of this law was to increase the number of nurses through financial assistance to nursing schools, students, and graduates taking advanced courses, and thus to help ensure more and better schools of nursing, more carefully selected students, a high standard of teaching, and better health care for the people. Signed into law by President Lyndon B. Johnson on September 4, 1964, the original law provided $287.6 million for 5 years.

The fight is constant to retain federal funding for nursing education and research. This has often meant overcoming substantial political obstacles, such as budget constraints, competition with other compelling health care needs and interests, lack of presidential support, and an absence of understanding among members of Congress about the importance of nursing research and graduate education. However, the profession has succeeded and even triumphed in gaining federal support and recognition.

In 1985, the renamed Nurse Education Act (NEA) reauthorized federal funding for nursing education for 3 years. President Reagan signed the new law (P.L. 99-92) primarily because it represented lower funding levels compared with previous bills. Although the authorization level of $54 million was considerably lower than funding levels in the 1970s, the bill was still a political success for nursing, given the tightly constrained budgetary environment.

Federal funding for nursing education was reauthorized in 1988 and 1992. In 1994, President Clinton proposed the consolidation of over 25 health profession programs, including nursing, into five categorical grants. Nursing organizations generally opposed such a move, arguing that it would force nursing to compete with other programs and would lower the funding levels for nursing. The consolidation proposal failed, but it is possible that it will reemerge in the future as a way of addressing the health care needs of the public, rather than the separate education programs of each profession.

In the meantime, federal funding for nursing education followed the precedents of previous years and has gradually increased since the late 1980s. In recent years, the major portion of these funds has supported graduate programs for NPs and CNMs, and advanced (mostly graduate) nurse traineeships. Other categories for funding included education for disadvantaged and minority health professionals, CRNAs, and student loan repayments. Given budgetary constraints, which limit the extent to which funding can be increased for discretionary programs such as nursing education, these funding levels are indicative of nursing's political success.

The NEA was again recast in 2001 as the Nurse Reinvestment Act (NRA), but died in committee. The NRA was subsequently reintroduced and passed in 2002. Its companion appropriation bill was passed in February 2003. The NRA represents a broader view on Title VIII of the Public Health Service Act than its predecessors. The NRA added new provisions to the Title VIII legislation resulting in a broad, comprehensive, and flexible legislative authority by which the federal government could help address the nursing shortage of the day. Specifically, the NRA includes a nurse scholarship program and a nurse faculty loan program—both of which provide support to individuals for nursing education with a payback provision following graduation. At the institutional/organizational level, the NRA provides grants for career ladders, internships, and residencies, and also addresses support for public service announcements to promote the nursing profession and funds to promote facilities to implement the Magnet Recognition Program of ANCC.

Until recently, nursing's political strategy had been to concentrate on a select package of legislation that was exclusive to its needs. If those bills failed, the loss was tragic. Currently, sources of funding for nursing and the health professions are included in a variety of places. Networking external to the field, incremental building from smaller funding sources, and education of the profession's leadership to search out new and more nontraditional sources may offer long-term protection.

In keeping with this philosophy, in November 2008, the nursing community approved the strategy to secure funding for Title VIII programs through the stimulus package

(American Recovery and Reinvestment Act [ARRA]), which was designed to help an economically hurting nation. In these difficult times, this was seen as a unique opportunity to act now, alleviating current funding concerns for nursing education and increasing appropriations for all the Nursing Workforce Development programs in FYs 2009 and 2010. Title VIII (Nursing Workforce Development) programs were subsequently funded as part of the omnibus ARRA and received a historic $243.872 million for FY 2010. This legislation includes dollars for advanced education including the nurse anesthetist, nursing workforce diversity, nurse education-practice and retention, loan repayment and scholarships, nurse faculty loans, and comprehensive geriatric education.[22]

The National Institute of Research

For nurses, 1985 was a landmark year because it marked the establishment of the *National Center for Nursing Research* (NCNR) at NIH. Nurses claimed the victory on November 20, when the Senate voted 89 to 7 to override President Reagan's veto of the NIH reauthorization bill. The House had already supported the bill in its 380 to 32 vote to override the veto the previous week. The bill culminated several years of negotiations among various interest groups, legislative chambers, and branches of government. It also was a compromise between House members advocating a National Institute of Nursing and senators who opposed any type of new national nursing research entity.

Within a short time, the center was up and running under the dynamic leadership of a distinguished nurse scientist, Ada Sue Hinshaw, RN, PhD, FAAN. In a short time, the center was conducting collaborative intramural research (within NIH) on topics such as the frail elderly, extramural grants to schools of nursing, a research program in bioethics and clinical practice, and research initiatives for low-birth-weight infants and patients with HIV infections (see Chapter 14).

In June 1993, the NCNR was upgraded to the *National Institute of Nursing Research*, following 2 years of lobbying and advocacy on behalf of nurses in Washington and across the country. Although the change in status from center to institute did not involve a change in budget, it did reflect an increase in status and visibility for nursing research.

Generally, federal funding for nursing research seems to have fared better than funding for nursing education. By 1991, funding for nursing research had increased to $40 million (from $10 million in 1985), and reached almost $145.66 million in FY 2010.[23] Despite these increases, many approved NINR applications go unfunded. Both the quality and quantity of grant applications has significantly increased.

■ HEALTH CARE REFORM

Starting in the 1980s, policy makers discussed various proposals to provide health coverage for the uninsured. The major obstacles to all of these proposals were that the burden of cost would fall on different groups, depending on the policy scheme, and that invariably the plans involved increased costs and spending. In addition, each plan targeted a different group, and unless Congress accepted some form of national health insurance, there was no way to provide coverage for everyone.

Underlying all of these proposals are unanswered questions about health care as a right or privilege. If one assumes that access to affordable health care is a right, then which level of government is responsible for it? Although health care is not explicitly stated in the Constitution as a right, the federal government does devote many resources to providing health care. On the other hand, many health programs are under state jurisdiction, and perhaps health care, like education, should be left to states' discretion. Finally, the issue of equity needs to be addressed. Are all individuals entitled to the same level and quality of health care, regardless of their ability to pay for that care? Or can we accept a two-tiered level of care, wherein those who can afford to pay more are entitled to the better quality and quantity of services their money can buy? Although the answers to these questions seem elusive, they raise important issues for nurses to consider as they become increasingly involved with the health care system.

In 1992, President Clinton was elected to office on a platform that included changes in the health care system. His first 2 years in office, 1993–1994, witnessed one of the most controversial and intense deliberations pertaining to health care in recent history. His *Health Security Act*, an ambitious bill of more than 1000 pages, covered every aspect of health care and proposed broad, sweeping reform, a virtual dismantling and reconstruction of the delivery system. Many nurses were part of the committees and task-forces that designed the bill, and ANA endorsed the Health Security Act shortly after it was formally introduced. An astute strategist could have predicted defeat, given that the proposal seemed to promise more bureaucracy than ever; aspects of the plan challenged the traditional and sacred province of states' rights; and in its entirety the proposal was too much too soon, jeopardizing 13 percent of the national economy.

The Clinton proposal did deliver a wake-up call to the nation's conscience, and there has been decisive movement of a nature that is typically American.

1. There has been significant movement toward universal health care coverage with disenfranchised and vulnerable populations being included first: women, children, the poor and aged, the uninsured, and the chronically ill and disabled. To some this represents a patchwork approach; to others it is the incrementalism that has characterized our public policy.

2. The evolving system continues to be built around a combination of public/private sector initiatives and state/federal partnerships.

3. The workplace remains an important source of health care insurance, but less often the exclusive source, and continued coverage is not dependent on continued employment.

4. No one can be denied coverage because of a preexisting condition or the risk he or she represents.

5. The public is being allowed to exercise more choice and subsequently share risk with government.

6. The traditional medical model is declining in its domination of the system and a social model is beginning to prevail.

7. Consumers are being expected to actively participate in decisions about the management of their illnesses and assume more responsibility for their personal health and self-care.

8. Integration and coordination of health care services on behalf of individuals is a necessity.

9. Cost will continue to be an issue, but quality is gaining ground as an issue.

10. Managed care, although continuing to dominate the health care scene, is being subtly reshaped to suit consumer preferences. Much of that shaping will come from consumer protections in the form of public policy.

Many states moved forward with creative models to help with decisions about the best use of scarce health care resources, or to provide universal coverage for their citizenry. Most health care industry groups and professional associations also contributed to the thinking, and organized nursing's proposal, *Nursing's Agenda for Health Care Reform*, was publicly commended for its solid recommendations.[24]

In the 111th Congressional session, an even more contentious struggle took place between the President, a Democrat-controlled Congress, and the Republican minority. The result was passage of the *Affordable Care Act* of 2010. Though currently in the dispute resolution and rule-making stage, it is possible to share some of the specifics. The Affordable Care Act would

- Expand coverage to 32 million Americans who are currently uninsured
- Create state-based insurance exchanges with subsidies available to individuals and families with income between 133 percent and 400 percent of poverty level
- Establish separate exchanges for small businesses to purchase coverage
- Pay for the plan through increasing Medicare payroll tax, a tax on investments, and a tax on insurers for "high end" policies
- Close the Medicare prescription drug "donut hole"
- Expand Medicaid to include 133 percent of the federal poverty level which is $29,327 for a family of four
- Require states to expand Medicaid to include childless adults
- Make illegal immigrants ineligible for Medicaid
- No longer deny anyone coverage based on a preexisting condition
- Allow children to stay on their parents' insurance plans until age 26
- Not require any health care plan to offer abortion coverage
- Eliminate federal funds for abortions except in the case of rape, incest, or health of the mother
- Require everyone to purchase health insurance by 2014 or face a $695 annual fine
- Require employers with more than 50 employees to provide health insurance or pay a fine of $2,000 per worker each year
- Not allow illegal immigrants to buy health insurance in the exchanges, even with their own money.[25]

These stipulations have different time periods when they become operational, and that has not been included here. The reader is referred to a more complete recounting for those details.

■ ABORTION AND FAMILY POLICIES

Since the 1973 Supreme Court decision *Roe v. Wade*, which legalized abortion, there have been many legislative and judicial battles over abortion. In the late 1970s, Congress prohibited federal funding for abortion when it appended the Hyde amendment to health services appropriations bills. However, approximately 14 states have been able to circumvent the Hyde amendment by allowing the use of state funds for publicly funded abortions.

Controversies over funding and the legality of abortions intensified in the 1980s with two consecutive conservative presidents and increases in like-minded federal court appointments. Several states enacted laws restricting access to abortions, and abortion rights activists questioned many of these new laws in courts. Often, the cases were referred as high as the Supreme Court. One of the most notable cases was the 1989 case of *Webster v. Reproductive Health Services*, in which the Supreme Court upheld the provisions of a Missouri law restricting access to abortions. Although the 1989 ruling left intact the *Roe v. Wade* decision legalizing abortion, it signaled the Court's willingness to reverse its previous decisions on abortion, which deemed other restrictive state laws unconstitutional. The three provisions of the Missouri law that the Court upheld in the 1989 case follow:

1. Prohibition of public employees from performing or assisting in abortions other than those necessary to save a pregnant woman's life
2. Prohibition of the use of public buildings or facilities for performing abortions
3. Requirements that physicians perform tests on fetal viability if they believe a woman to be at least 20-week pregnant

It is important to note that the *Webster* decision refers only to Missouri. However, the 1989 Supreme Court decision changed the scope and nature of abortion politics considerably. It seems to have set the stage for ferocious battles in state legislatures and exacerbated tensions within both political parties.

There have been other cases testing how far the Court will let states go in restricting access to abortion. Major issues have included the use of federal funds (usually meaning Medicaid) for abortions, how much information health providers must give women as part of informed consent for abortion, weighing fetal potential life against the well-being of the mother, and the right to require parental consent or notification when minors seek abortions. Specifically, in 1990, the Supreme Court ruled on cases from Ohio and Minnesota as to whether the Constitution allows minors to obtain abortions without first informing one or both parents, and upheld the constitutionality of parent notification.

In the aftermath of *Webster*, several proposals to restrict abortions at the state level emerged. However, over time, relatively few changes in state abortion policy were enacted. One could conclude from the outcomes of these events that in reality, the Court did not leave a lot of room to make major changes in abortion policy. In addition, public opinion polls indicated that the public overwhelmingly opposed severely restricting a woman's right to obtain an abortion.

Many members of Congress supported the *Freedom of Choice Act* (FOCA), first introduced in 1990, which would codify the *Roe v. Wade* decision. (The United States has been unique among countries in lacking legislation pertaining to abortion.) Hearings were held on the bill and it was given serious consideration. However, the controversy surrounding abortion, even under a more liberal president, impeded enactment. The one area on which Congress was able to reach consensus was the right to obtain access to abortion clinics. The Bill, enacted in 1994 with strong bipartisan support, makes it a federal offense to physically obstruct women's access to a clinic, or to use force, threats, or other tactics intended to intimidate women seeking abortion. The legislation was introduced in response to the rise in violent incidents at abortion clinics and killings of physicians who performed abortions. It also provides protection to abortion clinic employees, places of worship, and pregnancy counseling centers operated by groups that are against abortion.

On another front, a 1988 ruling, known as the *gag rule*, banned health care practitioners from providing abortion counseling in federally funded (Title X) clinics. In the following years, many legislators introduced legislation to overturn the gag rule, but they always were defeated. In the meantime, in May 1991, the Supreme Court declared the ruling constitutional, but its implementation was delayed, owing to political protests and squabbles over its implications. In 1992, DHHS announced that only physicians were allowed to counsel women regarding abortion as a health care option under Title X. Nurses were outraged and argued that this infringed on their rights to practice their profession and assist women to make informed choices. The uproar over the gag rule continued until early 1993, when, as one of President Clinton's first actions, he reversed it, relaxing the restrictions placed on all practitioners in Title X clinics.

In addition to abortion, there are other family-related issues that should be mentioned here—family leave and child care. The *Family and Medical Leave Act (FMLA)* went into effect on August 5, 1993. In previous years, Congress came close to enacting legislation on family and medical leave that would require employers to give unpaid time off to parents of newborn or sick children or dependents. Women's rights groups and organized labor supported such legislation. However, business groups opposed any type of parental leave bill that made benefits mandatory.

The 1993 law allows employees to take up to a total of 12 workweeks of unpaid leave during any 12-month period for the birth or care of a child born to an employee; placement of a child for adoption or foster care with the employee; care for an employee's immediate family member with a serious health condition; or a serious health condition that makes the employee unable to perform at work. FMLA applies to all public agencies, all public and private elementary and secondary schools, and companies with 50 or more employees. On returning from leave, the employer must give the employee the same position or an equivalent one in terms of benefits, responsibilities, and pay. FMLA also requires that group health benefits be maintained during the leave.[26] This legislation was very important for signaling the federal government's support for the millions of workers that shoulder responsibilities for caring for family members while also maintaining full-time jobs.

As for childcare, Congress enacted a landmark bill as part of the 1990 budget reconciliation act. It featured a new *Child Care and Development Block Grant* to assist states in improving the quality and availability of childcare facilities, and it expanded the earned income tax credit. Both the block grant and the tax credit target low-income working families with children.

■ FEDERAL POLICIES FOR PROTECTING CIVIL, PATIENT, PRACTITIONER, AND LABOR RELATIONS RIGHTS

Beginning in the 1960s, a number of laws were passed to prohibit discrimination based on sex as well as race, color, religion, and national origin. Many of these are particularly meaningful to women and are cited in Chapter 17. Some of the most important are the following.

The *Civil Rights Act of 1964,* called by some the most far-reaching social legislation since Reconstruction, intended to create a rule of law under which the United States could deal with its race problems peaceably through an orderly, legal process in federal courts. Title VII of the Civil Rights Act (the Equal Employment Opportunity Law) affected the job status of nurses because it includes a section forbidding discrimination against women in job hiring and job promotion among private employers of more than 25 persons. Executive Order No. 11246 as amended extended the law to include federal contractors and subcontractors. Hospitals and colleges are subject to this order because of their acceptance of federal grants of various kinds.

One year later, the *1965 Voting Rights Act*, with direct bearing on the Civil Rights Act, was passed, requiring that the procedure for registering persons to vote within a given county must be the same for everyone. Intended to ensure the right to vote promised in the Fifteenth Amendment, this law attempted to eliminate the practice of disqualifying potential voters on the basis of discriminatory literacy tests. This legislation represented an alteration in federal-state power, because the states had the authority for nearly two centuries to set, for the most part, the standards for voting eligibility within their own borders.

The *Educational Amendments of 1972* had three provisions of economic importance to women: (1) equal treatment of men and women in federally funded educational programs (especially admissions to programs); (2) minimum wage and overtime pay benefits to employees of nursery schools, private kindergartens, and other preschool enterprises; (3) extension of the federal Equal Pay Act of 1963 to executives, administrators, and professional employees. The same pay was guaranteed to men and women doing substantially equal work, requiring substantially equal skill, effort, and responsibility under similar working conditions in the same establishment. Comparable worth issues were discussed in Chapter 17.

The *Age in Employment Discrimination Act Amendments* of 1975 were intended to eliminate "unreasonable discrimination on the basis of age." Among other things, it banned certain kinds of mandatory retirement. The *Fair Labor Standards Act Amendments* of 1974 (originally 1938) increased the minimum wage and extended coverage to 7 million workers, including state, county, and municipal employees.

One of the most frequently cited provisions is Section 504 of the *Rehabilitation Act* of 1973. It reads, "no otherwise qualified handicapped individual in the United States shall, solely by reason of his handicap, be excluded from the participation in, be denied the benefit of, or be subjected to discrimination under any program or activity receiving federal financial assistance." The definition of *handicapped* includes drug addicts and alcoholics, as well as those having overt physical impairment such as blindness, deafness, or paralysis of some kind. A 1984 expansion of the definition relates to deformed newborns, as discussed in Chapter 22. Because most health facilities and health professional education programs have some federal support, this law applies both to admission to a nursing school, for instance, and to employment in a hospital.

The *Americans With Disabilities Act* was widely acclaimed at the time of its enactment in 1990 as providing broad protection against a range of discriminatory practices to the disabled. Discrimination is prohibited in areas such as public accommodations, transportation, and private employment. Firms may not deny jobs to individuals solely on the basis of disability, as long as reasonable accommodations can be made. The legislation is aimed at protecting the approximately 43 million disabled Americans including people infected with HIV. In the years since its enactment, however, courts frequently interpreted the Americans With Disabilities Act as affording far less protection than was initially anticipated. The Supreme Court's first case involving HIV and AIDS, *Bragdon v. Abbott*, addressed this trend by ruling that a woman with asymptomatic HIV infection is protected from discrimination in accessing dental services. In doing so, the Court endorsed an interpretation of the Americans With Disabilities Act that is broadly protective for individuals with disabilities. The Court also ruled that health care professionals might legally refuse to treat a patient because of concern that the patient poses a direct threat to their safety only if there is an objective, scientific basis for concluding that the threat to safety is significant.[27] In addition to the Americans With Disabilities Act, state laws frequently prohibit disability discrimination and apply to employers not regulated by federal law.

The *Civil Rights Act* of 1991 was a response to Supreme Court rulings in 1989 that were blows to civil rights enforcement. Specifically, in cases where employees experience job discrimination, the new rulings shifted the burden of proof from the employer to the employee. An earlier version of the civil rights bill came one vote short of a veto override in 1990. President Bush was motivated to reach a compromise in 1991. The Civil Rights Act of 1991 restored many employees' rights and left the most controversial issues open to court interpretation, thereby clearing the path toward enactment; however, it did not go as far as some civil rights advocates, including ANA, would have liked. Compromises were needed to enact the bill.

The 1991 law left to the judicial system the determination of whether an employer has set up requirements, such as educational or physical tests, that have an adverse impact on women or minorities. The law also imposed a cap on the amount of punitive damages that women, religious minorities, and the disabled can claim, and called for a commission to study the glass ceiling effect, referring to the lack of women and minorities in top corporate positions. Many groups, including ANA, are committed to fighting to reverse the caps as part of their civil rights agenda.

The right to privacy also affects nurses. Among the most important federal laws in this area are the *Freedom of Information Act* (FOIA) of 1966 and the *Privacy Act* of 1974. The purpose of the FOIA is to give the public access to files maintained by the executive branch of government. Recognizing that there were valid reasons for withholding certain records, the law exempted broad categories of records from compulsory public inspection, including medical records. To further clarify the situation, the FOIA of 1974 was passed to amend the 1966 law. It had been necessary to set some time and expense limits for federal agencies because, in their frequent reluctance to give up information, they tended to use bureaucratic red tape to delay transmission of the requested records and imposed high fees to photocopy them. The next question that arose was whether a person should not have the right to see all information about him- or herself in government files and to amend that information if it is incorrect. The result was enactment of the *Privacy Act*. Its purpose was to provide additional safeguards against invasion of personal privacy and misuse of records or information, and to establish liability for the violation of rights under the act without one's consent.

The *Health Insurance Portability and Accountability Act* (HIPAA) of 1996 is best known for creating a health insurance safety net for individuals moving from one job to another. Lesser known is the Act's sweeping mandates concerning the privacy rules of health information. HIPAA calls for either Congress or (in the absence of congressional action) the DHHS to develop national standards to protect the security and privacy of both electronic data transactions and personal health information transmitted in any format (electronic, paper, or oral) by insurers, managed care organizations, and federal health programs. In fact, this is the legislative basis for developing the computer-based patient record. Most covered entities must have implemented the HIPAA privacy rule provisions by April 2003. During rule making, the administration rolled back some of the major protections to privacy of medical records that had existed. The earlier requirement expected doctors, hospitals, and other health care providers to obtain written consent from patients before disclosing or using personal medical information for treatment or paying claims. Instead, providers will have to notify patients of their rights and only make a good faith effort to obtain written acknowledgment of receipt of the notice.[28]

Another step in providing access to one's own records was the enactment of the *Family Educational Rights and Privacy Act* of 1974, also known as the *Buckley Amendment*. The basic intent of this law was to provide students, their parents, and their guardians with easier access to and control over the information contained in academic records. Educational records are defined broadly and include files, documents, and other materials containing information about the student and maintained by a school. Students must be allowed to inspect these records within 45 days of their request. They need not be allowed access to confidential letters of reference preceding January 1975, records about students made by teachers and administrators for their own use and not shown to others, certain campus police records, certain parental financial records, and certain psychiatric treatment records (if not available to anyone else). Students may challenge the material, secure the correction of inaccurate information, and insert a written explanation regarding the content of their records. The law also specifies who has access to the records (teachers, educational administrators, organizations such as testing services, and state and other officials to whom certain information must be reported according to the law). Otherwise, the records cannot be released without the student's consent. The law applies to nursing education programs as well as others.

The rights of research subjects have also been incorporated in diverse federal laws, especially in recent years. The *National Research Act* of 1974 set controls on research, including the establishment of a committee to identify requirements for informed consent for children, prisoners, the mentally disabled, and those not covered by the federal regulations, and required an institutional committee to review a research project to protect the patient's rights. The 1974 Privacy Act required clear,

informed consent for those participating in research. The 1971 *Food and Drug Act* also gave some protection in regulating the use of experimental drugs, including notification to the patient that a drug is experimental. The *Drug Regulation Reform Act* of 1978 took further steps to protect the patient receiving research drugs. Before undergoing clinical testing, an *Investigational New Drug* (IND) Application must be submitted to the FDA, followed by three phases of clinical trials, which can take many years and require substantial funding to complete. Only 20 percent of all IND Applications progress to the point of New Drug Application eligibility with the FDA.

Rulings by the Federal Trade Commission (FTC) also have affected the rights of practicing nurses. The FTC, established pursuant to federal law in 1914, has extensive power. It can represent itself in court, enforce its own orders, and conduct its own litigation in civil courts, and it seems to have relative freedom from the executive branch of government. One of the most important FTC cases for nursing was in 1982, when an amendment attached to the FTC reauthorization bill exempted state-licensed professionals from its jurisdiction. A major supporter was AMA; an opponent was ANA. The underlying issue was, for instance, if professionals were exempted from fair trade practices, physicians could legally restrain the practice of competitors, such as CNMs. That time the FTC won, but the problem continues to resurface in various forms as more nurses engage in independent practice, obtain legislative rights to do so, and pose competitive threats to other medical professionals.[29]

Another FDA-related bill, the *Safe Medical Devices Act* of 1990, mandated that health care facilities report to the FDA and manufacturer (depending on the case) all incidents that could suggest that a medical device caused or contributed to the death, serious injury, or serious illness of a patient. Facilities that fall under the jurisdiction of this act include hospitals, ambulatory surgical facilities, nursing homes, and outpatient treatment facilities other than physician offices. The law was in response to the proliferation of medical devices and the need to protect patients and providers in the course of their use. This law has strong implications for nursing because nurses are typically the ones who monitor and are responsible for patient well-being, and who complete incident reports, whether or not they relate to medical devices. The regulations for the law were finalized in early 1992, and nurses working in facilities that are under the law should be knowledgeable about them and how they might affect nursing practice.

Also within the broad category of rights are those laws addressing labor relations. The first was the *National Labor Relations Act* (NLRA), one of several pieces of legislation enacted to pull the country out of the Great Depression. The logic was that labor unions could prevent employers from lowering wages, resulting in higher incomes and more available spending money. Initially, to allow the growth of unions, the power of employers had to be curtailed. For instance, they could no longer legally fire employees who tried to unionize. The *National Labor Relations Board* (NLRB), created by law, was empowered to investigate and initiate administrative proceedings against employers who violated the law. If these administrative actions did not curtail the illegal acts, court action followed. Only employer violations were addressed.

In 1947, the NLRA was substantially amended, and the amended law, entitled the *Labor Management Relations Act* (or *Taft-Hartley Act*), listed prohibitions for unions. Section 14(b), for instance, contained the so-called right-to-work clause, which authorizes states to enact more stringent union security provisions than those contained in the federal laws. More than 20 states have enacted such laws. Usually they prohibit union security clauses in contracts that make membership or non-membership in a labor union a requirement for obtaining or retaining employment. Such laws prohibit the closed shop, union shop, and sometimes (right-to-work states) the agency shop in which employees who do not join a union must pay a fixed sum monthly as a condition of employment to help defray expenses.

In 1959, a third major modification was made. One of the purposes of the law, the *Labor-Management Reporting and Disclosure Act* or *Landrum-Griffin Act*, was to curb documented abuses such as corrupt financial and election procedures. For this reason, it is sometimes called the union members' Bill of Rights. The result is a series of rights and responsibilities of members of a union or a professional organization, such as the constituent member associations of ANA, that engages in collective bargaining. Required are reporting and disclosure of certain financial transactions and administrative practices and the use of democratic election procedures. That is, every member in good standing must be able to nominate candidates and run for election and must be allowed to vote and support candidates; there must be secret ballot elections; union funds must not be used to assist the candidacy of an individual seeking union office; candidates must have access to the membership list; records of the election must be preserved for 1 year; and elections must be conducted according to bylaw procedures.

Highly significant for nurses is the 1974 repeal of the Tyding amendments to the Taft-Hartley Act (P.L. 93-360), the *Nonprofit Health Care Amendments*. This law made nonprofit health care facilities that, through considerable lobbying, had been excluded from the 1947 law, subject to national labor laws. These employees were now free to join or not join a union without employer retribution, a right previously denied to them unless they worked in a state that had its own law allowing them to unionize. It also created special notification procedures that must precede any strike action. Included in the definition of health care facility were hospitals, health maintenance organizations (HMOs), health clinics, nursing homes, extended care facilities (ECFs), or "other institutions, devoted to the care of sick, infirm, or aged persons." Employers of all kinds must abide by the various civil rights and other protective laws contained here.

The *Civil Service Reform Act* of 1978 also had an influence on the labor relations activities of nursing because its definition of supervisor allowed nurse supervisors to be included in collective bargaining units. The US Supreme Court visited the employee status of licensed nurses in May 1994 (see Chapter 30).

In 1988, the NLRB issued rules regarding appropriate bargaining units for the health care industry and determined that RNs constitute a separate bargaining unit and have a strong desire for separate representation. "The Board found LPNs to be appropriately included with technical employees." ANA had been an active participant in NLRB rule making. Other legislated workplace protections are included in Chapter 30.

The *North American Free Trade Agreement* (NAFTA) and the *General Agreement on Tariffs and Trade* (GATT) could create serious labor issues for American nurses. Our best information comes from observations of NAFTA, but GATT warrants similar precaution. Between 1994 and 1995, Canadian nurse entrants to the United States increased from 1286 to 5500 due to NAFTA, whereas Canadian immigration requirements have continued to be an obstacle to US nurses wanting to work in Canada. In the broader business community, there is proof that more than 400,000 US jobs were displaced, and workers' rights and workplace standards were generally compromised owing to these trade agreements. It is possible for nurses to be removed from a list of professionals eligible for temporary entry into the country under NAFTA, and this option is being explored. Physicians are not included. There is current government discussion about extending NAFTA to include South America. An additional issue in NAFTA is clarifying the differences in educational and practice standards, and credentialing for entry-level, specialty, and advanced practice that exist between the participating countries. The *Trilateral Initiative for North American Nursing* was established with Kellogg Foundation funding and leadership provided by CGFNS International (formerly the Commission on Graduates of Foreign Nursing Schools). The Trilateral Initiative has the Herculean task of building consensus among US, Canadian, and Mexican nursing interests.

As would be the case in any nursing shortage, interest has peaked within the industry about relaxing nurse immigration standards. Associations representing hospitals and nursing facilities argue that immigration offers an immediate response to the shortage and that current nurse immigration policies are burdensome and duplicative. Several pieces of legislation have been introduced that would eliminate quotas on the number of visas issued and the need for any prescreening by CGFNS. Neither would these alien nurses be guaranteed work hours commensurate with those of similarly employed American nurses. The industry would be flooded with nurses who would become second-class citizens. Organized nursing opposes looking abroad for nurses when the real problem is that the US health care industry has failed to maintain a safe, quality environment that retains American nurses in practice.

KEY POINTS

1. Compared with other industrialized nations, the United States has been reluctant to establish a government-sponsored social policy system.

2. The first social policy system was worker's compensation, which existed in almost every state by the late 1920s.

3. Old-Age, Survivors, and Disability Insurance and Medicare Part A are funded from equal contributions of the employer and employee.

4. For most retirees, Social Security benefits only represent a portion of their retirement income.

5. Supplementary Security Income is totally federally funded and awarded to Social Security recipients on a basis of need.

6. Medicare is a nationwide health insurance program for the aged and disabled who qualify for Social Security and those with end-stage renal disease.

7. The Balanced Budget Act of 1997 reshaped the face of health care by offering incentives for the aged on Social Security to join managed care arrangements, imposing new case mix requirements on long-term care, and decreasing the dollars available to public entitlement programs.

8. In the early 1980s, many categorical sources of funding at the federal level were converted into block grants with much of the political and administrative responsibility shifted to the states.

9. One of Congress' attempts to combine concerns about cost and quality was the Agency for Health Care Policy and Research, recently renamed the Agency for Health Care Research and Quality.

10. The health care of women continues to be of prime concern, most recently with the revealing research about estrogen combination drugs for the postmenopausal.

11. The major nursing presence in the federal government is the National Institute of Nursing Research and the Division of Nursing.

12. There has been significant movement toward universal health care coverage over the past 35 or 40 years, but progress has been incremental in a traditional American fashion.

13. The evolving system of health care continues to be built on public/private sector initiatives and federal/state partnerships.

14. The public is being allowed to exercise more choice and consequently assume more risk in health care and its financing.

15. Cost will always be an issue, but quality is gaining ground.

16. Managed care is dominating health care, but it is being reshaped to suit American preferences.

17. Although *Roe v. Wade* is still the law of the land, court decisions have severely restricted access to abortions.

REFERENCES

1. Social Security Administration. http://www.socsec.org/facts/basics_right_4.htm. Retrieved May 12, 2010.

2. Ibid.

3. InvestmentU. The Dependency Ratio. January 29, 2010. http://www.investmentu.com/2010/January/the-dependency-ratio.html. Retrieved May 3, 2010.

4. Social Security Administration, loc cit.

5. Employee Benefit Research Institute. Databook on Employee Benefits. October 2009. http://www.ebri.org/pdf/publications/books/databook/DB.Chapter%2007.pdf. Retrieved May 10, 2010.

6. Ibid.

7. The Henry J. Kaiser Family Foundation. Medicare. January 2010. http://www.kff.org/medicare/upload/1066-12.pdf. Retrieved May 13, 2010.

8. Medicare. Nursing Homes: Paying for the Care. May 8, 2009. http://www.medicare.gov/nursing/payment.asp. Retrieved May 3, 2010.

9. Ibid.

10. Medicare. Prescription Drug Coverage. January 27, 2009. http://www.medicare.gov/pdphome.asp. Retrieved May 10, 2010.

11. The Heritage Foundation. Medicare Administrative Costs. June 25, 2009. http://www.heritage.org/Research/Reports/2009/06/Medicare-Administrative-Costs-Are-Higher-Not-Lower-Than-for-Private-Insurance. Retrieved May 10, 2010.

12. First Health Services Corporation. https://pacecares.fhsc.com/. Retrieved May 14, 2010.

13. The Henry J. Kaiser Family Foundation. Medicaid and Managed Care: Key Data, Trends and Issues. February 2, 2010. http://www.kff.org/medicaid/8046.cfm. Retrieved May 10, 2010.

14. USA Today. Nursing Home Residents Get Aide to Move Out. April 22, 2010. http://www.usatoday.com/news/health/2010-04-21-nursing-homes_N.htm. Retrieved May 10, 2010.

15. Shi L, Singh D. *Essentials of the US Health Care System.* Sudbury, MA: Jones and Bartlett, 2005.

16. Leavitt M. Report to the Congress: Improving the Medicare Quality Improvement Organization Program—Response to the Institute of Medicine Study. 2006. https://www.cms.gov/QualityImprovementOrgs/downloads/QIO_Improvement_RTC_fnl.pdf. Retrieved May 14, 2010.

17. Anesthesia Progress. Medical Anesthesiologists Keep CRNA Supervision Rules Intact. November 20, 2009. http://www.anesthesiaprogress.com/medical-anesthesiologists-keep-crna-supervision-rules-intact.html. Retrieved May 10, 2010.

18. Knapp M. The Power of Paperwork. *Contemporary Long-Term Care* (Special Supplement on Subacute Care), 1998.

19. State Health Facts. Medicaid/CHIP Eligibility. December 2009. http://www.statehealthfacts.org/comparemapreport.jsp?rep=43&cat=17&sub=171&rgnt=5&sortc=1&o=a. Retrieved May 15, 2010.

20. Lamar J, Washington H, Hull J. Welfare to Workfare. http://www.time.com/time/magazine/article/0,9171,960554,00.html. Retrieved May 15, 2010.

21. HRSA. The HIV/AIDS Program. http://hab.hrsa.gov/law/leg.htm. Retrieved May 15, 2010.

22. All Nurses. American Recovery and Reinvestment Act Includes Funds for Nursing Education. February 20, 2009. http://allnurses.com/nursing-news/american-recovery-reinvestment-372032.html. Retrieved May 10, 2010.

23. AACN. FY 2010 Appropriations: Omnibus. http://www.aacn.nche.edu/Government/pdf/FY2010FundingChart.pdf. Retrieved May 16, 2010.

24. *Nursing's Agenda for Health Care Reform.* Washington, DC: American Nurses Publishing, 1991.

25. CBS News. Health Care Reform Bill Summary. March 21, 2010. http://www.cbsnews.com/8301-503544_162-20000846-503544.html. Retrieved May 10, 2010.

26. US Department of Labor. Family and Medical Leave. November 17, 2008. http://www.dol.gov/dol/topic/benefits-leave/fmla.htm. Retrieved May 15, 2010.

27. Gostin L, Feldblum C, Webber D. Disability discrimination in America: HIV and other health conditions. *JAMA* 281:745–752, February 24, 1999.

28. Bush rolls back rules on privacy of medical data. *The New York Times* pp A1, A8, August 10, 2002.

29. Antitrust Exemptions for Health Care Professionals. http://nursingworld.org/gova/federal/legis/107/antifcts.htm. Retrieved August 10, 2002.

Licensure and Health Personnel Credentialing

A major focus in the criticism of the health care system has been the undeniable fragmentation of services, accelerating costs, and poor utilization and maldistribution of health manpower. Therefore, credentialing of health manpower, as one of the factors that probably contributes to these problems, has been given special attention by legislative, governmental, and consumer groups. This pointed scrutiny has subsequently aroused new, or at least renewed, interest on the part of the health occupations and professions.

Licensing of individuals is the most authoritative mechanism of credentialing because it is a function of the police power of the state. Its primary purpose is to protect the public. Therefore, the state, through its licensure laws, sets standards and qualifications for the licensed practitioner and holds the power to punish those who violate the law. At the same time, licensure, as it currently stands, has definite advantages for the licensee: status, protection of title (RN, LPN/LVN, MD), and certain economic gains. Other methods of credentialing for individuals or institutions have also evolved. Whether official, quasiofficial, or voluntary, most purport to provide a certain assurance of quality or safety to the public as well as benefits for the credentialed. Therein lies the dilemma. The dangers inherent in credentialing and the potential for conflict of interest were eloquently expressed over 30 years ago and are still relevant today.

It is true that any professional society or group, no matter how socially oriented, will tend to develop barriers to protect itself. . . . Among the contemporary protective mechanisms for the health professions are accreditation, certification, licensure, and registration. All four of these mechanisms medicine has employed with excellent results, if not always for the benefit of society, at least for the benefit of most members of the profession. And now many of the numerous other health professions wish to adopt, if they have not already done so, the same steps which medicine had fashioned to meet the needs of society *and its own protection* (emphasis mine).[1]

This phenomenon has not escaped the notice of the consumer or the government. Because the health professions, as a whole, did not seem to show rapid progress in remedying the more questionable aspects of credentialing, particularly licensure, a series of blue-ribbon panels, high-level committees, and prestigious task forces at state and national levels were formed in the 1970s. There is clear evidence that the recommendations of these groups were a strong impetus to changes in the various forms of health manpower credentialing. These are reported in detail in the fifth edition of this book. Exhibit 20–1 contains a summary of the major credentialing processes that are used almost universally.

■ CREDENTIALING AND ITS ISSUES

Individual Licensing

As noted, licensure is a police power of the state; that is, the state legislative process determines what group is licensed and with what limits. It is the responsibility of a specific agency of state government to see that the law is carried out, including punishment for its violation. Although licensure laws differ somewhat in format from state to state, the elements contained in each are similar. For instance, in the health professions laws, there are sections

■ **EXHIBIT 20–1.** Variations on Credentialing

Approval: (Title may vary somewhat from state to state) **Mandatory** review to ensure that a **program** of study or health care has met the **minimum state standards**. In nursing education, this means recognition by their respective boards of nursing, and the subsequent right of graduates to take the licensing examination. Approving agencies derive their authority from the state.

Accreditation: The **voluntary** review process by which a **private-sector** organization evaluates and recognizes a **program** of study or health care as meeting predetermined standards that go **beyond minimum** state approval. Accrediting agencies often hold deemed status from the government.

Licensure: A credential awarded to an **individual** through the police power of the state that gives permission to engage in a given profession or occupation, verifying that she or he has attained the **minimal degree of competency** necessary to ensure that the public health, safety, and welfare will be reasonably well protected.

Certification: A credential awarded to an **individual** as a mark of **competence or specialization**, and not just safe practice. Certification has traditionally been defined as a voluntary, nongovernmental credential. This is no longer consistently true. Government agencies have begun to use this term.

Registration: The process by which **individuals** are listed on an official roster by either a **governmental or nongovernmental** entity. This status could attest to the individual's current or past competency or merely their participation in certain work. *Registered* nurses are more correctly *licensed* nurses.

Licensing of the health occupations was advocated in the early nineteenth century, but it was not until the early 1900s that a significant number of such licensing laws were enacted. They were generally initiated by the associations of practitioners that were interested in raising standards and establishing codes for ethical behavior.

Because voluntary compliance was not always forthcoming, the associations sought enactment of legislation. To some critics, this movement is also seen as a means of giving members of an occupation or profession as much status, control, and compensation as the community is willing to bear. It is true that as the health occupations proliferate, each group begins to organize and seek licensure. Because many of these occupations are subgroups of the major health professions or are highly specialized, licensure creates problems in further fragmentation and increased cost in health care—according to the critics.

In all of the proposals for changes in health manpower credentialing, criticism of individual licensure is implicit or explicit. Some of the key criticisms follow:

1. Many licensure laws for the health professions do not mandate continuing education (CE) or other requirements to prevent educational obsolescence. Therefore, the minimal standards of safety, theoretically guaranteed by granting the initial license, may no longer be met by some (perhaps many) practitioners.

2. Specific requirements for courses, roles, and so on are rigidly specified in statutes instead of relying on the administrative rule-making process. This makes timely responses to a changing environment difficult and slow. The result is that minimal standards and educational innovations in the health professions lag behind the practice realities.

3. Definitions of the area of practice are generally not specific, so that allocation of tasks is often determined by legal decisions or interpretations by laypeople. On the other hand, some limitations of practice—often ones that are not congruent with changing health care needs—are delineated.

4. Some licensing boards are dominated by members of the particular profession and may not have representation by competent lay members or allied health professions. This has been negatively viewed as a means by which the profession controls entry into the field.

There is the possibility of shutting out other health workers climbing the occupational ladder and also

on the definition of the profession that delineates the scope of practice; requirements for licensure, such as education; exemptions from licensure; grounds for revocation of a license; creation of a licensing board, including member qualifications and responsibilities; and penalties for practicing without a license.

Licensure laws are either mandatory or permissive. If *mandatory*, the law forbids anyone to practice that profession or occupation without a license, on pain of fine or imprisonment. If *permissive*, the law allows anyone to practice so long as she or he does not claim to hold the title of the practitioner (such as registered nurse) cited in the law.

limiting the number of practitioners for economic reasons. Moreover, the members of a one-profession board may lack overall knowledge of total expertise in the health care field, so that the scope of functions that could be delegated to other workers is not clearly determined. This creates the possibility that others capable of performing a particular activity may be prevented from doing so by another profession's licensing law. On the other hand, the inclusion of members of potentially competing health professions on licensing boards may result in the promotion of additional barriers to competition rather than growth and expansion of the profession being regulated.

5. There are always some licensed practitioners who are unsafe, and even if they lose their license in their own state, boards in other states are not notified and the individual simply crosses a state line and continues to practice. Physicians were particularly pinpointed, and in 1990 the government established a National Practitioner Data Bank (NPDB) to track serious disciplinary actions taken by medical boards and societies and hospitals, as well as settled malpractice cases. State boards and others are mandated to use these data before permitting a physician to practice. This also applies to other providers, including nurses, where they apply for a license or practice privileges.

The lack of geographic mobility that licensing causes for some health professionals is a concern. Nursing, with its state board examinations called the National Council Licensure Examination (NCLEX) that are used in every state, allows for licensure by endorsement in most states. That is, assuming that other criteria for licensure are met, a nurse need not take another examination when relocating from state to state. Even then, nursing does not completely escape the mobility criticism, because, in the last few years, various state boards of nursing have adopted rather idiosyncratic criteria, particularly for advanced practice nurses (APNs). A solution to this problem for both advanced practice and the entry-level credential or license may be the nurse licensure compact (NLC) as discussed later in this chapter.

Nevertheless, it seems that almost all of the established or fledgling health occupations, more than 250 at last count, consider licensing as a primary means of credentialing. The licensure problems of one health occupation obviously are not necessarily the same as those of all the others. Yet, because the majority of all kinds of health workers function in organizations, the various weaknesses of all health occupations' licensing laws, the inconsistencies and varying standards of those seeking licensure, and the sheer numbers involved appear to be the bases for whatever enthusiasm exists for alternatives to the individual license, such as institutional licensure.

Institutional Licensure

Institutional licensure is a process by which a state government regulates health institutions; it has existed for over 40 years. Usually, requirements for establishing and operating a health facility address administration, accounting requirements, equipment specifications, building construction and space planning, structural integrity, sanitation, and fire safety. In some cases, there are also minimal standards for occupancy, including square footage per bed and minimal nursing staff requirements. The issue in the new institutional licensure debate is whether personnel credentialing or licensing should be part of the institution's responsibility under the general aegis of the state licensing authority. There are various interpretations of what institutional licensing means and how it could or should be implemented.

One model advocates that the employing institution regulate institutionally based health workers within bounds established by state institutional licensing bodies. Further, a job description classification similar to that used in civil service should be developed. Personnel categories could be stated in terms of levels and grades, along with descriptive job titles. Under such a system, the individual's education and work experience would be taken into consideration by the employing institution for the individual's placement in a grade. Basic qualifications for the position, expressed in terms of education and experience, would be set by the state's hospital licensing agency.

Thus, professional nurses returning to work after 10 or 15 years might be placed in a nurse's aide or practical nurse (PN) position, moving on to a higher grade when they have regained their skills and become familiar with professional and technological advances through in-service programs. Not much is said about the role of the physician in this credentialing picture, implying that the current practice of hospital staff review was really a pioneer effort along the same lines and might as well continue to function. Presumably this model would apply to all institutions and agencies providing health services, such as hospitals, nursing homes, physicians' offices, clinics, and the all-inclusive *et cetera*.

There are many criticisms of institutional personnel credentialing. One concern is whether all agencies would be willing to initiate the expensive and extensive educational, evaluative, and supervisory programs necessary to fulfill the basic tenets of institutional licensure. With increasing pressure to control costs, extensive staff education programs seem even less likely. This raises the specter of a return to the corrupt apprentice system of early hospital nursing in the United States. Probably a hospital's own personnel would be used as preceptors. Who, then, would do their job? How would they be compensated? How long would students be expected to function in their current positions with the current salary while they practice the new role? With what kind of supervision? What kind of testing program for each level? Testing by whom? With what kinds of standards? Such a model may well cut manpower costs, but would also seem guaranteed to indenture workers instead of freeing them with new mobility.

Problems in specifying criteria to support a standard are also obvious. If 50 states cannot agree on criteria for individual licensure, why would institutional licensure be any different? Considering the thousands of profit and nonprofit hospitals with bed capacities ranging from the tens to the thousands, in rural and urban areas, with administrators and other key personnel prepared in widely varied ways, and the even larger number of extended care facilities, clinics, and home care agencies that are equally dissimilar, a state of confusion, diversity, and parochialism becomes an overwhelming probability.

Instead of facilitating interstate mobility, institutional licensure would more likely limit even inter-institutional mobility. A worker could qualify for position X in institution A, with absolutely no guarantee that this would be acceptable to institution B. Moreover, the disadvantages to those health professions that have fought to attain, maintain, and raise standards might be disastrous to patient safety.

Many of these practices may exist today (de facto institutional licensure), but it hardly seems progressive to legalize what is already considered an unsatisfactory situation. Let there be no mistake, under this proposed system the institution would determine the specific tasks and functions of each job and indicate the skill and proficiency levels required, regardless of the employee's licensure, certification, or education. Control would be almost complete.

However, would not the state guidelines protect the consumer, if not the employee? Presumably, the state licensing agency would be empowered to review the institution's utilization and supervision of health personnel to determine whether employees are performing functions for which they are qualified. How feasible would such an evaluation be? No one believes that an army of experts knowledgeable in all the subcategories of health care could be recruited, employed, and dispersed to check the hundreds of thousands employed in the multiple subcategories of workers in the thousands of caregiving facilities in any state. Therefore, one more paper tiger would be created—inspection by paperwork—and a complementary bureaucracy. Nursing has historically opposed institutional licensure, and the issue continues to surface, taking a variety of forms.

It is conceivable that with the trend toward multi-institutional ownership, especially by for-profit groups, and the concomitant trend for physicians to become employees, corporate-wide credentialing may be sought. It is speculative whether professional groups would have the political clout to prevent it.

Nurse Licensure Compact (NLC) States

The licensing of nurses is a demonstration of the police power of the state and is thus handled on a state-by-state basis. This has become burdensome in recent years because of practice models such as telenursing, which raise questions of practice across state lines, and the growing presence of multistate health care systems. In response to these circumstances, the National Council of State Boards of Nursing (NCSBN) has proposed a mutual recognition system of nurse licensure. This system would be largely based on the driver's license model, requiring a primary license in the state of the licensee's residence. That individual could then practice in any other (remote) state that had entered into an interstate compact with the state of the primary license. The one-license concept could provide a number of advantages, including

1. Reduces barriers to interstate practice
2. Improves tracking for disciplinary purposes
3. Promotes cost-effectiveness and simplicity for the licensee
4. Acts as an unduplicated listing for licensed nurses
5. Facilitates interstate commerce[2]

In practicing in a remote state, the licensee is subject to that state's practice laws and discipline. Therefore, even though practice rights and responsibilities may vary from state to state, this need not serve as an impediment to entering into an interstate compact. However, it is expected that the process that precedes finalization of any such agreement would promote some movement toward standardization. The licenses in question at this time are the registered nurse (RN) and licensed practical nurse/licensed vocational nurse (LPN/LVN). The advanced practice credential represents much more state-to-state variation and will be much more difficult to move to goal. On March 14, 1998, Utah became the first state to adopt into law the concept of the NLC state. This legislation allows Utah to enter into negotiation with any other state with legislation supportive of this model. As of May 2010, 24 states have NLC laws. The reader is referred to Exhibit 20–2.

A similar design is pending for an advanced practice registered nurse (APRN) compact. The APRN Compact will offer states the mechanism for mutually recognizing APRN licenses/authority to practice. This is a significant step forward for increasing access to qualified APRNs. A state must either be a member of the current NLC for RNs and LPNs, or choose to enter into both compacts simultaneously to be eligible for the APRN Compact. No date has been set for the implementation of the APRN Compact, but Utah, Iowa, and Texas have already passed laws authorizing their participation.[3]

Movement toward agreement on the regulation of advanced practice has been facilitated by the work of the NCSBN with APRN stakeholders. The Advanced Practice Nursing Consensus Work Group and the National Council of State Boards of Nursing APRN Committee, working independently, came together in what was labeled the APRN Joint Dialogue Group. Their goal was to reach agreement on elements of a consensus model for advanced practice, which could eventually be cast into the APRN Compact. These elements were to include licensure, accreditation, certification, and education.

While education, accreditation, and certification are necessary components of an overall approach to access the APRN to practice, the licensing boards—governed by state regulations and statutes—are the final arbiters of who is recognized to practice within their jurisdiction. Currently, there is no uniform APRN regulatory system. In the APRN model of regulation proposed by the Dialogue Group, there are four roles: certified registered nurse anesthetist (CRNA), certified nurse-midwife (CNM), clinical nurse specialist (CNS), and certified nurse practitioner (CNP). These four roles are all considered APRNs. APRNs are educated in one of the four roles and in at least one of six population foci: family/individual across the lifespan, adult-gerontology, pediatrics, neonatal, women's health/gender-related, or psych/mental health.

APRN education programs must be accredited and housed within graduate programs that are nationally accredited. Their graduates must be eligible for national certification, which is used for state licensure. APRN certification programs will be accredited by a national certification accrediting body, and will require a continued competency mechanism. APRNs may specialize but they cannot be licensed solely within a specialty area. Education programs preparing individuals with this additional knowledge in a specialty, if used for entry into advanced practice registered nursing and for regulatory purposes, must also prepare individuals in one of the four nationally recognized APRN roles and in one of the six population foci. As nursing practice evolves and health care needs of the population change, new APRN roles or population foci may evolve. Competence at the specialty level will not be assessed or regulated by boards of nursing, but rather by professional organizations. All APRNs are educationally prepared to provide a scope of services across the health wellness-illness continuum to at least one population focus. However, the emphasis and implementation within each APRN role varies. The services or care provided by APRNs is not defined or limited by setting but rather by patient care needs. The title Advanced Practice Registered Nurse (APRN) is the licensing title, and it is protected. Preparation in a specialty area of practice is optional, but if included must build on the APRN role/population-focused competencies. In addition, for licensure purposes, one exam must assess the APRN core, role, and population-focused competencies.[4] The reader is referred to the NCSBN for more detail.

■ **EXHIBIT 20–2. Nurse Licensure Compact States, May 2010**

Arizona	Maryland	Rhode Island
Arkansas	Mississippi	South Carolina
Colorado	Missouri	South Dakota
Delaware	Nebraska	Tennessee
Idaho	New Hampshire	Texas
Iowa	New Mexico	Utah
Kentucky	North Carolina	Virginia
Maine[a]	North Dakota[a]	Wisconsin

[a]By administrative rules.

In the years since the introduction of the NLC, the American Nurses Association (ANA) has continued to advocate for credentialing systems that best support the needs of both the consumer and the profession. ANA had voiced concern about a potential loss of control over disciplinary actions, the potential for diminished revenue to boards of nursing, the threat to the confidentiality of those nurses who are investigated but not necessarily charged, the erosion of states' rights, and the ability to move nurses in large numbers across state borders to dilute the effectiveness of job actions. Many of these criticisms are being addressed. The reality is, the NLC is achieving success.

Sunset Laws and Other Public Actions

Besides considering alternatives, improving the licensure process has become a state priority. Although the speed of the action has varied from state to state, steps taken almost universally include adding consumers and sometimes other functionally related health professionals to each board, giving more attention to disciplinary procedures, and gradually developing proficiency and equivalency examinations. Boards may function under committees of laypeople (or at least a majority of consumers), who make the decisions about licensing, with the individual boards acting in an advisory capacity. Other states have been restructured to form multidisciplinary boards, or at the least investigative and administrative functions have been consolidated. One reason given is improved efficiency, but some nurses fear that this is an indirect approach attenuating nursing's control over its practice.

For some professions, improving the licensure laws to protect the public was a new experience. A motivating factor was the enactment of *sunset laws* that require the periodic reexamination of licensing agencies to determine whether particular boards or activities should be maintained. Most states have this provision. These laws were a result of a lobbying campaign by Common Cause, a consumer group, to bring about legislative and executive branch oversight of regulating boards and agencies of all kinds. An evaluation was to allow for public input, as well as that of the boards and occupations involved. Consolidation and responsible pruning were encouraged. Although appropriate legislative and executive committees would do the review, safeguards were to be built in to prevent the arbitrary termination of boards and agencies. These principles are generally adhered to, but states do vary in their management of sunset reviews. If a sunset law is in effect,

the data and justification for existence are a joint staff–board responsibility, although the professional organizations are also closely involved. Nursing was no more ready for sunset review than other disciplines, but nurses learned, sometimes the hard way.

Over time, most nursing boards had undergone sunset reviews, and the new or amended laws usually reflected changes in practice and society. Most practice acts have broadened the scope of practice, added consumers to their boards, and sometimes required evidence of current competence through various means, including continuing education. State boards have given increased attention to removing or rehabilitating incompetent nurses. Meanwhile, educators are working seriously on equivalency and proficiency examinations and other methods of providing flexibility and upward mobility for nursing candidates. Nurses in the field have continued to improve techniques of peer evaluation, implement standards of practice, and encourage voluntary continuing education.

Assurances of Continued Competency

The rapidly changing scientific and technological environment has given new meaning to the image of the health care professions as being dynamic. It is no longer a simple responsibility to stay on top of your field.

Concerns over the continuing competence of provider professionals is not new, but both licensing boards and the professions are being pressured by consumers to provide assurances about their constituencies. Continuing education, either mandatory or voluntary, has served as an interim measure, but its efficacy has been largely undemonstrated. There are other options, but they are largely talk and untested: self-assessment, readministration of a licensure exam, peer review, simulations, and individual portfolios, to name a few.

This whole area has been moved to center stage by the recommendations of the Pew Health Professions Commission's Taskforce on Health Care Workforce Regulation and pressures from the Citizen Advocacy Center (CAC) (see Chapter 5). The literature on the subject raises many questions. The practitioner goes through inherent changes from the point of new graduate to established provider of services. Where on this developmental continuum do we find the measure of competence? What is the cost of these assurances, and who should bear that cost? Is competence the actual ability to perform, the cognitive artfulness, or both?

One particularly sensible suggestion is that candidates for reassessment be chosen through a random selection process, or that triggers be used to identify practitioners who merit more careful scrutiny. Such triggers may be recent disciplinary action, return to work after a significant hiatus, independent or isolated practice, and multiple job changes in a short period of time or a radical shift in a specialty area of practice. This is an area for careful thought.

Certification

Traditionally *certification* has been defined as a voluntary, nongovernmental credential awarded to individuals after they prove their ability as experts in their field. It signifies competence or specialization, not just safe practice, and requires such qualifications as (1) graduation from an accredited or approved program; (2) acceptable performance on a qualifying examination or series of examinations; and/or (3) completion of a given amount of work experience. This is no longer consistently true. Government agencies have begun to use this term more loosely in a number of situations where they either conduct the entire credentialing process or accept some private sector evidence as part of that process. We have Certified Home Health Aides (CHHAs) and Certified Nursing Assistants (CNAs) who are prepared in educational programs approved by the state, and the educational program is obligated to verify the safety of their practice. Many Boards of Nursing are certifying APNs, and national professional certification is one requirement to qualify. In summary, neither terms nor processes are sacred or even stable today.

The distinction between *public* and *private* credentialing needs full explanation. Public credentialing (licensure) can legally prohibit unlicensed practice. Those who lack private credentials still have the legal right to practice, although they may be at a disadvantage in the marketplace because independent decision makers, such as consumers, hospitals, and public or private financing plans, value their services less highly. The major purpose of private credentialing to the public is informational, a recognition or seal of approval from the professional group that awards it. It gives the consumer an opportunity to make more informed decisions, in that certification indicates that the certified person has voluntarily met certain standards that similar caregivers have not. Accreditation of educational programs, as done by National League for Nursing Accrediting Commission (NLNAC) and the Commission on Collegiate Nursing Education (CCNE), or of health care facilities, as done by the Joint Commission, are other examples of private credentialing. The reader is referred to Exhibit 20–1.

Because the public needs to know that the certifying group and its standards have some legitimacy, there are second-tier credentialing organizations, like the National Commission for Certifying Agencies (NCCA), that can be either voluntary or governmental. Their general purpose is to certify the certifiers. NCCA includes the organizations that certify allied health professionals and sets certain uniform standards and guidelines. The American Board of Nursing Specialties (ABNS) is also a second-tier credentialing organization that specifically addresses nursing certification and is discussed later in this chapter.

Criticisms of certification are remarkably like those of licensure. One is that some individuals as well qualified as those who are certified are denied certification and are thus disadvantaged in the marketplace. The denial may be owing to the lack of a certain educational background or failure to pass an examination. The latter is a common certification mechanism. Examinations for all types of credentialing are under constant scrutiny, with continual involvement of test experts. Nevertheless, some persons question whether any examination can really identify the competent practitioner.

Second, there is the question of *grandfathering,* also a licensure problem. Usually those who were certified in a specialty before an upgrading of educational or practice requirements are grandfathered into the new status, that is, permitted to hold the certification without fulfilling the new requirements. Thus, the information given the public—that these persons fulfill certain criteria—is not accurate. Here the answer may lie in requirements to demonstrate ongoing competency through the recertification process—providing that the measure is valid. Recertification as a requirement has become standard.

Finally, there is the concern that certification may be done by the professional organization that also accredits the educational program from which the candidate must graduate to qualify for certification. Clearly, that mechanism provides complete control by the occupation and can also shut out potential candidates. This problem was resolved, to a large extent, by the Federal Trade Commission (FTC) rulings that such arrangements were the illegal restraint of trade. Another variation on this same theme is certification done by the professional society that evolves standards and represents the profession. NCCA frowned on this arrangement as well, and the professions gradually moved certification functions into separate organizational structures. Many examples exist, some being the Council on Certification of Nurse Anesthetists and the American Nurses Credentialing Center (ANCC), both of which were once structural units of the American Association of Nurse Anesthetists, and the American Nurses Association, respectively. Despite these criticisms, certification is generally advocated as a way to assist the consumer in making choices.

Accreditation

Both educational programs and institutions and health care organizations often seek accreditation because it is presumably a mark of excellence, that is, it indicates that higher standards are maintained than those required by the government. Quite often, accreditation is necessary for health care facilities, as a requirement for federal reimbursement and to have medical residency programs. Educational institutions find that accreditation is required to receive federal or state funds for scholarships or other purposes. Accreditation is not only a consumer attraction, but also a necessity.

State boards of nursing often use the term *accreditation* because they approve nursing education programs. In this instance, it does not signify a standard of excellence, but indicates that graduates have completed a program that permits them to sit for the licensing exam. This approval is mandatory. We are not speaking to this public function here, but to accreditation as a voluntary mechanism.

The major accrediting organization for diploma, associate degree, and practical nursing education programs is the NLNAC. Both the NLNAC and the CCNE accredit baccalaureate and graduate programs in nursing. The Joint Commission, or in the case of home health agencies either the Joint Commission or the Community Health Accreditation Program (CHAP), commonly accredits health care organizations. The issues involved here relate in part to the accrediting process and in part to who should do the accrediting.

Standards are set by the profession, and the degree to which a program or institution conforms to these standards is determined through the accreditation process, which includes significant consumer input. By way of example, standards for nursing services are established by the ANA, but the ANCC in the process of awarding magnet status applies them to the nursing services of a particular agency or institution. It is required that the accrediting agency be autonomous and that those who make credentialing decisions be free of conflict of interest and protected from any external coercion that might affect those decisions.

The ANCC Magnet Recognition Program and Pathway to Excellence designations are accreditation mechanisms to recognize health care organizations that provide nursing excellence. They are included here because of their relevance as accreditation mechanisms, and are again discussed in Chapter 25. Recognizing quality patient care, nursing excellence, and innovations in professional nursing practice, these programs provide consumers with the ultimate benchmark to measure the quality of care that they can expect to receive. When *U.S. News & World Report* publishes its annual showcase of "America's Best Hospitals," being an ANCC Magnet organization contributed to the total score for quality of inpatient care. ANCC is one of only a few organizations providing outside data to the *U.S. News & World Report* ranking methodology. Fifteen of the top 21 medical centers (71 percent) featured in the prestigious Honor Roll were Magnet-recognized organizations in 2009. In the Children's Hospital Honor Roll, 9 of the top 10 (90 percent) were ANCC Magnets. The Magnet Program and Pathway to Excellence are similar, but not identical. Pathway to Excellence is more suited to the small and mid-sized institution, but not exclusive to them. These surveys only look to the quality of nursing. The Magnet concept derives from the ANA and research conducted by the Academy of Nursing. The ANCC was made a freestanding subsidiary of ANA in 1991.[5]

In most situations, the accreditor maintains a close relationship with the professional association that created it. There are philosophical and power issues: Should the NLN (and NLNAC), which was given the responsibility at the reorganization of the major nursing organizations in 1952, continue to be the major force in educational standard setting and accreditation in nursing education? Should the American Association of Colleges of Nursing (AACN), which represents the interests of the academic deans and directors and is associated with the CCNE, become the major force in standard setting for baccalaureate and higher degree programs? There is also the obvious matter of control and income. Considerable income is derived from activities related to accreditation: organizational memberships, consulting, and the accreditation process itself. These resources provide attractive incentives to enter the business of accreditation or to participate in an allied association that drives standards. A final issue is the fact that the NLNAC offers a comprehensive service with all programs having the ability to seek accreditation under the same auspices. The CCNE's scope of interest is narrower, thus sacrificing consolidation.

Accreditation is not a simple process. Certain fees are required, and the program must complete a self-study report. If the report indicates that the criteria have been met, there is a site visit by a team of peers whose work is to clarify, verify, and amplify the report, and report back to the board that decides on the credential. After consideration by the accreditation board, recommendations are made to accredit for a certain period of time or not, a decision that may be appealed. (This is a very brief overview; changes in procedure are made periodically.)

Besides the criticisms of accreditation in general, another in nursing is that a university or college already goes through a regional accreditation process and that a nursing accreditation is duplicative and costly, a point that is being made by academic administrators about other kinds of specialty accreditation, too.

■ NURSING ACTIONS IN CREDENTIALING

Nursing has always been in the thick of credentialing activities. Since the beginning of organized nursing, finding ways to assure the public of high-quality nursing was given a high priority by nursing leaders (see Chapter 5). A major study of credentialing sponsored by ANA made some daring proposals in 1979, including suggesting the establishment of a national nursing credentialing center, run by a federation of organizations with "legitimate interests" in nursing and credentialing "as the means of achieving a unified, coordinated, comprehensive credentialing system for nursing."[6] A follow-up taskforce affirmed the study's recommendations, particularly about establishing a credentialing center with a coalition of other organizations. This recommendation was not accepted by nursing, except "in principle." Then, with the increase of nurse specialists and the confusion in licensing laws, the question of the best way to credential specialists became urgent. The ANA decided that voluntary certification rather than recognition of specialists by licensing was the best choice. *Nursing's Social Policy Statement* reaffirms that position.

> The credentialing boards that are associated with ANA and specialty nursing organizations develop and implement certification examinations and procedures for nurses who want to have their specialty practice knowledge recognized by the profession. Certification is a judgment of competence made by nurses who are themselves practicing within the area of specialization.[7]

By 1980, the ANA had already established 15 specialty practice certifications, and many of the specialty organizations also offered certification. In 1982, a meeting was convened for the purpose of discussing a multiorganization credentialing center, but there was little interest, each player fearing a loss of control over its practice area. In 1985, the ANA House of Delegates endorsed the establishment of the Center for Credentialing Services as an administrative unit within the Association, and in 1991, the ANCC became a separately incorporated subsidiary of ANA. Interest in the development of a comprehensive system for credentialing remained an ANA priority, but with the cooperative relations between ANA and NLN, no overt action was taken by ANA to accredit formal nursing education programs (ANA does accredit CE programs). House of Delegates resolutions about the need for ANA to become involved in accreditation of nursing services were finally honored in the establishment of the magnet programs. These programs set the gold standard for systems of nursing service.

In 1986, the ANA published the first of a monograph series on credentialing in nursing, which, along with the Credentialing Study, gives information about nurse credentialing that is as comprehensive and provocative as that in any publication. In this first monograph, Dr. Margretta Styles, who had chaired the original Credentialing Study, made some in-depth comparisons between the credentialing of nurses in the United States and in the rest of the world. She had been commissioned by the International Council of Nurses (ICN), which also had many concerns about nurse credentialing, to help them develop a position on credentialing and regulation in nursing. The position paper she developed included 12 principles of regulation equally applicable to American nursing, other countries, and professionals beyond nursing.

Basically these principles warn against over-regulation, propose a flexibility that allows practice to respond sensitively to the changing times, recognize the temptation for regulation to be self-serving and protect the fiefdoms among professionals, and urge consumer input, universal standards, and the broadest practice role commensurate with the ability of the provider and social need.[8] These principles are presented in detail in the seventh edition of *Dimensions of Professional Nursing.*

In viewing US patterns of regulation, Styles commented on our uniqueness: the mix of public and private, mandatory and voluntary mechanisms; the decentralization of authority to the state and local level, but with some federal controls retained. Styles considered a second license for specialists to be duplicative and recommended national certification. In 1989, Styles completed an extremely comprehensive study on nursing specialties, including a survey of characteristics of specialties in nursing summarized in a voluminous appendix. She defined the characteristics of mature specialty areas.[9] These indices were eventually expanded and became the initial standard for the American Board of Nursing Specialties (ABNS).

Clear distinctions between areas of specialty practice are particularly important in certification, where we are trying to communicate with the public. Styles believed that to empower nurse specialists, specialty credentials must be strengthened through a national board of nurse specialties created to review and approve specialties and their certification programs. As a corollary process, marketing may have financial as well as professional implications; once certification is fully recognized, the person holding board certification may be reimbursed for services at a higher rate than a nurse without these credentials.

In 1991, the ABNS was established after generous developmental funding from the Josiah Macy Foundation. Its objectives include setting standards for the formal recognition of professional nursing specialties, establishing policies and procedures for the review and approval of certification programs, recognizing specialty nursing certification that meets ABNS standards, informing the public about this credential, and supporting national certification for professional regulation. Twenty certification boards comprise the membership of the ABNS, collectively representing nearly 500,000 RNs currently certified in the United States.[10] The standards for membership in the ABNS are as follows:

- The certification is based on a distinct and well-defined field of nursing practice that subscribes to the overall purpose and functions of nursing. The nursing specialty is distinct from other nursing specialties and is national in scope. There is an identified need for the specialty and nurses who devote most of their practice to the specialty.
- A tested body of research/data-based knowledge related to the nursing specialty exists. Mechanisms are established for the support, review, and dissemination of research in the specialty. Activities within the specialty contribute to the advancement of nursing science within the specialty.
- The certification board is an entity with organizational autonomy. However, a collaborative relationship exists between the certification body and a national or international nursing specialty association that supports the nursing specialty and the standards for specialty practice.
- There is a provision for public consultation/representation on the certification board.
- The eligibility criteria for the basic certification of nurses include RN licensure and educational and experiential qualifications as determined by the individual specialty certification organization.
- The eligibility criteria for the advanced certification of nurses include RN licensure and a minimum of a graduate degree in nursing or the appropriate equivalent, including content in the specified area of specialty practice.
- Certification tests are constructed and evaluated using methods that are psychometrically sound and fair to all candidates.
- The certifying body has conducted validation studies to assure that inferences made on the basis of test scores are appropriate and justified.
- The certifying body assures that test scores, including subscores, are sufficiently reliable for their intended uses.
- The certifying body does not discriminate among applicants as to age, gender, race, religion, ethnic origin, disability, marital status, or sexual orientation.
- Certification tests are administered in a manner that minimizes construct-irrelevant variance.
- Procedures are in place to maximize the security of all certification test materials.
- Passing scores for the certification examination are set in a manner that is fair to all candidates using methods that are psychometrically sound.
- The certifying body has mechanisms in place to encourage certificate holders to maintain and to periodically document knowledge necessary to maintain competence in the specialty.
- The certifying body provides information that clearly describes the certification process to candidates and other stakeholders.
- The certifying body assures that confidential information about candidates and certificate holders is protected.
- The certifying body has an appeal process in place for nurses who have been denied access to an examination or renewal of certification or who have had certification revoked.
- The certifying body has a mechanism in place to respond to instances of misrepresentation and noncompliance with eligibility criteria or certification board rules; this mechanism includes reporting cases of misrepresentation to appropriate authorities.

- Once accredited, certifying organizations shall adhere to ABNS Accreditation Council Standards. The ABNS Accreditation Council is to be informed in writing of any changes to an accredited certification that may affect compliance with ABNS Standards.
- The certification agency shall have an internal audit and review system in place including a provision for continuous corrective and preventive actions for quality improvement.[11]

Understanding the balance between internal and external regulation is important for professionals because their regulatory systems are based on a subtle balance between these systems of control. The purpose of internal regulation (within the profession) is to ensure the advancement of nursing while serving the public interest; external regulation (outside the profession) exists chiefly to protect the public. It makes sense, then, that internal regulation is based on expert opinion and may attempt to move the profession on to new, yet unachieved frontiers of practice. External regulation is based on a combination of expert opinion and role delineation studies that portray practice as it currently exists. Related reading is also located in Chapter 9.

■ LICENSURE: THE LEGAL BASIS OF NURSING PRACTICE

Enactment of nurse licensure laws was the most common reason for the formation of the state nurses' associations. The first permissive nursing practice law in this country was enacted in North Carolina on March 3, 1903. Weak though it was compared with present-day laws, it represented a great achievement for nursing leaders who had been working toward this goal for a decade. Within a month, New Jersey passed a state nursing practice act, followed closely by New York and Virginia. In 1904, Maryland was the only state to pass such an act, but in each succeeding year from 1905 until 1917, state legislation was enacted to govern the practice of nursing. By 1917, 45 states and the District of Columbia had nursing practice acts; by 1923, the last of the 48 states in existence adopted such an act. In 1952, all states and territories had such laws. Hawaii's first nursing practice act was passed in 1917 and Alaska's in 1941.

In every instance, the original state law was permissive. The first mandatory licensure statute was enacted in New York in 1938, but it was not put into effect until 1947. One of the real dangers of permissive licensing was the use of graduates of schools with poor curricula and inadequate clinical experience. These workers could legally use the title

nurse, although they were potentially dangerous practitioners. Such programs also tend to defraud unsuspecting students who do not know that they are ineligible for licensure. A school must maintain minimum standards set by the state board before graduates may sit for licensing examinations.

As of 1990, all states had mandatory licensure laws for professional and practical nurses. However, some states are permissive in their interpretation of *mandatory*. States that have such global exemption clauses in licensure laws stating that almost anyone can be a "nurse," provided that there is some kind of "supervision," are sometimes seen as permissive states regardless of a mandatory clause.

Objections to making licensure laws mandatory come from many sources. Some feel that mandatory laws are used to keep out individuals who might be capable but lack the formal education and other requirements for licensure. It is true that some laws are rigid in these requirements, but more and more states are beginning to consider the use of equivalency and proficiency examinations and other means of demonstrating knowledge and skills.

Another concern is that those already practicing in the field will be abruptly removed and deprived of their livelihood. This is, however, untrue because mandatory laws are forced, for political and constitutional reasons, to include a grandfather clause. A *grandfather* or *waiver* clause is a standard feature when a licensure law is enacted or amended. The grandfather clause allows persons to continue to practice the profession or occupation when new qualifications are enacted into law. Although the concept goes back to post–Civil War days, it is also related to the Fifth and Fourteenth amendments to the Constitution. The US Supreme Court has repeatedly ruled that the license to practice a profession or occupation is a property right and that the Fourteenth Amendment extends the due process requirement to state laws. All nurses currently licensed and in compliance with state law are protected by the grandfather clause when a new law is passed or new requirements are instituted, although most probably never realize it. For instance, when the Wyoming Nursing Practice Act was repealed in 1983, the new law had a grandfather clause, and all nurses holding a valid license continued to be licensed. When the grandfather clause is enacted in relation to mandatory licensure, those who can produce evidence that they practiced as, say, a practical nurse (PN), if applying for LPN status, must be granted a license. However, grandfathering does not guarantee employment. Thus, some employers chose not to employ waivered PNs, just as they had not employed them as unlicensed practitioners.

Because of these problems, and often because of their need and desire to be safe, many competent practitioners took courses to fill the gaps in their knowledge and chose to take the state board examinations later. One interesting exception was attempted with the Wyoming law: a limited grandfather clause for previously approved nurse practitioners (NPs), giving them 2 years to meet the new NP qualifications. The legislature disagreed because NPs were being treated differently from other RNs. The Mississippi Supreme Court made a similar decision.[11]

■ CONTENT OF NURSING PRACTICE ACTS

Unfortunately, many nurses know no more about the law that regulates their practice than that it requires them to take state board examinations to become licensed. More details about the procedure for obtaining a license will be given later; however, it is vital that nurses understand the components of their licensure law and how these affect their practice. (CNMs and CRNAs may be included within a nursing practice act, a medical practice act, separately, or totally ignored legislatively. If mentioned, certification is usually a prerequisite for legal practice.)

Because each state law differs to a degree in its content, it is important to have available a copy of the law of the state in which you practice and the regulations that spell out how the law is carried out. These may be obtained from the state board or an agency in state government or on the Internet. The language in all laws often seems stilted because they are written in legal terms. However, a little effort or discussion with someone familiar with the law will soon enable you to become almost as familiar with legal jargon as with nursing jargon. This is particularly important, because this is the public policy that spells out your rights and responsibilities.

Most nursing practice acts have basically the same major components, although not necessarily in the same order: legislative mandate (why have this law?), definition of nursing, requirements for licensure, exemption from licensure, grounds for revocation, suspension or conditioning of the license, provision for endorsement for persons licensed in other states, creation of a board of nurse examiners, responsibilities of the board, and penalties for practicing in violation of the act or without a license. All states do not, unfortunately, have the same requirements in these categories. Some follow the ANA guidelines, some the model act of the NCSBN, others enact what is politically feasible or necessary in their particular state.

The ANA guidelines and the NCSBN Model Act are basic resources. The question is often raised as to why two influential groups involved in nurse licensure should have separate recommendations for legislation. This is not difficult to answer; they operate from different mandates. Each group has its own constituents: NCSBN, with its representatives from all the state boards of nursing, works from the perspective of elected or appointed state officials, with an overriding responsibility to ensure that licensure protects the consumer, whereas ANA, with its diverse group of nurses and state associations, is committed to setting standards for nursing. There are useful elements in both the ANA and NCSBN documents. ANA is oriented to a philosophy that expects the provisions of the practice act to drive the reality of the future, and NCSBN is firmly focused on the present reality. Neither document has any legal clout, and states tend to use what suits their needs, but those involved in nurse legislation generally study both documents. This would be a worthwhile exercise for interested nurses as well, providing provocative and stimulating food for discussion on how we see nursing.

By 1991, some form of regulation had become common for advanced practice in almost every state. This was predictable; government tends to become involved in consumer protection at the point of reimbursement for services. For nurses that point was most commonly advanced practice, whereas for physicians it is the MD/DO, with specialization being informative for the public, but not always essential for reimbursement.

Leadership in both nursing and medicine has historically opposed governmental regulation of specialty practice. Internal regulation has been overwhelmingly favored based on the clinical complexity of specialized practice and the fact that the science advances through research conducted in specialty areas. The reasoning continues that for the discipline to advance and change at a pace commensurate with the science, the specialty edge must remain unencumbered by public policy and the inevitable bureaucracy it attracts.

Logical or not, it was too late for nursing to hold to this classic standard. Because all states address advanced practice in public policy, it was a question of achieving some standardization and creating harmony between form and function.

State boards of nursing hold the formal authority and many require a national certification in the specialty as a minimum requirement to qualify for APN governmental recognition. They had already begun to commingle the domains of professional and public recognition. However, there was not complete comfort that the certification process as provided by professional groups guaranteed competency, and guarantees of competency became the driving force. In 1994 at their annual meeting, the NCSBN membership called to move forward and investigate the development of a national certification mechanism under its own aegis for NPs. This ignited a flurry of activity to verify the credibility of the profession's certification mechanisms. This included scrutiny of the psychometric measures of adequacy as well as reconsideration of the role of expert opinion and role delineation studies in constructing the examinations. The expectations of the NCSBN must have been adequately addressed, given that in 1995 the NCSBN membership tabled their intention to develop their own examinations in favor of working toward consensus with the major existing certifying bodies.[12]

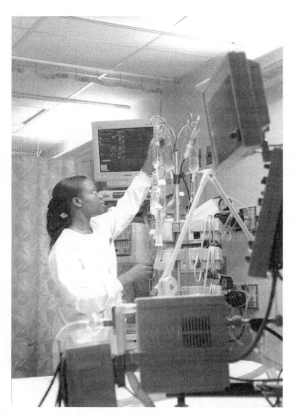

It is each nurse's responsibility to honestly assess his or her competence in clinical practice. This is what the individual license is all about. (Courtesy of Robert Wood Johnson University Hospital, New Brunswick, New Jersey)

Definition and Scope of Practice

The definition of nursing in the licensure law determines both legal responsibilities and the scope of practice of nurses. Inevitably, the definition of nursing in all nursing practice acts is stated in terms that are quite broad. This is generally frustrating to nurses who turn to the definition to determine if they are practicing legally. The definition does not spell out specific procedures or activities. Often such activities are not even spelled out in the regulations of the laws. However, a broad definition is usually preferable because being too specific excludes other options. Additionally, changes in health care and nursing practice often move more rapidly than a law can be changed; the amending process can be long and complex. If particular activities were named, the nurse would be limited to just those listed. Not only would the list be overwhelmingly long, but also it is conceivable that any new technique performed by a nurse would require an amendment to the law. An occasional state law does specify certain procedures, but it always includes the phrase "not limited to."

A practicing nurse soon finds that the nursing functions taught in an educational program may differ from those expected by an employer. The differences may be small and caused by variations in the settings of nursing care. Nursing in a medical center may require knowing more sophisticated techniques or assuming more comprehensive responsibilities in nursing care. Sometimes, whether in a large or small agency, there are procedures performed that the nurse has not learned. If the nurse has not practiced for some time, this is even more likely to happen. In other cases, the responsibilities expected in the nursing role are not nursing care but clerical and administrative tasks. Although this may not be desirable, it is not illegal. What concerns nurses is whether the direct patient care expected in the employment situation is legal or in the domain of another health profession. Many of the activities in health care overlap. A common example might be the administration of drugs, which could be done by the physician, RN, LPN, and various technicians in other hospital departments if related to a diagnostic procedure or treatment. Yet, dispensing a drug from the hospital pharmacy, still done by many nursing supervisors at times when no pharmacist is on duty, is in most states a violation of the pharmacy licensing law.

Obviously, one of the greatest concerns for nurses is the possible violation of the Medical Practice Act. Nurses have gradually been performing more and more of the technical procedures that once belonged exclusively to medicine, but often these are delegated willingly by physicians. Whether nurses are always properly prepared to understand and perform them well is seldom questioned. However, as some nurses have assumed more comprehensive overall responsibilities in the care, cure, and coordination of patient care, both nurses and physicians have raised questions. Some are resistant to such changes; others are supportive but concerned about the legality of such acts. There are few data on nurses being disciplined for practicing medicine without a license. It should be noted that the boundaries between the professions do change over time, and that where there are questions, the board of nursing should be asked for an interpretation. An official change in public policy is not frequently needed.

In the now-classic DHEW report, *Extending the Scope of Nursing Practice*, there is a statement that an identical act or procedure "may be the practice of medicine when carried out by a physician and the practice of nursing when carried out by the nurse" (see Chapter 5).

> There is an ever-widening area of independent nursing practice entailing nursing judgment, procedures, and techniques. This is due to natural evolution, commencing with the nurse's assumption of certain activities carried out under medical direction, and the subsequent relaxation or removal of that direction.

Concomitant with increasingly complex nursing practice is the continual realignment of the functions of the professional nurse and physician. The boundaries of responsibility for nurses are not shifting more rapidly simply because of increased demands for health services. The functions of nurses are changing primarily because nurses have demonstrated their competence to perform a greater variety of functions and have been willing to discontinue performing less important functions that were once performed only by nurses.[13]

The same report stated that there are no legal barriers to extending the scope of practice because the statutory laws governing nursing practice (the licensing laws) are broad enough to permit such extension, provided that the nurse has the proper skills and necessary knowledge of the underlying science. The report did acknowledge that at times there have been declaratory decisions of the courts about some aspect of nursing that is not included in statutes. When this happens, the profession should consider whether the statutes need to be changed. That is exactly what happens.

Until 1974, the nursing practice acts of most states had, as their definition of nursing, one similar to a model suggested by ANA in 1955:

> The practice of professional nursing means the performance for compensation of any act in the observation, care, and counsel of the ill, injured, or infirm, or in the maintenance of health or prevention of illness of others, or in the supervision and teaching of other personnel, or the administration of medications and treatments as prescribed by a licensed physician or dentist; requiring substantial specialized judgment and skill and based on knowledge and application of the principles of biological, physical, and social science. (The foregoing shall not be deemed to include acts of diagnosis or prescription of therapeutic or corrective measures.)[14]

The definition distinguished between *independent acts* that the nurse might perform, but also identified certain *dependent acts*, and prohibited diagnosis and treatment (not preceded by the word *medical*). In the 1970s, with expanded functions being assumed by nurses, state nurses' associations (SNAs) increasingly became concerned about the adequacy of this definition. Therefore, the first states to change their laws concentrated on broadening the definition to encompass these changing roles and functions.

Professional nursing literature had been distinguishing between the independent acts that a nurse must undertake and the dependent acts that must be carried out under the supervision or orders of the physician. The problem in the 1955 definition, in terms of the needs of the 1970s, was that although the first sentence did not prohibit the nurse from carrying out medical acts or making diagnoses, the last sentence effectively prohibited a broad interpretation by the courts.

As nurses in their expanded role seemed to be moving into the gray areas between medicine and nursing, it was evident that, if a state had a licensure law with a dependent clause, nurses might be seen as practicing medicine. The 1971 and 1973 credentialing reports suggested extending the delegation of authority in all fields, but nursing was concerned that such delegation might mean including nurses specifically in the exception clause of medical practice acts, thus permitting the practice, but placing control totally in the hands of physicians. Perhaps as a compromise or in the hope that medicine and nursing could work together as they should in providing new health care options to the public, ANA counsel at the time suggested that a new clause be added to the ANA model definition. This became known as an "additional acts" amendment:

> A professional nurse may also perform such additional acts, under emergency or other special conditions, which may include special training, as are recognized by the medical and nursing professions as proper to be performed by a professional nurse under such conditions, even though such acts might otherwise be considered diagnosis and prescription.[15]

Later, after various states had amended their laws with this phrase or changed it altogether, with varying success, an ANA ad hoc committee revised the definition entirely in 1976. This model law, recommending one nursing practice law with provisions for licensing all practitioners of nursing, used the terms *registered nurse* and *practical/vocational nurse*. This definition differentiated between the independence of the RN's functions and the dependence of the LPN/LVN. It also placed the responsibility for what the RN can legally do in the hands of the nursing profession, always considered a hallmark of professionalism.

The changes in practice act language are a reflection of the times. In 1990, the ANA held firm for one practice act and strained to keep any mention of advanced practice out of the public domain. In that same era, the ANA spoke of technical and professional nurses, whereas the NCSBN document was silent on any distinction between RNs, an obvious attempt on the part of ANA to reflect its preferred future for nursing. Later, model practice acts achieved more consistency in language. Both versions included clear delegatory language. ANA used bolder words about medical diagnosis and treatment, and introduced the responsibility for research. The NCSBN is clearer on the collaborative nature of the role.

The title *Advanced Practice Registered Nurse* (APRN) is protected in both renditions. This goes beyond title protection and verifies the existence of nurses who bring a specialized knowledge and skill to the public. Both also accept the umbrella title of APRN and define the term as inclusive of NP, clinical nurse specialist (CNS), CRNA, and CNM. The need for this language became all too apparent when practice rights were denied NPs and CNSs (CRNAs and CNMs were already commonly mentioned in public policy) in some states because these practitioners hypothetically did not exist, there being no recognition of their existence anywhere in public policy. Further, there is common agreement that some detail has to exist in public policy about the rights and responsibilities of APRNs, and their educational background. At what level of policy and in what detail remains to be debated, and is probably more dependent on politics than legal necessity. Although the requirement for physician collaboration/joint practice/supervision remains in many states, it is absent in both model acts. (The terms *APRN* and *APN* are used interchangeably in this book.)

APRNs are recognized in public policy in every state. This represents significant progress. The earliest approaches to formalizing the expanding role of the nurse were joint statements between nurses', medical, and hospital associations. These statements offered no legal protection, but documented mutual acceptance of an evolving pattern of practice. Lawyers found such statements helpful in mounting a defense on behalf of both nurses and physicians if their joint practices were challenged. Both ANA and NCSBN agree that the board of nursing should be the sole authority to regulate advanced practice, but multiple board (nursing, medicine, pharmacy for the most part) involvement has resulted in some states, probably finding justification in those early joint statements.

Although there has been some significant movement toward agreement about advanced practice, other disagreements continue. ANA persists in its contention that state boards of nursing should accept the profession's standards and certifications, whereas NCSBN holds that they should establish the criteria for competence, and then the profession can have the opportunity to prove that they examine for those criteria.

The greatest differences between the ANA and NCSBN documents are in the preferred vehicle for explication and change. ANA relies on administrative statements for detail, whereas NCSBN is either silent on the vehicle or looks for codification in statutes. The ANA addresses other issues (the impaired nurse, prescriptive authority) in separate acts. ANA's caution is to avoid opening the Nursing Practice Act wherever possible, and to keep practice act language broad, using administrative statements or rule making for amplification. The intent is both to protect the practice act and to allow easier routes for change where it is necessary. The reader is referred to the seventh edition of *Dimensions of Professional Nursing* for a detailed description of the evolution of advanced practice in public policy.

Creation of a Board of Nursing

The name of the state administrative agency for the Nursing Practice Act varies from state to state, as does the number of board members. Traditionally, this board had been made up entirely of nurses, who may or may not be designated as to area of practice and education. In most states, members are appointed by the governor from a list of names submitted by the SNA and others. Because of some public outcry against control by professionals, gradually the addition of non-nurses, either public members or other health professionals, has become legally required and common. Although some nurses have considered this a danger to the profession, it can be to the advantage of nursing to have the input and support of the public and others on the health team because these public members can be educated to understand and appreciate the problems of the profession. The danger exists when political pressure seeks to force the creation of a board with a majority of non-nurses, so that nursing practice and education can be totally controlled by others. Most states had consumers or other professionals as members by 1977. The ANA supports consumer participation, as does the NCSBN. There is also increasing interest in having APNs on boards. Where the board of nursing regulates the practice of LPNs/LVNs, this constituency has representation. Board sizes range from 5 to 19 appointed members. Staff employed by the board carry out the day-to-day activities.

Responsibilities of the Board of Nursing

The major responsibility of a board is to see that the nursing practice act is carried out. This involves establishing rules and regulations to implement the broad terms in the law itself and setting minimum standards of practice. Usual responsibilities include the approval of educational programs for nursing and the development of criteria (minimum standards) that address the clinical placements used for educational purposes, curriculum, faculty, and so on; evaluating the personal and educational qualifications of applicants for licensure; determining by examination applicants' competence to practice nursing; issuing licenses to qualified applicants; and disciplining those who violate the law or are found to be unfit to practice nursing, sometimes holding hearings. (Investigations and hearings are often conducted by another arm of the state government.)

Other responsibilities include developing standards for continuing the competency of licensed practitioners; issuing limited licenses to those who cannot practice the full scope of nursing, perhaps owing to a handicap; interpreting the scope of practice as codified in the statutes; and developing policy for other purposes such as prescriptive authority, pronouncement of death, and so on, to the extent that the

law allows. Nursing boards may hold educational programs, collect data, and cooperate in various ways with other nursing boards or the boards of other disciplines. If they operate under an overall board (one professional board representing many disciplines), certain administrative responsibilities will be carried out centrally.

The power of the board should not be underestimated. For instance, it was simply by changing regulations that the North Dakota Board established new educational requirements for RN and LPN licensure.

Requirements for Licensure as a Nurse

Licensure is based on fulfilling certain requirements. The following points are usually included:

1. The applicant must have completed an educational program in a state-approved school of nursing and received a diploma or degree from that program; usually the school must send the student's transcript. There is some legislative pressure that the applicant not be required to have completed the program, particularly if the uncompleted courses are in a non-nursing area such as liberal arts. This is not looked on favorably by either ANA or NCSBN.

2. The applicant must pass an examination given by the board. This examination is currently the NCLEX-RN, developed under the aegis of the NCSBN and given in every state. The examination is now offered using a computerized adaptive testing (CAT) approach.

3. Some states require evidence of good physical and mental health, but this is not recommended by either ANA or NCSBN. Actual practice varies a great deal from state to state. Handicapped students have been admitted, graduated, and taken state boards in some states; in others, this is denied. Court cases often result.

4. Most states maintain a statement that the applicant must be of good moral character, as determined by the licensing board, but this, too, is impractical. The model act suggests terminology that refers to acts that are grounds for board disciplinary action if the nurse is licensed.

5. A fee must be paid for admission to the examination.

6. A temporary license may be issued to a graduate of an approved program pending the results of the first licensure exam.

7. Demonstrated competence in English is recommended. It has been declared unconstitutional to make requirements of age, citizenship, and residence.

Provisions for Endorsement of Persons Licensed in Other States

Nurses, with the exception of nurses in advanced practice, have more mobility than any other licensed health professionals because of the use of a national standardized examination. However, usually the individual must still fulfill the other requirements in the state in which he or she seeks licensure and must submit proof that the license has not been revoked. The candidate's nursing school record is usually evaluated to determine whether the program is generally equivalent to the state's program requirements of the same time period. If it is not, the nurse may be required to take the courses that are lacking and the examination.

If all requirements are satisfactorily fulfilled, the nurse is granted a license without retaking the state board examination. A fee is also required for this process of endorsement. *Endorsement* is not the same as *reciprocity*, which means acceptance of a licensee by one state if the other state does likewise.

Endorsement is the interstate mechanism that currently exists, but the Nurse Licensure Compact, as discussed earlier in this chapter, is growing in use (see Exhibit 20–2).

Renewal of Licensure

Until the early 1970s, nursing licenses were renewed simply by sending in the renewal fee when notified, usually every 2 years. For nurses licensed in more than one state, as long as the license was not revoked in any state, the process was the same. Theoretically, the individual might be denied relicensure for certain physical or mental handicaps or drug abuse, but there was no organized way to check on this. Usually the form asked for information about employment and the highest degree completed (and still does), but no attempt was made to determine if the nurse was competent, or if the information was correct. At about that time (also the time of the credentialing reports), there was increased concern about the current competency of practicing health professionals, and an estimate was made that perhaps 5 percent of all health professionals were not competent for some reason. Moreover, there was some question as to whether the professions made any real effort either to rehabilitate or retool these people or to revoke their licenses. The credentialing reports emphasized the need for CE as a requirement for relicensure. One outcome was the enactment of a mandatory CE clause in some state licensing laws; that is, a practitioner's license would not be renewed unless she or he showed evidence of CE. A number of health disciplines have such legislation.

By 1977, a number of states had made mandatory CE a requirement for relicensure (or a legal practice requirement) for about 20 health occupations. Even where they exist, such requirements are not always well enforced. Some states do have permissive legislation for possible later implementation. In addition, most certifications require continuing education for renewal.

Actually, any state could use regulations to require CE without changing the law because all practice acts give the licensing boards the authority to determine standards of competence, and these are usually delineated in regulations. Nevertheless, in the 1970s, a number of state nurses' associations introduced legislation either requiring CE or specifically directing the state board to study or plan such a requirement. Realistically, this action may have been attributable as much to the fear of externally introduced legislation that might remove control of the issue from nursing as to the conviction that this was a necessary amendment. Some of these states recognize only CE offerings approved by their boards or given by an agency, group, or institution that has been given a provider (or approval) number. This may create problems for those licensed in more than one state or living in a state other than where licensed. In the latter situation, some states permit the nurse to maintain the license on an inactive status, which can be reactivated when evidence of CE is shown.

Forms of CE accepted by states include various formal academic studies in institutions of higher learning converted to continuing education units (CEU credit); college extension courses and studies; grand rounds in the health care setting; home study programs; in-service education; institutes; lectures; seminars; workshops; audiovisual learning systems, including educational television, audiovisual cassettes, tapes, and records with self-study packets; challenge examinations for a course or program; self-learning systems such as community service, controlled independent study, delivery of a paper, preparation and participation in a panel; preparation and publication of articles, monographs, books, and so on; special research; and Internet courses. When continuing education is mandatory for relicensure, the required number of hours varies considerably. More is included on mandatory CE in Chapter 13 and Exhibit 13–3. In 2009, 29 state boards had CE requirements for the renewal of licenses for the RN and LPN/LVN.[16]

No law requires formal education directed toward advanced degrees. In fact, although additional formal education is acceptable, the emphasis is on continuous, updated competence in practice. The fears and anger of many nurses have been misdirected because they assumed that advanced degrees would be required. Obviously, there are innumerable ways in which an individual can maintain competence and increase knowledge and skills. How to measure achievement for the large number of nurses concerned is the real problem.

Objections to mandatory CE focus on the difficulty of assessing true learning; the question of whether learning can be forced (attendance does not mean retention or change in behavior); the danger of breeding mediocrity; the lack of research on the effectiveness of CE in relation to performance; limitation of resources, particularly in rural areas; the cost to nurses; the cost to government; the usual rigidity of governmental regulations; the problems in record keeping; and the lack of accreditation or evaluation procedures for many CE programs.

But the issue is far from resolved. Although the trend toward mandatory CE slowed considerably in the 1980s for all occupations, the call for continued competence has intensified. It is possible that another trend, peer evaluation, and other kinds of performance evaluation may provide a more effective answer to continued competence.

Exemptions from Licensure

This may also be called an *exception clause*. Generally exempted from RN licensure are basic students in a nursing program; anyone furnishing nursing assistance in an emergency; anyone licensed in another state and caring for a patient temporarily in the state involved; anyone employed by the US government as a nurse (Veterans Administration, public health, or armed services); any legally qualified nurse recruited by the Red Cross during a disaster; anyone caring for the sick if care is performed in connection with the practice of religious tenets of any church; anyone giving incidental care in a family situation; and any RN or LPN from another state engaged in consultation as long as no direct care is given.

In all these cases, the person cannot claim to be an RN of the state concerned. Over strong nursing protests, some states have also incorporated in the exemptions nursing services of attendants in state institutions, if supervised by nurses or doctors, as well as other kinds of nursing assistants under various circumstances. This, of course, weakens the mandatory aspect of the law.

Grounds for Revocation of Licensure

The board has the right to revoke or suspend any nurse's license or otherwise discipline the licensee. The reasons most commonly found in practice acts for revoking a license are acts that might directly endanger the public, such as practicing while one's ability is impaired by alcohol, drugs, or physical or mental disability; being addicted to or dependent on alcohol or other habit-forming drugs or a habitual user of certain drugs; and practicing with incompetence or negligence or beyond the scope of practice. Other reasons are obtaining a license fraudulently, being convicted of a felony or crime involving moral turpitude (or accepting a plea of *nolo contendere*); practicing while the license is suspended or revoked; aiding and abetting a nonlicensed person to perform activities requiring a license; and committing unprofessional or immoral acts as defined by the board. The refusal to provide service to a person because of race, color, creed, or national origin may also have been added in some states.

The most common reasons that nurses lose their licenses are the same as those that apply to physicians—substance use and abuse or theft. Criteria for reinstatement are based on a statement from the board showing that the nurse has been evaluated and is able to function. Eventually state nurses' associations recognized this as a professional responsibility and created programs of peer assistance, including counseling and support (see Chapter 10). It is probably for this reason that the ANA suggests a separate law (*Nursing Disciplinary Diversion Act*) that mandates that the board of nursing seek ways to rehabilitate impaired nurses and to establish a voluntary alternative to traditional disciplinary actions. Alcohol abuse or intemperance interfering with practice is also part of what is considered substance abuse.

As is true in obtaining or renewing licenses, a nurse could also lose his or her license because of physical or mental impairment. Legal blindness is the most common physical condition involved, but there are many exceptions, especially since the passage of the Rehabilitation Act described in Chapter 19.

With the exception of substance abuse, it is rare that specific conditions for revocation or suspension of license are detailed in legislation or even regulations. Rather, disciplinary action may be authorized by the ubiquitous "unprofessional behavior" clause. A number of states already have regulations defining unprofessional conduct, and depending on how the licensure laws are structured, the regulations may define unprofessional behavior as it applies to all licensed health professionals (New York) or may be written into each separate law.

The courts have also played a major role in shaping interpretation. They have been opposed to trivializing unprofessional conduct and have held to the criteria of behavior that intellectually or morally creates jeopardy through practice. An example exists where the District Court in Nebraska reversed the Board of Nursing's denial of license, finding that the plaintiff may be difficult to get along with and resistive to directions, but not unprofessional. Criteria used by the state of Utah date back to 1991, but remain especially clear and provide a good example:

1. Failing to utilize appropriate judgment in administering safe nursing practice based on the level of nursing for which the individual is licensed

2. Failing to exercise technical competence in carrying out nursing care

3. Failing to follow policies or procedures defined in the practice situation to safeguard patient care

4. Failing to safeguard the patient's dignity and right to privacy

5. Violating the confidentiality of information or knowledge concerning the patient

6. Verbally or physically abusing patients

7. Performing any nursing techniques or procedures without proper education and preparation

8. Performing procedures beyond the authorized scope of the level of nursing and/or health care for which the individual is licensed

9. Intentional manipulation or misuse of drug supplies, narcotics, or patients' records

10. Falsifying patients' records or intentionally charting incorrectly

11. Appropriating medications, supplies, or personal items of the patient or agency

12. Violating state or federal laws relative to drugs

13. Falsifying records submitted to a government agency

14. Intentionally committing any act that adversely affects the physical or psychosocial welfare of the patient

15. Delegating nursing care, functions, tasks, and/or responsibilities to others contrary to the laws governing nursing and/or to the detriment of patient safety

16. Failing to exercise appropriate supervision over persons who are authorized to practice only under the supervision of the licensed professional

17. Leaving a nursing assignment without properly notifying appropriate personnel

18. Failing to report, through the proper channels, facts known to the individual regarding the incompetent, unethical, or illegal practice of any licensed health care professional[17]

It should be noted that many state nursing practice acts and the NCSBN Model Nursing Practice Act contain lists of unprofessional practices, but they are less clear than the example offered above. The absence of very specific language in statutes or regulations is purposeful to avoid foreclosure on unanticipated types of behavior. This problem is sometimes resolved by using the phrase "not limited to," but if the legislature has a particular concern, this may be written into the law. Some states have also adopted the ANA standards of practice as criteria for incompetence.

A particular problem in both statutory and regulatory language concerns such terms as *moral, ethical,* and *moral turpitude,* because these can be interpreted in various ways. Model acts use phrases such as "has engaged in any act inconsistent with standards of nursing practice as defined by Board Rules and Regulations" and "a crime in any jurisdiction that relates adversely to the practice of nursing or to the ability to practice nursing."

Another issue is what a nurse should do about reporting incompetence or unprofessional conduct on the part of physicians or other health professionals. Because the nurses' code of ethics requires that she or he safeguard the patient, incompetent or unprofessional practitioners should be reported. Most surveys indicate that a large percentage of nurses would take some sort of action, usually speaking with the doctor, head nurse, or supervisor, if the patient was endangered by medical action. Few would report the physician to a peer review or licensing board. In part, this is because they fear a lawsuit. All but a few states have laws giving immunity from civil action to any person who reports to a peer review board if there is no malice, but this does not preclude being sued, even though malice is very difficult to prove. In New York, a statute was enacted requiring physicians to report other physicians' misconduct on penalty of being cited for unprofessional conduct themselves; nurses and others are also encouraged to report such misconduct. (Some have interpreted the law as requiring such reporting by all licensed professionals.) Other states have similar statutes, including states requiring nurses to report nurses. There is another problem; some nurses who have reported a physician have either been dismissed from their jobs or harassed, a situation that is more difficult to resolve. *Whistle blower laws* can provide some protection here and are discussed in Chapter 30. A supportive working environment can also make a difference.

Although the law seems to protect the public, data show that relatively few nurses have had licenses revoked or suspended. In part, the reason is believed to be the reluctance of other nurses to report and consequently testify to these acts by their colleagues before either the nursing board or a court of law. Nursing associations and state boards are now emphasizing the responsibility of professional nurses to report incompetent practice. Most current model acts make nonreporting a disciplinary offense.

When a report is filed with the state board charging a nurse with violation of any of the grounds of disciplinary action, he or she is entitled to certain procedural safeguards (*due process*). After investigation, the nurse must receive notice of the charges and be given time to prepare a defense. A hearing is set and subpoenas are issued (by the board, attorney general, or a hearing officer). The accused has the right to appear personally or be represented by counsel, who may cross-examine witnesses. If the license is revoked or suspended, it may be reissued at the discretion of the board. (Sometimes the individual is only censured or reprimanded.)

Consumers have questioned whether health care professionals are vigilant in monitoring their own against charges of incompetence and illegal behavior. To ensure the public's safety, legislation created the *National Practitioner Data Bank (NPDB)*. The intent of the NPDB is to collect and release information about the conduct of health care practitioners. Effective March 1, 2010, the scope of the NPDB was expanded to include adverse licensure information on all licensed health care practitioners and health care entities. It also includes certain final actions or recommendations to sanction that have been taken by Private Accreditation Entities and Peer Review Organizations. The NPDB must, by law, be consulted by any health care institution seeking to hire a new provider and by certifying bodies, insurance companies, and federal and state licensing agencies when they are going to certify, credential, or license a provider, including a nurse, for the first time. Hospitals must then recheck the NPDB every 2 years for every provider's records. Information is required to be reported to the data bank by these same bodies about all providers, including nurses, related specifically to

- Malpractice payments made by or for the nurse, including judgment, arbitration, decisions, and out-of-court settlements (but not the amount spent on the defense)

- Licensure actions such as revocation, suspension, reprimand, censure, or probation[18]

The *Health Care Integrity and Protection Data Bank* (HIPDB) is another data source provided by the federal government (for a fee) to organizations that goes further than the NPDB. The HIPDB is a flagging system that serves as an alert to its users that a particular provider or supplier may warrant additional, more comprehensive review. NPDB does not collect data on all health care practitioners, providers, and suppliers on all legal charges and complaints of fraud or abuse.[19]

The pieces of legislation that led to the creation of the NPDB and the HIPDB were enacted because the US Congress believed the need to improve the quality of care had become a nationwide problem that warranted greater efforts than any individual state could undertake. The intent is to improve the quality of health care by encouraging state licensing boards, hospitals, other health care entities, and professional societies to identify and discipline those who engage in dangerous behavior, and to restrict the ability of incompetent practitioners to move from state to state without disclosure or discovery of previous adverse action history. These databases are an alert or flagging system intended to encourage a more diligent review of past history. The information contained in the NPDB/HIPDB should be considered together with other relevant data and is intended to augment, not replace, traditional forms of credentials review. Both the NPDB and HIPDB are prohibited from disclosing specific information on a practitioner, provider, or supplier to the general public.

Penalties for Practicing Without a License

Penalties for practicing without a license vary from a minimum fine to a large fine or imprisonment. Usually legal action is taken. Penalties are being strengthened to deter illegal practice.

■ HOW TO OBTAIN A LICENSE

Almost all new graduates of a nursing program apply for RN licensure, because it is otherwise impossible to practice. Although there is nothing to prohibit you from postponing licensure, it is generally more difficult psychologically and because of lack of clinical practice to take the state board examination (NCLEX-RN) much later.

As a rule, your school makes available all the data and even the application forms necessary for beginning the licensure procedure. Should you wish to become licensed in another state, because of planned relocation, request an application from that nursing board. Correct titles and addresses of the nursing boards of all states are found in the *Career Guide of the American Journal of Nursing*, which is published annually. The board advises you of the proper procedure, cost, and data needed.

NCLEX-RN is administered year-round using CAT. Applications for the examination are made to the board of nursing in the jurisdiction where you want to be licensed. Once the licensure application has been reviewed and your eligibility approved by the board of nursing, you will receive an Authorization to Test (ATT). A bulletin, *Scheduling and Taking Your NCLEX*, will also be forwarded that describes the examination, procedures for making an appointment, a list of available test center locations and telephone numbers, and a toll-free number to call for information on any newly opened centers. The NCLEX is administered by Pearson Professional Centers, with at least one site located in each state and territory. The individual candidate schedules his or her own date and time for the examination. For more information on specific application procedures and requirements, contact your board of nursing.

The CAT provides for each candidate to have a unique examination because it is assembled interactively as the individual is tested. The computer calculates a competence estimate based on all earlier answers as the candidate answers each question. A large question bank stores all the examination questions and classifies them by test plan area and level of difficulty. The questions are then searched and the one determined to measure the candidate most precisely in the appropriate test plan area is shown on the computer screen. This process is then repeated for each question, thus forming an examination unique to the candidate's knowledge and skills. Grades are reported simply as a pass-fail score. Both NCLEX-RN and -LPN are based on periodic job analyses.

The tests are the same for all nurses seeking an RN, whether graduating from a diploma, associate degree, or baccalaureate program. This has been the subject of controversy because the stated goals of all three programs are different. However, proponents of a single licensing exam state that the purpose is to determine safe and effective practice at a minimal level, and that this criterion applies equally to all levels of nurses.

Nurses who pass the licensing examination receive a certificate bearing a registration number that remains the same as long as they are registered in that state. The certificate (or registration card) will also carry the expiration date—usually 1, 2, or 3 years hence. Failure to renew

promptly may mean that you must pay a special fee to be reinstated.

It is advisable to keep your registration in effect, whether actively engaged in nursing or not. The expense is nominal. All nurses continue to have the responsibility (and sometimes the legal requirement) to keep their nursing knowledge updated through CE.

To become licensed or registered by endorsement, applicants must already be registered in one state, territory, or foreign country. They must apply to the state board of nursing in the new state and present credentials, as requested, to prove that they have completed preparation equal to that required. A temporary permit is usually issued to allow the nurse to work until the new license is issued.

Nurses who wish to be reregistered after allowing their licenses to lapse should contact their state board for directions. An RN wishing to practice nursing in another country also needs to investigate the country's legal requirements for practice. The sponsoring group will advise members of the armed forces or the Peace Corps, or those under the auspices of an organization such as the World Health Organization or a religious denomination. Registration in one state is usually sufficient.

Since 1993, the United States has entered into two major trade agreements that have significant ramifications for nurses and nursing. These are the *North American Free Trade Agreement* (NAFTA) and the *General Agreement on Tariffs and Trade* (GATT). The trade pact between the United States, Canada, and Mexico (NAFTA) removes most trade barriers among these nations. This creates the world's largest free-trade zone and permits the unencumbered movement of nurses across borders for employment opportunities given that they are qualified. ANA, partnering with the Office of the US Trade Representative and a coalition of licensed professionals, worked hard to ensure state primacy and autonomy in matters related to licensing and credentialing under NAFTA by obtaining language in the Statement of Administrative Actions clarifying that NAFTA does not permit Mexican or Canadian professionals to practice a licensed profession in the United States without meeting all applicable state licensing criteria.

The Commission on Graduates of Foreign Nursing Schools

In the late 1960s, the United States experienced an increase in nurses migrating to the United States to practice nursing. Immigration officials were having difficulty identifying which of the nurses educated abroad and applying for nursing occupational visas would actually be eligible for licensure as RNs in the United States. At that time, only about 15 to 20 percent of the nurses educated out of the United States were passing the US registered nurse licensing exam. This led the Division of Nursing to contract for two studies regarding RN licensure of foreign-educated nurses in the United States. The findings of these landmark studies on foreign nurse immigration were presented at a 1975 Department of Health, Education, and Welfare conference attended by representatives from governmental and private organizations, including the US Department of Labor, the Immigration and Naturalization Service, the ANA, and the NLN.

The outgrowth of the conference was that in 1977, ANA and NLN agreed to cosponsor the establishment of an independent nonprofit organization for the purpose of developing an equitable system through which nurses educated outside the United States could gauge their chances of becoming licensed as RNs in the United States. Such an organization would have as its mission to establish an orderly process for assessing the individual knowledge and level of preparation of each nurse applicant. These efforts would also help serve to protect the public health by ensuring that nurses educated outside the United States meet standards that are comparable to those of RNs educated in the United States. The organization created and chartered with this mission was the *Commission on Graduates of Foreign Nursing Schools* (CGFNS), most recently known as CGFNS International.

Currently, the Commission provides a variety of services, including the CGFNS Certification Program and the Credentials Evaluation Service, for nurses and other health professionals educated outside the United States who wish to practice in the United States. To support these services, CGFNS conducts studies and surveys, and is an active participant in policy discussions concerning international education, licensure, and practice.

To obtain either a permanent or temporary occupational preference visa from the Department of Homeland Security, a nurse will need a CGFNS certificate or a full, unrestricted license to practice as an RN in the state where she or he will be employed, and additionally an offer of employment from a US health care organization.

◼ ISSUES, DEVELOPMENTS, AND PREDICTIONS

It seems that almost every month brings information about changes in nurse practice acts or challenges as to what they permit. The scope of practice issue will go on forever.

The topic of the educational standards for entry into nursing practice has generated spirited discussion among nurses and legislators alike. Recently, the Carnegie National Nursing Education Study has joined the debate, calling for a "radical transformation" in educating nurses.[20] Because nurses spend the most time caring for patients, it is critical that they are well educated in patient care. Studies show that when nurses possess a BSN or more advanced nursing degree, patient care is enhanced with better outcomes.[21]

That discussion is heating up once again as legislation is pending in 18 states that would require newly licensed RNs to earn a BSN within 10 years of the date of initial licensure to retain their RN status.[22] This proposal, known as the "BSN in 10," if signed into law, would have a lasting impact on the nursing profession. What are the pros and cons? Schools are already turning potential candidates away because of faculty shortages. Concern over the fate of associate degree in nursing and diploma programs is a major issue, as is the potential monetary burden that could be placed upon nurses to fulfill the BSN educational requirement. From another perspective, some argue that the new requirement would be worth it to ensure that nurses are equipped to handle the ever-increasing complexity of patient care. In addition, they say nursing needs to step up its game and remain viable and equally competitive in the health care arena. Making the baccalaureate degree the minimal requirement to maintain licensure moves us toward this goal. The "BSN in 10" could become a reality through legislation, rule making, or even an executive order in some states. Only time will tell.

With the accelerated change in the delivery of health care, and national and state health care reform efforts, the boundaries of advanced practice nursing are being rapidly expanded. Recommendations have been offered to solve the quagmire of confusion related to the regulation of nurses in advanced practice so that they can truly enhance the nation's health care delivery system. The movement toward the NLC, although it does not directly address the APN, might eventually standardize the advanced practice environment. Nursing has made great strides in the area of prescriptive authority; all 50 states award APNs some variety of authority. The prescriptive authority may be through statutes, regulations, or delegation of authority from another practice act. Gains in reimbursement have been as successful, but progress has been slow, tedious, and incremental. APNs are to some degree recognized in every federal program, but there are still gaps here and there. State-based programs and commercial and indemnity plans have been slower to respond and depend on the political strength and governmental sophistication of organized nursing on a state-specific basis. More detail is provided in Chapters 15 and 19.

At the other end of the educational scale is the growing concern about the competency of nurse's aides and the increased use of unlicensed assistive personnel (UAP). As the least expensive and least prepared nursing person, the aide is still expected to detect physical and behavioral changes that may signal a serious health problem—and is not always trained to do so. Yet, state governments, health care facilities, payers, and even some boards of nursing see an advantage in allowing nurses to delegate more extensively to a variety of assistive personnel. Safeguards must be meticulously built into legislation and regulations for a delegatory process that places authority with the RN to determine if the task and setting are appropriate and if the UAP is competent to perform the task. A frightening trend to trivialize care of the elderly has been noted in recent years, and is probably linked to the general shortage of nursing personnel. In the spring of 2001, the Secretary of DHHS waived the CNA training requirement for aides who transport residents inside nursing homes, and in May 2002 a similar waiver was instituted for aides who feed nursing home residents. This is the beginning of a slippery slope. This tendency to use single-task workers in the care of our frailest and most compromised Americans threatens the quality of nursing home care.

Equal concern can be directed at the growing responsibilities of LPNs. Many state boards are put under tremendous pressure by employers to approve procedures for LPNs that are not in their curricula, such as venipuncture. Some boards approve and demand that LPN programs include these procedures in their course of studies. Schools say there is already enough to cover in 1 year. The impact is uncertain. What of the responsibility of nurses who supervise LPNs? Might these new demands escalate the move toward associate degree education for LPNs?

The credentialing issues in health care will not be easily resolved, and they involve much more than nursing. More health occupations will continue to seek licensure or other legal status. All these groups will have problems similar to those of nursing with definition, scope, discipline, and testing methods. Resolution of the problems posed here could set the stage for cooperative action. If someone must take the lead, it may as well be nursing.

KEY POINTS

1. There are a variety of mechanisms for credentialing nurses and other health care workers, all of which have some problems.

2. Mandatory licensure means that an individual cannot practice without a license and safeguards the public more than permissive licensure.

3. Among the criticisms of licensure is too much control by the profession or occupation, a tendency for practice requirements to be rigid and out of date, and primarily that the public has no guarantee of competence.

4. The Nurse Licensure Compact seems to be growing in favor, and over time may move nursing in the direction of more standardization.

5. Institutional licensure, although favored by some for economic reasons, would not guarantee improved care, but would limit the autonomy and mobility of nurses who now have individual licenses.

6. Nursing practice acts may vary from state to state, but they generally have the same components that define and control practice.

7. Nursing practice acts must change with the times, but the currently licensed individuals are protected by a grandfather clause.

8. The most common reasons for revocation of a license are substance abuse or other failure to meet the standards of the profession.

9. The purpose of nursing certification is to recognize advanced practice.

10. The approaches to authorizing advanced nursing practice are a combination of public/private sector partnership.

11. Sunset legislation, which requires a review of existing governmental agencies to determine if they are fulfilling their purpose, has resulted in some good revisions of nursing practice acts.

12. A major problem with CE as a requirement for relicensure is that there is little evidence that it results in the maintenance of competence.

KEY POINTS

13. Continued competency has become a concern of the American public that may call for more careful scrutiny of select RNs, that is, those holding disciplinary actions, a significant hiatus in their work history, or a change in their clinical or functional work role.

14. CGFNS was created to safeguard the interests of both the foreign trained nurse and the American public.

15. Meticulous safeguards must be built into legislation, regulation, and workplace policies for using nursing assistants in direct care functions.

REFERENCES

1. Study of Accreditation of Selected Health Education Programs. *Part I: Staff Working Papers: Accreditation of Health Educational Programs.* Washington, DC: National Committee on Accrediting, 1972, p A6.

2. NCSBN. Nurse Licensure Compact. May 2010. https://www.ncsbn.org/2002.htm. Retrieved May 15, 2010.

3. NCSBN. APRN Compact. https://www.ncsbn.org/917.htm. Retrieved May 17, 2010.

4. APRN Consensus Work Group and the National Council of State Boards of Nursing APRN Advisory Committee. Consensus Model for APRN Regulation. July 7, 2008. http://nursingcertification.org. Retrieved May 10, 2010.

5. U.S. News & World Report. America's Best Hospitals. July 20, 2009. http://www.nursecredentialing.org/Magnet/ProgramOverview.aspx. Retrieved May 10, 2010.

6. The Study of Credentialing in Nursing. *A New Approach,* Vol. 1. *Staff Working Papers,* Vol. 2. Milwaukee: ANA, 1979.

7. ANA. *Nursing's Social Policy Statement.* Washington, DC: American Nurses Publishing, 1995.

8. Affara F, Styles M. *Nursing Regulation Guidebook: From Principle to Power.* Geneva: ICN, 1993.

9. Styles M. *On Specialization in Nursing: Towards a New Empowerment.* Kansas City, MO: American Nurses Foundation, 1989.

10. American Board of Nursing Specialties. Consensus Model for APRN Regulations. July 8, 2008. http://nursingcertification.org/pdf/Approved%20Consensus%20Document%20-%207-2008.pdf. Retrieved May 10, 2010.

11. Ibid.

12 Joel L. Advanced practice nursing in the current sociopolitical environment. In Sheehy C, McCarthy M (Eds.): *Advanced Nursing Practice.* Philadelphia: FA Davis, 1998, pp 48–67.

13. The Department of Health, Education, and Welfare. *Extending the Scope of Nursing Practice.* Washington, DC: The Author, 1971, p 12.

14. ANA. *Suggestions for Major Provisions to Be Included in a Nursing Practice Act.* Unpublished report. New York: The Author, 1955.

15. Kelly L. Nursing practice acts. *Am J Nurs* 74:1314–1315, July 1974.

16. Annual CE Survey. *Journal of Continuing Education in Nursing,* January 2010. http://www.jcenonline.com/survey.asp. Retrieved May 17, 2010.

17. Heinecke V. *Department of Commerce, Division of Occupational and Professional Licensing.* 810 P.2d 459 (Utah App 1991).

18. NPDB/HIPDB. http://www.npdb-hipdb.hrsa.gov/hipdb.html. Retrieved May 20, 2010.

19. Ibid.

20. Benner P, Sutphen M, Leonard V, Day L. *Educating Nurses.* San Francisco, CA: Jossey-Bass, 2010.

21. Van den Heede K, Lasaffre E, Diya L, Vleugels A, Clarke SP, Aiken LH, Sermeus W. The relationship between inpatient cardiac surgery mortality and nurse numbers and educational level: Analysis of administrative data. *Int J Nurs Stud* 46(6):796–810, 2009.

22. Nursing Spectrum. NY and NJ Consider BSN Requirement. September 9, 2009. http://news.nurse.com/article/20090907/NATIONAL02/309070028. Retrieved May 10, 2010.

Updates can be found at **www.kellysnursing.com**

Nursing Practice and the Law

US citizens who enter schools of nursing of any type take with them all of a citizen's legal rights and responsibilities. As nursing students, however, they gradually take on duties and responsibilities that may involve them in litigation, directly or indirectly, trivial or serious, that would not concern them as citizens only. On graduation and licensure they may be held liable for actions that apply only to registered nurses (RNs), as well as for other acts of a more general nature. With nursing experience and knowledge, responsibilities will increase still further, because a court of law takes these facts into consideration.

There are numerous ways in which nurses become involved with the law in their practice. The impact of statutory law has been previously discussed in Chapter 17. In this chapter, other legal aspects will be considered, primarily within the common law of torts, that is, an intentional or unintentional civil wrong. This is the kind of law that relates to the daily practice of most nurses. When cases are used to illustrate a legal principle, it is important to remember that even a landmark decision may be overturned. As one attorney said:

> Nurses cannot learn all the laws, even if it were desirable to do so. Even if they could be learned, they would be out of date immediately. Indeed, even as this . . . is being read, American lawmakers are enacting thousands of new regulations, statutes, and case law in state capitals and courthouses across the United States and in Washington, D.C.[1]

Although this chapter includes a variety of legal topics, the emphasis is on malpractice in the clinical setting.

■ LITIGATION TRENDS IN HEALTH CARE

Part of the doctrine of common law is that anyone can sue anyone if she or he can get a lawyer to take the case or is able to handle it personally (as is common in small claims court). This does not necessarily mean that there is just cause or that the person suing (plaintiff) has a good chance of winning; in fact, the defendant might be protected by law from being found liable, as when someone, in good faith, reports child abuse.

Most people are reasonably decent in their dealings with others, and unless a person sustains a serious injury, they will not institute legal proceedings. Sometimes this is because legal services are expensive, perhaps more so than paying the medical bills, and the offended person is realistic enough to know this. Often the person inflicting the injury is also realistic and prefers to settle the matter out of court, knowing that it will be less costly in the long run, or insurance may pay for the damage inflicted. One or both parties may settle their difficulties out of court because one or the other or both want to avoid publicity and do not want to have a court record of any kind.

Once people seemed particularly reluctant to make trouble for nurses, doctors, or health agencies such as certain nonprofit or voluntary hospitals, either out of respect for the services offered or because they presumably had so little money that it seemed unfair or pointless. The latter was probably always an inaccurate generality, but today patients and families who feel aggrieved are considerably more likely to sue any or all concerned, sometimes for enormous sums. Health care is big business. The number of claims and the value of awards began to increase in the

1930s, declined during World War II, and then rose again, with the 1990s and 2000s seeing multi-million-dollar awards where the injuries were serious. Malpractice suits against hospitals, especially, have increased.

A variety of reasons have been cited: the litigious spirit of the general public, what seems to be a "sue if possible; I'm entitled" attitude; changing medical technology that brought new risks, with a potential for exceptional severity of injury; sometimes high, unrealistic public expectations; the increase in specialization that has resulted in a deterioration of the physician–patient relationship; and patient resentment of depersonalized care and sometimes rude treatment in hospitals and anger at the high cost of care. Moreover, in recent years, the highly publicized notion (and some evidence) that managed care might be depriving people of necessary care has stimulated the introduction of bills that would allow patients to sue health maintenance organizations (HMOs). Certainly, this has added to the growing distrust of the health care system and its workers. (Many of these corporate concerns are receiving attention in nursing journals, some of which are listed in the bibliography.)

When faced with a bad outcome, it has been documented that patients and families are more likely to sue if they feel that the physician was not caring and compassionate. Quality of care was not the main determinant. The main positive factors were spending a little more time with the patient, explaining or teaching about what to expect, using some humor, encouraging patients to talk and ask questions, and checking understanding—all of which sounds like rather basic communication. Certainly, nurses can also consider these points in their practice. Nevertheless, there is no question that if there is severe disability, not only will there be a malpractice suit, but the award won will probably be larger for patients who have been permanently disabled.

However, there is also some evidence that people are being socialized into thinking that if something goes wrong, they should sue. One factor is seen to be the influence of the ubiquitous advertisements of attorneys on radio and television, promising legal help for a multitude of injuries and accidents. An American Medical Association (AMA) report also identifies other health professionals or workers as encouraging patients or families to sue because they feel that there was malpractice.

Most suits are settled out of court. The dramatic multi-million-dollar suits seldom result in awards anywhere near the original figure; sometimes they are not won at all, and almost always progress to the appellate level. The largest awards have the largest elements of compensation for pain and suffering, almost exclusively occurring after some negligently caused catastrophic injury, such as severe brain damage or paralysis, which obviously has an enormous effect on the victim's life. The frequent suits and large awards were part of the reason for the mid-1970s and 1980s malpractice crisis, when many physicians could not get malpractice insurance, and neither hospitals nor physicians felt that they could afford it if they could get it. In 1990, malpractice fees were being reduced; state laws limiting awards and physicians' increased caution were cited as reasons. By 1992, a study of medical malpractice cases indicated that unjustified payments were rare.

The vast majority of malpractice cases are against physicians or hospitals. Do nurses get sued? Absolutely. As noted later, a good percentage of hospital and physician suits include nurses and may be based on the nurse's negligence. Because of the various legal doctrines also explained later, the aggrieved patient has the option of suing multiple defendants. The *deep pocket theory* of naming all those who can pay has become traditional tort law strategy, as has the method of *casting a broad net* to sue every defendant available. Thus, the likelihood of recovery from one or more defendants is greater, and a favorite defense of admitting negligence but blaming an absent party, the so-called *empty chair defense*, is defeated. Because presumably either or both the physician and the hospital have more money than the nurse, either may have to pay the award or at least more of the award, even if it is the nurse who is clearly at fault. The hospital whose liability and responsibility may be only secondary (*vicarious liability*) may recover damages from the employee primarily responsible for the loss. This is not common, but has been done.

In 1986, as the result of federal legislation, the National Practitioner Data Bank (NPDB) was established to encourage the identification of health care practitioners who are found guilty of unprofessional conduct: malpractice claims paid, disciplinary action by a licensing board, clinical privilege suspension or revocation, or professional society action. By April 2010, the NPDB reported RNs had only been cited in 8225 medical malpractice reports and 122,038 actions regarding licensure, professional societies, peer review organizations, or clinical privileges over the entire history of the NPDB (from September 1990).[2] More detail is available in Exhibit 21–1. Claims for obstetrical and surgical cases were prominent.

■ **EXHIBIT 21–1. NPDB Summary Report (September 1, 1990 to April 17, 2010)**

Profession/Provider	Medical Malpractice Reports	Licensure, Clinical Privileges, Professional Society, Peer Review Organization Reports	Remarks
Clinical nurse specialist	12	18	From 9/9/02
Doctor of osteopathy	16,261	7,530	
Licensed practical/ vocational nurse	612	74,083	
Nurse's aides	101	13,112	Includes CNAs from 10/17/05, but not home health aides
Nurse anesthetist	1,390	305	
Nurse midwife	788	80	
Nurse practitioner	1,033	748	
Pharmacist	1,821	13,693	
Physician (MD)	253,523	77,185	
Registered nurse	5,010	120,900	

Source: Adapted from the NPDB Summary Report. April 17, 2010. http://www.npdb-hipdb.com/pubs/stats/NPDB_Summary_Report.pdf.

Because of the cost of going to court, both in time and money, not to mention emotional stress, alternatives have been suggested that are quicker and less costly. One is *alternative dispute resolution* (ADR). In 1993, Washington State passed a law requiring participants involved in a health care claim to try *mediation*, one form of ADR, before proceeding with a lawsuit. Some other jurisdictions are also moving in this direction. This process will be described later in this chapter. Another option is no-fault insurance. The attraction of no-fault insurance is the increasing public tendency to believe that if someone is hurt, someone must pay, whether or not negligence is clearly evident. How costly this would be remains to be seen; no-fault auto insurance has been much more costly than ever contemplated. It has also been noted that physicians, through self-owned insurance companies, are more stringently controlling the practice of their peers. Actually, the majority of malpractice suits are decided in favor of the physician. Still, with the continual discussions of health care reform, tort reform is also on the agenda.

Besides encouraging ADR procedures, tort reform bills are tending to look at

1. Limiting noneconomic damages
2. Limiting attorney's fees
3. Requiring that the loser pay the court costs and attorney fees
4. Modifying rules of evidence
5. Eliminating joint and several liability
6. Reducing defensive medicine
7. Restrictions on punitive damages
8. Diminishing statutes of limitation

■ BASIC LEGAL CONCEPTS AND TERMS

As in any profession, law has its own terminology. Short definitions and illustrations of key words and phrases used in tort law follow:

Abandonment—failing to continue to give services to a patient without notice; refusal to treat after accepting the patient. (Example: a nurse leaves the unit at the end of a shift without reporting off or determining that there is another RN to cover his or her assigned patients.)

Borrowed servant—an employee temporarily under the control of someone other than the employer (a hospital operating room or scrub nurse placed under the direction of a surgeon).

Breach of duty—under the law of torts, not behaving in a reasonable manner where such is required; in the legal sense, causing injury to someone. (Example: careless administration of drugs.)

Captain of the ship doctrine—similar to the borrowed servant concept that physicians are responsible for all those presumably under their supervision. The trend is now to hold the individual responsible for their own acts, quickly making this doctrine obsolete where the nurse and doctor are concerned. (Example: incorrect sponge count done by nurses.) However, this does not preclude the hospital being sued under the doctrine of respondeat superior.

Charitable immunity—(originating in English common law) holds that a hospital will not be held liable for negligence to a patient receiving care on a charitable basis. In 1969, the Massachusetts Supreme Court prospectively abolished the immunity of charitable institutions. In other states it varies, but the trend is toward recognizing the liability of charitable institutions. However, some states put a limit on how much money can be recovered from a hospital, and the plaintiff can collect the difference in the award from the negligent nurse or doctor. For government hospitals, the old doctrine of sovereign immunity granted them freedom from liability (the-government-cannot-be-sued concept). However, the Federal Tort Claims Act (1946) partially waived sovereign immunity of the federal government, and a US Supreme Court ruling in 1950 made the government liable for harm inflicted by its employees. Immunity of state and municipal hospitals varies, but the trend is toward liability. Immunity does not include the individual's liability. (Example: a clamp was left in a patient's abdomen during surgery in a state hospital. Although this occurred before the state lifted the doctrine of sovereign immunity, both the physicians and OR nurses were held liable for gross negligence.)

Damages or monetary damages—redress sought by a plaintiff for injury or loss. *Nominal damages* (sometimes $1) are token damages when the plaintiff has proved his or her case but actual injury or loss could not be proven or is minor. *Compensatory damages* are the actual damages, with amounts awarded for proven loss. These include *general damages* (pain, suffering, loss of limb) and *special damages* that must be proved (wage loss, medical expenses). *Punitive or exemplary damages* may be awarded when the defendant has acted with

wanton, reckless disregard, or has acted maliciously. Because awards may be large for pain and suffering, this is an object of tort reform.

Defendant—person accused in a court trial.

Employee—someone who works for a person, institution, or company for pay.

Employer—one who selects, pays, and can dismiss the employee, and controls his or her conduct during working hours.

Expert witness—someone with special training, knowledge, skill, or experience who is permitted to offer an opinion in court. The expert witness gives *expert testimony.*

Foreseeability—holds the individual liable for all consequences of any negligent act that could or should have been foreseen under the circumstances. (Example: a suicidal patient is left unattended near an open window and jumps.)

Indemnification—if the employer is blameless in a negligence case but must pay the plaintiff under respondeat superior, the employer may recover the amount of damages paid from the employee in a separate action.

Subrogation—the employer can sue the employee for the amount of damages paid because of the employee's negligence. This may also occur if the award is more than that covered by either the employer's or the nurse's insurance. It is not yet common, but does happen.

Liability—being held legally responsible for negligent acts. The rule or doctrine of *personal liability* means that everyone is responsible for his or her own acts, even though someone else may also be held legally liable under another rule of law. *Vicarious liability*—liability imposed without personal fault or without a causal relationship between the actions of the one held liable and the injury (usually a case of respondeat superior), not a situation where individuals work as colleagues as in the case of CNM and physician. *Corporate liability* relates to the legal duty of a health care institution to provide appropriate facilities (staff and equipment) to carry out the purpose of the institution and to follow established standards of conduct.

Locality rule or community rule—first enunciated in 1880 in *Small v. Howard*, in which a small-town doctor unsuccessfully performed complex surgery and was held not liable. The rationale was that a physician in a small or rural community lacks the opportunity to keep abreast of professional advances. Gradually, courts took into account such facts as accessibility of medical facilities and experience. Beginning in the 1950s, various state supreme courts abandoned the locality rule on the basis that modern communications, including the availability of professional journals, TV, the Internet, and rapid transportation, made the rule outdated. The proper standard considered is whether the practitioner is exercising the care and skill of the average qualified practitioner, taking into account advances in the profession, as well as national standards.

Long tail—the lag between the time when an injury occurs and the claim is settled. Insurance companies say that because of this lag, it is difficult to determine reasonable premiums for a malpractice insurance risk.

Negligence—conduct that falls below the standard established by law for the protection of others against unreasonable risk of harm. This includes the concept of foreseeability. It is measured by an objective standard of what an ordinary, reasonable, and prudent person would do in the same circumstances.

Malpractice—is negligence applied to the acts of a professional. Malpractice results when the professional, a nurse in our case, fails to act as a reasonably prudent nurse would have acted under the same circumstances. Malpractice, professional negligence, may occur by omission or commission and does not have to be intentional.

Professional negligence—conduct of professionals that falls below the standard of care. If nurses are not charged with malpractice, in those venues where only physicians are considered "professional" in health care, they may be charged with professional negligence. The difference? Malpractice claims have a shorter statute of limitations. Both malpractice and negligence claims can be judged on the basis of statutory law, but primarily on case law.

Criminal negligence and gross negligence—(sometimes used interchangeably) refer to the commission or omission of an act, lawfully or unlawfully, in which such a degree of negligence exists as may cause a serious wrong to another. Almost any act of negligence resulting in the death of a patient would be considered *criminal negligence.*

Comparative negligence—takes into consideration the degree of negligence of both the defendant and the plaintiff. This allows the possibility of the plaintiff

having some redress, which often is not possible if there has been contributory negligence.

Contributory negligence—a rather misleading expression used when the plaintiff has contributed to his or her own injury through personal negligence. This may occur accidentally or deliberately. Some authorities assert that a plaintiff who is guilty of contributory negligence cannot collect damages; others state that he or she may collect under certain conditions. As in most legal matters, decisions vary widely. Because contributory negligence must be proved by the defendant, as much written evidence as possible is needed. (Example: a patient died of burns when he smoked in the hospital bed, although the nurse had taken away his cigarettes and told him not to smoke.)

Corporate negligence—the health care facility or an entity is negligent. This is a concept based on the landmark decision *Darling v. Charleston Community Memorial Hospital*, discussed later. It is based on two responsibilities: monitoring and supervising all professional personnel and investigating physicians' credentials before granting staff privileges.

Outrageous conduct doctrine or tort of emotional distress—allows the plaintiff to base his or her case on intentional or negligent emotional distress caused by the defendant. This is quite hard to prove as described in a hypothetical case where a woman suffered a miscarriage and the nurses involved made extremely insensitive statements about disposal of the fetus. The courts would probably find the behavior unprofessional and bizarre, but not as justifying damages.

Plaintiff—party bringing a civil suit seeking damages or other legal relief.

Proximate cause or causation—the immediate or direct cause of an injury in a malpractice case. The plaintiff must prove that the defendant's malpractice caused, precipitated, or aggravated his condition. For example, in a case where a patient's baby was stillborn, the medical expert testified that although the nurses did nothing wrong prior to the cessation of the fetal heart tone, they should not have waited 21 minutes before calling the doctor. Because it could not be proved that this delay, although negligent, would have changed the outcome, the court found the hospital and nurses not liable.

Reasonably prudent man theory—standard that requires an individual to perform a task as any reasonably prudent person with comparable education, skills, and training under similar circumstances would perform that same function. It is often described as requiring a person of ordinary sense to use ordinary care and skill. This concept is the key to determination of the standard of care.

Res gestae—all of the related events in a particular legal situation, which may then be admitted into evidence.

Res ipsa loquitor—("the thing speaks for itself") a legal doctrine that gets around the need for expert testimony or the need for the plaintiff to prove the defendant's liability because the situation (harm) is self-evident to even a layperson. The defendant must prove, instead, that he or she is not responsible for the harm done. Before the rule of res ipsa loquitor can be applied, three conditions must be present: the injury would not ordinarily occur unless there was negligence; whatever caused the injury at the time was under the exclusive control of the defendant; and the injured person did not contribute to the negligence or voluntarily assume the risk. A common example involving nurses occurs when sponges have been left inside an abdomen after surgery, and the nurse had made an inaccurate sponge count.

Res judicata—once a final decision has been made by a court having jurisdiction (often an appellate court at the top level), it is binding on all parties, and there is a bar to further legal action, damages, or claims.

Respondeat superior—("let the master answer") the employer is responsible for what employees do within the scope of their employment. This is a part of the vicarious liability doctrine. Independent contractors such as private duty nurses may or may not be included. Almost all cases involving nurses come under respondeat superior, because the vast majority of nurses are employed. However, they are usually also named in the suit.

Standard of care—the skill and learning commonly possessed by members of the profession. How the standard of care is determined is discussed in detail later.

Stare decisis—("let the decision stand") legal principle that previous decisions made by the court should be applied to new cases. Also called *precedent*. The decisions cited are usually made at the appellate level, including the state supreme court or the US Supreme Court, highest appellate court in the land.

Statute of limitations—legal limit on the time a person has to file a suit in a civil matter. The statutory period usually begins when an injury occurs, but, in some cases, as with a sponge left in the abdomen, it starts when the injured person discovers the injury (*discovery*). In the case of an injury to a minor, the statute will usually not start to run or *toll* until the child has reached age 18. The statute of limitations that relates to malpractice actions has not been applied to nurses in all states; instead, the longer periods for statutes of limitations for negligence are applied to them (thus not considering them as professionals). However, along with other new legislation related to the NP and physician assistant (PA), several states have revised their statutes of limitations to include nurses. Court decisions about the inclusion of nurses in malpractice statutes of limitations have varied, with a previous but changing tendency to hold them liable for negligence, not malpractice, because they were seen as performing under specific directions. The shorter time is intended to ensure a professional a "fair chance to defend on merit and not find his defenses eroded by lapse of time." This apparently was not seen as necessary for anything less than malpractice, or depending on how it is defined, *professional negligence*. Although the length of time involved varies from state to state, it ranges between about 2 years for malpractice and 4 years or more for negligence by others.

Statute of repose—places an outer limit on the time frame within which a suit can be filed. It is often incorporated into a statute of limitations to provide some mitigation of hardship on defendants exposed to potential suits under the discovery rule.

Tort—civil wrong against an individual.

To have a cause of action based on malpractice or negligence, four elements must be present:

1. There was a duty owed to the plaintiff by the defendant to use due care (reasonable care under the circumstances).
2. The duty was breached (the defendant was negligent).
3. The plaintiff was injured or damaged in some way.
4. The plaintiff's injury was caused by the defendant's negligence (proximate cause or causation).

No matter how negligent the health provider was, if there was no injury, there is no case. The plaintiff must also establish that a health practitioner–patient relationship existed and that the practitioner violated the standard of care.

■ APPLICATION OF LEGAL PRINCIPLES

With the added responsibilities nurses have assumed over the years, they are much more likely now to be involved in negligence actions by their patients. Not only must nurses respond to the prescription of the doctor and other provider professionals, but they must use their own professional judgment in assessing a patient, reporting signs and symptoms, and taking appropriate action, sometimes very quickly. Yet, most are not directly in charge of the patients' care and treatment. In addition, nurses supervise other nursing personnel, not all well trained, and agency nurses. This work is not done in a vacuum, for patients are sicker and staff is often reduced. The conflict and mixed messages are obvious.

Particularly in times of downsizing, when health care institutions tend to use less-prepared personnel with whom the nurse is required to work, there are inevitable problems. Three types of liability must be recognized in supervising any non-RN, but especially unlicensed assistive personnel (UAP). These are

1. Inappropriate delegation, that is, delegating a series of tasks for which that person does not have the skills. If the nurse does not know what level of skills that person has, she or he should check any documentation of competencies, ask the person what he or she is able to do, and supervise closely—not easy if the unit is short staffed. There should be policies about what UAPs can and may do.

2. Inappropriate delegation of tasks contrary to the state's Nurse Practice Act. It is possible that the person can actually do certain tasks, for instance, foreign nurses not licensed in the United States. But even without a problem, this is violating the practice act, and the RN is held responsible. Any nursing intervention that requires independent, specialized nursing knowledge, skill, or judgment cannot be delegated.

3. Inadequate supervision. This comes under the easier-said-than-done category, but the nurse must take extra precautions.

Even in the greatest turmoil, a nurse is required by licensure law to give, at a minimum, safe and effective care. It is useful to begin by understanding how at least some of the legal principles mentioned translate into real cases involving nurses. Some of the examples that follow are classic cases that are repeatedly cited in nursing law; others are more recent. At times, when two similar cases are judged in quite different ways, both are given. The findings may change with the changing role of the nurse and a court's concept of what a nurse is and does. For instance, in a nurse liability case of 40 years ago, a nurse giving the wrong medication ordered by a physician was probably not held responsible, even if she knew it was wrong, because it was thought a nurse simply needed to follow the doctor's orders. Today, both the nurse and the doctor would be held responsible, if the nurse should have known, or suspected, but did not check, that the medication was wrong. The nurse is expected to use nursing judgment.

Assuming that you are at little risk because you do not work in the intensive care unit (ICU), the emergency room (ER), or some other high-pressure unit is a mistake. In reviewing cases in which nurses were found liable, the sad news is that most of the incidents are everyday situations in which nurses not only did not use judgment, but sometimes did not even use common sense. Quite often they neglected basic principles that they learned in their first year of nursing, such as how to give medications, or were careless about communication. Not only are RNs found liable, but also students. The following hypothetical case provides a useful illustration as well as several other legal principles.

A first-year student nurse was assigned by the instructor to care for a thin, very ill patient who required an intramuscular injection. The student had only practiced the procedure in the school laboratory. She injected the medication in the patient's sciatic nerve and caused severe damage. The patient sued the doctor, hospital, head nurse, faculty members, and school of nursing. This was a case of res ipsa loquitor. The student was clearly negligent because she should have known the correct procedure and should have taken special precautions with an emaciated patient. The student is held to the standards of care (standards of reasonableness) of an RN if she is performing RN functions. If the student is not capable of functioning safely unsupervised, she should not be carrying out those functions. The doctor may or may not be held liable, depending on the court's notion about the captain of the ship doctrine. However, this would have nothing to do with the drug and injection itself, assuming that it was an appropriate order. The hospital will probably be held liable under respondeat superior, because students, even if not employed, are usually treated legally as employees. In addition, because the head nurse is responsible for all patients on the unit and presumably should have been involved in the student's assignment or should have assigned an RN to such an ill patient, she too would be liable, because she did not make an appropriate assignment (appropriate delegation of duties).

The instructor might be found liable, not on the basis of respondeat superior—just as the head nurse or supervisor would not be liable if the student had been an RN, because these nurses are not employers in the legal sense—but on the basis of inadequate supervision. If a supervisor or other nurse assigns a task to someone not competent to perform that task and a patient is injured because of that individual's incompetent performance, the supervising nurse can be held personally liable because it is part of her or his responsibility to know the competence and scope of practice of those being supervised. Although theoretically this nurse could rely on the subordinate's licensure, certification, or registration, if any, as an indication of competence, if there is reason to believe that that individual would nevertheless perform carelessly or incompetently and the nurse still assigns that person to the task, the nurse is held accountable (as is the employer under the doctrine of respondeat superior). The school might be found liable in the case of the student if the court believed the dean/director had not used good judgment in employing or assigning the faculty member carrying out those teaching responsibilities.

In another situation, the outcome would be different. A student gave an electric heating pad, per the doctor's order, to a patient who was alert and mentally competent and demonstrated to the nurse her ability to adjust the temperature and her knowledge of the potential hazards. The patient fell asleep on the pad, set at a high temperature, and burned her abdomen. In this case, there would seem to be sufficient evidence of contributory negligence on the part of the patient, with the student having good reason to assume that the patient was capable of managing the heating pad. Therefore, even if the patient sued, her case would be weak. If the court used the doctrine of comparative negligence, some liability might be assigned to the student if, for instance, she or he did not check on the patient within a reasonable amount of time. If the heating pad were faulty, the hospital would probably be liable, not the nurse.

Another case involving a student reinforces the principle of individual and teacher responsibility. In *Central Anesthesia Associates v. Worthy* (173Ga.App.150 [325 SE2d 819]), a senior student nurse anesthetist was accused of administering anesthesia improperly, causing the patient

to have a cardiac arrest and brain damage. The student was under the supervision of a PA employed by the professional corporation that had the nurse anesthetist program. The Supreme Court of Georgia held the student, the PA, and the three anesthesiologist teachers liable. It rejected the student's argument that she should be held to the student standard; she was held to the standards of a CRNA. The teachers were not on the scene and had not delegated supervision properly. The PA either did not supervise adequately or was himself not capable. This case has implications for nursing students and their staff nurse preceptors when faculty are absent.

The captain of the ship doctrine was negated by a case that cost the hospital $5 million in *Nelson v. Trinity Medical Center* (419 N.W. 2d 886 [S.Ct. N.D. 1988]). The physician of a woman in active labor ordered the assessment of fetal heart tones, an IV, and analgesia. Standing orders in that labor unit called for continuous fetal heart monitoring, but the nurse, without checking, assumed the monitors were all in use and did not place one on the patient until an hour later. It indicated fetal distress, and despite an immediate cesarean, the infant had severe brain damage. According to the expert who testified, the damage was caused by placenta abruptio, which could have been diagnosed by earlier fetal monitoring. The defendant hospital tried to invoke the captain of the ship doctrine to cover the nurse's negligence. The court ruled that even though the doctor was in charge of the case, he had no direct control over what the nurse did (as opposed to an OR situation) and that the nurse was performing a routine act.

A particularly useful example from many points of view is the landmark decision of *Darling v. Charleston Community Memorial Hospital* (33 Ill.2d 326, 211 N.E. 2d 253). A minor broke his leg playing football and was taken to Charleston Community Memorial Hospital, a hospital accredited by the Joint Commission. There a cast was put on the leg in the ER, and he was sent to a regular nursing unit. The nurses noted that the toes became cold and blue, charted this fact, and called the physician, who did not come. Over a period of days, they continued to note and chart the deteriorating condition of the exposed toes and continually notified the physician, who came once but did not remedy the situation. The mother then took the boy to another hospital, where an orthopedist was forced to amputate the leg because of advanced gangrene. The family sued the first doctor, the hospital, and the nurses involved. The physician settled out of court; he admitted he had set few legs and had not looked at a book on orthopedics in 40 years. The hospital's defense was that the care provided was in accordance with the standard practice of like hospitals, that it had no control over the physician, and that it was not liable for the nurses' conduct because they were acting under the orders of a physician. However, the appellate court, upholding the decision of the lower court, said that the hospital could be found liable either for breach of its own duty or for breach of duty of its nurses. The court reasoned that there was a commitment that the hospital did not fulfill. The court held that the hospital had failed in its duties to review the work of the physician or to require consultation when the patient's condition clearly indicated the necessity for such action. This is corporate negligence. For nurses, the crucial point was the duty to inform hospital administration of any deviation in proper medical care that poses a threat to the well-being of the patients. (The hospital was also expected to have a sufficient number of trained nurses capable of recognizing unattended problems in a patient's condition and reporting them.) Specifically, the court said,

> the jury could reasonably have concluded that the nurses did not test for circulation in the leg as frequently as necessary, that skilled nurses would have promptly recognized the conditions that signalled a dangerous impairment of circulation in the plaintiff's leg, and would have known that the condition would become irreversible in a matter of hours. At that point, it became the nurses' duty to inform the attending physician, and if he failed to act, to advise the hospital authorities so that appropriate action might be taken (*Darling v. CCMH*, 211 N.E. 2d 253).

Because Darling-type situations are not rare, it is essential for nurses to know their legal responsibilities (and rights) in such cases, so that they can act accordingly. That this kind of notification problem may still exist is shown by another $2 million award. Nurses in a Department of Veterans Affairs (VA) hospital were found liable because they failed to recognize the emergent condition of a post-operative patient and failed to take prompt steps to notify attending physicians. When the physicians were slow to respond, the nurse made no effort to call another physician or anyone else because she said she thought no one else was capable of handling the situation (which was not so). This case also points out the importance of a patient's chart, which the judge called "a mess"—sketchy and unreliable with important data missing. The court stated that the lack of charting contributed to the decision against the nurses. Actually, because physicians and nurses working in

a VA hospital cannot be sued separately, under the Federal Tort Claims Act, the United States was the defendant.

■ MAJOR CAUSES OF NURSING LITIGATION

The number of legal suits involving nurses has increased significantly. It is difficult to say whether this is because there is actually more negligence, the public's litigious spirit now extends to nurses, or people simply are more aware of nurses' increased responsibilities, and nurses are now seen as professionals responsible for their own actions. It may be that all these factors are involved.

Failure to Use Adequate Precautions to Protect the Patient Against Injury

This broad category covers almost any aspect of nursing care because the precautions are often such that all nurses generally learned them early in their education. Patient falls are the most frequent basis for malpractice suits against nurses. For instance, in a Connecticut case, a 74-year-old woman with Alzheimer's disease was admitted to the hospital after a fall at home. Left unattended on a gurney, the patient attempted to get up and fractured her left wrist. Because the nurses failed to take precautions to protect the patient, despite warnings by the family, the jury awarded the plaintiff more than $100,000 in damages. There are similar cases, often involving the elderly.

A particularly egregious case is found in *NX (New York) v. Cabrini Medical Center* (97 N.Y.2d 247, 765 N.E.2d 844, 739 N.Y.S.2d 348). Nurses ministering to a patient within a few feet and with an unobstructed view (no drawn curtains) of the plaintiff failed to protect her from the sexual assaults of a surgical resident. The court found that the nurses unreasonably disregarded that which was readily there to be seen and heard, and which could have been prevented.

The nurse's role in protection resounds in *Chin v. St. Barnabas* (160 N.J. 454, 734 A.2d 778). A patient's death was caused by the incorrect hook-up of a hysteroscope that introduced gas into her uterus and blood stream during a surgical procedure. Two nurses who had no experience, familiarity, or training on the Hystero-flow Pump were assigned to the procedure as scrub nurses. A third nurse, having some experience with the equipment, acted as circulating nurse. At the beginning of the procedure, the circulating nurse removed the pack containing the sterile tubing from the operating room cabinet, opened it, and presented it to the scrub nurse. The circulating nurse was responsible for hooking up the gas line to the nitrogen gas regulator and the exhaust tube to the suction. One scrub nurse asked the other for a suction tube, and received the sterile end while the nonsterile end of the tube was to be connected to a suction canister. Through negligence, either the nonsterile end of the suction tube was improperly connected to the exhaust hose or the sterile end of the suction tube was improperly connected to the outflow part of the hysteroscope. Either of these connections could have caused the closed circuit that resulted in the patient's death. The jury awarded the plaintiff $2 million in damages, assessed as 20 percent against the physician, 20 percent against one of the inexperienced scrub nurses, 25 percent against the circulating nurse, and 35 percent against the hospital. The rule of res ipsa loquitor was applied.

Medication errors are a particularly serious problem. A recent report from the Institute of Medicine (IOM; a private nonprofit entity providing health policy advice to the National Academy of Sciences under a Congressional mandate) revealed that between 44,000 and 98,000 people in the United States die every year from medical errors. Even at the lower limit, this is more people than die from highway accidents, breast cancer, or acquired immunodeficiency syndrome (AIDS).[3] The Institute for Safe Medication Practices (ISMP) claims that it is impossible to know the exact number of medication errors, projecting that only 5 to 7 percent of errors are even reported.[4] The whole issue of medication errors has created some intense debate. One dispute is between those who favor mandatory reporting systems that are inherently punitive and others who support non-punitive systems as an approach to identifying problems and focusing on prevention.

There are many legal cases based on medication errors, but actually it is generally agreed that those reported are the tip of the iceberg. Unless a patient has a serious adverse reaction, errors may not be reported or recorded. Common errors include wrong drug, wrong dose, wrong route, and wrong time. In nursing school, correct administration of medications emphasized the *five rights*, instead of these wrongs, plus making sure that you have the right patient, verifying the name by checking his or her ID bracelet and asking the patient his or her name, if possible. There are many, many examples of how the wrongs led to trauma and sometimes death, almost always resulting in legal suits involving nurses. These include a child receiving an adult dose of a potent drug; a nurse injecting a drug into the hip of an obese patient with too short a needle; a nurse delaying an anti-psychotic drug for 2 hours, with the result that the patient jumped out a window; and a student nurse giving a patient Maalox IV instead of orally.

An eight-figure settlement was recently secured in *Johnson v. Weiss Memorial Hospital* (Cook County Cir. Ct.,

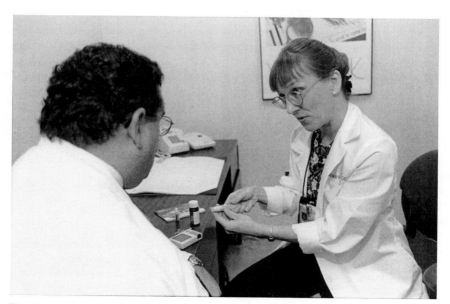

Teaching patients thoroughly can help avoid medication errors and malpractice claims. (Courtesy of Robert Wood Johnson University Hospital, New Brunswick, New Jersey)

No. 01 L 6581). A woman was left in a persistent vegetative state after suffering a cardiac arrest and subsequent brain damage while hospitalized for treatment of an intestinal condition. The plaintiff alleged that nurses had negligently overdosed her on an IV version of the narcotic Dilaudid, additionally medicated her with two drugs that are contraindicated when giving Dilaudid, failed to ensure that the patient was carefully monitored after receiving this potent sedation, and neglected to ensure that resuscitative equipment was readily available to her.

Naturally, there is much good advice given to prevent medication errors, especially as new techniques and equipment, such as automated dispensing systems, unit dose, and electronic wrist bracelet identification, become common. There are also warnings to stop storing dangerous drugs in clinical areas; decrease access to the pharmacy for nonpharmacy personnel (having nurses dispense drugs violates the pharmacy practice act); have clinical information readily available; and encourage manufacturers to check their labels and packaging, since there are too many lookalike drugs and labels. The reader is referred to Exhibit 21–2 for suggestions offered by the American Society of Hospital Pharmacists.

Patients can also be put in harm's way due to short staffing. In the case of *Adams and the Youville Health Care Center* (*Youville Health Care Center v. NLRB*, 526 F.2d 3), a nurse employed on a subacute care unit blew the whistle on unsafe health care practices. As the hospital instituted staffing cuts and cost-containment measures, safety and quality suffered. There were increased falls, serious medication errors, and instances where patients were left to lie in their own urine and feces for extended periods of time. For 3 months, there was an earnest attempt to communicate concerns to the administration through the designated channels. The administration offered no response, and when the nurse decided to document his observations and report to the proper governmental authority, he was fired, despite a history of excellent performance reviews. The nurse sued and won his case with the National Labor Relations Board. The hospital appealed and lost.

Physician–Nurse Communication Problems

Do you have a responsibility to take action when a doctor writes an order that you think is incorrect or unclear? When he or she does not respond to a patient's worsening condition? When he or she does not come to see a patient

---

■ **EXHIBIT 21–2. Recommendations to Help Nurses Stop Medication Errors**

- Review the medications of all patients, assessing drug interactions. If you have questions, get the information from pharmacists or other resources. If you're not satisfied, don't administer the medication until you've checked with the physician ordering it.
- Verify all new drug orders before you carry them out by checking the original order, the medication itself, and the patient's ID.
- Inspect the medication, checking expiration date and general appearance. If it doesn't look right, check with the pharmacist.
- Confirm calculations with another nurse or the pharmacist for drug dosage, flow rate, and anything else that requires a mathematical formula.
- Administer medications at the scheduled time. Don't remove identifying information until just before administration. Chart immediately.
- Follow up after administering a drug like an analgesic or antihypertensive to be sure it has had its intended effect.
- Check with the pharmacy if the patient's medication hasn't arrived. Don't substitute or borrow from another patient's medication. Return all unfinished or discontinued drugs to the pharmacy.
- Question unusual orders, particularly for large dosages.
- Counsel patients and their caregivers about the prescribed medications, making sure they understand the purpose, how taken, side effects to watch for, and the physical appearance of the medication itself.
- Listen to patients who question or object to the use of a particular drug. If concerns remain after you explain the medication's purpose, double check the order and the dispensed medication with the doctor and pharmacy before giving it.

even if you think it's urgent? When he or she does not follow accepted precautions in giving a treatment? What if he or she becomes angry and abusive? Even if he or she was right? According to court decisions in the last few years, the answer to all these questions is that it is the nurse's responsibility to take action. Medications seem to be a major problem. When an order is incomplete or written illegibly and the nurse does not question it, the results can be tragic.

A classic case is *Norton v. Argonaut Insurance Company* (144 So. 2d 249 [La. Ct. App]). A nursing supervisor thought she would help out in a pediatrics unit when it was short staffed, even though she was not familiar with current pediatric nursing practice. An order of medication for an infant did not state the appropriate route of administration and, after asking nearby physicians whether the dose was appropriate (not the route), the nurse gave it by injection. By this route, the amount given was a massive overdose and the child died. The nurse was not aware that the drug came in an oral solution and had not called the physician who wrote the order. Both were found liable. (This case also demonstrates the dangers of not having current knowledge.)

A nurse who follows a physician's orders is just as liable as the physician if the patient is injured because, for instance, a medication was the wrong dose, given by the wrong route, or was actually the wrong drug. If the order is illegible or incomplete, it is necessary to clarify that order with the physician who wrote it. If you doubt its appropriateness, check with a reference source or the pharmacist, and always check with the physician who wrote the order.

You have a right to question the physician when in doubt about any aspect of an order, and the nursing service administration should support any nurse who does so. In fact, there should be a written policy on the nurse's rights and responsibility in such matters, so that there is no confusion on anyone's part and no danger of retribution to a justifiably questioning nurse faced with an irate physician. What if the physician refuses to change the order? You should not simply refuse to carry out an order because you may not have the most recent medical information and could injure the patient by not following the order. You should report your concern promptly to your administrative supervisor. The supervisor or other nurse administrator is often expected to act as an intermediary if there is a problem. However, a good collegial relationship and mutual courtesy can prevent or ease a doctor–nurse confrontation and should be cultivated by both.

Verbal or telephone orders are another part of this problem. Although they are considered legal, the dangers are evident. In case of patient injury, the doctor, the nurse, or both will be held responsible. There frequently are or should be hospital, and sometimes legal, policies to serve as guides. Nurses should be very familiar with these, because adherence to such policies may protect them from liability. If telephone orders are acceptable, precautions should be taken that they are clearly understood (and questioned if necessary), with the doctor required to confirm the orders in writing as soon as possible. Some hospital policies require a repetition of the order; it is not unheard of to have two nurses listen together to a telephone order with the second nurse cosigning the order. In any case, most hospitals require the nurse to record the date and time of the communication.

If the doctor's order comes by fax and it is not clearly legible, the physician should be called for a new transmission. When there is no immediacy, it is better to wait for the original. In states where PAs' orders have been declared legal (as an extension of the physician), the same precautions must be taken, with the physician again confirming the order as quickly as possible. If a UAP relays a verbal order, it is best to verify it with the physician. The hospital should have a policy about this.

An incident that repeatedly shows up in litigation is the failure of a physician to see a patient either on the unit or in the ER. Often the nurse is held liable for not following through. More and more often, it is suggested that a system (or a policy) be set up specifying whom the nurse then contacts. If you neglect to call a doctor when the patient needs help or simply because you are not aware of the seriousness of the patient's condition, simply charting is not enough. This was clearly demonstrated in the *Darling* case. In another frequently cited case, *Goff v. Doctor's General Hospital of San Jose* (166 Cal.App.2d 314), the nurse did not call the physician when a pregnant woman continued to bleed excessively, "because he wouldn't come." The patient died, and the hospital was held vicariously liable because of the nurse's negligence.

Another failure in communication occurs when a nurse does not report a situation because she or he does not fully investigate or fully assess it. A 22-year-old suffered multiple fractures as a result of a motorcycle accident. The report of blood gases revealed that the patient was hypoxemic, but the nurse did not report it, nor did she report that the patient had vomited after being given medication ordered by the surgeon. After shift change, other nurses found the patient with unequal pupils, but it took several hours for the patient to be put on oxygen. He suffered severe brain damage. A settlement of $1.2 million was reached. This shows serious deficiencies in both communication and assessment.

Still other judgments against nurses have been given when a doctor has not followed through on appropriate technical procedures, such as the timely removal of an endotracheal tube. If you know that a particular procedure is being done incorrectly or a wrong medication is ordered (because it is within the scope of your knowledge) and do nothing about it, you can be held liable as well as the physician. A nurse may also refuse to administer a drug or treatment because it is against hospital policy. However, it is important to have support from nursing management if discussion with the physician ends with an impasse. If the supervisor refuses to help, it will be necessary to go up the chain of command.

At times, a nurse suspects that a physician is mistaken in his or her diagnosis of a patient. Although medical diagnosis is not within a nurse's purview, she or he does have a duty to speak up. In one case, a physician, doubting that a patient could have tuberculosis because he depended on outdated information, did not bother to order an x-ray and simply diagnosed the patient as having emphysema based on his physical exam. The nurse, with 30 years of experience, suspected that the patient did have TB and documented her assessment carefully as well as telling her charge nurse. The charge nurse never questioned the doctor. Without appropriate treatment, the patient's condition deteriorated. Later, the patient and his family sued. The physician settled out of court, but the nurse and hospital were found liable. The jury found that the nurse had a responsibility not just to record her observations, but to speak up and follow up.

An incident that occurred in a New York City hospital illustrates the vulnerability of nurses when communication is inadequate. Two gynecologists/obstetricians were trying new equipment in surgery for what was supposed to be a simple procedure. The equipment salesman was also in the operating room assisting them. Mistakes were made, and the patient died. The OR nurse supervisor was fired immediately and other OR nurses were formally punished, presumably for not stopping the salesman and doctors or not apprising administration promptly of the participation of the salesman. (Newspaper reports were not specific about the reasons.) The physicians had already been subject to complaints, but had been permitted to continue their hospital practice and surgery. After this publicity they lost their hospital privileges, but it was the nurse who was fired immediately. She may also be included in the legal suit that the patient's husband said he would file, which, if it follows the usual "casting the broad net" approach, will include everyone involved.

These examples reinforce the need for nurses to recognize their accountability to the patient, even if it means disagreeing with physicians and reporting them if the patient appears to be endangered. Some hospitals that appreciate how difficult the nurses' situation can be in such a potential confrontation have set policies that clarify everyone's responsibilities. Nurses need to take precautions even if there is formal administrative backup.

There are a number of actions you can take. Do not hesitate to call a physician; be persistent in tracking down the attending or substitute physician; stay on the phone until you get the information you need (use nursing judgment). Be especially careful about telephone orders. Make sure you and the physician are both talking about the same patient. Make certain you understand what the doctor is saying even if it requires repetition. Repeat the order. Document the order, noting the physician's name, time, date, and name of the third party if there was a witness.

On the other hand, failing to keep a physician fully informed, when there is little question about clarity, leaves a nurse liable for violating the standard of care. In one case, ICU nurses failed to keep the physicians apprised of a patient's seizures, despite specific orders. The patient suffered permanent brain damage and a malpractice suit was brought against the hospital and physicians. The jury verdict found the physicians not liable, but the nurses and therefore the hospital (under respondeat superior) liable. An expert witness said that failing to notify the physicians of continued seizure activity contributed to the patient's brain damage and violated the standard of care.

Legal Problems in Record Keeping

It is almost impossible to overemphasize the importance of records in legal action, especially nurses' notes. They hold the only evidence that orders were carried out and what the results were; they are the only notes written with both the time and date in chronological order; and they offer the most detailed information on the patient. Nurses' notes, like the rest of the chart, can be subpoenaed. No matter how skillfully you practice your profession, if your actions and observations are not documented accurately and completely, the jury can only judge by what is recorded. If you are subpoenaed, comprehensive notes will not only give weight to your testimony, but also will help you to remember what happened. A case may not come up for years, and unless there was a severe problem at the time, it is difficult to remember exact details about one patient. General, broad phrases such as *resting comfortably*, *good night*, and *feeling better* are totally inadequate. How could a jury interpret them? How could even another professional who did not know that patient interpret them? Although today's tendency is to limit the amount of charting, skimpy nurses' notes can lose a case for a nurse or hospital.

The correct way to chart, with legal aspects in mind, is probably charting as you were taught and following good nursing practice: use black or blue ink; avoid spelling and grammatical errors; be legible; be objective—write what you see, hear, smell, feel; do not make flip or derogatory remarks; and use acceptable hospital or agency abbreviations. Be as accurate as possible, but if a mistake is made, recopy or cross out with the original attached and still legible but marked *error* or *mistaken entry*, and say why, as in *wrong chart*, and do this as soon as possible. Do not use correction fluid. Never alter a record in any way; this has been shown to influence a jury negatively. Every good malpractice attorney calls on experts to examine charts for alterations, erasures, and additions. Computer records have changed charting and correction procedures significantly, because corrections can be made immediately. Computerized patient records do allow for more accurate, timely, and legible charting, but the issue of confidentiality discussed in Chapter 22 may present a problem. All too often, a nurse makes a change or an omission in the chart to protect a physician or the hospital. This can lead to criminal charges.

Some of the most serious problems arising from poor charting concern lack of data, such as omission of a temperature reading or other vital signs, lack of observations about a patient's condition, or no record of oxygen liter flow in a newborn infant; these and others have resulted in liability judgments against nurses and hospitals, although in each it was contended that the right thing had been done.

Although it is often inaccurate, the statement *if it wasn't charted, it wasn't done* has evolved into a legal standard. Because of this, new attention is being given to the shortcuts in charting such as a flow chart and charting by exception, which reverses that statement. The flow chart should be consistent with the nurses' notes. You cannot simply check off what the nurses on the previous shift checked off. If you were sued, such discrepancies would damage your credibility. Moreover, you should not depend too heavily on flow charts; it is still important to record the patient's response to care in your notes. There have been several cases where failure to perform even one step of the protocol may appear to be falsifying the record. In *Lama v. Barras* (16 F.3d 473 [1st Cir]), the hospital was held negligent because, although Mr. Lama developed an infection after herniated disk surgery, not enough qualitative information was charted about his symptoms of persistent pain, drainage, and bleeding. It was not required by institutional policy. Care should also be taken if clinical pathways are included in the chart. These are considered legal if the record meets the standard of accuracy concerning the patient's care and condition. Whether documentation of the patient's care is in a traditional chart or otherwise, errors and omissions are major factors in juries finding for the plaintiff in all nursing settings (see Exhibit 21–3).

This does not mean that you should withhold pertinent information, because withholding information is no different from altering information. It is important to record accurately oral conversations with physicians, family, and others. If there is a later dispute about who said what and if the patient is injured, a clear description of the conversation recorded at the time it was held will generally be considered accurate by the court.

Information in the patient's record that is particularly important from a legal point of view includes names and signatures of the patient, nurses, and doctors; notations of the patient's condition on admission, with progress notes on changes for the better or worse while in the hospital; accounts of injuries sustained accidentally while in the hospital, if any; a description of the patient's attitude toward the treatment and personnel; medications and other treatments given (what, when, how); vital signs; visits of doctors, consultants, and specialists; and receiving the patient's permission for therapy and all special procedures such as surgery. Gaps in documentation can be as dangerous as errors. Another potentially dangerous practice occurs when a nurse must chart what an aide says he or she did or what occurred when the nurse had not personally seen it (as is usual). Some lawyers advise adding a statement that clarifies the facts to protect yourself. Also, nurses should never sign for another RN.

■ **EXHIBIT 21–3. Dos and Don'ts of Charting**

1. Avoid using labels to describe your patient's behavior, such as *noncompliant* or *combative*. Describe what happened instead.
2. Don't refer to staffing problems.
3. Refrain from mentioning that an incident report has been filed.
4. Don't try to explain a mistake or use words like *accidentally* or *somehow*, which opposing attorneys look for. Just record what was done.
5. Avoid airing your dirty laundry—disputes with, or criticism of, your colleagues, both nurses and physicians.
6. Never chart that you've *informed* a colleague of a certain event if you really only mentioned it. *Informing* means to clearly state why she or he is being notified.
7. Never refer to another patient by name. Use roommate, initials, or bed number.
8. Document any nursing action taken in response to a problem. There should always be an action to respond to a problem.
9. Document all safeguards used, such as side rails, splints, and so on.
10. Never backdate or add to a previous entry.
11. Record on every line; do not leave spaces and sign every entry.
12. Follow the prescribed procedure for an error; never erase or in other ways try to cover an error.

Other Common Acts of Negligence

Among the acts of negligence a nurse is most likely to commit in the practice of nursing are the following (not in order of importance):

1. *Failure to respond to or ask someone else to respond promptly to a patient's call light or signal* if, because of such failure, a patient attempts to take care of his or her own needs and is injured. This might happen when he or she attempts to get out of bed to go to the bathroom or reaches for a bedpan in the bedside stand. Sometimes the bedpan or urinal is not even at hand.

   Or the patient may simply be looking for help. In *Adams v. Cooper Hospital* (684 A. 2d 506–NJ), the jury awarded $1.5 million against the hospital and nurse defendant. After a severe auto accident and placement in ICU, the patient was transferred to a medical-surgical unit. The patient had a tube inserted in his throat and started to have trouble breathing and coughed up thick yellow mucus. The nurse left to do something else and the patient tried to reach the call bell and fell out of bed. He fractured his hip and sustained severe head trauma, requiring several additional surgeries. The nurse breached the reasonable standard of care by leaving the choking patient unattended.

2. *Inadequate or dated nursing knowledge.* Because having current knowledge is a professional responsibility, there

seems to be little excuse for this kind of negligence. However, on occasion, even the most competent nurse has a problem. If an entirely new type of treatment or piece of equipment is introduced on your unit, it is your responsibility, as well as that of the head nurse or supervisor, to get the appropriate information on it. Further problems can come from floating and short staffing. In these cases, you may be placed in a specialty area with which you are not familiar, with or without a more experienced nurse. There is no clear answer to this dilemma; some courts have ruled that shifting staff is the employer's privilege and refusal can be considered insubordination. The supervisor, of course, is also responsible for any damage done because he or she is supposed to delegate safely. The float nurse must be especially careful and report any change in a patient's condition. To protect yourself, it is also worthwhile to go to your immediate supervisor, express your concerns, and perhaps ask for a list of duties you are expected to carry out. Keep a record of your conversation. If floated to an area with which you are completely unfamiliar, such as telemetry, someone who is knowledgeable should be working with you. Go up the chain of command, if necessary, to have the situation resolved for safe practice. If floating is a regular occurrence, the hospital would do well to have at least basic training programs for specialty areas. You can be held responsible for an error, but it can also cost the hospital a hefty malpractice claim.

Even when you are practicing in your area of specialization, there will be times when the standard of care is challenged. In *Hollar v. Cain* (36 Fed. Appx. 846, 2002 WL 1291793 [6th Cir.Ky.]), a 20-year-old college student was seen in an ER after a soccer injury to his right leg. After a thorough examination by two ER nurses and a certified emergency medicine physician, he was diagnosed as having a sprained knee. During the course of the physical, normal pedal pulses were verified, but a Doppler stethoscope was not used. He was discharged, because the hospital's policies did not justify admission. After many intervening events, the plaintiff sustained an amputation of the right leg due to an arterial transection and subsequent gangrene. The plaintiff contended that if a Doppler had been used at the time of the initial emergency treatment, the arterial transection might have been detected, had it existed at that time. No negligence was found on the part of the ER nurses, because they had not violated the prevailing standard of care and competence in examining the plaintiff. An expert witness testified that when a medical examination detects a pedal pulse in a damaged limb, due care does not require the use of a Doppler.

3. *Abandoning a patient. Abandonment* simply means leaving a patient when your duty is to be with him or her. One example would be leaving a child or incompetent adult without the protection you would have offered. There is also actual abandonment. A New York nurse, when told she needed to stay overtime, said she would stay several hours until relieved. A short time later, she left the unit to speak to the manager and then went home without telling her staff. There were very ill patients on that unit, and the other staff consisted of nursing assistants and a respiratory therapist. She was found guilty of unprofessional conduct and her license was suspended. The state Supreme Court upheld the penalty (*Husker v. Commissioner of Education of the State of New York*).

In another variation on this theme, a quadriplegic brought suit against the county health department and its private contractor of home health care, seeking to enjoin them from terminating services. The patient was only able to move his head, although his mental condition and intellect were unaffected. His physical disability was progressive. He developed a stage 4 decubiti that signaled an increasing need for assistance that home care services could not address. The court found for the defendants stating, "When the plaintiff selects a course which the professional nurses feel inappropriate or unsafe, they are free to refuse to participate and to withdraw from the case upon providing reasonable assurances that basic treatment and care will continue." In this situation, nurses continued to service the plaintiff, but with the right to terminate service if they furnished the plaintiff with appropriate inpatient care or provided the plaintiff with a reasonable period of time in which to make his own alternative arrangements (*Couch v. Visiting Home Care Services of Ocean County*, 329 N.J.Super.47, 746 A.2d 1029).

4. *Failure to teach a patient.* Nurses sometimes neglect to teach a patient in preparation for discharge, either because of the time it takes or because the physician objects. Nurses are responsible for providing appropriate teaching to the patient or caregiver. An increasing number of suits are being filed because such teaching was not done or not done thoroughly or understandably. Written instructions are often considered necessary to help the patient and family remember the information. It is wise to chart exactly what was taught and how the patient responded.

5. *Failure to make sure that faulty equipment is removed* from use, that crowded corridors or hallways adjacent to the nursing unit are cleared, that slippery or unclean floors are taken care of, and that fire hazards are eliminated. This is an area of negligence that, in most instances, would implicate others just as much as, or more than, the professional nurse. For example, the hospital administration would certainly share responsibility for fire hazards and dangerously crowded corridors, and the housekeeping and maintenance departments would not be blameless either. This does not lessen your responsibility for reporting unsafe conditions and following up on them, or in checking equipment you use. Report persistent hazards in writing and keep a copy for personal protection.

A *medical device* is broadly defined to include everything from gauze to pacemakers. Whenever a device user becomes aware of information that reasonably suggests that a device might have contributed to the death of a patient, the facility must report this to the FDA and the device manufacturer. Reports of adverse events are required within 10 days, with penalties of up to $1 million for violations. Nurses and other medical personnel should be aware of the kind of incidents that are reportable, not all of which are limited to patient injury. However, if an injury is caused by misuse of the equipment or if a nurse has not checked to make sure that the equipment is not faulty, the nurse and the institution (under respondeat superior) are liable.

■ SPECIALTY NURSING

As nurses assume more responsibility in nursing, particularly in specialty areas, they often seek help in determining their legal status. Frequently their concern has to do with the scope of practice: Are they performing within legal bounds? Negligence, whether in a highly specialized unit, an ER, or a self-care unit, is still a question of what the reasonably prudent nurse would do. Therefore, although a nurse might look for a specific answer to a specific question, the legal dangers lie in the same set of circumstances described earlier, simply transposed to another setting. Nevertheless, there are some areas such as OR, psychiatric, and obstetric units, which have been mentioned, that merit some special attention.

ER nurses have particular problems in these days of overcrowding and lack of beds for emergent patients. Policies and procedures for admitting or transferring patients should be in place, but this is not always so. Using nursing judgment is particularly important when hospitals or doctors order the arriving patient to be sent to another hospital without seeing the patient. The *Emergency Medical Treatment and Active Labor Act* (EMTALA) protects patients requiring emergency care, and they should never be told that they could not be examined or treated unless they pay or have health insurance.

Even in the best of circumstances, the ER is considered a target area for liability. In one study analyzing adverse events in ERs, 70 percent were owing to negligence, particularly lack of proper communication or assessment resulting in injury or death. In *Ramsey v. Physician's Memorial Hospital* (373 A2d 26 [Md. Ct. Spec. App. 1977]), two boys with high fever and rash were brought to the ER by their mother. She said that she had removed two ticks from one of her sons, but the nurse did not inform the physician and he failed to diagnose Rocky Mountain Spotted Fever. One child died. In another case, the nurse failed to properly assess the patient's heart condition and told him to drive himself to another hospital. He, too, died. The vast variety of conditions that bring people to the ER, and how these can be handled most effectively, are a challenge for the ER staff and offer patients the opportunity for litigation. Another case, *Affinity Hospital,*

L.L.C. v. Willford (2009-AL-0420.002), raised the question of whether a nurse was liable for the suicide of a waiting ER patient. A patient who was experiencing suicidal thoughts sought treatment at the emergency department of the hospital. He was initially interviewed by an RN and was asked to sit in a waiting area. He was later found dead in a restroom, having hanged himself. It appeared that the nurse merely interviewed the patient. There is no indication in the case whether the nurse made any effort whatsoever to evaluate the patient's condition. If the nurse had attempted to evaluate the patient, it would have been obvious that he was in need of immediate examination and treatment. Since the nurse did nothing more than secure basic information, name and address, this allowed the patient to have the time to finalize his intention to commit suicide and carry out his suicide to completion. The case does not get into the issue of the negligence of the nurse in failing to see to it that the patient received the necessary treatment for which his condition called. Was the patient so close to committing suicide that the nurse should have recognized the need for the immediate evaluation and treatment? Undoubtedly, this will be the issue with which a trial judge and jury will be confronted when the case is tried. Nurses who participate in determining who will be told to wait for treatment and who needs immediate attention should make every effort to see to it that those who need immediate emergency care get it. In addition, nurses must often deal with police investigations, which have their own peril. For instance, a nurse may hesitate to obey a police demand to draw blood on an unwilling prisoner when drunkenness or rape is suspected. Often the laws of the state regulate if, when, and how this can be done.[5]

APNs practicing in the ER or some other ambulatory care facility may be especially vulnerable. Their practice is judged by the standard of care of other APNs, even if they are employed in the status of a staff nurse. APNs practicing in the areas of anesthesia and obstetrics are in particularly delicate positions, because these are known as high areas of litigation. One CRNA administered anesthesia improperly, delayed giving necessary blood, and delayed notifying the anesthesiologist about problems until too late. The patient was seriously hurt and died later of her injuries. The CRNA was found liable, but not the surgeon, although the hospital tried the borrowed servant defense. Nevertheless, on appeal to the State Supreme Court, the surgeon was also found liable, because the policy manual established the surgeon's responsibility to control anesthesia (*Harris v. Miller*, 407 S.E.2d 556).

In a case involving a CNM, the staff, including the CNM, was held liable for failing to diagnose and treat a mother's preeclamptic condition. The baby was seriously disabled. Because this occurred in the Indian Health Service, the United States was held liable for about $3.4 million and a trust was established for the care of the child (*Anderson v. United States*, 731 F. Supp. 391). An important note is that APNs working for the government are not immune from lawsuits. Another interesting case is that of an NP working for Kaiser Permanente, an HMO. The NP and two physicians were found liable for failure to diagnose a patient's heart attack. This case (*Fein v. Permanente Medical Group*, 34. 38 Cal. 3d 137, 696 P. 2d 665, 211 Cal. Rptr. 368) is considered a precedent in California because it addressed the standard of care of NPs. However, a physician, not an NP expert, testified about the NP standard of care, and that should have been challenged.

Another specialty area that has its own hazards is school nursing. At a time when disabled children who require some medical or nursing attention are in regular classrooms, the school nurse must be knowledgeable about not only medical tests, but laws relating to the kind of care that must be given.

With the increased interest in home health care, more attention is being given to the nurse's liability in providing such services. Among the concerns are the use of equipment (knowing how to operate it, monitor it, and provide associated care, such as suctioning) and teaching the family to use it properly and to be alert for specific problems. Still another concern is knowing how to get action if the patient has an emergency and must be seen by a physician promptly. What can be even more serious is having the family threaten to sue you because of something the home health aide has done, like letting the patient fall out of bed. In this case, it is particularly important that aides have proper training, that the duties performed are within the scope of that training, and that the aides are properly supervised.

There are several other factors in home care that need to be considered. Teaching patients and families should be done with care, with demonstrations if possible, written directions, and thorough documentation. Documentation is always very important should a patient sue. When nurses feel as though they are doing the same thing on every visit, writing details may seem unnecessary; however, because this may be the only evidence of care given and a patient's condition and response to care, accurate and complete documentation is even more important in court or when giving a deposition. Honest documentation is also extremely important today, because fraud investigation is a top priority of the federal government and home health is particularly suspect. Recording a visit when a telephone call is made instead or falsifying the need for skilled care (for Medicare reimbursement) are both areas of fraudulent documentation that have already been identified. Fraud, of course, is a criminal act.[6]

Another long-term care (LTC) setting often suspected of fraud and abuse is the nursing home or the skilled nursing facility (which may be the nursing home). Nurses and the institution have been judged liable for neglect of the elderly, as when decubiti are not treated. In one case, a patient died because of multiple infected decubiti. The jury awarded $2 million. One factor was inadequate documentation of treatment; 23 patients had decubiti and nursing notes did not indicate care or condition. Policies were also inadequate.[7]

Mistreating a patient can result in additional penalties of punitive damages, as occurred when an aide slapped a resident. Sexual abuse of patients, often those who are confused or helpless, is still another situation that leads to litigation or assault and battery charges. If the attacker is an employee, the latter certainly applies, although this might also be true if the alleged perpetrator is another patient, if that patient is competent. In one case where the nurse did not document or report a rape of a patient by another patient, the Board of Nurse Examiners revoked her license.[8]

Whether to apply restraints and how to monitor patients is another concern of LTC nurses, as it is in acute care facilities. Because falls are the number one reason LTC facilities are sued, there is always the question of whether restraints should be used as prevention, especially if there is not enough staff to monitor each patient who is liable to fall. Generally, it is said that restraints should be applied only under the most extreme situations, because there are often adverse medical sequelae to restraint use. (Many hospitals and nursing homes are now working toward a restraint-free environment, especially because the Joint Commission considers this desirable.) It should also be remembered that the Omnibus Budget Reconciliation Act of 1987 and its Nursing Home Reforms established strict policies for the use of both chemical and physical restraints with residents.

Nurses working in psychiatric units or institutions have special problems. Sometimes patients are abusive, even violent, and just how they can be restrained is also an issue here. In addition, some are suicidal, and maintaining a safe environment is essential. One patient managed to suffocate himself with a plastic garbage bag, and the jury awarded the widow $1.6 million. There are also delicate legal problems in treating patients against their will. This is ultimately a state-by-state issue and debate rages around depriving someone of their right to choose (see Chapter 22).

Office nurses also have special problems. The most frequent cause for liability is the patient who falls, often from an examining table, and is injured. Equally important is what information the nurse gives to a patient over the phone and how it is given. The nurse and physician should agree on the type of information that is appropriate.

As these examples show, nurses in specialty practice face specific liabilities related to that particular area. Many more could be listed. Nurses must apply the same principles of care that prevent negligence, no matter where they work. And as nurses deal with new technology, regardless of the setting, they must be particularly alert, because laws and legal cases are just emerging. Telecommunications and interactive television where information is transmitted across miles, actually sometimes worldwide, bring issues of licensure, informed consent, confidentiality, and reimbursement as well as liability.[9]

■ STANDARD OF CARE

The standard of care basically determines nurses' liability for negligent acts. If this standard is based on what the *reasonably prudent* nurse would do, who makes that judgment? In litigation, it is the judge or jury, based on testimony that could include the following:

1. *Expert witness.* Did the nurse do what was necessary? A nurse with special or appropriate knowledge testifies on what would be expected of a nurse in the defendant's position in like circumstances. The expert witness would have the credentials to validate his or her expertise, but because the opposing side would also produce an equally prestigious expert witness to say what was useful to them, the credibility of that witness on testifying is critical.
2. *Professional literature.* Was the nurse's practice current? The most current nursing literature would be examined and perhaps quoted to validate (or invalidate) that the nurse's practice in the situation was totally up to date.
3. *Hospital or agency policies.* Were hospital policies, especially nursing policies (in-house law), followed? Example: If side rails were or were not used, was the

nurse's action according to hospital policy? On the other hand, if a nurse followed an outdated policy or followed policy without using nursing judgment (according to the expert witness), it could be held against her or him.

4. *Manuals or procedure books.* Did the nurse accurately follow the usual procedure? Example: If the nurse gave an injection that was alleged to have injured the patient, was it given correctly according to the procedure manual? However, these manuals, too, must be up to date.
5. *Drug enclosures or drug reference books.* Did the nurse check for the latest information? Example: If the patient suffered from a drug reaction that the nurse did not perceive, was the information about the potential reaction in a drug reference book, such as the *Physicians' Desk Reference* (PDR) or a drug insert?
6. *The profession's standards.* Did the nurse behave according to the published ANA or a specialty group's standards?
7. *Licensure.* Did the nurse fulfill her or his responsibilities according to the legal definition of nursing in the licensure law or the law's rules and regulations? Example: Did she or he teach a diabetic patient about foot care?

If the judge or jury were satisfied that the standards were met satisfactorily, even if the patient has been injured, the injury that occurred would not be considered the result of the nurse's negligence. Different judgments in different jurisdictions must be expected. Nevertheless, a nurse who knows the profession's standards and practices accordingly is in a much firmer position legally than one who does not.

■ OTHER TORTS AND CRIMES

The average nurse probably will not get involved in criminal offenses, although in the last several years, a number of nurses have been accused of murder. Nurses, like anyone else, may steal, murder, or break other laws. Crimes most often committed are criminal assault and battery (striking or otherwise physically mistreating or threatening a patient); murder (sometimes in relation to right-to-die principles); and drug offenses. If found guilty of a felony, the nurse will probably also lose her or his license, or suffer other non-disciplinary action.

Sometimes nurses will be involved in litigation as *accessories*; that is, they are connected with the commission of a crime but did not actually do it themselves, although they were present and promoting the crime or were near enough to assist if necessary.

An *abettor* encourages the commission of a crime but is absent when it is actually committed. The term *accomplice* is similar in meaning to both accessory and abettor, although a distinction may be made in some jurisdictions. A nurse (or anyone else, for that matter) found guilty of any of these crimes might be held equally guilty with the person who commits the crime. However, whether the nurse is a perpetrator, a victim, or simply has to deal with people who are, it is useful to know the definition and scope of the most common criminal offenses. These can be found in most nursing law texts. Several will be discussed here. Not discussed but worth noting are some torts and crimes in which nurses occasionally are involved in their professional lives: *forgery*—fraudulently making or altering a written document or item, such as a will, chart, or check; *kidnapping*—stealing and carrying off a human being; *rape*—illegal or forcible sexual intercourse; and *bribery*—an offer of a reward for doing wrong or for influencing conduct.

Intentional Torts

Intentional torts are meant to cause a specific outcome that unlawfully assails the interest of another. The injured party need not show that damages were incurred. Those most often seen in health care are *assault, battery, false imprisonment, intentional infliction of emotional distress*, and *conversion of property*. Of these, assault and battery and false imprisonment are also discussed in detail in Chapter 22. An overview of intentional torts follows:

- **Assault**—A threat or an attempt to make bodily contact with another person without that person's consent; it causes the person to fear that battery is about to occur. There is no requirement of actual touching the plaintiff.
- **Battery**—The impermissible unprivileged touching of one person by another. Actual harm may or may not occur; contact is necessary. However, the victim does not need to be aware of it, as with an unconscious patient.
- **False imprisonment**—This tort protects a person from restriction of one's choice of movement, for any length of time, no matter how short. The victim is unable to leave confinement, whether by physical barriers or use of force.
- **Intentional infliction of emotional distress**—If a person's conduct is extreme and outrageous, "exceeding the bounds of common decency," and causes or is fairly certain to cause severe emotional distress with or

without physical results, this tort is satisfied. The plaintiff could also be someone observing another being treated offensively.
- **Conversion of property**—This tort involves actual interference with the right of a person to possess his or her own property, either by exercising control over it, transferring it, altering it, or disposing of it. An example might be searching a patient's suitcase and removing prescription drugs. The practitioner may be free from liability if there is adequate justification for the action.

Quasi-Intentional Torts

A tort is **quasi-intentional** when intent is missing, but there is a willful action directly causing suffering. Damages are not at issue. Quasi-intentional torts include *defamation, libel, slander, breach of confidentiality*, and *invasion of privacy*. Brief explanations follow:

- **Defamation, libel, slander**—*Defamation* includes *libel* (written word) and *slander* (spoken word). For this tort, there must be (1) communication about the individual to a third party or parties, (2) the communication will harm the victim's reputation, (3) this will lower others' estimation of the person so that they may not wish to associate with him or her. The defamation is personal, not group—"She's a promiscuous nurse" versus "All nurses are promiscuous." The latter is not actionable. Slander must be proved by the plaintiff because it is not in a permanent state as written communications are. Perhaps a taped statement would qualify, but to be admissible, generally the person taped must be aware of it.
- **Breach of confidentiality**—This tort protects a patient's sharing information with someone involved with his or her care. Once it referred only to physicians, but now it includes nurses and others. Many states have protected patient confidentiality, but a problem arises if the information involves danger to others. There are also mandatory reporting requirements, such as in child abuse.
- **Invasion of privacy**—Here the interest protected is that of an individual's right to be free from unreasonable intrusion into his or her private affairs. Exceptions here are also the mandatory reporting requirements.

There are a variety of defenses that are used in all these torts, depending on the circumstances. These can be quite complex or relatively simple and generally require the assistance of counsel.

Homicide and Suicide

Homicide means killing a person by any means whatsoever. It is not necessarily a crime. If it is unquestionably an accident, it is called *excusable homicide*. If it is done in self-defense or in discharging a legal duty, such as taking a prisoner, putting a condemned person to death, or preserving the peace, it is termed *justifiable homicide*. The accused must be able to prove justification, however.

Criminal homicide is either murder or manslaughter. *Murder* is the unlawful killing of one person by another of sound mind and with malice aforethought. It may be by *direct violence*, such as shooting or strangling, or by *indirect violence*, such as slow poisoning. Murder is usually divided into two degrees: *first degree* when it is premeditated and carried out deliberately, and *second degree* when it is not planned beforehand but is nonetheless performed with intent to kill. In both, there must be a design to cause death. *Manslaughter* is defined as a homicide not bad enough to be murder but too bad to be no crime whatsoever. Categories of manslaughter include *voluntary manslaughter* (killing another in the heat of passion or when provoked), *involuntary manslaughter* (killing another when committing a crime or when criminally negligent), or *criminally negligent involuntary manslaughter* (conducting oneself in a lawful manner but without proper care or necessary skill).

Suicide is considered criminal if the person is sane and of an age of discretion (usually 14 years)[10] at the time of his or her action. An unsuccessful attempt to commit suicide is a misdemeanor under the law. If there is doubt as to whether a person has committed suicide, a court of law usually presumes that he or she has not, although this judgment may be reversed by evidence to the contrary. A person who encourages another to commit suicide is guilty of murder if the suicide is affected. Statutes vary from state to state.

As a professional, it is not unusual for a nurse to become implicated in cases of murder and suicide, usually associated with patients. Following are a few suggestions for keeping as free of legal involvement as possible:

1. Any indication on the part of any patient or employee that she or he has suicidal tendencies should be taken seriously and be reported to the appropriate person.
2. Generally, a patient with known suicidal inclinations should not be left alone unless completely protected from self-harm.
3. Items that a depressed person might use for suicidal purposes should be kept out of reach.
4. Observations should be accurately reported on the patient's chart.
5. Help should be sought for individuals or their families immediately on becoming aware of suicidal tendencies.
6. Cooperation with the police and hospital authorities guarding a patient who is accused of homicide is important.
7. Unethical discussions of a homicide case involving a patient or employee should be avoided.
8. Complete and accurate records of all facts that might have a bearing on the legal aspects of the case should be kept.

■ IS ERROR A CRIME?

Negligence or malpractice by nurses or other health professionals usually ends up in a civil court, even if the patient has died. It is assumed that there is no intent to harm, and although the defendant may pay a heavy price financially, in damage to his or her professional reputation and loss or suspension of the professional license, the circumstances are not considered criminal. There have been a few exceptions, but they are rare.

It was a different story when criminal charges were brought against three nurses in Colorado. There were numerous articles in the nursing press condemning the behavior of the district attorney (DA), which was seen as punitive and politically motivated. Perhaps the nurses had such support because they were trying to protect the patient, because they were open about what happened, and because they followed correct reporting procedures. In St. Anthony Hospital North, near Denver, CO, a baby boy was born to a mother whose blood work indicated that she might have or have had syphilis. The physician decided to treat the infant for congenital syphilis and ordered one dose of 150,000 units of penicillin G benzathine to be given intramuscularly. The pharmacist misread the order and prepared two syringes containing a total of 1,500,000 units, 10 times the ordered dose. The primary care nurse was concerned about how many times she would have to jab the baby, who had already had a lumbar puncture. She conferred with an APN and a neonatal NP. The two researched the drug and determined that it could be given IV. (This was an incorrect conclusion based on not-very-clear information in the source consulted, which was later changed after the neonatal NP wrote to the publisher.) The drug was then given IV, and in a few minutes the baby went into respiratory failure; he died later in the day. The nurses reported their actions through correct channels, and the neonatal NP met with the Colorado Board of Nursing and answered all police questions. Five months later, the Adams County DA decided to criminally indict all three nurses for criminally negligent homicide. The DA took the case to a grand jury, rather than filing for information—a process where the evidence against the accused is presented to a judge at a preliminary hearing and the defense can cross-examine the witnesses. The judge then decides whether enough evidence exists to establish probable cause. In a grand jury, only the prosecution can present evidence without the presence of anyone for the defense. The grand jury indicted all three nurses; a trial date was set. Shortly before the scheduled trial the APN and the NP pleaded guilty on the advice of their attorneys, knowing that a guilty verdict would mean loss of their nursing licenses and perhaps prison. The primary nurse, who had not been directly involved after conferring with the other nurses, chose to stand trial. The jury took only 45 minutes to return a not guilty verdict. Golz and Fitchett received strict sanctions from the Board of Nursing, including suspension of their licenses for 1 year and required counseling and formal re-education in neonatal pharmacology.

They received deferred judgment when sentenced in criminal court, meaning that they would not face any jail time, and if they do not violate the terms of their sentence, their records will be clean. The terms included 2 years' probation and 24 hours of public service, in which the nurses would educate nursing students by discussing the case. They did so, but as they have stated, this does not erase their emotional trauma at the death of the baby. Interestingly, the pharmacist who made the original fatal error, although fired by the hospital, was never charged for anything by the DA. When asked why, the DA said experts claimed that the child would not have died if the medication route had not been changed. As to the nurses, he said, "I wanted the community to decide what the standard of care should have been." It was noted that a newspaper had been running articles about errors made by doctors, hospitals, and nurses. This case was one of them. No one else was indicted for anything, and there was a strong feeling in the nursing community that this was a political act.

There was a great uproar in the nursing world concerning this situation. Because there are already disciplinary procedures in place to deal with negligence, particularly with each state's Board of Nursing, the question arose: Is this a wave of the future? It could be. In another case, five nurses were indicted in New Jersey, based on a statute that made it a crime for any person responsible for the care of an elderly or disabled person to unreasonably neglect their charge. The nurses, three RNs and two LPNs, had cared for a 74-year-old patient who was recovering from a stroke and a blood clot in his leg in the Roosevelt Care Center, a county-owned nursing home.

One night he began to have trouble breathing and his condition rapidly deteriorated. The prosecutor alleged that the nurses had done nothing to help the patient over two shifts and did not attempt to contact an on-call physician until the next morning. The patient was then rushed to a hospital where he died of internal bleeding. The accusations turned out to be false. The nurses placed two telephone calls to a physician's answering service, neither of which was returned. Other problems were an unclear policy about calling in extreme emergencies and tremendous cuts in staffing, leaving only one on-call physician during off hours. Even the family's lawyer stated that the nurses should not shoulder all the blame, although the family filed civil suits against the nursing home, the nurses, and several doctors. It was eventually recommended that the nurses, who apparently had spotless records, would be enrolled in a pretrial intervention program that would allow them to avoid a trial and possible jail time without admitting any guilt. Their records would eventually be cleared of all charges. Why were they indicted? One LPN's attorney speculated that it was a message to all nurses: Don't automatically expect immunity from prosecution if you're negligent.

■ GOOD SAMARITAN LAWS

The enactment of Good Samaritan laws in many states exempts doctors and nurses (and sometimes others) from civil liability when they give emergency care in good faith with due care or without gross negligence. The first state to pass such a law was California in 1959; in 1963, California enacted such legislation specifically for nurses. By 1979, all states and the District of Columbia had Good Samaritan laws, not all including nurses in the coverage. The law is intended to encourage assistance without fear of legal liability. As far as the law is concerned, there is no obligation or duty to render aid or assistance in an emergency, except in a few states.[11] Only by statutory law can the rendering of such assistance be made obligatory.

RNs engaged in occupational health nursing are likely to be called on to give first-aid treatment to patients with wounds and other injuries as part of their job responsibility. Such emergency treatment in a health care setting is not covered under the Good Samaritan laws. These nurses, just like nurses in an ER, should take every precaution to make sure they are operating within the bounds of legally authorized practice for nurses in their position.

Because of the lack of clarity of terms and the many differences in the law from state to state, many health professionals are still reluctant to give emergency assistance. Some cautions may help: Don't give aid unless you know what you're doing; stick to the basics of first aid; offer to help, but make it clear that you won't interfere if the victim or family prefers to wait for other help; don't draw any medical or diagnostic conclusions; don't leave a victim you've begun to assist until you can turn his care over to an equally competent person; whether you do or do not volunteer your services, be absolutely certain to call or have someone else call for emergency medical service immediately. Generally, where an unconscious victim cannot respond, a good Samaritan can help the victim on the grounds of implied consent.

■ LIABILITY (MALPRACTICE) INSURANCE

Nurses should carry their own malpractice or professional liability insurance, whether or not their employer's insurance includes them. The employer's insurance is intended primarily to protect the employer; the nurse is protected only to the extent needed for that primary purpose. It is quite conceivable that the employer might settle out of court, without consulting the nurse, to the nurse's disadvantage. The nurse has no control and no choice of lawyer. There are a number of other limitations. The nurse is not covered for anything beyond the job in the place of employment during the hours of employment. If the nurse alone is sued and the hospital is not, the hospital has no obligation to provide legal protection (and may choose not to). Moreover, if the nurse carries no personal liability insurance, there is the possibility of subrogation (the nurse is sued by the insurance company to recoup its loss). Should there be criminal charges, the employer or insurance carrier may choose to deny legal assistance, or the kind offered could be inadequate. A nurse must remember that no matter how trivial or how unfounded a charge might be, a legal defense is necessary and often costly, aside from the possibility of being found liable and having to pay damages. However, it is important to know that punitive damages are generally not covered by any insurance company. Punitive damages are monetary compensation

awarded to an injured party that goes beyond that which is necessary to compensate the individual for losses and that is intended to punish the wrongdoer.

Professional liability insurance should be bought with some care so that adequate coverage is provided. The most important distinction to be made in selecting insurance is whether it is on an occurrence-based or a claims-made basis. If the insurance policy is allowed to lapse, an incident that occurred at the time of coverage will be covered in an occurrence-based policy, but not in a claims-made policy. Claims-made policies cover injuries only if the injury occurs within the policy period and the claim is reported to the insurance company during the policy period or during the tail. A *tail* is an uninterrupted extension of the policy period and is also known as the *extending reporting endorsement*.[12] The claims-made policy may be less expensive but will require almost continuous coverage, which might be a problem for a nurse planning to take time out for child rearing or for one close to retirement. Benefits usually include paying any sum awarded as damages, including medical costs; paying the cost of attorneys; and paying the bond required if appealing an adverse decision. Some policies also pay damages for injury arising out of acts of the insured as a member of an accreditation board or committee of a hospital or professional society, or when a nurse gives advice or care to a neighbor or friend; personal liability (such as slander, assault, and libel); and personal injury and medical payments (not related to the individual's professional practice).

Whether you pay for your own policy or your employer does, here are some questions you should ask:

- Is it occurrence based or claims made? What does it cover and for what amount? (One million dollars is reasonable coverage today—more if you are an APN.)
- What, if any, is the deductible?
- Is there a subrogation clause?
- Are you covered for personal liability?
- Will you be covered off the job?
- What, if any, are the exclusions?

Generally speaking, an ANA or state association policy is the best buy for most nurses. ANA has made arrangements with an insurance carrier that covers all nurses, including NPs and nurses in private practice. For the relatively low cost of personal liability insurance, it is sensible to buy it.

Today's managed care environment, with reduction in staffing and often a bottom-line mentality, has eliminated much of the family atmosphere that was once present in many workplaces. There is currently no record of indemnification or subrogation suits (action to make parties whole who paid on a claim) against nurses.

■ IN COURT: THE DUE PROCESS OF LAW

Yes, you can be sued. What happens if you become involved in litigation? What steps should you take to try to make sure that the case will be handled to your best advantage throughout? The answers to these questions will depend on whether you

1. Are accused of committing the tort or crime;
2. Are an accessory, through actual participation or observance;
3. Are the person against whom the act was committed; or
4. Appear as an expert witness.

Assuming that it is a civil case, five distinct steps are taken:

1. the filing of a document called a complaint by a person called the *plaintiff* who contends that his legal rights have been infringed by the conduct of one or more other partners (could be the hospital) called *defendants*;
2. the written response of the defendants accused of having violated the legal rights of the plaintiff, termed an *answer*;
3. pretrial activities of both parties designed to elicit all the facts of the situation, termed *discovery*;
4. the *trial* of the case, in which all the relevant facts are presented to the judge or jury for decisions; and
5. *appeal* from a decision by a party who contends that the decision was wrongly made.

The majority of persons who are asked to appear as witnesses during a hearing accept voluntarily. Others refuse and must be subpoenaed. A *subpoena* is a writ or order in the name of the court, referee, or other person authorized by law to issue the same, which requires the attendance of a witness at a trial or hearing under a penalty for failure to appear. Cases involving the care of patients often necessitate producing hospital records, x-rays, and photographs as evidence. A subpoena requiring a witness to bring this type of evidence with him or her contains a clause to that effect and is termed a *subpoena duces tecum*.

The plaintiff, defendant, and witnesses may be asked to give a *deposition*, an oral interrogation answering various questions about the issue concerned. It is given under oath and taken in writing by a court reporter or attorney. The deposition is an opportunity to examine a witness under oath about the facts of a case. Although you may be asked the same questions on the witness stand, the examining (opposing) attorney sometimes asks questions that would not be permitted in court. Also, if you contradict in court what was said in the deposition, this might *impeach* you as a witness. Usually the examining attorney inquires into the background of the witness, facts related to the patient's claims and defenses, and any injuries or damages incurred. The examining attorney asks the majority of questions; the witness' attorney monitors and responds to questions through the use of objections; there is no impartial party to rule on objections. The court reporter notes that the objection has been made. Sometimes, after the depositions of key witnesses, the factual issues may have been narrowed enough for one of the parties to file for a summary judgment. This occurs in cases where the relevant material facts are not in dispute and only a question of law remains. If the case proceeds to court, other rules apply.

A witness has certain rights, including the right to refuse to testify as to privileged communications[a] and the protection against self-incrimination afforded by the Fifth Amendment to the Constitution. The judge and jury usually do not expect a person on trial or serving as a witness to remember all of the details of a situation. Witnesses in malpractice suits are permitted to refer to the patient's record, which, of course, they should have reviewed with the attorney before the trial.

Only under serious circumstances is someone accused (and convicted) of *perjury*, which means making a false statement under oath or one that she or he neither knows nor believes to be true.

There are certain guidelines on testifying, at a deposition or in court, that are the same whether serving as an expert or other witness or if the nurse is the defendant.

1. Be prepared; review the deposition, the chart, and technical and clinical knowledge of the disease or condition; discuss with the lawyer potential questions; educate the

---

[a]Be alert that the right to privileged communications varies from state to state. This right has only very selectively been extended to nurses. APNs have this privilege in some states, as do some registered nurses in psychiatric practice. The reader should be sensitive to the difference between confidentiality, which is an ethical obligation, and privileged communication, which is based in the law. They may sometimes be in conflict in the real world.

lawyer as to what points should be made. Trials are adversarial procedures that are intended to probe, question, and explore all aspects of the issue.

2. Dress appropriately; enunciate clearly.

3. Behave appropriately: keep calm, be courteous, even if insulted; don't be sarcastic or angry; take your time (a cross-examining attorney may try to put you in a poor light).

4. Give adequate and appropriate information: if you can't remember, notes or the data source, such as the chart, can be checked. Answer fully, but don't volunteer additional information not asked for.

5. Don't use technical terminology, or, if use is necessary, translate it into lay terms.

6. Don't feel incompetent; don't get on the defensive; be decisive.

7. Don't be obviously partisan (unless you're the defendant).

8. Keep all materials; the decision may be appealed.

In the *expert witness role*, the same precepts hold, but in addition the nurse should present her or his credentials, degrees, research, honors, and whatever else is pertinent without modesty; the opposing expert witness will certainly do so. Expert witnesses are paid for preparation time, pretrial conferences, consultations, and testifying. Nurses are beginning to act officially in this capacity more frequently, and several state nurses' associations accept applications for those interested in placement on an expert witness panel, screen applicants in a given field for a specific case, submit a choice of names to attorneys requesting such information, and have developed guidelines and continuing education (CE) courses for nurse expert witnesses and consultants.

In most malpractice cases, a jury of laypeople makes the judgment. If it is financially feasible, attorneys try to learn as much as possible about potential jurors and what they think. Jurors can be dismissed for a variety of reasons. To get a perspective on how potential jurors feel about nurses' legal accountability, a small study was done over a 3-year period. The jurors felt that when mistakes are made and someone is injured, particularly by a professional, someone should be held liable—even if that person was following standard acceptable practice. They felt particularly strong about negligence and violation of patient confidentiality. Most also thought that both employer and the RN should bear the cost. It appears that jurors feel that the employer was responsible for providing high-quality care, as well as the nurse (see Exhibit 21–4).

As noted, ADR is being increasingly encouraged, as opposed to going to court. Instead of months, sometimes years, before a legal case goes to court, the situation can be settled in much less time at much less cost. Of course, should a patient injury be very severe, an ADR probably would not be considered. Using an ADR process, the disputants decide on the time, place, and length of the hearing, as well as whether the resolution will be advisory or binding. They choose their own "judge" or mediator, a roster of which is available through the American Arbitration Association at 800-778-7879 or at www.adr.org. The two sides usually split the cost. Each person may still have an attorney present, if desired (and if one does, the other should). Although most malpractice companies do not provide attorneys for ADR proceedings unless a lawsuit has already been filed, the carrier should be notified that ADR is being used. An ADR process might be welcomed, but if you do not notify your insurance company, you might lose coverage, including payment for any settlement.

The idea of mediation is that the independent third party, the mediator, helps the two sides to negotiate. If they both agree in advance to abide by the mediation, the decision has the force of a contract. Failing to abide by its terms could result in litigation based on breach of contract. It is also possible to have Med/Arb, in which the disputing parties agree to arbitration if the mediation does not bring mutual agreement. The mediation process works something like this:

1. Under the guidance of the mediator, both sides openly and candidly discuss their sides of the conflict.

2. Both listen and react frankly, getting a better understanding of the other's point of view. The mediator prevents this from getting rancorous.

3. They come to some conclusion about a fair settlement.

4. The whole proceeding is confidential, with no one recording it, even on paper; the final agreement is the only written record.

Arbitration is more formal. A neutral third party (or it may be a panel of three) trained in the process listens to both sides of the dispute and then decides the case, usually in favor of one or the other. If both sides have agreed to *binding arbitration*, the decision is final, but can be appealed to a court under limited circumstances.

The process is like an informal court, with both sides able to give opening statements, provide evidence, and cross-examine witnesses. A court reporter is present, but transcripts are not available to the public. If you choose

■ **EXHIBIT 21–4. Suggestions for Your Own Defense**

1. Cut off all communication with the claimant; simply tell whoever contacts you that your insurer will be in touch. (Then find out why they haven't been already.)
2. Educate the insurer; claims adjusters may know little about nursing.
3. Keep tabs on the claim. Don't be afraid to ask questions.
4. Be sure that your claim is supervised adequately. You have a right to ask that an experienced and attentive professional handle it.
5. Seek input on settlement decisions. You might not have the right, but you can ask your insurer to check with you before making an offer.
6. Remember that the defense attorney is your attorney. If you really think his or her qualifications are inadequate, ask for a change.
7. Dictate all memories of the patient to the attorney. Do it as soon as possible, but not until an attorney has been assigned to your case, or your information may not be considered privileged.
8. Retrieve medical records. You have access if you still work at the same place and can get access before the attorney does.
9. Review the records.
10. Compile a list of experts; the case may hinge on getting the best. (Although in some courts, physicians have been allowed as expert witnesses on a nursing case, ordinarily it should be the nurse[s] who is most knowledgeable about the type of situation involved.)
11. Have a reference list available on the topics related to nursing care of the patient involved so that you have backup for your actions.
12. Speak up in court; you must project self-confidence.
13. Be cautious not to speak to anyone at your place of employment about the case, except the risk manager.
14. Do not speak about the case with anyone involved in any way with the plaintiff or to reporters.
15. Don't hide information from your attorney, and never alter the patient record.

arbitration, prepare to defend yourself as you would in any courtroom. Arbitration differs from a formal court proceeding because each side has a chance to present all relevant information, some of which would not be allowed in a formal court. It is also much quicker because a court calendar need not be considered.

Med/Arb is a creature of both negotiation and arbitration, and can thus have whatever precise meaning is given to it in a given situation. The essence of Med/Arb is to allow a softer mediation process to occur first, thus taking every opportunity of achieving a resolution to a dispute, which is not imposed and to which each party to the dispute subscribes voluntarily. In this initial phase, the presiding neutral third party acts as a mediator and coaches or encourages the parties toward a settlement, taking into account the information received from both at a mediation hearing. *Med/Arb* motivates the participants at the mediation given the shadow of the instant conversion to arbitration. If no progress is shown, the presiding officer assumes the role of arbitrator and is no longer mediator.

The arbitrator is enabled to proceed as if the hearing was one of arbitration and to impose a resolution, a final and binding award.[13]

■ RISK MANAGEMENT

No matter how strong the defense, everyone agrees that prevention is better than any suit. Therefore, hospitals have now adopted *risk management programs* to which nurses are very well suited as part of the team, or sometimes in one of the risk management positions, including patient representative or advocate. Risk management must be a team effort involving everyone.

Risk management initiatives are now required by the Joint Commission and more and more by state legislation. The purpose is not only to protect the interest of the hospital and its personnel, but also to improve the quality of patient care. Risk management means taking steps to control the possibility that a patient will complain and minimizing any risks before complaints are filed.

The Joint Commission urges facilities to voluntarily file reports of *sentinel events*, defined as "an unexpected occurrence involving death or serious physical or psychological injury, or the risk thereof," and to conduct a *root-cause analysis* within 30 days. However, there is some fear that such a report is discoverable and could lead to lawsuits.

Nurses are all involved in risk management, which includes focusing on the review and improvement of employee guidelines, personnel policies, incident reports, physician–nurse relationships, safety policies, patient records, research guidelines, and anything else that might be a factor in legal suits.

Nevertheless, patient injuries do occur. In case of patient injury, most hospitals and health agencies require completion of an incident report. The purpose is to document the incident accurately for remedial and correctional use by the hospital or agency, for insurance information, and sometimes for legal reasons. The wording should be chosen to avoid the implication of blame and should be totally objective and complete: what happened to the patient, what was done, and what the patient's condition is. The incident report may or may not be discoverable, depending on the state's law. It is considered a business record, not part of the patient's chart, but some courts rule that it is not privileged information. The incident must be just as accurately recorded in the patient's chart. This kind of omission casts doubt on the nurse's honesty if litigation occurs. However, the fact that an incident report was filed should not be charted. (There is also some suspicion that not all incidents are being reported.)

Appropriate behavior by nurses and other personnel is often a key factor as to whether or not the patient or family sues after an incident, regardless of injury. Maintaining a good rapport and giving honest explanations as needed is very important.

However, one attorney advises the following:

1. Before meeting with the family, get your facts straight.
2. Try to meet with the family as soon as possible.
3. Be careful not to accept unnecessary responsibility for the incident. You need to discuss the event with caution.
4. Express your sympathy to the family.

All of this involves nurses. For individual nurses who have specific concerns about the legal aspects of their practice, it may be possible to get some information from the employing agency's legal counsel or the state licensing board. Keeping abreast of legal trends is always necessary. Observing some basic principles will also help to avert problems:

1. Know your licensure law.
2. Don't do what you don't know how to do (learn how, if necessary).
3. Keep your practice updated; CE is essential.
4. Use self-assessment, peer evaluation, audits, and supervisor's evaluations as guidelines for improving practice and follow up on criticisms, and knowledge and skill gaps.
5. Don't be careless.
6. Practice interdependently; communicate with others.
7. Record accurately, objectively, and completely; don't erase.
8. Delegate safely and legally; know the preparation and abilities of those you supervise.
9. Help develop appropriate policies and procedures.
10. Carry liability insurance.

KEY POINTS

1. Malpractice suits of any kind are often stimulated by how the patient and family were treated, as well as by the possible injury.
2. The standard of care by which a nurse is judged in a malpractice case is based on what the reasonably prudent nurse of the same background and in the same situation would do.
3. The most common reason for legal suits against nurses is negligence.
4. Negligence frequently occurs in giving medication and treatments because the nurse has inadequate knowledge or is careless.
5. Torts are private civil wrongs, in contrast to crimes, which are wrongs against the state.
6. *Darling v. Charleston Community Memorial Hospital* is a landmark case pinpointing the corporate liability of hospitals for the actions of their employees and physicians. For nurses, it underlines the legal responsibility to follow through and ensure that patients get competent care.

KEY POINTS

7. Poor communication between doctors and nurses, and among nurses themselves, can endanger patients and result in litigation.

8. Advances in technology have increased the possibility for legal actions involving nurses.

9. To avoid problems in law, be accurate, complete, and objective in charting. Never falsify a record for any reason.

10. When selecting professional liability (malpractice) insurance, among the points to consider is whether it is occurrence based or claims made.

11. When testifying in a court of law, be prepared and calm; give appropriate information without jargon, and be accurate and honest.

12. To avoid malpractice, it is especially important to know your licensure law, stay up to date in your practice, communicate with others adequately, be careful, and practice humanistic nursing.

REFERENCES

1. Hall J. *Nursing Ethics and Law*. Philadelphia: Saunders, 1996, p 4.

2. NPDB-HIPDB. NPDB Summary Report. April 17, 2010. http://www.npdb-hipdb.com/pubs/stats/NPDB_Summary_Report.pdf. Retrieved May 24, 2010.

3. Editor's Memo. Medical errors are making headlines. *Nurse Pract* 25:12–13, May 2000.

4. ISMP. Medication Safety Tools and Resources. 2010. http://www.ismp.org. Retrieved May 25, 2010.

5. Lawrence N. *Role of Forensic Nurse As an Integral Part of the Criminal Investigative Team*. May 29, 2010. http://www.ehow.com/facts_6317502_role-part-criminal-investigative-team.html. Retrieved May 29, 2010.

6. American Association for Home Care. Help Us Stop Medicare Fraud and Abuse. http://www.aahomecare.org/displaycommon.cfm?an=1&subarticlenbr=496. Retrieved May 20, 2010.

7. University of Maryland School of Medicine. Neglect: The Most Frequent Abuse in Long-Term Care. http://www.videopress.org/elder_abuse/frequentneglect_AB404.html. Retrieved May 10, 2010.

8. National Center on Elder Abuse, Administration on Aging. Major Types of Elder Abuse. September 28, 2007. http://www.ncea.aoa.gov/ncearoot/Main_Site/FAQ/Basics/Types_Of_Abuse.aspx. Retrieved May 10, 2007.

9. Walker J. Telehealth: A complex issue being addressed by state and federal governments. *AORN Journal*, October 1997.

10. The 'Lectric Law Library. Discretion. http://www.lectlaw.com/def/d175.htm. Retrieved May 3l, 2010.

11. American Heart Association. Good Samaritan Laws. http://www.americanheart.org/presenter.jhtml?identifier=3024007. Retrieved May 30, 2010.

12. Chitty K, Black B. *Professional Nursing: Concepts and Challenges*, 6th ed. Philadelphia: Saunders, 2011.

13. Med-Arb. http://www.duhaime.org/legaldictionary/M/MedArb.aspx. Retrieved May 31, 2010.

Updates can be found at **www.kellysnursing.com**

Health Care and the Rights of People

The civil rights movement of the late 1950s and early 1960s had a profound effect on American society. Not only were there major and obvious changes in public policy, but also it seems American citizens learned to *think* differently: We learned to think and speak much more in terms of individual *rights*.

The consumer movement was an outgrowth of the civil rights movement. It further led us to think in terms of our *rights* as purchasers or users of goods and services. Especially as health care has come to be perceived as an essential public good on which all members of the community have legitimate claims, it seems natural that Americans increasingly speak about health care in the language of *rights*.

Until recently, people felt helpless in their patient role—and no small wonder why. Stripped of their individuality as well as their belongings (if the hospital or nursing home is central to their care), they are thrust into an alien environment where they feel that they have little control over what happens to them. Unidentified faces and unidentifiable equipment surround them. Their privacy is invaded. Their dignity is lost. They hesitate to complain or criticize for fear of reprisals from the staff. They may be reluctant to press for answers to their questions because, too often, the idea that the doctor or nurse is too busy is conveyed. Underlying all is fear for their health, and even their lives.

Now, an increasing number of consumers are no longer willing to put up with this state of affairs, will no longer accept the traditional role of the good patient: the one who does as he or she is told and asks no awkward questions. The frequent denial of patients' fundamental rights—among them rights to courtesy, privacy, and, most of all, information—has brought about the ultimate form of patient rebellion: malpractice suits. Almost 30 years ago, a national Commission on Medical Malpractice declared that "to ignore these and other rights of the patient is both to betray simple humanity and to invite dissatisfaction that may lead to malpractice suits."[1]

■ PATIENT RIGHTS

Most of the rights about which patients are concerned are theirs legally as well as morally and have been so established by common law. They are also stated in the codes of ethics of both physicians and nurses (although, to be honest, much is stated by implication and thus open to considerable personal interpretation). Moreover, they closely reiterate the four basic consumer rights President John F. Kennedy enunciated in his consumer message to Congress in 1962:

1. The right to safety
2. The right to be informed
3. The right to choose
4. The right to be heard

Since the well-publicized American Hospital Association's (AHA's) "A Patient's Bill of Rights" was first presented in 1973 (revised in 1992), a plethora of such rights statements has followed: for the disabled, the mentally ill, the retarded, the old, the young, the pregnant, the handicapped, and the dying. By the end of the 1970s, many state legislatures had made these statements the basis of new statutory law.

In fact, the *Patients Bill of Rights* legislation that has been stalled in Congress since 1998 is modeled after this document. Besides other protections, this law would allow for limited suits against health maintenance organizations (HMOs). By 2002, different versions of the bill had been passed by the House and the Senate and were in the House-Senate Conference Committee awaiting some resolution, which never came. See Exhibit 22–1 for excerpts from the AHA document.

In 1974, new Medicare regulations for skilled nursing facilities included a section on patients' rights. Just how disgraceful the violation of rights of this captive group was might be judged when reviewing the rights: the right to send and receive mail; the right to have spouses share rooms if both are patients, or allow privacy for visits; the right to have restraints used only if authorized by the physician and only for a limited time; the right to use one's own clothes and possessions, as space permits; and the right to require written permission by the patient for management of his or her funds. And, as in other laws, patients had to be told what their rights were.

Since that time the continuing scandals involving the violation of patients' and residents' rights in so many long-term care (LTC) facilities have resulted in legislation in various guises, usually requirements under Medicare and Medicaid. For the LTC facilities that are not certified, there is still some control by state regulation. The regulations on rights are enacted and enforced erratically, sometimes depending on the political climate. However, now nursing home residents have the right to talk directly to state surveyors, who ensure that the facilities meet the standards set by the Centers for Medicare and Medicaid Services (CMS), which include rights statements. Nursing homes also may have a volunteer ombudsman, and teaching nursing homes have students and faculty who observe what goes on. Such facilities are not usually problem sites. Some states have also given legal attention to the rights of residents in continuing care communities and assisted living, including such aspects as complete disclosure of costs and other financial data, posting of the last state examination report, freedom to form a residents' organization, and other mechanisms to avoid fraud and deception.

Many rights advocates have little enthusiasm for most of these declarations, particularly the AHA statement, because they tend to hedge about some or many of the rights, ethical or legal. This is probably because few, if any, evolved out of some massive "goodness of heart" by the institutions or by government. The AHA bill, for instance, came about because of pressures from consumer advocates in health centers affiliated with larger general hospitals where their clientele, mostly black and Hispanic, were mistreated even when treated. They were subjected to long waiting times, never seeing the same physician twice, and had little or no explanation of their diagnosis or no confidentiality of records, no real effort to get informed consent, multiple student access without consent, involvement in research without consent, and overall loss of dignity. This history is clearly reflected in the AHA statement. The stage was set for a consumer assault on health care. The various arms of government followed, sometimes for political purposes.

■ INFORMED CONSENT

For years, when patients have been admitted to hospitals, they signed a frequently unread universal consent form that almost literally gave the physician, his or her associates, and the hospital carte blanche in determining the patient's care. There was some rationale for this because civil suits for battery (unlawful touching) could theoretically be filed as a result of giving routine care such as baths. Patients undergoing surgery or some complex, dangerous treatment were asked to sign a separate form, usually stating something to the effect that permission was granted to the physician or his or her colleagues to perform the operation or treatment. Just how much the patient knew about the hows and whys of the surgery, the dangers, and the alternatives depended on the patient's assertiveness in asking questions and demanding answers and the physician's willingness to provide information. Nurses were taught never to answer those questions, but to suggest, "Ask your doctor." Health professionals, and especially physicians, took the attitude, "We know best and will decide for you."

Many patients probably still enter treatment and undergo a variety of tests and even surgery without a clear understanding of the nature of the condition they have and what can be done about it. Although they may very well be receiving care that is medically acceptable, they have no real part in deciding what that care should be. Most physicians have believed that anything more than a superficial explanation is unnecessary, for the patient should trust the doctor. Yet, the patient has always had the right to make decisions about his or her own body. A case was heard as early as 1905 on surgery without consent, and the classic legal decision is that of Judge Cardoza (*Schloendorff v. The Society of New York Hospital*, 211 N.Y.

1. The patient has the right to considerate and respectful care.

2. The patient has the right to and is encouraged to obtain from physicians and other direct caregivers relevant, current, and understandable information concerning diagnosis, treatment, and prognosis.

   Except in emergencies when the patient lacks decision-making capacity and the need for treatment is urgent, the patient is entitled to the opportunity to discuss and request information related to the specific procedures and/or treatments, the risks involved, the possible length of recuperation, and the medically reasonable alternatives and their accompanying risks and benefits.

   Patients have the right to know the identity of physicians, nurses, and others involved in their care, as well as when those involved are students, residents, or other trainees. The patient also has the right to know the immediate and long-term financial implications of treatment choices, insofar as they are known.

3. The patient has the right to make decisions about the plan of care prior to and during the course of treatment and to refuse a recommended treatment or plan of care to the extent permitted by law and hospital policy and to be informed of the medical consequences of this action. In case of such refusal, the patient is entitled to other appropriate care and services that the hospital provides or transfer to another hospital. The hospital should notify patients of any policy that might affect patient choice within the institution.

4. The patient has the right to have an advance directive (such as a living will, health care proxy, or durable power of attorney for health care) concerning treatment or to designate a surrogate decision maker, with the expectation that the hospital will honor the intent of that directive to the extent permitted by law and hospital policy.

   Health care institutions must advise patients of their rights under state law and hospital policy to make informed medical choices, ask if the patient has an advance directive, and include that information in patient records. The patient has the right to timely information about hospital policy that may limit its ability to implement fully a legally valid advance directive.

5. The patient has the right to every consideration of his or her privacy. Case discussion, consultation, examination, and treatment should be conducted so as to protect each patient's privacy.

6. The patient has the right to expect that all communications and records pertaining to his or her care should be treated as confidential by the hospital, except in cases such as suspected abuse and public health hazards when reporting is permitted or required by law. The patient has the right to expect that the hospital will emphasize the confidentiality of this information when it releases it to any other parties entitled to review information in these records.

7. The patient has the right to review the records pertaining to his or her medical care and to have the information explained or interpreted as necessary, except when restricted by law.

8. The patient has the right to expect that, within its capacity and policies, a hospital will make reasonable response to the request of a patient for appropriate and medically indicated care and services. The hospital must provide evaluation, service, and/or referral as indicated by the urgency of the case. When medically appropriate and legally permissible, or when a patient has so requested, a patient may be transferred to another facility. The institution to which the patient is to be transferred must first have accepted the patient for transfer. The patient must also have the benefit of complete information and explanation concerning the need for, risks, benefits, and alternatives to such a transfer.

9. The patient has the right to ask and be informed of the existence of business relationships among the hospital, educational institutions, other health care providers, or payers that may influence the patient's treatment and care.

10. The patient has the right to consent to or decline to participate in proposed research studies or human experimentation affecting his or her care and treatment or requiring direct patient involvement, and to have those studies fully explained prior to consent. A patient who declines to participate in research or experimentation is entitled to the most effective care that the hospital can otherwise provide.

11. The patient has the right to expect reasonable continuity of care when appropriate and to be informed by physicians and other caregivers of available and realistic patient care options when hospital care is no longer appropriate.

12. The patient has the right to be informed of hospital policies and practices that relate to patient care, treatment, and responsibilities. The patient has the right to be informed of available resources for resolving disputes, grievances, and conflicts, such as ethics committees, patient representatives, or other mechanisms available in the institution. The patient has the right to be informed of the hospital's charges for services and available payment methods.

Source: Excerpted from *A Patient's Bill of Rights*. Chicago: American Hospital Association, 1992.

125, 105 N.E. 92): "Every human being of adult years and sound mind has a right to determine what shall be done with his own body."[2]

Informed consent is the process by which fully informed patients can participate in choices about their health care. It originates from the legal and ethical right patients have to direct what happens to their body and from the ethical duty of the physician to involve patients in their health care.[3] In what is still considered the most important study of informed consent, the President's Commission concludes that "ethically valid consent is a process of shared decision making based upon mutual respect and participation, not a ritual to be equated with reciting the contents of a form that details the risks of particular treatments."[4] The most important goal of informed consent is that the patient has an opportunity to be an informed participant in his or her health care decisions.

The increasing number of malpractice suits that involve an element of informed consent highlights the patient's need for and right to this kind of knowledge. (Some lawyers are advocating the use of the term *authorization for treatment,* implying patient control.) For many years, in such suits, courts tended to rule that the physician must provide only as much information as is general practice among his colleagues in the area, as determined by their expert testimony. Later decisions, however, changed this attitude, most of them hinging on informed consent. The landmark decisions have involved situations in which the surgery was done effectively but patients sued because of complications or results about which they had not been warned. In one such case, *Canterbury v. Spence* (464 F.2d 772 D.C. Cir. 1972), a 19-year-old man became paralyzed following a laminectomy and a subsequent fall. The family sued because they were given only partial information without the options for alternative treatment and the risks of surgery were not disclosed. In another, *Butler v. South Fulton Medical Center* (452 S.E.2d 768—GA 1994), a patient was given a neurolytic block with phenol instead of the epidural injection listed on the consent form. He had not read the consent form. The court ruled that even if the patient is given legal and proper disclosure, he or she must understand what is said or written, so that the permission given is *voluntary.* In these and other cases, judges disallowed the right of the medical profession to determine how much the patient should be told, once called the *reasonable physician standard*; rather, they said, the patient should be told enough, in understandable lay language, to make a decision. The relative importance of the risk or facts to be disclosed by the physician is to be determined by applying the standards of a reasonable man, not a reasonable medical practitioner. This reasonable patient standard asks the question, "What would a reasonable person in similar circumstances need to know to make an informed decision?" The trend now is for the courts to view the doctor–patient relationship as a partnership in decision making.

Principles of Informed Consent

Consent is defined as a free, rational act that presupposes knowledge of the thing to which a person who is legally capable of consent gives consent. *Informed consent* is not expected to include minutiae but to delineate the essential nature of the procedure and the consequences. The disclosure is to be reasonable, without details that might unnecessarily frighten the patient. The patient may, of course, waive the right to such explanation, or any teaching, and that right should be honored. This does not affect his or her right to decide about the medical regimen. Consent is not needed for emergency care if there is an immediate threat to life and health, if experts agree that it is an emergency, if the patient is unable to consent and a legally authorized person cannot be reached, and when the patient submits voluntarily.

It is generally accepted that complete informed consent includes a discussion of the following elements:

1. The nature of the decision/procedure
2. Reasonable alternatives to the proposed intervention
3. The relevant risks, benefits, and uncertainties related to each alternative
4. Assessment of patient understanding
5. The acceptance of the intervention by the patient[5]

Consent must, of course, not be obtained fraudulently—for example, a patient being told that he is signing some other necessary paper. In addition, the patient should always be invited to ask questions and be free of coercion and unfair persuasions or inducements. The key is *voluntarism*—freedom of choice without duress.

The last statement has special significance, because the legal concept of informed consent really became viable with the Nuremberg Code, originating from the trials of Nazi physicians who were convicted of experimenting on prisoners without their consent. The principles were formalized in the Declaration of Helsinki, adopted by the

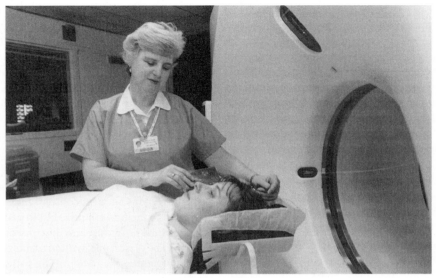

Ultimately it is the patient's right to choose whether or not to submit to diagnostic and therapeutic procedures. (Courtesy of the Valley Hospital, Ridgewood, New Jersey)

Eighteenth World Medical Assembly in 1964 and revised in 1975. Informed consent is *a process, not a form*. A consent form is a piece of physical evidence that the process took place and is evidence in case of a legal suit. However, one can have true informed consent without producing a form and a form without true informed consent, and as noted by the legal cases, a written consent does not necessarily protect the health care provider or institution if the patient maintains lack of understanding. Also, it does not protect the provider or health care agency against a malpractice suit if an error is made.

Informed Refusal

There is generally a presumption of decision-making capacity for the adult—without this consent is not valid. Refusal of the treatment or procedure does not imply that this capacity is limited. It may be that further clarification is necessary, as well as think time. Yet, when a patient consents, often the assumption is that the patient is competent, and if the patient refuses, he or she is incompetent.

There are various definitions of competency. If the court declares incompetency, perhaps because of advanced Alzheimer's disease, it is *de jure incompetency*. A person may also be considered incompetent without a court ruling—*de facto incompetency*.[6] Sometimes incompetency is transitional, owing to trauma, drugs, or environment.

Even in cases of the "confused" elderly, mentally retarded, or those committed involuntarily to a mental institution, it must still be decided as to what effect, if any, the patient's current mental/emotional status has on the ability to decide about treatment. Research suggests that the terms *decision-making capacity or incapacity* are better than *competency*. If decision-making capacity is compromised, resorting to the courts may be necessary for an adjudication of legal disability. The hospital administrator, an attorney, or a state ombudsman may be designated a *guardian ad litem* (just for the purpose of these decisions) to make medical decisions for the patient, presumably looking after his or her best interest. At other times, a proxy decision maker, often the spouse, children, parents, siblings or other family members, and occasionally a close friend, can give consent. This situation becomes more complex in the right-to-die situations discussed later. It also becomes a problem if those most closely involved disagree about what is to be done.

Children and young people are frequently considered unable to give informed consent, but there are a number of exceptions and changes emerging, also discussed later.

In cases involving the elderly, there are varied outcomes when their ability to consent is questioned (usually when they *do not* agree). Sometimes the elderly person gives in to the tears or anger of a child. There are also cases when that child wishes to be made guardian and decide, but the court determines that the person may be old but is perfectly able to make a health care decision and refuses guardianship.

Other refusals often relate to religious convictions. For example, a Jehovah's Witness may refuse a blood transfusion, even though it might be life saving, because taking such transfusions is against religious beliefs. The Witnesses and the American Medical Association (AMA) in 1979 agreed on a consent form requesting that no blood or blood derivative be administered and releasing medical personnel and the hospital for responsibility for untoward results because of that refusal. This particular problem has been lessened to some extent as better blood substitutes and bloodless surgery have become available.[7] However, a Jehovah's Witness sued a major medical center and five physicians because he was given blood after a serious automobile accident. Although he was unconscious and it was an emergency situation, he claimed his rights were violated. In other situations, if a minor child of a Witness needs the blood and the parent refuses, a court order requested by the hospital usually permits the transfusion. This is based on a 1944 legal precedent when the Supreme Court ruled that parents had a right to be martyrs, if they wished, but had no right to make martyrs of their children. Conversely, if the child is deemed a *mature minor* able to make an intelligent decision, regardless of chronological age, the child has been allowed to refuse the treatment.[8]

In another religion, Christian Science, the official doctrine, is opposed to medical diagnosis and treatment. Seeking medical care is in opposition to the religion. Such refusal quite often upsets health care personnel when, by chance, a Christian Scientist is brought to a health care facility, but it is an adult's choice. With children, it is a different matter. A well-publicized case was that of Robyn Twitchell, a 2-year-old girl who died because the prayers of the family and others, including a Christian Scientist nurse, did not correct a bowel obstruction, which could have been corrected surgically. This became a case of child neglect, and the parents were arrested (*Commonwealth v. Twitchell*, 416 Mass. 114 1993). There are similar cases, and according to the American Academy of Pediatrics (AAP), parents should not be allowed to refuse to accept medical intervention for a child—a position that some find difficult to reconcile with the features of a pluralistic society.[9]

Under any circumstance, refusal of treatment should be carefully and comprehensively documented (as should

consent). Moreover, health professionals must remember that the competent person has a legal and ethical right to refuse, and that right is firmly established.

The Nurse's Role in Informed Consent

What is the nurse's role in informed consent? To provide or add information before or after the doctor's explanation has been given? To refer the patient to the doctor? To avoid participation? The advice given varies. Some suggest that getting involved in informed consent is simply not a nurse's business and is best left to the doctor; others consider it an ethical responsibility.

It is generally agreed that nurses do not have the primary responsibility for getting informed consent; that is the physician's responsibility. However, the President's Commission noted that "nurses as a practical matter . . . typically have a central role in the process of providing the patients with information,"[10] and advanced practice nurses (APNs) are responsible for obtaining informed consent prior to performing any risky or invasive procedure that falls within their scope of practice. This includes informing patients about their conditions, tests, and treatment. Nurses at the bedside are responsible for explaining all nursing procedures to the patient. Consent is implied when the explanation has been given and the patient allows the nurse to begin nursing care. Procedures that are not invasive or risky do not require formally executed informed consent. Of course, "risky" or "invasive" needs to be defined. A nurse should never be delegated the work of obtaining an informed consent for the physician or someone else.[11] It has also been stated that any medical professional exercising his or her own professional judgment when treating a patient may have the duty to obtain consent from that patient. However, if a dependent practitioner who is subject to the independent professional, usually a doctor, APN, or nurse, performs a procedure ordered by that other, it is not his or her responsibility to get consent. This principle may also apply to a registered nurse (RN) (not considered a dependent practitioner) who carries out a complex procedure ordered by a physician. But that nurse should be sure that the consent is informed. There have been cases when both doctor and nurse were sued because the patient claimed that information about a procedure was withheld. Nevertheless, the question asked by most nurses is how much can be told, especially if the physician chooses not to reveal further information. The American Nurses Association (ANA) has stated that the nurse has a responsibility to facilitate informed decision making. Perhaps both patient and family are frightened, confused, and overwhelmed by the barrage of information from the physician, and they simply are not clear about the how, what, where, and when of the proposed procedure. If the doctor does not follow through, inviting questions, the nurse may do so. Lack of clarity can be determined, in part, by asking the patient and/or family if there are any questions or by asking them to repeat what the doctor said. They should also have enough time to think about the situation, and, if practical, be given clearly written information, not in legalese or medical language. (If the person does not speak or understand English, or is a deaf mute, a capable interpreter is required by law.) Often this follow-up is best pursued by the nurse, with whom the patient and family may be more comfortable.

Sometimes a knowledgeable nurse can answer some of the questions or clarify points; however, if questions remain, the nurse should inform the physician about the confusion. He or she should be grateful and follow through, but if not, the nurse must go through the chain of authority to report that the patient is not giving an informed consent—a legal danger for all if the procedure is done anyhow. At any rate, the patient and family should always be reassured of their right to a full, lucid explanation. If the patient withdraws consent, even verbally, the nurse is responsible for reporting this and ensuring that the patient is not treated. This is a legal responsibility not only to the patient, but also to the hospital, which, again, can be held liable. Such was the case in *Issac v. Jameson Memorial Hospital* (59 PaD&C 4th 375, 2002). The patient verbally withdrew her informed consent for sterilization to the nurse, who neglected to inform the physician. The court held the hospital liable for negligence under respondeat superior, not the physician who performed the procedure.

The patients' questions may range over a variety of topics, from what you are doing to the patient and your qualifications (which you should answer honestly) to interpreting what the doctor said (explain in lay terms) to, "What's wrong with me?" (which you should not answer directly) or, "Is my doctor any good?" (tell the patient that he or she has a right to ask the doctor for his or her qualifications and experience or to get a second opinion). The nurse's specific responsibility is to explain nursing care, including the whys and hows. An interesting idea to contemplate is whether you should tell patients about the risks of nursing procedures you do, even though this is not a legal requirement. (Nor does it prevent you from doing so.) The answer seems to be—maybe, but carefully.

It has been suggested that the nurse's role in informed consent is threefold: to perform a patient assessment to evaluate the patient's readiness to understand and respond intelligently to the consent form; to determine the best approach to obtain informed consent (time, environment, presence of a supportive person); and patient and staff follow-up (reaffirmation that the patient understood), supporting the patient's decision, reinforcement of information, and apprising staff and physician of the patient's understanding.

Hospitals are beginning to use a clerk to witness the consent form, after the physician provides an explanation, on the theory that only the signature is being witnessed, not the accuracy or depth of the explanation. Other hospitals ask the physician to bring another physician, presumably to validate the explanation. Where nurses witness the form, it should be made clear what they are witnessing—the signature or the explanation. Hospital policy can clarify this.

Is Informed Consent Practical?

Some physicians do not believe that it is feasible to obtain an informed consent because of such factors as lack of interest or education and high anxiety level, in which case a patient might refuse a necessary treatment or operation. The physician may decide to invoke *therapeutic privilege*, in which disclosure is not required because it might be detrimental to the patient.

The circumstances in which evoking therapeutic privilege can be justified are very rare—on the order of once or twice in a career. Most times, when physicians plead that full disclosure (and hence truly informed consent) would be too distressing, it is evidence of an old-fashioned (i.e., pre–Civil Rights era) notion that patients' rights are relatively less important than physicians' responsibility to do good.

Most often, failures of informed consent seem to be a communicating function of physicians who simply are not good at talking or not inclined to take time to talk with patients or family members. As is true of nurses, those physicians who enjoy or otherwise derive rewards from genuine personal interaction at an intimate level are those who will be the most effective teachers, counselors, and advocates for their patients.

Although the President's Commission avoided recommending legal alternatives, the members came out in unequivocal support of shared decision making and full disclosure to patients except in unusual circumstances. Their surveys (like others before) indicated that people do want full information even when they trust their doctor completely and will probably go along with the physician's recommendations. They may not always remember the details later, but with a full explanation given in lay terms, and with enough time for questions and answers, they can understand. However, many patients are still reluctant to ask for fear of appearing stupid or bothering the doctor.

The written consent form that is generally accepted as the legal affirmation that the patient has agreed to a particular test or treatment has undergone a number of changes in the last few years. The patient rights movement has motivated hospitals, especially, to review and revise their consent forms. The catchall admissions consent has already been ruled as legally inadequate for anything other than avoiding battery complaints, because it does not designate the nature of the treatment to be given. What have emerged are forms that contain all the required elements for the informed consent process, usually individualized by the physician for each patient. Often they are available in the foreign languages most prevalent in the area. One of the key points is having a form that avoids unnecessary technical terms or compound–complex sentences.

Communications specialists who have developed and tested such forms conclude that, although a comprehensible form will not guarantee adequate communication between patient and provider, it is at least an indication of good faith on the provider's part and an effort to help the patient understand.

The emphasis on the entire topic of informed consent has focused on the hospital. In current health care, more and more treatments, including surgery, are being done on an outpatient basis, including in clinics and doctors' offices. If anything, with fewer practitioners around, the temptation toward shortcuts in explanations could be great. On the other hand, the staff may know the patient better and handle explanations more adroitly. Regardless, the ethical and legal principles remain.

■ THE RIGHT TO DIE

Because of new technology that can keep a patient's heart beating and lungs breathing, people who once would have been considered dead because those organs no longer functioned can be kept alive. Whether or not the brain is functioning is another question. To some, this new technology was a miracle that saved lives; to others it was a nightmare that kept a body "alive," when in another sense it was really dead. Ordinary people, often older people, dreaded the thought of having their bodies kept alive in this manner and sought ways to have some control of their dying in this new age. Scientists sought ways to identify

and define death that would take into consideration what technology could do.

Consequently, in the United States, there are three definitions of death from a theoretical perspective. The traditional *heart–lung definition* that has been a standard for centuries is the "irreversible cessation" of spontaneous respiration and circulation. This was the generally accepted criterion until the 1960s. In 1968, an Ad Hoc Committee of the Harvard Medical School defined *brain death*, which caused considerable scientific, philosophical, ethical, and sometimes legal discussion—among other things, what qualities were necessary to be alive and human. In 1980, the President's Commission for the Study of Ethical Problems in Medicine and Biomedical and Behavioral Research drafted the *United States Uniform Determination of Death Act*, which permitted brain death to become part of the legal standard. *Brain death* was defined by the Commission as "the irreversible cessation of all functions of the entire brain, including the brain stem." In 1981, the operational definition and criteria needed to determine brain death were added.[12]

Unfortunately, the term *brain death* has perpetuated the mistaken notion that there are two kinds of death—brain death and real death. The more accurate term, and the one less likely to confuse both professionals and the general public, is *death as determined by neurologic criteria*. Such semantic precision is important.

The determination of death by neurologic criteria is a common diagnosis in specialized units, particularly trauma centers. Staff recognize that the diagnosis, although painstaking and time-consuming, is rarely difficult. They speak to family members in terms of death as they continue to test for signs of brain stem responsiveness. Finally, when they are convinced that death has occurred, they turn off the ventilator rather than asking family permission to do so. This also allows transplant teams to procure organs (with permission). In summary, all 50 states and the District of Columbia have adopted brain death as determined by neurological criteria to be the a legal definition of death. If brain death is diagnosed in an individual, there is no legal duty to provide continuing treatment because that person is clinically dead.[13]

Still, to some, this *whole-brain* definition causes problems because of the continued physiologic functioning of the body. Looking further, a group of ethicists feels that this definition of death is too limited and have proposed using *higher-brain death* as a better definition of death: irreversible loss of all higher brain functions, that is, the cognitive function. This would include the individual's personality, conscious life, uniqueness, and capacity for remembering, judging, reasoning, acting, enjoying, and so on—all activities requiring cerebral functioning. Naturally, there is disagreement about this concept, which would include those patients in a persistent vegetative state (PVS). Even in whole brain death, there have been objections by religious and conservative groups. Both New York and New Jersey have enacted statutes recognizing this. In New Jersey, physicians are prohibited from declaring brain death in persons who have some firm religious traditions not accepting this concept. Another proposal is the *bounded zone* definition of death, with the cardiopulmonary standard as the lower bound and neurologic dysfunction, including PVS, as the higher bound, and allowing individuals to choose their definition (presumably before death). However, that presents other problems.[14]

The popular label of *right to die* has been applied to a long series of famous court cases in which patients and, more often, their surrogates have fought to have life-sustaining treatment discontinued. The label is misleading because, strictly speaking, there is no right to die. The rights to which these patients and their families have actually appealed are either (1) the right to freedom from undue state interference, often called the right to privacy, or (2) the right to self-determination. The first of these rights involves an appeal to constitutional guarantees. The second is based on our long tradition of common law.

At one time, most of the right-to-die cases were heard exclusively in state courts because they did not entail legal questions appropriate to federal judicial review. Thus, it is not surprising that different states have evolved different standards. A review of selected landmark cases will illustrate the point.

In the Saikewicz case (*Superintendent of Belcherton State School v. Saikewicz*, 370 N.E. 2d. 417 1977), the high court in Massachusetts upheld a decision not to give a severely retarded 67-year-old man more chemotherapy than would be unpleasant for the sake of a short extended lifespan. (He died a month later of pneumonia.) The court ruled that such decisions on behalf of incompetent patients should be made only with explicit permission of the courts. A very different procedure was established by the New Jersey Supreme Court in the *Quinlan* case (In re *Quinlan*, 70 N.J. 10, 355 A.2d 647 NJ 1976). In this case, a 22-year-old woman received severe and irreversible brain damage that reduced her to a PVS. Her father petitioned the court to be made her guardian with the intention of having all extraordinary medical procedures sustaining her life removed. The court ruled that the father could be the guardian and have the life support systems discontinued with the concurrence of her family; the attending physicians, who might be chosen by the father; and the hospital ethics committee. After disconnection of the respirator, Karen Quinlan continued to live another 10 years, sustained by fluids and other maintenance measures, in a nursing home. In a long series of subsequent cases the New Jersey Supreme Court held to its initial stance that such decisions belong in the traditional control of family and primary caregivers. However, courts in some other jurisdictions have continued to insist on a role for judicial review.

One might suppose that nonemergency cases involving competent patients would be clearer. In such cases, there can be no question about whether the elements of informed consent have been satisfied. When someone wants to discontinue kidney dialysis today because the quality of life is unacceptable, there is relatively little objection. That may be because the patient is ambulatory and may simply choose not to come back for treatment.

Other cases are not so simple, and legal processes can take a long time. The Paul Brophy case in Massachusetts is an example (*Brophy v. New England Sinai Hospital*, 497 N.E.2d 626 Mass 1986). It took 2 years and the refusal of the US Supreme Court to review the case (which would have taken even longer) before, after many contrary rulings, his wife, who was a nurse, could have him transferred to a hospital that was willing to do what he wished—remove his feeding tube. He died 8 days later, kept comfortable but not fed and cared for by his wife.

People like Mrs. Brophy and the parents of Karen Ann Quinlan, although motivated by the plight of their own family member, have gone on to do a service for the entire community. These cases are called *landmark* because the decisions had implications far beyond the persons whose names they bear.

In the 1980s, as health care institutions and the courts were struggling with a number of *right-to-die* situations, which so often were taken to the courts for resolution, there were a variety of decisions, and they were infrequently consistent from state to state. Sometimes the decision was made to allow withdrawal of food and fluids or respiratory support, sometimes not. Courts did or did not feel that families or surrogates provided enough evidence that their request would have been the patient's. A particular problem still occurs when families disagree, as in the *Martin* (In re *Martin*, 538 N.W. 2d 399 Mich.1995) case where the Michigan Supreme Court, in 1995, chose to side with the patient's mother and sister and to reject the request of his wife, who was also his legal guardian, who requested withdrawal of Mr. Martin's gastrostomy tube. This despite the fact that two lower courts and the hospital ethics committee found "clear and convincing evidence" that the patient would refuse treatment in his current situation. Sometimes it seems that personal values affect a judge as much as evidence or points of law.

Why *clear and convincing evidence*? It was inevitable that, given the controversy on these issues and the fact that there may be several hundred thousand PVS patients, a case would eventually reach the US Supreme Court, probably as a privacy (Fourth Amendment) issue. The first right-to-die case to go before the court was that of Nancy Cruzan (*Cruzan v. Director of Missouri Department of Health*, 497 U.S. 261 [1990] 497 U.S. 261), a 32-year-old woman who was injured in an auto accident in 1983 and was eventually determined to be in a PVS. In 1988, her case was the first in Missouri to raise the question of whether feeding tubes can be equated with other life-sustaining medical treatments, and whether patients in Nancy's condition have any rights regarding their care. The parents, stating that this would have been Nancy's wish, wanted to have the implanted gastrointestinal tube removed. A probate judge ruled that they could remove the tube, but this was overruled by the Missouri Supreme Court, which relied on a Missouri statute requiring clear and convincing evidence of a patient's prior wish that life support be removed.

The US Supreme Court's decision in *Cruzan* is complex. The court upheld the general concept, implied or asserted in so many cases from Quinlan onward, that there is a constitutional right to refuse life-sustaining treatment. Moreover, the court ruled that artificially delivered nutrition and hydration are not legally distinct from other kinds of medical intervention and thus may be withheld or withdrawn in the same way as other treatment. Finally, the court upheld the right of the Missouri legislature to insist on clear and convincing evidence of prior wishes. Although clearly not requiring other states to adopt such a strict standard, the court ruled that Missouri's statute does not violate the US Constitution. (Only New York and Missouri have laws insisting on clear and convincing evidence, a test difficult to meet by any means short of a *living will*.) Eventually, the family came up with enough clear and convincing evidence to satisfy the Missouri legal system, and Nancy was allowed to die.

There were two other interesting cases post-*Cruzan* that tested the Supreme Court decision. In the matter of Sue Ann Lawrence (In re *Lawrence*, Indiana Supreme Court, No. 29504-9106-CV-00460 1991), the Indiana Supreme Court upheld the parents' request to consent to removal of artificial food and fluid from their 42-year-old daughter. An accident when she was 7 had left her mentally retarded; a second injury and surgery had left her in a PVS. This case is interesting because Indiana had no prior right-to-die case law and the case dealt with proxy/surrogate decision making as opposed to the use of an advance directive. *Cruzan* was never mentioned. This case supports the substituted judgment rationale, because certainly the Lawrence family only considered the best interest of their never-competent daughter.

The other case shows that, because the Supreme Court allowed states to set their own standards on removal of death-delaying medical treatments, a *patchwork* effect may occur. Mr. Busalacchi (In re *Busalacchi*, No. 59582, 1991 WL 26851, 1991 Mo. App. LEXIS 315) had been appointed guardian of his daughter, Christine, who had been in a serious accident in California. PVS was diagnosed and a gastrostomy tube implanted. (In a PVS, the patient is unaware of self or surroundings. There is no voluntary movement, emotion, or cognition. Some patients cough or gag, or their eyes move. They seem to have periods of sleeping or waking.) Placement in a skilled nursing facility was recommended, but Mr. Busalacchi could not find a place for her in California or in Missouri, where he resided. When he found a place in Minnesota, the governmental agency changed Christine's diagnosis to something less severe than PVS and filed legal papers to prevent the transfer, maintaining that Mr. Busalacchi only wanted to move her to a place where the gastrostomy tube could be removed legally. After numerous appeals (and expenses) back and forth from the Missouri Supreme Court, the Court finally dismissed the case. Then a right-to-life advocate, with no connection to Christine, filed for a temporary restraining order, which was granted. In 1993, 6 years after the accident that left her in a PVS, her tube was removed and she died.

Many of these cases revolve around the issue of *medical futility*, generally a medical determination, but not one without its critics. There is not always a clear definition. Clinicians may focus on *quantitative* or *physiologic futility*, which says that because an intervention has failed many times, using it will be futile. *Qualitative futility* means that an "intervention only sustains unconsciousness or doesn't end a patient's total dependence on intensive medical care," and it may be assumed that the patient would not want such treatment. The issues include whether this should be purely a medical decision or whether community standards should be taken into consideration. For instance, families may simply not understand or accept such a definition because their values are different. Some have gone to court when advised by a physician that aggressive care is futile, stating that the physician or institution did not think that their loved one deserved the care being given. Patient care conferences and considerate explanations may help here. Needless to say, court decisions have had an impact, as has the media, which have been providing more information on the topic of futility acceptance.

Even when the concept of medical futility is accepted by all concerned, the actual removal of life-sustaining devices is always difficult for a patient's significant others—families or close friends. In some ways, removal of respiratory assistance devices is more easily accepted, because this is clearly an artificial aid to breathing. An enduring problem still seems to be discontinuing artificial nutrition and hydration, usually given by a gastrostomy tube. The idea of allowing a loved one to die of thirst or starvation, as pro-life groups often describe it, is naturally repugnant to families. Although there is little evidence that a patient in a PVS has such sensations, the pressure on the family and caregivers can be great, particularly because they are not sure that removal of the tube is either ethical or legal. However, there have been a number of court decisions on this issue, and it is legal. A case in point is the story of Emilio Gonzales (*Gonzales v. Seton Family of Hospitals*, No. A07CA267 W.D. Tex. Apr. 4, 2007), an 18-month-old boy with a progressive and fatal neurometabolic disorder. National attention was focused on his mother's struggle to prevent the Children's Hospital of Austin from withdrawing life support from the child. Emilio had been on life support in the intensive care unit for 5 months. The hospital had invoked the Texas Advance Directives Act, which authorized it to withdraw life support if an ethics committee determined that further life support was medically futile and providing that the hospital gave the family 10 days' notice, and attempted to transfer Emilio to an alternative facility. This is one such futility law in the United States, the other being in Virginia.[15] With the support of lawyers and a coalition of advocacy groups, Ms. Gonzales had successfully obtained extensions of the deadline, but Emilio died before the judge issued a final ruling on the case.

The Gonzales case is the most recent in a series of famous "futility" cases. All are stories about families insisting on the continued use of life-sustaining treatments that are considered to be medically inappropriate. Many of these cases are the product of a severe breakdown of trust in the relationship between the clinicians and the patient's family. Even in the best circumstances, providers may communicate poorly, and this deficiency is exacerbated when the communication must occur across the gaps created by language, class, and culture. Improvement of communication and conflict-resolution skills would no doubt go a long way toward preventing such cases from occurring.[16]

The ANA issued a position statement on "Foregoing Nutrition and Hydration" in 1992. It states, "The decision to withhold artificial nutrition and hydration should be made by the patient or surrogate with the health care team. The nurse continues to provide expert care to patients who are no longer receiving artificial nutrition and hydration."[17] This stance is in essential agreement with that of the AMA and the Hastings Center's "Guidelines on the Termination of Life-Sustaining Treatment."

Advance Directives

Advance directives is the generic name embracing both instruction directives (living wills) and proxy directives (medical power of attorney, appointment of someone to act when the directive maker is incapacitated). Living wills are written documents or statements by competent persons setting forth how they wish to be cared for at the end of their lives. The beginning statement of a living will generally says that the maker is emotionally and mentally competent and that he or she directs the physician and other health care providers, family, friends, and any surrogate appointed by him or her to carry out the stated wishes if the maker is unable to do so. The intent is to withhold life-sustaining treatment if there is no reasonable expectation of recovery from a seriously incapacitating or fatal condition. The directive also has space for specific directions about treatments the individual may refuse, such as electrical or mechanical resuscitation of the individual's heart when it has stopped beating; nasogastric tube feedings when the individual is paralyzed or unable to take nourishment by mouth; and mechanical respiration if the individual is no longer able to sustain his or her own breathing. If such a list is already present in the document, the person is directed to cross out all that do not reflect his or her wishes or to add others. Two witnesses sign the document; sometimes it must be notarized. Of course, the maker can withdraw the living will at any time, but otherwise it stands as a clear indication of the person's wishes.

In 1977, California enacted a *Natural Death Act*, the first legal state living will. The next year, Arkansas, Idaho, Nevada, New Mexico, North Carolina, Oregon, and Texas followed with similar statutes. By 1990, at the time of the Supreme Court decision in the Cruzan case, 41 states and the District of Columbia had enacted such laws and others were being debated. All granted civil and criminal immunity for those carrying out living will requests. All states now have such laws.

In 1984, California enacted a law entitled the *Durable Power of Attorney for Health Care*, which was the first of its kind. This law allowed terminally ill patients to designate another individual to make life-or-death decisions in the event that the patient was unable to do so. The agreement conveys the authority to consent, refuse, or withdraw consent to any care, treatment, service, or procedure to maintain, diagnose, or treat a mental or physical condition. Like living wills, durable power of attorney provisions are now recognized throughout the United States. They are also known as *proxy directives*, and the person who has been designated may variously be known as the *proxy*, the *health care representative*, or the *person with durable power of attorney for health care*. Some forms include designation of an alternate surrogate, "should my surrogate be unwilling or unable to act in my behalf." The document must also be witnessed. Sometimes both components, will and proxy, are combined in one document.

Although probably a generic living will, that is, not the official state document, would be seen as a clear indication of a person's intent, legally the forms specific to the particular state in which the individual lives should be used. These can be obtained from Caring Connections at

http://www.caringinfo.org/index.cfm?

Federal law now requires all health care institutions receiving Medicare or Medicaid reimbursement to maintain policies and procedures regarding advance directives. The *Patient Self-Determination Act* of 1989 (PSDA) applies to hospitals, nursing homes, hospices, and home health agencies. It further requires that each newly enrolled patient be asked whether he or she has an advance directive. If the answer is *yes*, a copy is to be placed in the patient record. If the answer is *no*, the patient must be offered information about the right to execute such a document. The PSDA also requires institutions to provide education on advance directives both to staff and to the community.

Much has been written about both advance directives in general and the PSDA. Both are intended to protect the right to self-determination for people while they are still able to make such decisions. Yet, even if people know about advance directives and approve of the concept, few people ever execute one. The major reasons seemed to be lack of prior discussion with their provider; lack of understanding of an advance directive; lack of understanding of their condition and prognosis; and incongruence with personal beliefs. It is recommended that nurses, physicians, and social workers educate patients about the need for advance directives. One study confirmed that even a simple educational intervention significantly increased the completion of forms for durable powers of attorney, yet experts still claim that only 20 to 30 percent of adults have executed advance directives. Surprisingly, even in a hospice, only 35 percent of the patients had an advance directive.[18] Many choosing not to issue one claimed to know all about them. The ANA, supporting patient self-determination in its position statement on the topic, states that it is the responsibility of nurses to facilitate decision making for patients making choices about end-of-life care, which could imply teaching about the advance directives. Going over the advance directive with a person can be helpful because there is some evidence that most advance directives, especially the state documents, are difficult to understand; therefore, a person either cannot complete it or leaves major omissions, usually specifics. In part, this may be because the situations mentioned in the advance directive are only those the person thought of or knew about at the time. Therefore, when an unlisted option comes up, the health care professional cannot interpret the person's wishes, and the proxy decision maker may make a choice according to his or her own values.

The congruence of decisions between surrogate and patient varies, sometimes being quite diverse, if the two have not discussed the advance directive thoroughly. For instance, in one study, although the two, when asked separately, agreed on most matters as to what the patient would want, in one exception, the surrogates were much more likely to choose chemotherapy for cancer when the patient would have them refuse. Other barriers include the fact that patients may verbally change their minds about something in the advance directive, but not change the document. If this happens in the hospital, it should be recorded. Also, there are misconceptions by some ethnic groups who fear that advance directives are vehicles for discrimination, whereas cultural beliefs by others may preclude addressing end-of-life decisions.[19] It should also be remembered that the PSDA requires hospitals to verify whether a new admission has an advance directive, and if not, to provide information. Quite often, though, the admissions clerk, who is not very knowledgeable about advance directives, brushes over this requirement and sometimes gives false information. Nurses on the unit should always follow through, attaching the advance directive as soon as possible and flagging the chart in whatever way hospital policy requires, so that everyone is aware of its presence. From another perspective, an "old" advance directive may raise questions on the part of both the proxy and the medical staff. Would different directives have been executed if the patient had more current information about treatment?

Do all these precautions assure that a patient's advance directive is honored? Unfortunately not. Although the vast majority of the public indicates that they want their end-of-life decisions obeyed, there is some evidence that these are overridden about 25 percent of the time. Family preferences are often a decisive influence, and frequently, the advance directive has not been discussed with the doctor. The media have reported on many examples, usually the most disturbing, and indeed there have been a number of lawsuits against the medical community for ignoring right-to-die requests.

When an individual has no living will and has not designated a specific surrogate, physicians have traditionally consulted the "next of kin" or close friends. With increased litigation, they are becoming more reluctant to use such an informal process. Currently over 39 states and the District of Columbia have passed laws that establish a prioritized list of surrogate decision makers with authority to make medical decisions for patients who cannot make such decisions for themselves and did not or could not record their treatment preferences in advance. In all but six of these states, statutes give priority to the spouse as decision maker for an incapacitated person. If the surrogate does not know what the patient would have wanted, the surrogate must base his or her decision on what, in the surrogate's judgment is in the patient's best interest.[20]

Where patients are invited to execute advance directives unexpectedly, such as on admission to a hospital, they may be tense and only hearing part of your message. You could postpone the living will, but encourage the designation of a health care proxy/surrogate. Try to get some sense of how objective and knowledgeable of the patient's preferences this person is. Further, if this person is not a family member, how acceptable will he or she be to the family?

It is important that nurses are knowledgeable about advance directives, hospital policy, and state law. On the whole, nurses who are thus aware and knowledgeable feel empowered in their roles as patient advocates. For example, the laws of many states require that a physician who will not or cannot in good conscience honor an advance directive withdraw from the case. Nurses who know this feature of the law can break, and often have broken, a decisional stalemate by simply reminding the physician or the proxy of this legal requirement. However, nurses must also come to terms with their own moral and ethical beliefs. If these conflict with a patient's wishes, the nurse too can ask to be removed from that assignment, as long as the patient is not hurt.

Of Principles and Practice

In what is probably the most comprehensive part of their 1983 report, *Deciding to Forgo Life-Sustaining Treatment*, the President's Commission supported the patient's right to refuse treatment and the right of the family of an incapacitated patient to make that decision with the physician. (The data presented are unusually detailed.) The next year, a group of experienced physicians from various disciplines and institutions came to the conclusion that in relation to these issues, "the patient's role in decision making is paramount, and a decrease in aggressive treatment when such treatment would only prolong a difficult and uncomfortable process of dying" is acceptable.[21] In summary, several important points were made. In dealing with a competent patient, the treatment should "reflect an understanding between patient and physician and should be reassessed from time to time." Patients who are determined to be brain dead require no treatment. With patients in a PVS, "it is morally justifiable to withhold antibiotics and artificial nutrition and hydration, as well as other forms of life-sustaining treatment, allowing the patient to die. (This requires family agreement and an attempt to ascertain what would have been the patient's wishes.)" Severely demented and irreversibly demented patients only need care to make them comfortable. It is ethically appropriate not to treat intercurrent illness. Again, the patient's previous desires and the family's wishes must be considered. With elderly patients who have permanent mild impairment of competence—the "pleasantly senile"—emergency resuscitation and intensive care should be provided "sparingly." Yet, with all the professional pronouncements and the legal right for a person to refuse treatment, why the demand by much of the public for professionally assisted suicide?

Professionally Assisted Suicide

On both the ethical and the legal fronts, the most current right-to-die issue is physician-assisted suicide, sometimes called professionally assisted suicide (PAS). This subject has been under discussion for some time and is usually brought into open debate after highly publicized PASs. One created considerable discussion in the health care community in 1988 after the physician involved wrote about it anonymously in *JAMA*. In New York State, Dr. Timothy Quill had cared for a young woman with terminal ovarian cancer for some time. When she asked, he gave her a large dose of morphine that enabled her to die peacefully. A grand jury refused to indict him and, indeed, many praised him. In fact, he is still practicing, with his patients fully understanding his philosophy. He says, "A physician's aid in dying should be legal, but a rare step." He was a major figure in a 1997 Supreme Court case, discussed later.[22] More dramatic was Dr. Jack Kevorkian, who campaigned for the right for physicians to aid people who wanted to die because their illness made life unbearable to them. He designed a device that allowed patients to kill themselves painlessly, while he and/or their significant others attended them. He did this openly with a great deal of publicity. He was prosecuted a number of times, but juries came back with a not guilty verdict each time. By mid-1998, he had assisted 120 people to die. However, in late 1998, he actually gave a fatal injection (at the request of the person) and allowed this to be seen on national television. He said that he was inviting prosecution for murder as a test and was indeed indicted in Michigan. In April 1999, retired pathologist Dr. Jack Kevorkian was sentenced in Michigan to two terms of imprisonment for helping a man suffering from amyotrophic lateral sclerosis or Lou Gehrig's disease (ALS) to die. For the second-degree murder of Thomas Youk he received a sentence of 10 to 25 years, and for using a controlled substance (lethal drug) he was given 3 to 7 years in jail, the sentences to run concurrently.

Earlier, the Hemlock Society, which advocates euthanasia (as desired by an ill person), published a how-to-do-it book that became a bestseller. At the same time, newspapers and popular magazines carried stories by prominent and anonymous individuals who had helped a loved one to die one way or another (or killed the person, depending on your point of view). Some were prosecuted on criminal charges. Some were freed; others served prison sentences based on individual circumstances, such as whether the victim had asked for help in dying. Except for Kevorkian, no physician has ever been prosecuted for assisting a patient to commit suicide, but such actions have seldom been publicized. The debate continues (see Exhibit 22–2).

How frequently does euthanasia or assisted suicide occur? Passive euthanasia is said to be the norm in US hospitals. According to the AHA, about 70 percent of the deaths in hospitals occur after a decision has been made to withhold treatment. Other patients die when medications they are given to ease their pain stop their breathing. There are fewer data concerning deaths in nursing homes

---

■ **EXHIBIT 22–2. A Definition of Terms to Explain Euthanasia**

1. **Euthanasia (good death)**—Those acts that have the specific goal of ending another's life
2. **Passive euthanasia**—Decision to cease or not start treatment in the case of (probably) dying patients
3. **Voluntary active euthanasia**—Intentional administration of medications or other interventions to cause the patient's death at the patient's explicit request and with full informed consent
4. **Involuntary active euthanasia**—Intentional administration of medications or other interventions to cause the patient's death when the patient is competent but without the patient's explicit request and informed consent
5. **Nonvoluntary active euthanasia**—Intentional administration of medications or other interventions to cause the patient's death when the patient is incompetent and mentally incapable of explicitly requesting it
6. **Indirect euthanasia**—Administration of narcotics or other medications to relieve pain, with the incidental consequence of the possibility of causing respiratory depression, which might result in the patient's death; also called *double effect*
7. **Professionally or physician-assisted suicide**—A physician or health professional supplies a person with the means of committing suicide

or at home, but patients are often sent home with a self-regulated morphine drip for pain or to prevent overzealous care. For instance, an old, fragile man is sent home with the understanding that he will not return to the hospital in case of a fever. This is what most would prefer.[23]

Several surveys have documented that nurses receive requests for aid in dying. Asch reported that approximately 17 percent of the 852 critical care nurses who responded to an anonymous, mailed survey said that they had received requests from patients or family members to perform euthanasia or assist in suicide.[24] Matzo mailed anonymous surveys to a random sample of 600 RNs who were Oncology Nursing Society members. Thirty percent of the 441 respondents (75 percent response rate) reported that they had received at least one request for assisted suicide and 25 percent indicated that they had received at least one request for euthanasia.[25] In Oregon, approximately 40 percent of hospice nurses responding to a questionnaire stated that since November 1997, when the Death with Dignity Act went into effect, they had cared for a patient who had explicitly requested assisted suicide.[26] Ferrell et al. received 2333 responses to an anonymous survey that was completed by a random sample predominantly comprised of oncology nurses. They reported that most respondents opposed the legalization of assisted suicide (70 percent opposed) and euthanasia (77 percent opposed). Since becoming a nurse, 20 percent had received one or more requests to assist patients in obtaining a prescription to end their lives, and 22 percent had received requests from patients to administer a lethal injection to end their life.[27] Only some of the more recent studies are mentioned here, and the reader is referred to the ninth edition of this book for a more inclusive summary.

These studies highlight important issues. First, nurses are witness to tremendous suffering; they must be supported and educated in the ways to ameliorate suffering. They must also explore and identify their own responses to this suffering and practice self-care. If nurses do not identify their own distress, they will be unlikely to assess accurately those whose suffering is being addressed through assistance in dying.

Physicians face the same dilemma, and their positions are discussed in the medical and related literature, as well as the public media. There were reports that many receive requests from patients for aid in dying, and a certain percentage complies. Anywhere from a quarter to half of doctors in other surveys say that they would be willing to prescribe a lethal dose of medication, if it were legal.

Some insist that the number of PASs is exaggerated and, at any rate, the AMA, like the ANA, officially opposes PAS.[28]

Legalizing assisted suicide has been an issue in a number of state court cases and in the US Supreme Court. Two cases, *Washington v. Glucksberg* (1977) and *Vacco v. Quill* (1997), advanced to the Supreme Court. On June 26, 1997, the Supreme Court ruled that there is no constitutional right to assisted suicide. This spoke to assisted suicide at the federal level, but left the door open for a later look at the issue through state courts, state legislatures, and referenda.

The other result of the Supreme Court decision was that because "state's rights" were upheld, Oregon, whose voters had supported a Death with Dignity Act and refused to overturn it by a 60 percent margin, could proceed with implementing the PAS law. Basically, the law allowed doctors to prescribe drugs that a person might *self-administer* (a requirement) to end life. The patient must be a resident of Oregon, be competent, have a life expectancy of less than 6 months, and make a formal request. Physicians are not required to participate in PAS, nor are they required to refer the patient to another doctor who will. There were also a number of other restrictions to protect the public.[29]

The Oregon law survived other challenges. Acting on a request from two Republican Congressmen, the Federal Drug Enforcement Agency (FDEA) warned that physicians prescribing drugs, with the intent of aiding the terminally ill to die, could face serious sanctions. However, by June 1998, the US Attorney General ruled that these physicians would not be prosecuted. In addition, the state panel running Oregon's health plan agreed to spend tax money to pay for PAS. Despite the fear that people would rush to Oregon to get help to die, this did not happen. In the spring of 2002, the US Attorney General claimed the authority to punish physicians in Oregon who were writing lethal prescriptions. A federal judge ruled that he had overstepped his authority,[30] but the battle is far from over.

Oregon reported 460 assisted suicides between 1997, when the Death With Dignity Act (DWDA) became legal, and 2009. During 2009, 95 prescriptions for lethal medications were written under the provisions of the DWDA. Of these, 53 patients took the medications, 30 died of their underlying illness, and 12 were alive at the end of 2009. In addition, six patients with earlier prescriptions died from taking the medications, resulting in a total of 59 DWDA deaths during 2009. As in prior years, most participants were between 55 and 84 years of age (78.0 percent), white

(98.3 percent), well educated (48.3 percent had at least a baccalaureate degree), and had cancer (79.7 percent). Most patients died at home (98.3 percent), and most were enrolled in hospice care (91.5 percent) at the time of death. Compared to previous years, the number of patients who had private insurance (84.7 percent) was much greater than in previous years (66.8 percent), and the number of patients who had only Medicare or Medicaid insurance was much less (13.6 percent compared to 32.0 percent). As in previous years, the most frequently mentioned end-of-life concerns were loss of autonomy (96.6 percent), loss of dignity (91.5 percent), and decreasing ability to participate in activities that made life enjoyable (86.4 percent). Prescribing physicians were present at the time of ingestion for three (5.1 percent) patients compared to 22.6 percent in previous years. There was another provider in attendance in over 80 percent of cases at ingestion and at the time of death.[31]

In 2008, Washington and Montana became the second and third states to adopt a Death With Dignity Act or such provisions through court decisions.[32] Whether others will follow suit remains to be seen. There are still those who feel that such a law has a slippery slope aspect, and that it will begin to include those not ready or willing to die.

The Netherlands was the first country in the world to legalize euthanasia and PAS. The Dutch legislation allows doctors to euthanize patients with terminal disease who are suffering "unbearably" if they request it. The bill regulates a practice discreetly used in Dutch hospitals and homes for decades, turning guidelines adopted by Parliament in 1993 into legally binding requirements. These require a long doctor–patient relationship and exclude euthanasia for nonresidents. Doctors are not supposed to suggest euthanasia as an option and a patient must be aware of all other medical options and have sought a second professional opinion. The request would have to be made voluntarily, persistently, and independently while the patient is of sound mind. Patients can, however, leave a written request for euthanasia, giving doctors the right to use their own discretion when patients become too physically or mentally ill to decide for themselves.[33] The example of the Netherlands was followed by Belgium and Luxemburg, whereas PAS alone is legal in both Germany and Switzerland.

Certainly the legalization of PAS affects nursing. In Oregon, the Oregon Nurses Association requested specific standards within which nurses can operate without fear of disciplinary action. For instance, because the Act focuses only on physicians, if a qualified patient is unable to administer the medication without assistance, who is most likely to be called on to help? Is it the nurse who must stay with a patient until he or she dies if the doctor stays only until the patient is unconscious, at best? Although, because of the *conscience clause* included in the law, the nurse may be excused from participating. Other groups, such as the hospice programs, which opposed the law, must also find ways to balance their traditional approach with the rights of patients.

One aspect of end-of-life care that may now receive more attention is palliative care. An expert Institute of Medicine (IOM) panel reported that studies show that a majority of patients die with severe, untreated pain, which is one of the reasons they wish for PAS. The panel called for better physician education on the issue and a revision of drug laws that endanger a physician's license if large amounts or high doses of narcotics are ordered. Another investigation, called the Study to Understand Prognoses and Preferences for Outcomes and Risks of Treatment (SUPPORT) involved 9000 people in five different US hospitals. The researchers, who were nurses, identified many shortcomings in the cases of intensive care unit (ICU) patients. For instance, less than 50 percent of physicians knew when their patients wanted a do not resuscitate order (DNR). At least 50 percent of patients, some of whom were dying, suffered moderate to severe pain at least half of the time. When the SUPPORT study nurse reported the wishes of patients and families concerning their preferences for end-of-life care to physicians, and especially about the need for pain control, the interventions were not successful. In other words, the physicians' behavior was unchanged and they did not change their orders for pain relief, even though they were inadequate. A medical ethicist reviewing the data noted that the situation might have been different if the study had been under the direction of a physician, noting that "doctors are notoriously reluctant to take advice from nurses."[34]

Nevertheless, nurses must continue to fight for the patient to be free of pain, and if additional treatment is not warranted, to provide comfort measures, and some would say spiritual support, if desired by the patient. The ANA position statement on the topic notes that "the increasing titration of medication to achieve adequate symptom control, even at the expense of maintaining life or hastening death secondarily, is ethically justified."[35] This requires adequate collegial communication among nursing colleagues and physicians.

■ TRANSPLANTS AND ARTIFICIAL PARTS

Since Dr. Christiaan Barnard performed the first human heart transplant in 1967, the question of tissue and organ transplants has become a point of controversy. Tissue may be obtained from living persons or a dead body. In recent years, improvement in immunosuppressive therapy has lessened the need for close tissue matches in most cases, thus permitting most transplants to shift from living donors to cadaver donors. As that shift occurred, the need to clarify brain death became more apparent. Thus, the rising need for cadaver organs accelerated the process of legal acknowledgment discussed previously, the development of medical standards for the determination of death by neurologic criteria, and the growth of a nationwide network for tissue and organ sharing.

Although newly bereaved families from hospitals everywhere donate cadaver organs, the largest numbers come from regional trauma centers. Not only do such centers tend to concentrate those patients who are prime candidates for donation, but also it is in such centers where the staff develop the familiarity with and expertise in recognizing potential donors and asking the next of kin for permission to harvest organs. Such hospitals are also apt to approach the determination of death by neurologic criteria with relatively greater efficiency and more near to established standards.

Many potential opportunities for harvesting organs are missed because physicians and nurses are reluctant to broach the subject of organ donation or even to acknowledge in a timely and forthright fashion that their patient is or may soon be brain dead. A reluctance to be the bearer of bad news or a belief that grieving family members are best served by indirect communication and maintenance of hope is almost surely the major factor in the avoidance of a timely determination of death and hence of requests for donation.

Timing is everything. This often repeated statement is especially applicable here. Highly vascularized organs are lost if the blood supply is interrupted for any significant period. Meanwhile, the ethically correct and psychosocially sensitive behavior is not to ask for organ donation until after the next of kin has been told that death has apparently occurred. (*Apparently* because the standards require repeat examinations and/or confirmatory tests.) Nurses and physicians with the most extensive experience in securing family consent for organ donation insist that ethically correct and psychosocially sensitive timing also ensures the highest yield of donation from newly bereaved family members.

Common law once prevented the decedent from donating his or her own body or individual organs if the next of kin objected, and statutes prohibited the mutilation of bodies. However, all 50 states and the District of Columbia have adopted, in one form or another, the Uniform Anatomical Gift Act, approved in 1968 by the National Conference of Commissioners on Uniform State Laws. The basic purposes are to permit an individual to control the disposition of his or her own body after death, to encourage such donations, and to eliminate unnecessary and complicated formalities regarding the donation while safeguarding the interest of all those involved.[36] As a practical matter, however, organs are ordinarily not harvested without the explicit permission of the next of kin, regardless of the decedent's prior wishes. Of course, such permission is very likely to be granted if the newly dead family member had previously expressed a desire to donate.

Since 1987, hospitals have been required by CMS to ask the next of kin of all potential donors whether or not they wish to donate. This *required request* law has resulted in widespread changes in hospital policies and stimulated some staff education, because it is also required for the Joint Commission accreditation. Most importantly, it resulted in the designation of a person or set of persons who could be called when a prospective donor is identified. Such designated requesters are often both more knowledgeable about donation and more psychologically skilled than the primary physicians and nurses.

In some states, amendments to the Uniform Anatomical Gift Act require notification to an organ procurement organization (OPO), qualified by the US Secretary of Health and Human Services, at the first indication of brain death and prior to the cessation of mechanical ventilation, if the patient is considered a suitable candidate for donation. Usually this does not include those who are infected with human immunodeficiency virus (HIV) or have AIDS. A representative from the procurement group, experienced in organ solicitation and knowledgeable about the kinds of concerns and questions families may have, then approaches the family. Generally, the priority order of decision making is

1. Spouse
2. Adult son or daughter
3. Either parent
4. Adult brother or sister

5. Grandparent
6. Guardian of the person at the time of death
7. Any other person authorized or under obligation to dispose of the body

If the family agrees, a qualified *transplant recovery specialist*, who is a licensed medical professional or technician, may remove the organs according to a protocol that may be developed by the state. However, when such arrangements with an OPO are not in place, it may fall within a nurse's responsibility to work with the families. It should be the physician, but some physicians are not comfortable asking for organ donations, do not know how, or do not want to become involved.

Whoever makes the request needs to take the time to give accurate information to the family and develop their trust. Maximizing access to the patient enables them to see that their loved one is unresponsive. Frequent visits also assist the grief process. It is important to

1. Allow time for sequenced grieving.
2. Provide opportunities for questions.
3. Avoid the use of medical jargon.
4. Introduce the idea of donation and allow time for family discussion.
5. Tell them that organ donation and transplant is generally approved by the major Judeo-Christian traditions.
6. Explain that they may donate as many or as few organs as they wish.
7. Clarify terms (if asked) such as *organ* and *tissue* and their use.
8. Let them know that all tissues and organs are recovered in the OR (except corneas), and that the donor is reconstructed in such a way that traditional funeral preparations, including viewing, can be carried out.
9. Have the appropriate organ donor card ready, if the family agrees.
10. Give the family time to discuss the matter if members disagree, then return and see if you need to clarify questions.
11. Support their decision if the family still opposes the donation.

Clearly, this entire approach requires knowledge and finesse. However, in seeking donations, the nurse also serves on behalf of the unknown patients who receive the organs. Only a short overview is presented here, and it is well worth the effort to learn all that you can about organ transplantation.

For more than a quarter of a century, various attempts to get people to donate organs have been generally disappointing. The need for organs continues to far exceed the supply. Even now, consent rates for organ donations are not more than 50 percent, and are even lower for tissues and corneas. Ten people die each day waiting for a transplant. Yet, it is said that one tissue donor can provide transplantable tissue for 55 people.[37]

Although most people express positive attitudes toward organ donation, few take specific steps to make it more likely that their own organs will be harvested. Chief among those steps would be repeated, open conversations within families about organ donations and other aspects of end-of-life care. The problem for those who seek quick solutions to the persistent shortage of organs is that legislative initiatives and institutional rule making do not readily address the discomfort of professionals and the public.

Still another ethical and rights issue relates to who gets the organs needed when. Potential heart transplant recipients must undergo rigorous screening and a decision is based, in part, on how well the patient will do and can manage, and the patient's life expectancy after transplantation. If the transplant will not benefit the patient sufficiently, or the risks outweigh the benefits, the treatment is considered futile. However, separating futility from rationing is not always easy.

The transplant community is joined under a nationwide umbrella. The United Network for Organ Sharing (UNOS), a nonprofit charitable organization, maintains the nation's organ transplant waiting list under contract with the Health Resources and Services Administration of the US Department of Health and Human Services. UNOS members include every transplant program, organ procurement organization, and tissue-typing laboratory in the United States. For transplantation purposes, the United States is divided into 11 geographic regions. These regions play a role in organ allocation. With the exception of perfectly matched donor kidneys, organs are offered to sick patients within the area in which they were donated before being offered to other parts of the country. This policy originated because, at one time, there was a risk in having an organ outside the body for very long while it was taken elsewhere. Although this situation has changed to a great extent, staff in transplant centers, who are more sophisticated in soliciting organs, may want to keep as many organs as possible for their own patients both for altruistic reasons and to stay in business. In early 1998, the Secretary of Health and Human Services said that the existing regional system for distributing organs would be dismantled and replaced with one in which the sickest patients would go to the top of the list, no matter where in the country they lived. UNOS argued that the current system was working well and hired lobbyists to influence Congress. The system has remained the same.[38]

Given the scarcity of organs, there are many other issues to consider. The various sources of organs and tissue, including live human donors, cadavers, mechanical devices, fetuses, anencephalic infants, and brain-dead donors, all bring their own ethical and legal problems. In one case, a Florida court determined that parents could not consent to the removal of organs from an anencephalic infant who was technically alive. This is contrary to a 1994 AMA position that maintains that the infant is not really alive because it cannot and will not experience consciousness, and that the donation of organs could save other infants. There are also voiced or unvoiced fears that, in the effort to harvest organs, resuscitation of an unconscious person might be stopped prematurely, or that medical personnel might subject a brain-dead person to a prolonged deathlike existence until potential donors are located. Whether these concerns are or are not real, the legal and ethical issues in the entire organ transplant situation are incredibly complex.

■ THE RIGHTS OF THE HELPLESS

Children, the mentally ill, the mentally retarded, and certain patients in nursing homes are often seen as relatively helpless, because they have been termed legally incompetent to make decisions about their health care for many years. Often the rights overlap, as when a child or elderly person is mentally retarded. Some of the rights of the elderly are protected by a legalized bill of rights.

The Mentally Disabled

For mental patients, state laws and some high court decisions have served the same purpose. Both have focused on mental patients' rights in the areas of voluntary and involuntary admissions; kind and length of restraints, including seclusion; informed consent to treatment, especially sterilization and psychosurgery; the rights of citizenship (voting); right of privacy, especially in relation to records; rights in research; and especially, the right to treatment.

Although rulings have varied, the trend is toward the protection of rights. The landmark decision of *Wyatt v. Stickney* (344 F. Supp. 373—Dist. Court, MD, Alabama, 1972) clearly defined the purposes of commitment to a public hospital and the constitutional right to adequate treatment. The case of *Wyatt v. Stickney* came to a conclusion after 33 years, through the tenure of nine Alabama governors and 14 state mental health commissioners, the longest mental health case in national history. The State of Alabama estimates its litigation expenses at over $15 million.

Later, a Massachusetts court's decision in *Rogers v. Okin* (478 F.Supp.1342 [D.Mass.1979], 634) that gives a voluntary mental patient the right to refuse psychiatric medication created a furor. The appeals court modified the ruling, holding that voluntary patients could be forced to choose between leaving the hospital or accepting the prescribed treatment. Later, a Massachusetts court ruled that an incompetent person could refuse medication if he or she was able to express a "sensible" opinion, unless there was a proven danger to the public. For certain extraordinary medical treatments, the courts would have the ultimate authority to decide whether treatment is given. However, a number of states have enacted legislation protecting the right of the mentally ill to refuse medication.[39]

In some situations, a structured internal review system in which patients could appeal treatment decisions has seemed to work. On the other hand, follow-up on patients who refused treatment has shown a deterioration in their functioning when they were released to the community. In large and small cities, the evening television news shows disquieting pictures of apparently under-medicated, mentally ill persons whose lives are endangered by harsh environments that they are not equipped to negotiate safely.

When an individual refuses admission to a psychiatric facility, that refusal may not be honored if he or she fits the criteria in the state mental health code for an involuntary unit admission (commitment). A 1975 US Supreme Court case, *O'Connor v. Donaldson* (422 U.S. 563 1975), was a landmark decision in mental health law. The US Supreme Court ruled that states could not confine citizens to an institution (or similar) without treatment if they were non-dangerous and capable of living by themselves or with the aid of responsible family or friends.

Children and Adolescents

The legal status of young people is presented in Chapter 17. The rights of young people and children in health care relate primarily to consent for treatment or research and protection against abuse. It is a general rule that a parent or guardian must give consent for the medical or surgical treatment of a minor (under age 18) except in an emergency when it is imperative to give immediate care to save the minor's life. Legally, however, anyone who is capable of understanding what he or she is doing may give consent, because age is not always an exact criterion of maturity or intelligence. Many *mature minors* are perfectly capable of deciding for themselves whether to accept or reject recommended therapy and, in cases involving simple procedures, the courts have refused to invoke the rule requiring the consent of a parent or guardian. If the minor is married or has been otherwise emancipated from his or her parents, there is likely to be little question legally. In addition, states cite different ages and situations in which parental permission is needed for medical treatment. The almost universal exception is allowing minors to consent to treatment for sexually transmitted diseases, drug abuse, and pregnancy-related care. Although it has been understood that health professionals have no legal obligation to report to parents that the minor has sought such treatment, a few states are beginning to add statutes that say that the minor does not need parental permission, but that parents must be notified. In 1983, the Reagan administration issued a rule that would require parents to be notified whenever children under 18 received any contraceptives from federally funded family planning clinics. After a number of court challenges, this was overruled as infringing on a woman's right to privacy.

In 1972, the Supreme Court ruled that state statutes prohibiting the prescription of contraceptives to unmarried persons were unconstitutional because they interfere with the right of privacy of those desiring them. However, it did not rule on a minor's right to privacy in seeking or buying contraceptives. This was left to the states, and a number of states still set age limitations from 14 to 21. In many states, however, doctors and other health professionals may provide birth control information and prescribe contraceptives to patients of any age without parental consent. Changes in federal and state laws also required welfare agencies to offer family planning services and supplies to sexually active minors. In general, there had been a national trend toward granting minors the right to contraceptive advice and devices, but the political power of conservative groups who oppose this trend is being felt, and state legislatures frequently attempt to put limits on young people in these areas.

An even more dramatic change has occurred in relation to abortion. In 1976, the Supreme Court held that states may not constitutionally require the consent of a girl's parents for an abortion during the first 12 weeks of pregnancy. In addition, parents could not either prevent or force an abortion on the part of a daughter who, in the eyes of the court, was "a competent minor mature enough to have become pregnant."

Since that time the reproductive rights of teenagers have been gradually eroded by state legislation and federal edicts influenced by conservatives and right-to-life groups. More than half the states have laws requiring teenagers to notify one or both parents, even if divorced, or to get permission from them before an abortion.

The Justices of the Supreme Court ruled five to four in June 1990 that states had a right to make such a requirement of unmarried women under 18 as long as there was an alternative of judicial bypass (speaking to a judge instead) if the law requires notice to both parents. The five conservative justices did not allow for the fact that one or both parents might be abusive, alcoholic, or drug addicted, or even that the pregnancy might be a result of incest.

In one study of parental involvement laws, it was found that there was indeed a decrease in the number of abortions, but no indication that the laws drove up birth rates for minors. Instead, it appears that minors traveled out of state for abortions or possibly received illegal or undocumented abortions. There is already evidence that minors seek illegal abortions and, as in pre–*Roe v. Wade* days, they have been fatal. Should the young woman decide against an abortion and elect to bear the child, she can receive care related to her pregnancy without parental consent in almost every state. An unwed mature minor may also consent to treatment of her child. Meanwhile, state laws on parental consent and notification are still a hodgepodge, differing from state to state. Undoubtedly, pro-choice forces will continue to work to overturn these restrictive state laws.

Groups such as the American Academy of Pediatrics (AAP), the Society for Adolescent Medicine, and the National Association of Children's Hospitals and related institutions have taken stands on protecting the rights of minors in health care. For example, the AAP Committee on Youth has presented a model act for the consent of minors for health services, recommended for enactment in all states. The *Pediatric Bill of Rights* may also be a forerunner to legal action, as was the AHA Patient's Bill of Rights. (Unless such a statement is incorporated into law, the effect is that of a professional guideline to encourage the protection of rights, with no enforcement powers.)

In its recommendations, the AAP categorizes children as (1) those who lack decision-making capacity; (2) those with a developing capacity; and (3) those who have decision-making capacity for health care decisions. For the first, the parents should make decisions, unless the decisions are abusive or neglectful. For the second, the physician should seek parental permission and the child's assent. The latter should be binding, or at least the physician should seek third-party mediation for the parent–child disagreement. If the child dissents from life-saving treatment, he or she could be overruled, but attempts should be made to persuade the child to assent. In the third case, the child has the right to give informed consent, and the parents should be seen as consultants.[40] One author sees a problem with these recommendations, because an assumption is made that decision-making capacity can be measured, and pediatricians do not necessarily have that training. She notes that if a 14-year-old child is capable of making life and death decisions, why not the legal right to smoke or drop out of school? Equal rights for children would mean "dissolution of child labor laws, mandatory education, statutory rape laws, and child neglect statutes."[41]

Actually, cases in which mature minors are permitted to make life-and-death decisions are increasing. Scott Rose, a talented 14-year-old from Oklahoma, had a cellular immunodeficiency disease similar to the famous bubble boy in Houston. He refused to live in a similar enclosure, preferring to live a normal life as long as he could. With his lungs deteriorating and his suffering increasing, he refused further life-sustaining treatments. With his parents' tacit approval, but against his doctor's wishes, he disconnected himself from the ventilator and died.[42]

Benito Agrela, born with an enlarged liver and spleen, had a liver transplant at age 8 and another at 14. He then stopped taking his medications, because he could not tolerate all the side effects. The Florida Department of Social Services had him forcibly removed from home and admitted to a hospital transplant floor. When he refused further treatment, his case was taken to court. After consultation with Benito and his physicians, the judge ruled that Benito had a right to refuse the medications and could return home. Before he died at age 15, he reiterated that he had a right to make his own decisions and that he understood the consequences.[43] There are a number of similar cases.

The legal principles involved in many of these cases are *parental autonomy*, a constitutionally protected right; *parens patriae*, the state's right and duty to protect the child; the *best interest doctrine*, which requires the court to determine what is best for the child; and the *substituted judgment doctrine*, in which the court determines what choice an incompetent individual would make if he or she were competent. (The last could be applied properly only to a once-competent person, and thus not to young children or severely retarded persons of any age.)

Another unresolved issue is whether the grossly deformed neonate should be allowed to die. Few judges will rule to let it die, but often parents and health care personnel quietly make the decision. These situations are especially difficult for a nurse who cares for the infant. Ethical and moral considerations weigh strongly.

The so-called Baby Doe case began with a child born in Indiana with Down syndrome and a correctable esophageal fistula. The parents refused surgery, and the courts upheld their decision. The child was deprived of artificial nutritional life support and died. Although similar action had been taken in other cases, this one came to the attention of President Reagan. It resulted in a DHHS regulation that threatened hospitals that neglected such children with loss of funds under Section 504 of the Rehabilitation Act of 1973 (which protects the handicapped). Large signs had to be posted alerting people to a hot-line number to call to report such incidents. After a series of legal challenges, this regulation was ruled unconstitutional—arbitrary and capricious—among other things. Eventually, an alternative suggestion by the AAP was agreed on: establishment of *infants bioethics committees* (IBCs) with diverse membership whose responsibility, in part, would be to advise about decisions to withhold or withdraw life-sustaining measures. This was encouraged in the Baby Doe law, the federal Child Abuse Amendment of 1984, which labeled withdrawal or withholding of medically indicated nutrition as child abuse. However, the regulation basically left the decision as to whether such nutrition might be "virtually futile" up to the physician. There are specific guidelines.[44]

In 1983, a child known as Baby Jane Doe was born in New York with multiple serious congenital conditions, one of which required immediate surgery. The family was told that even if she lived, she would be in a vegetative state, so after consultation with a physician and religious adviser, they opted for conservative treatment. A right-to-life attorney from Vermont learned of the case and managed to be appointed guardian by a like-minded judge, but an appeals court overruled this. Other right-to-life groups attempted to intervene; so did the federal government, which demanded the child's medical records to see if Section 504 (see previously) was being violated. After considerable time, effort, and money had been spent, the government finally gave up. The child survived on conservative treatment and went home, where she required constant care for some time because of her paralysis and lack of mental development. Years later, she was reported as slightly retarded but generally all right.

Follow-up on the Baby Doe law indicates that many who are concerned about these infants agree that the federal regulations are an ethically inadequate response to the complex needs of the handicapped child, the family, the health care professions, and society as a whole. An ethics committee, if functioning well, can be helpful to the physician and family in making decisions, but the decisions lean toward preserving life.

It is a tragedy that the lives of some infants will be prolonged and they will suffer a fate worse than death because the physicians are afraid of the legal consequences of letting them die. On balance, the situation is similar to the so-called right-to-die situation for elderly adults. Although often cited as a reason for indecision and questionable treatment, the law rarely requires life-sustaining treatment contrary to the wishes of loving and sensible parents.

■ RIGHTS OF PATIENTS IN RESEARCH

The use of new, experimental drugs and treatments in hospitals, nursing homes, and other institutions that have a captive population—for example, prisons or homes for the mentally retarded—has been extensive. Nurses are often involved in giving the treatment or drugs. As noted earlier, DHHS regulations require specific informed consent for any human research carried out under DHHS auspices, with strong emphasis on the need for a clear explanation of the experiment, possible dangers, and the subject's complete freedom to refuse or withdraw at any time.

An interesting trend is toward including very young children in making decisions about research in which they are asked to participate. In the past, as a rule, parents were asked whether they consented to their child's participation in research—medical, educational, psychological, or other. There has always been some concern as to whether children should be subjected to such research if it was not at least potentially beneficial to them (such as the use of a new drug for a leukemic child). The child was seldom given the opportunity to decide whether or not to participate. New knowledge of the potential harm that could be done to the child, however innocuous the experiment, and appreciation of the child as a human being with individual rights have now resulted in recommendations that even a very young child be given a simple explanation of the proposed

research and allowed to participate or not, or even to withdraw later, without any form of coercion. In 1983, the DHHS published rules requiring children's consent to participate in research.

Research involving incompetent patients presents another problem of consent. Obviously that person cannot give an informed consent, if any at all. Occasionally, a guardian is allowed to give consent, which is inconsistent with the ethical standard of informed consent, but if the research protocol will benefit the guardian's ward, it may be acceptable. Regulations outlining Institutional Review Board (IRB) procedures say that consent may be sought from the prospective subject's authorized representative; some protocols allow for the consent of a responsible person, who may not have a legal standing. If the research is minimally harmful, this too may be acceptable, but the IRB must oversee the process. Newspapers are still reporting on research done on incompetent people that was certainly not minimally harmful and had no positive effect on the subject.

When a nurse is participating in research, at whatever level, ensuring that the rights of patients are honored is both an ethical and a legal responsibility. Nurses should know the patients' rights: self-determination to choose to participate; to have full information; to terminate participation without penalty; privacy and dignity; conservation of personal resources; freedom from arbitrary hurt and intrinsic risk of injury; as well as the special rights of minors and incompetent persons previously discussed. For instance, nurses have been ordered to begin an experimental drug knowing that the patient has not given informed consent. The nurse is then obligated to see that the patient does have the appropriate explanation. This is one more case in which institutional policy that sets an administrative protocol for the nurse in such a situation is helpful. If the nurse is the investigator, she or he must observe all the usual requirements, such as informed consent and confidentiality.

Any institution that applies for research funding from the DHHS is required to have an IRB in place. Multidisciplinary panels are charged with protecting human subjects from both unduly dangerous procedures and from abuses of their rights. These IRBs vary widely in the rigor of their processes, despite being tightly regulated. Some IRBs subject proposals for research to very careful scrutiny; others are much less effective.

Some boards may be less protective of patients' rights than they should be, especially in the area of informed consent. There is usually no follow-up to determine whether the plans to preserve subjects' rights that are presented in the proposals are really carried through. There is also criticism about lack of consistency in proposal approval. However, the IRB is generally seen as a safeguard to patients.

There is no requirement that there be nurses on these boards, even if the boards are in hospitals or other health care agencies. Nurses can bring a useful perspective and should probably propose themselves for membership where not already invited. However, they should be properly prepared and knowledgeable about research.

■ PATIENT RECORDS: CONFIDENTIALITY AND AVAILABILITY

There is some evidence that, in situations other than the legally required ones, the confidentiality of patients' records is frequently violated. From birth certificates to death certificates, the health and medical records of most Americans are part of a system that allows access to insurance companies, student researchers, and governmental agencies, to name a few. It is not realistic for patients to think that medical information about them will be kept confidential, even when staff follows all the basic rules about not discussing patients except in clinical situations. Confidentiality is even less likely since the advent of electronic information processing, huge data banks, and advancements in record linkage. The public is generally unaware of this threat and of the serious consequences of a loss of confidentiality in the health care system.

The Health Insurance Portability and Accountability Act of 1996 (HIPAA) has established rules to ensure that all patient account handling, billing, and medical records are protected. But HIPAA only applies to medical records maintained by health care providers, health plans, and health clearing-houses, and only if the facility maintains and transmits records in electronic form. A great deal of health-related information exists outside of health care facilities and the files of health care plans, and thus beyond the reach of HIPAA. The reader is referred to HIPAA basics at www.privacyrights.org/fs/fs8a-hipaa.htm for more comprehensive information. The extent of privacy protection given to medical information often depends on where the records are located and the purpose for which the information was compiled. The laws that cover the privacy of medical information vary by situation. And confidentiality is likely to be lost in return for insurance coverage, an employment opportunity, an application for government

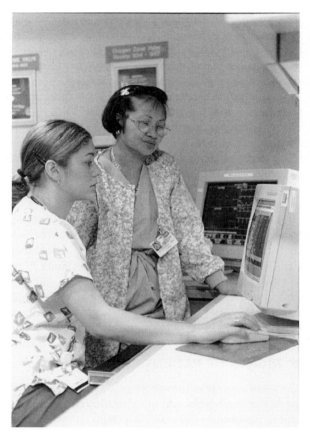

With the use of electronic patient records comes the responsibility to assure confidentiality. (Courtesy of Robert Wood Johnson University Hospital, New Brunswick, New Jersey)

benefits, or an investigation of health and safety at a work site. In short, individuals may have a false sense of security.

Some provisions of HIPAA demand that patients must be able to access their records, be able to correct errors, and be informed of how their personal information will be used. These requirements have led to a new vigilance in record keeping that dramatically affects the day-to-day practice of the nurse. Though passed by Congress and signed by the President in 1996, the provisions did not become mandatory until 2003. An orientation to HIPAA is part of any workplace orientation. The important message is that patients' records are personal and confidential, and that this confidentiality is scrutinized intently.

Although HIPAA was passed first by Congress, the federal Freedom of Information-Privacy Act (FOIA) was operational first. FOIA denies access to an individual's medical records without that person's consent. Additionally, the Fair Health Information Act of 1994 addresses the need for federal law to protect confidential material. Still, there was consensus that these laws would not be sufficient to protect individuals in an electronic age. And so HIPAA took shape, with all of its provisions for security in an era of computer-based patient records. There have indeed been some frightening violations of privacy, with clerks releasing confidential information, hospital personnel snooping, and others selling patient information to anyone who will buy. Patients, who are usually required to sign releases of their medical records for insurance purposes, lose all control of those records, practically speaking. The National Research Council, the research arm of the National Academy of Sciences, formed a 15-member panel (with one distinguished nurse), to look at the potential misuse and abuse of electronic records. The panel concluded that electronic health information was essential to improving health care while controlling costs, but that more safeguards were needed to protect patient privacy. One issue of concern was an aspect of HIPAA that called for *universal patient identifiers* or codes providing a nationwide link of all patients' files. The DHHS was to devise a security system to protect these computerized records. The universal patient identifier is the key to enabling a universal computerized patient record. Although such a system would have endless benefits for the American people, and the technology exists, the issues of confidentiality are still in dispute.

Physicians and health administrators have historically been hostile toward the concept of sharing the record with the patient. Some attorneys serving health care facilities tend to share that feeling, often because they fear that patients may detect errors or personal comments that will result in a legal suit. (Actually, patient access has been mandated in Massachusetts since 1946 without a single reported adverse incident.) Whether or not any person involved in health care still feels that way is immaterial. Almost without exception, the patient's medical record is available to him or her.

It is interesting to review the literature over the last 30 years to see the changes in attitudes and legislation. There were always physicians and others who saw sharing the record with the patient as not only fair, but sensible. Rather than worry that a patient would be too frightened or too stupid to understand, these practitioners had a philosophy of openness.

Choice in the matter of sharing the record has ended. Whereas it is legally recognized that the patient's record is the property of the hospital or physician (in his or her office), the information that the record contains is not similarly protected. Both states and the federal government have legislated access—either direct patient access, with or without a right to copy, or indirect access (physician, attorney, or provision of a summary only). States may differentiate between doctors' and hospital records and have other idiosyncratic qualifications. Of course, one certain way in which the patient can gain access is through a malpractice suit in which the record is subpoenaed, a costly process for both provider and consumer.

Does the nurse have any legal responsibility to be an intermediary? The answer is more complex than just yes or no. A nurse generally would not hand a patient the chart at request; that would be inappropriate. Most states and health care agencies have a protocol to be followed when patients request to access their records. This usually involves providing both privacy and an opportunity for the physician or another person to explain the content. Nurses should know the specific procedure in their agencies so that they can advise patients properly.

Privacy

Nurses and others who work with patients must be especially careful to avoid invading the patient's right to privacy. There are a number of special concerns. For instance, consent to treatment does not cover the use of a picture without specific permission, nor does it mean that the patient can be subjected to repeated examinations not necessary to therapy without express consent. Undue exposure during examination should also be avoided.

Exceptions to respect for the patient's privacy are related to legal reporting obligations. The nurse may be obligated to testify about otherwise confidential information in criminal cases. All states have laws requiring hospitals, doctors, nurses, and sometimes other health workers to report on certain kinds of situations, because the patient may be unwilling or unable to do so. The nurse often has responsibility in these matters because, although it may be the physician's legal obligation, the nurse may be the only one actually aware of the situation. Even if such reporting is not explicitly required by law, regulations of various state agencies may require such a report. Common reporting requirements are for communicable diseases, diseases in newborn babies, gunshot wounds, and criminal acts, including rape.

Every state requires that suspected child abuse or neglect be reported to the child protective agency. Although other kinds of reporting are relatively objective, there are problems in reporting abused children because of the varying definitions of *child* and the question of whether there was abuse or an accident, with the consequent fear of parents suing. Usually, however, the person reporting is protected if the report is made in good faith, that is, without malice and honestly. It is not necessary that one be sure that abuse has taken place; the obligation is to report suspected abuse. The responsibility to prove abuse belongs with the child protection agency. In some states, there are penalties for not reporting. Spousal abuse and elder abuse are also reportable in most states. In most states, the abuses covered are physical abuse, fiduciary abuse, neglect, and abandonment.

As the AIDS epidemic grew, new reporting problems arose. By 1987, all states had added AIDS to the list of reportable diseases. Many, but by no means all, require reporting of AIDS carriers, that is, the reporting of positive test results for HIV. Physicians have been willing to make these reports because of the virulence of the disease and the need to maintain the best possible epidemiologic records. However, the problem arises of whether to notify the family, especially a wife or lover, of a person with AIDS. Many patients object to notification and therefore will not come for testing; creating a situation that may be even more serious. State laws vary regarding a provider's legal "duty to warn" potentially exposed partners, when HIV-infected clients clearly indicate that they will not notify their partners or make the necessary information available for health department staff to make the notification. In cases related to other infectious diseases, judges have ruled that the physician had a duty to inform the third party. Theoretically the third party could sue the physician if they were infected and not warned. As a rule, this kind of reporting is a public health department's responsibility, but it has not yet been determined whether, for instance, a home health nurse with information on AIDS-related conditions has a duty to tell the family. Release of unauthorized records could lead to legal suits for invasion of privacy and breach of confidentiality. Agencies should have policies that support the prevention of disclosure of patient information and records without the patient's consent. Any exceptions to the policy should be included. Hospitals and other institutions generally have these policies.

Another type of sensitive health information is the results of genetic testing. Currently, no special protection exists to prevent revealing this information. Some people are afraid that such information could cause employer discrimination and ask their physicians not to record it. Confidentiality is of major importance. If a genetic disease is discovered,

health professionals probably should not contact other relatives without the consent of the person being screened, even if it would benefit those relatives. However, one can easily think of a clinical example in which the Tarasoff principle (explained later) would seem to require that a relative be told. Imagine, for instance, a patient newly diagnosed as a carrier of a serious congenital disorder whose estranged sibling is now 4 months pregnant. If the specific inheritance pattern indicates that there is a high likelihood of the fetus being affected, and if efforts fail to persuade the patient to disclose, what is the nurse's obligation to warn? As genetic testing becomes more common, more legal protection of the information can be expected.

Ethical and legal practice prohibits the professional person from divulging any confidential information to anyone else, unless possibly to a nurse or physician involved in the patient's care. Neither does the ethical person engage in gossip based on this information, trivial and harmless though it may seem at the time. Moreover, the professional nurse has an obligation to set a good example for others in nonprofessional groups who may be less aware of their responsibilities in this respect.

Confidential information obtained through professional relationships is not the same as *privileged communication*, which is a legal concept providing that a physician and patient, attorney and client, and priest and penitent have a special privilege. Should any court action arise in which the person (or persons) involved is called to testify, the law (in many states) will not require that such information be divulged. Not all states acknowledge that nurses can be recipients of privileged communication, but there are specific cases in which the nurse–patient privilege has been accepted, especially in the case of advanced practice nurses. Another issue is that psychiatric nurses, like other psychotherapists, have a responsibility to warn potential victims about their homicidal clients (the *Tarasoff principle*, named after a case in which a psychiatrist did not do so). Other than such a situation, however, a new ruling by the Supreme Court in 1996 has recognized the therapist–patient privilege, including as *therapists* psychotherapists and other mental health professionals.[45]

■ ASSAULT AND BATTERY

Assault and battery, although often discussed with emphasis on the criminal interpretation, also has a patients' rights aspect that is related to everyday nursing practice, especially when dealing with certain types of patients. Grounds for civil action might include the following:

1. Forcing a patient to submit to a treatment for which he or she has not given consent either expressly in writing, orally, or by implication. Whether or not a consent was signed, a patient should not be forced; resistance implies a withdrawal of consent.

2. Forcefully handling an unconscious patient.

3. Lifting a protesting patient from his or her bed to a wheelchair or stretcher.

4. Threatening to strike or actually striking an unruly child or adult, except in self-defense.

5. Forcing a patient out of bed to walk postoperatively.

6. In some states, performing alcohol, blood, urine, or health tests for presumed drunken driving without consent. There are some *implied consent* statutes in motor vehicle codes that provide that a person, for the privilege of being allowed to drive, gives an implied consent to furnishing a sample of blood, urine, or breath for chemical analysis when charged with driving while intoxicated. However, if the person objects and is forced, it might still be considered battery. This may also be true in relation to taking blood or DNA samples from unwilling individuals in potential criminal cases. Several states, acknowledging this, have enacted legislation to insulate hospital employees and health professionals from liability.

As a rule, intentional torts, such as assault and battery, are not covered by malpractice insurance.

■ FALSE IMPRISONMENT

As the term implies, *false imprisonment* means "restraining a person's liberty without the sanction of the law, or imprisonment of a person who is later found to be innocent of the crime for which he was imprisoned." The term also applies to many procedures that actually or conceivably are performed in hospital and nursing situations if they are performed without the consent of the patient or his or her legal representative. In most instances, the nurse or other employee would not be held liable if it can be proved that what was done was necessary to protect others.

Among the most common nursing situations that might be considered false imprisonment are the following:

1. Restraining a patient by physical force or using appliances without written consent, especially in procedures where the use of restraints is not usually necessary. This is, or may be, a delicate situation because if you do not use a restraint such as side rails to protect a patient, you may be accused of negligence, and if you use them without consent, you may be accused of false imprisonment. This is a typical example of the need for prudent and reasonable action that a court of law would uphold.

2. Restraining a mentally ill patient who is dangerous neither to him or herself nor to others. For example, patients who wander about the hospital division making a nuisance of themselves usually cannot legally be locked in a room unless they show signs of violence.

3. Using arm, leg, or body restraints to keep a patient quiet while administering an intravenous infusion may be considered false imprisonment. If this risk is involved—that is, if the patient objects to the treatment and refuses to consent to it—the physician should be called. Should the doctor order restraints for the patient, make sure that the order is given in writing before allowing anyone to proceed with the treatment. It is much better to assign someone to stay with the patient throughout a procedure than to use restraints without authorization.

4. Detaining an unwilling patient in the hospital. If a patient insists on going home or a parent or guardian insists on taking a minor or other dependent person out of the hospital before his or her condition warrants it, hospital authorities cannot legally require the patient to remain. (An exception can be made, in some states, for a *hospital hold* in the case of a child thought to be in imminent danger of abuse or neglect.) If a patient insists on leaving, the doctor should write an order permitting the hospital to allow the patient to go home *against advice*, and the hospital's representative should see that the patient or guardian signs an official form absolving the hospital, medical staff, and nursing staff of all responsibility should the patient's early departure be detrimental to his or her health and welfare. If the patient refuses to sign, a record should be made on the chart of exactly what occurred and an incident report probably should be filed. Take the patient to the hospital entrance in the usual manner.

5. Detaining a patient who is medically ready to be discharged for an unreasonable period of time. The delay may be due to waiting for the delivery of an orthopedic appliance or other service. It is never appropriate to delay a patient because of an inability to pay a bill. In such instances, the nurse or nursing department may or may not be directly involved, but it is always wise to

know the possibility of legal developments and to exercise sound judgment to be completely fair to the patient and avoid trouble.

■ LEGAL ISSUES RELATED TO REPRODUCTION

Laws permitting abortion have varied greatly from state to state over the years. In early 1973, the Supreme Court ruled that no state could interfere with a woman's right to obtain an abortion during the first trimester (12 weeks) of pregnancy. During the second trimester, the state may interfere only to the extent of imposing regulations to safeguard the health of women seeking abortions. During the last trimester of pregnancy, a state may prohibit abortions except when the mother's life is at stake (*Doe v. Bolton*, 410 US 190 1973, and *Roe v. Wade*, 410 US 113 1973).

Because of religious and moral reasons, some institutions are exempted from complying with the abortion law, and individual doctors and nurses have refused to participate in abortions. Individual professionals or other health workers may make that choice, and there is legal support for them (*conscience clause*). This does not preclude the right of the hospital to dismiss a nurse for refusing to carry out an assigned responsibility or to transfer her or him to another unit. There have been some suits by nurses objecting to transfer, but rulings have varied.

Almost 40 years after the *Roe v. Wade* decision, opinions are still strong on abortion issues, and generally the same arguments are heard. Immediately after *Roe v. Wade*, with a liberal Supreme Court, the rulings were almost consistently directed at freedom of choice, in opposition to restrictions on abortion being put by the states and later by the conservative Reagan administration. The rulings changed dramatically with later appointments of conservative judges by President Reagan, until there was a five-to-four conservative majority with the only woman Justice, Sandra O'Connor, considered the sometime swing vote. (However, she tended to be conservative on abortion issues.)

The following list shows the tilt of the court and the diversity of cases, generally brought by states. It is important to remember that the US Supreme Court rules only on issues related to the Constitution. In these cases, the Court rules that the state or other petitioner does or does not have a constitutional right to conduct itself in a particular way.

- **1973**—The Court struck down restrictions on places where abortions could be performed, allowing for abortion clinics.
- **1976**—The Court said that states could not give husbands veto power over their wives' decision to abort their pregnancies. It also said that parents of minor unwed girls could not be given an absolute veto over abortions.
- **1977**—The Court ruled that states have no constitutional obligation to pay for non-therapeutic abortions (referring to Medicaid patients).
- **1979**—The Court said that states may seek to protect a fetus that has reached viability, but the determination of viability is up to doctors.
- **1979**—The Court implied that the states might be able to require a pregnant unmarried minor to obtain parental consent to an abortion as long as the state provides an alternative procedure, such as a judge's permission.
- **1980**—The Court said that neither federal nor state government was constitutionally obligated to pay for even medically necessary abortions of women on welfare.
- **1981**—The Court ruled that states might require doctors consulted by immature or dependent minors to try to notify their parents before an abortion.
- **1983**—The Court heard three abortion-related cases, ruling that states and communities cannot require that all abortions for women more than 3 months pregnant be performed in a hospital. Also struck down were regulations requiring a 24-hour waiting period between consent and procedure.
- **1986**—The Court said that states could not require doctors to tell women seeking abortions about potential risks and available benefits for prenatal care and childbirth.
- **1987**—The Court split four to four, invalidating an Illinois law restricting access to abortion for some teenagers.
- **1989**—In *Webster v. Reproductive Health Services*, considered a turning point, the Court provided the states with new authority to limit a woman's right to abortion by upholding a Missouri law that banned abortions in tax-supported facilities except to save the mother's life, even if no public funds are spent; banned any public employee (doctors, nurses, others) from performing or assisting with abortions except to save a woman's life;

and required testing for viability of any fetus thought to be at least 20 years old.

- **1990**—The Court ruled constitutional the Ohio and Minnesota laws requiring parental notification by unmarried teenagers.
- **1992**—In *Planned Parenthood v. Casey*, the Court upheld most of the restrictions passed by the Pennsylvania legislature, and in doing so, established a new legal standard: Restrictions are constitutional so long as they do not impose undue burdens on a woman's right to choose.
- **1996**—The Court chose not to hear a case reopening the abortion issue, although Rehnquist, Scalia, and Thomas dissented.
- **1997**—The Court banned demonstrations within 15 feet of the entrance to abortion facilities (*fixed buffer zone*), but did not offer similar limitation protection for persons or vehicles seeking access to such facilities.
- **2000**—The Court ruled on the constitutionality of *partial birth abortion* when necessary to save the life of the mother, and any state ban on partial birth abortion is unconstitutional.

The aim of many of these cases was to force the overturn of *Roe v. Wade*. That did not quite happen, but some state legislatures passed increasingly restrictive laws (even forbidding abortion in cases of incest and rape), in part to try to force the Supreme Court to hear the cases. The most widespread are restrictions on minors or a mandatory waiting period for all pregnant women seeking an abortion. The big issue at the end of the 1990s was the so-called partial-birth abortion, done in the last trimester. Not a pretty procedure at best, but done rarely (less than 1 percent of abortions), it was touted as murdering a living child. Congress tried several times to pass a bill forbidding it, but President Clinton vetoed it. The effort continues. Discouraged by the federal outlook, over 40 states have taken up the matter and several have made the ban law, demonstrating the strength of the anti-abortion movement. Governors veto some of the more restrictive rulings, but the very fact that they got through two Houses is appalling to many men and women alike. Some young women have already sought back-alley abortionists with the expected dire results. Both pro-choice and pro-life forces have concentrated their efforts on legislators and candidates to bring about state laws that supported their particular point of view. The end is not in sight.

How does this affect nurses? Nurses support both sides of this issue, as was clear by the anger or joy expressed by nurses when ANA took a pro-choice stand. But despite their personal feelings they will care for women and young girls regardless of their choices. Ethically, nurses must give all patients good care, but who gets what care and why, as in the Webster case, may affect nurses professionally as well as personally. As citizens, nurses must stay abreast of such important issues. For instance, many pro-life groups also object to sex education and contraceptive use, yet an astounding number of teenagers get pregnant every year. It is important to see how some of these issues interrelate. For instance, groups opposed to abortion are now becoming involved in right-to-die issues, taking a *life-is-sacred* stand.

There have already been court rulings that bar women from jobs (usually higher paying) that might endanger the fetus of a pregnant woman, even if the woman is not pregnant and does not plan to have children. In another case, a dying woman was forced to have a cesarean to "save" her fetus. Both died, and later the action was ruled illegal. In still another case, a woman in a coma was denied an abortion, but later, in a similar case, one was permitted—even though a right-to-life lawyer who did not even know the woman tried to become her guardian to prevent it. And what of the Baby Doe–saved children? Who will be responsible for them? Will the family be forced to care for and pay for a severely deformed child? What of all the issues related to the fetus? Will new technology that has been successful in intrauterine surgery save some of these babies? Cure them? How will new techniques of birth control change the family planning scene?

There are a number of other reproduction-related rights that are also important, such as sterilization, artificial insemination of various kinds, and surrogate parenthood. *Sterilization* means termination of the ability to produce offspring. Laws and regulations both have been in the process of change. If the life of a woman may be jeopardized if she becomes pregnant, a therapeutic sterilization may be performed with the consent of the patient and sometimes her husband, although the latter rule is being challenged. If there is no medical necessity, the operation is termed *sterilization of convenience* or *contraceptive sterilization*. In some states, this is illegal; in others, it is arguable. Only a few states regulate non-therapeutic sterilization. Here, too, consents are often required from the individual and spouse and there may be a mandatory waiting period. The consequences of the operation must be made clear to all concerned, and often a special consent form is required. Some physicians have been advised not to perform sterilizations if the law is not clear. There seems to be little legal concern about male sterilization, *vasectomy*, which is being done with increasing frequency. The legal consequences of unsuccessful sterilization, both male and female, have resulted in suits. Called *wrongful birth*, these suits usually seek to recover the costs of raising an unplanned or unwanted child, normal or abnormal—but usually the latter. Judgments have varied, but are more likely to favor the plaintiff if the child is abnormal. The tort, *wrongful life*, refers to the birth of babies with serious diseases and disabilities. Wrongful life suits claim that the infant plaintiff was harmed by being born. It is maintained that when a child's existence is so miserable that he or she would have been better off unborn, the child has been both wronged and harmed.[46]

Eugenic sterilization is the attempt to eliminate specific hereditary defects by sterilizing individuals who could pass on such defects to their offspring. Once, approximately half the states authorized eugenic sterilization of the mentally deficient, mentally ill, and others, but since the case mentioned earlier, only a few do so; in fact, judges have refused to grant permission in the absence of a law. There have also been suits after sterilization. Legality where no law exists is questionable; civil or criminal liability for assault and battery may be imposed on anyone sterilizing another without following legal procedure or specific legal guidelines.

Laws on family planning, in general, also vary greatly. Some laws appear to be absolute prohibitions against information about contraceptive materials, but courts usually allow some freedom. It is important, however, that the information be complete and accurate. Nurses are particularly involved; they do much of this counseling, either as specialists or as part of their general nursing role. Moreover, new contraceptive drugs require continual updating. Because there are still some state limitations and, as noted, the federal government is becoming more involved, it is important for the nurse to keep up to date in this area of policy.

Artificial insemination, the injection of seminal fluid by instrument into a female to induce pregnancy, has evolved into an acceptable medical procedure used by childless couples. (Consent by the husband and wife is generally required.) Homologous artificial insemination (AIH) uses the semen of the husband and appears to present no legal dangers for doctors or nurses. Heterologous artificial insemination (AID) uses the semen of someone other than the husband and does raise the question of the child's legitimacy. On occasion, the question of adultery also arises in the courts if the husband's consent has not been obtained. Few states have enacted statutes to deal with the AID situation. When a woman, for a fee, is artificially inseminated with a man's sperm and bears a child, who is then turned over to the man and his wife, this is termed *surrogate motherhood*. It has already created some legal problems, such as when the woman decided not to give up the child and again when neither wanted a baby born with a birth defect.

One case in which the surrogate refused to give up the baby became a news sensation and stimulated some legislatures to introduce bills that, more often than not, would make surrogate motherhood for profit illegal. In the Baby M case, the New Jersey Supreme Court eventually awarded custody of the child to the natural father and his wife who had contracted for the baby, but the natural mother was given visiting rights somewhat like those in a divorce case. Not everyone thought that was best for the baby, but other decisions appear to be going in that direction as well. Equitable laws seem to be slow in coming, although badly needed.[47]

Among the most controversial legal concerns related to reproduction are the issues of in vitro fertilization and surrogate embryo transfer, each of which is intended to enhance the fertility of infertile couples. Other questions are being raised, such as, will the government put restrictions on such techniques as embryo freezing? (There has already been a case in which frozen embryos were awarded to a woman in a divorce settlement, somewhat like a child!) What about collecting sperm from a brain-dead patient? What of the trend of (very) multiple births?

■ RIGHTS AND RESPONSIBILITIES OF STUDENTS

Most legislation and judicial decisions affecting education can be applied to nursing education as well. Every approved school of professional nursing must meet the criteria for approval set by the state board of nursing, a legally appointed body found in every state, sometimes under a different name. The state-approved school must conduct an educational program that will prepare its graduates to take state board examinations and become licensed to practice as RNs. No matter where the students receive education and experience, the nursing school is still responsible for the content of the course of study.

The board's minimum standards require the school to provide a faculty competent to teach students to practice nursing skillfully and safely. Students are expected to be under the supervision of a faculty member who is also an RN, and the school and teacher are responsible, with the student, for the student's errors. As discussed in Chapter 21, most legal experts hold that when students give patient care, they are, for legal purposes, considered employees of the hospital or agency. They are liable for their own negligence if injury results, and the institution and faculty will also be liable for the harm suffered. Carrying malpractice insurance is a wise precaution, and many schools recommend or require its purchase by all students. Many state student nurses' associations offer low-cost insurance with membership.

State laws governing the practice of nursing vary widely and are subject to misinterpretation by the employing agency. Most laws classify students working part time as employees. In this capacity, students performing tasks requiring more judgment and skills than the position for which they are employed are subject not only to civil suits, but also to criminal charges for practicing without a license.

Traditionally, the relationship of institutions of higher education to a student under 18 years of age had been that of *in loco parentis*, which means that the school stands "in the place of the parent" and has the right to exercise similar authority over the student's physical, intellectual, and moral training. Since the early 1960s, courts have overturned this concept, and it is no longer considered to have much legal validity. However, the student's enrollment in a particular college generally is an implied contract, which requires that the student live up to the reasonable academic and moral standards of the college, with the school also having certain responsibilities. For instance, if the student lives in a dormitory associated with the school, it must meet safety and sanitation standards established by local regulations. However, the school rarely assumes responsibility for the student's loss of personal property.

Undesirable student conduct may result in some discipline, including suspension or expulsion, and there has been considerable disagreement on the school's power in such circumstances. Generally, it is expected that the school's rules of conduct are made public and that the student has the right to a public hearing and due process. Legal rulings may be different when applied to private or public universities. Private universities have greater power in many ways, particularly if they do not accept federal

monies directly, which then exempts them from certain federal laws such as the Rehabilitation Act of 1973.

Students most frequently cite Constitutional rights in complaints: the First Amendment (freedom of speech, religion, association, expression); the Fourth Amendment (freedom from illegal search and seizure); and the Fifth and Fourteenth Amendments (due process of law). The courts recognize the student first as a citizen, so that they will consider possible infringements of these rights. Most commonly, First Amendment rights involve dress codes and personal appearance. Although schools do not possess absolute authority over students in this sense, some lower court rulings have approved the establishment of dress codes necessary for cleanliness, safety, and health. Beginning with *Dixon v. Alabama State Board of Education* in 1961, random, unannounced searches that schools had carried out previously were no longer allowed without student permission or a search warrant; otherwise, evidence found is inadmissible in court. In addition, searches made for drugs, if reasonable, have been permitted in certain cases, as has drug testing.

Due process has been a major issue of legal contention, especially since the landmark case of *Dixon v. Alabama State Board of Education* (1961), where several black students were expelled during civil rights activities. They sued and the court held that they had a right to a notice and disciplinary hearings. This ruling was solidified before the US Supreme Court in *Goss et al v. Lopez* (419 US 565 [1975]). In essence, this means that the purpose of the rule or law must be examined for fairness and reasonableness. Is the student and faculty understanding of the rule the same? Did the student have the opportunity to know about the rule and its implications? What is the relationship between the rule and the objectives of the school? A decade ago, few schools had a grievance procedure, and this situation was believed by students to be a serious violation of rights. In 1975, the National Student Nurses' Association (NSNA) developed grievance procedure guidelines as part of a bill of rights for students. This was revised in 2006 and is available at www.nsna.org. Besides suggesting the makeup of the committee (equal representation of students and faculty) and general procedures, such issues as allowing sufficient time, access to information and appropriate records, presentation of evidence, and use of witnesses were included.

The usual steps in any grievance process are also followed for academic grievances, with the formal process consisting of a written complaint and suggested remedy by the student grievant, followed by a written reply, a choice between a private or public hearing, permission for the student to have counsel present, a student's right to remain silent, a hearing with presentation of evidence on both sides, a decision by the committee within a specific time, right of appeal, and sometimes arbitration. With students, the right to continue with classes during the total process is considered necessary, although in nursing, if the situation relates to a clinical problem and the safety of patients is considered at risk, further clinical experience may be put on hold until the matter is settled. In any case, a full and complete record of the hearing should be made. Due process is considered crucial for students who are expelled or suspended for disciplinary reasons or who feel that they are discriminated against because of race, religion, sex, or sexual preferences.

Going through the motions of due process is not enough. In *Jones v. The Board of Governors of the University of North Carolina*, Nancy Jones, a student in the nursing program, allegedly cheated in two different incidents. She went through a number of formal proceedings from a Student Court to the Vice-Chancellor of Academic Affairs, involving also the university's legal counsel. Her original *guilty of academic dishonesty* ruling was variously overturned and reaffirmed. When she was told that she could not return to classes because she now had an F in the course and rules forbid her continuing until it was removed, she filed suit in the federal district court, alleging violation of due process and requested reinstatement until the suit was settled. This was granted, despite the University appealing the decision.

There seem to be an increasing number of grievances filed or legal complaints made because of academic concerns, especially grades. The courts have been reluctant to enter this area of academic freedom. There has yet to be a definitive ruling on curriculum and degree requirements. This attitude is evident as one court issued a highly significant statement (45 Federal Rules Decisions, 133[1968], 136):

> Education is the living and growing source of our progressive civilization, of our open repository of increasing knowledge, culture and our salutory democratic traditions. As such, education deserves the highest respect and the fullest protection of the courts in the performance of its lawful missions. . . . Only when erroneous and unwise actions in the field of education deprive students of federally protected rights or privileges does a federal court have power to intervene in the educational process.[48]

This statement has a number of counterparts in other jurisdictions. A major case involved a female fourth-year medical student who, after receiving many documented warnings, was dismissed because of her attitude in the clinical area, unacceptable personal hygiene, inappropriate bedside manner, and tardiness. However, she had an excellent academic record. She fought this issue to the Supreme Court (in *Board of Curators of the University of Missouri v. Horowitz*) charging violation of her constitutional rights to liberty and property. She lost, in part because her clinical evaluations had been consistently unsatisfactory, she had been given sufficient warning, and the court accepted the faculty's judgment.[49] This was considered an academic case, as opposed to a dismissal for disciplinary reasons. It has implications for nursing. For instance, a nursing student was dismissed in her second year of a community college program for unsafe clinical behavior. After a grievance procedure, in which her dismissal was upheld, she sued, alleging bad faith on the part of the faculty. The court refused to overturn the decision.

Most colleges now have grievance procedures for students who think that they have received unfair grades, and these procedures must be followed first before any lawsuit can be filed. It is generally advised that before the student wages an all-out battle, the situation should be considered practically. The student must prove that the grade is arbitrary, capricious, and manifestly unjust, which is generally very difficult. Furthermore, unless that particular grade is extremely important to a student's career, the cost and time involved are greater than even a favorable result might warrant.

Cases in which the results have been more favorable to the student are related to inadequate advisement and the school catalog as a written contract. In the latter situation, a case that went to the Supreme Court (*Russell v. Salve Regina*) related to an obese woman who was admitted to a nursing program and did well. However, because she did not lose weight as agreed to in a *side contract*, she was asked to withdraw before her senior year. She transferred to another college, eventually graduated, and attained licensure. Then she sued with a variety of allegations, including contract violation. After a number of appeals, she was awarded a year's salary and additional costs for obtaining her baccalaureate. The court also commented negatively on how the faculty had treated her about her obesity. This case had a number of other interesting points of law. Earlier, also in relation to a contract issue, a landmark case was heard by the Supreme Court, which ruled that an all-women's nursing school could not refuse to admit a male student.

(In a non-nursing situation, two military schools of higher education were forced to admit women.) There were also a number of other nursing cases related to discrimination in admission and readmission.[50]

Because those schools receiving federal money directly are subject to federal laws, the Americans with Disabilities Act of 1990, the Civil Rights Restoration Act of 1987, and Section 504 of the Rehabilitation Act of 1973 created rights for students with disabilities. In one case, a prospective student with a severe hearing problem sued because she was not admitted to a community college nursing program. The court upheld the school's decision because the applicant's hearing disability made it unsafe for her to practice as a nurse. At another school, an applicant with Crohn's disease was refused because her disease process would probably cause her to miss too many classes. Although the court required the school to admit the student, the decision was later overturned on a procedural issue. In other disciplines, students have been dismissed because of contracting tuberculosis, AIDS, and other diseases; this may yet occur in nursing.

Another type of student right involves school records. The types of student records kept by schools vary. They may consist of only the academic transcript, or they may include extracurricular activities and problem situations, which are kept in an informal file. The enactment of the Buckley Amendment, described in Chapter 19, has clarified the issue of student access to records. The individual loses the right to confidentiality by waiving the right or by disclosing the information to a third person. A student's academic transcript is the most common document released, particularly to other schools and employers.

KEY POINTS

1. Patients are beginning to assert themselves in demanding their legal rights, and generally courts are supporting them.
2. To have a legal informed consent, the patient must be competent and not coerced; the process must include an explanation of the condition, the proposed treatment, alternatives, and dangers or benefits.
3. Nurses are not legally responsible for getting consents, but they should try to be sure that the patient knows to what he or she has consented.
4. When witnessing a document, it is important for the nurse to know if she or he is attesting to the signature or the content of the document.
5. Confused, retarded, or mentally ill patients may still have the ability to decide whether to consent to or refuse treatment.
6. Court decisions, statutory and administrative law, and organizational actions seem to be favoring the patient's right to die.
7. The living will is designed to allow individuals to express to their families, health care providers, and institutions in advance their desires about their care if they are later not able to do so.
8. Effective palliative care requires relief from pain, human support, and attention to the spiritual needs of the patient.
9. Death is determined by *brain death*, which indicates the unresponsiveness of the brain stem.
10. Legal issues related to abortion, sterilization, family planning, and artificial insemination are becoming more complex as technology offers new options and as advocates for or against certain points of view become more aggressive.
11. The law is changing rapidly in relation to the rights of children and the mentally ill.
12. Even though an action is intended for the patients' own good, forcing them to do something can be considered assault or battery.
13. The grievance procedure is necessary in settling disputes in the educational setting.

REFERENCES

1. President's Commission for the Study of Ethical Problems in Medicine and Biomedical and Behavioral Research. *Making Health Care Decisions.* Washington, DC: Government Printing Office, 1982, pp 2–3.
2. Douglas S, Green D, MacJenzie C. Nuances of informed consent. *Hospital for Special Surgery Journal* 3(1):115–118, February 2007.
3. The University of Washington School of Medicine. Ethics in Medicine. April 11, 2008. http://depts.washington.edu/bioethx/topics/consent.html#ques1. Retrieved June 1, 2010.

4. President's Commission, loc cit.

5. Ethics in Medicine, loc cit.

6. Berg J, Appelbaum P, Lidz C, Parker L. *Informed Consent*, 2nd ed. New York: Oxford University Press, 2001.

7. Center for Bloodless Medicine and Surgery. Understanding *Jehovah's Witnesses* and Their View of Blood Products. http://www. bloodlessmedicine.org/professionals/jehovahs-witnesses-blood-products.php. Retrieved June 1, 2010.

8. Elger B, Harding T. Terminally ill patients and Jehovah's Witnesses: Teaching acceptance of patients' refusals of vital treatments. *Med Educ* 36(5):479–488, May 2002.

9. American Academy of Pediatrics, Committee on Bioethics. Religious exemptions from child abuse satutes. *Pediatrics* 81(1):169–171, January 1988.

10. President's Commission, op cit, p 147.

11. Westrick S, Dempski K. *Essentials of Nursing Law and Ethics*. Dudbury, MA: Jones and Bartlett, 2009.

12. Veatch R. The evolution of death and dying controversies. *Hastings Center Report* 39(3):16–19, May–June 2009.

13. Morenski J, Oro J, Tobias J, Singh A. Determination of death by neurological criteria. *J Intensive Care Med* 18(4):211–221, 2003.

14 Truog R. Is it time to abandon brain death? *Hastings Ctr Report* 27(1):29–37, January–February 1997.

15. Moreno. Case puts Texas futile treatment law under a microscope. *The Washington Post*. April 11, 2007. http://www.washingtonpost.com/wpdyn/content/article/2007/04/10. Retrieved June 1, 2010.

16. Truog. Tackling medical futility. *New Engl J Med* 357(1): 1–3. July 5, 2007.

17. ANA. Position Statements: Foregoing Nutrition and Hydration. http://nursingworld.org/readroom/position/ethics/etnutr.htm. Retrieved May 20, 2010.

18. Sedensky M. Five years after Terri Schiavo. *The Miami Herald*. March 30, 2010. http://www.miamiherald.com. Retrieved June 1, 2010.

19. Mitty E. Ethnicity and end-of-life decision-making. *Reflect Nurs Leadership* 27(1):28–31, 46, 2001.

20. American Bar Association. Who Gets to Decide? http://www.abanet.org/adminlaw/midyear2005/tab9.pdf. Retrieved June 1, 2010.

21. Wanzer S, Federman D, Adelstein S, et al. The physician's responsibility toward hopelessly ill patients. *N Engl J Med* 310:955–959, April 12, 1984.

22. Gross J. Quiet doctor finds a mission in assisted suicide court case. *The New York Times*, January 2, 1997, pp B1, B4.

23. Rachels J. Active and passive euthanasia. *N Engl J Med* 292(2):78–80, January 9, 1975.

24. Asch DA. The role of critical care nurses in euthanasia and assisted suicide. *New Engl J Med* 334:1374–1379, 1996.

25. Matzo ML, Schwarz JK. In their own words: Oncology nurses respond to patient requests for assisted suicide and euthanasia. *Appl Nurs Res* 14:64–71, 2001.

26. Ganzini L, Harvath TA, Jackson A, Goy ER, Miller LL, Delorit MA. Experiences of Oregon nurses and social workers with hospice patients who requested assistance with suicide. *N Engl J Med* 347:582–588, 2002.

27. Ferrell B, Virani R, Grant M, Coyne P, Uman G. Beyond the Supreme Court decision: Nursing perspectives on end-of-life care. *Oncol Nurs Forum* 27:445–455, 2000.

28. Euthanasia, Suicide and Physician-Assisted Suicide: Assisted Suicide's Detractors. http://www.libraryindex.com/pages/3123/Suicide-Euthanasia-Physician-Assisted-Suicide-ASSISTED-SUICIDE-S-DETRACTORS.html. Retrieved June 1, 2010.

29. State of Oregon. Death with Dignity Act: Records and Reports. http://oregon.gov/DHS/ph/pas/index.shtml. Retrieved June1, 2010.

30. Federal Judge Upholds Oregon's Assisted Suicide. April 17, 2002. http://www.cnn.com/2002/LAW/04/17/oregon.assisted.suicide/. Retrieved August 20, 2002.

31. State of Oregon, loc cit.

32. State Laws on Assisted Suicide. January 4, 2010. http://euthanasia.procon.org/view.resource.php?resourceID=000132. Retrieved June 1, 2010.

33. International Task Force on Euthanasia and Assisted Suicide. http://www.internationaltaskforce.org/holland.htm. Retrieved June 1, 2010.

34. Pritchard R, Fisher E, Teno J, Sharp S, Reding D, Knaus W, Wennberg J, Lynn J. Influence of patient preferences and local health system characteristics on the place of death. SUPPORT Investigators. Study to Understand Prognoses and Preferences for Risks and Outcomes of Treatment. *J Am Geriatr Soc* 46(10):1320–1321, October 1998.

35. ANA. Position Statements: Pain Management and Control of Distressing Symptoms in Dying Patients. http://nursingworld.org. Retrieved June 1, 2010.

36. Uniform Anatomical Gift Act. Enactment Status. May 6, 2010. http://www.anatomicalgiftact.org/DesktopDefault.aspx?tabindex=2&tabid=72. Retrieved June 1, 2010.

37. Childress J. The failure to give: Reducing barriers to organ donation. *Kennedy Inst Ethics J* 11(1):1–16, March 2001.

38. United Network for Organ Sharing. http://www.unos.org. Retrieved June 1, 2010.

39. Cole R. *Rogers v. Okin*: A lawsuit to guarantee patients' right to refuse anti-psychotic medication. *Am J Forensic Psychiatry* 1(1):104–173, May 1978.

40. Ross L. Health care decision-making by children: Is it in their best interest? *Hastings Ctr Report* 27:41–42, November–December 1997.

41. Ibid, pp 41–45.

42. Weir R, Peters C. Affirming the decisions adolescents make about life and death. *Hastings Ctr Report* 27:30, November–December 1997.

43. Ibid.

44. Morrow J. Making mortal decisions at the beginning of life: The case of impaired and imperiled infants. *JAMA* 284:1146–1147, 2000.

45. Greenhouse L. Justices uphold patient privacy with therapist. *The New York Times*, June 14, 1996, pp A1, A25.

46. Steinbock B, McClamrock R. When is birth unfair to the child? *Hastings Ctr Report* 24:15–21, November–December 1994.

47. Capron A. Horton hatches the egg. *Hastings Ctr Report* 25:30–31, September–October 1995.

48. Forsyth D, Rubin Z. Conducting research on academic dishonesty. *Ethics Behav* 11(3):356–363, March 2001.

49. Ibid.

50. Kinma M. Discrimination in nursing. *Int Nurs Rev* 46(3):87–90, January 2003.

HELPFUL WEBSITES FOR PART II, SECTION FIVE

ANA: http://www.nursingworld.org

Cleveland Clinic, Department of Bioethics: http://www.clevelandclinic.org/bioethics

CNN News: http://www.cnn.com

FirstGov (gateway to government information): http://www.firstgov.gov

National Student Nurse Association: http://www.nsna.org

Partnership for Caring (Help with End-of-Life Decisions): http://www.partnershipforcaring.org

Physicians for Compassionate Care: http://www.pccef.org/press

Reuters (International News): http://www.reuters.com

Supreme Court of the United States: http://www.supremecourtus.gov

United Network for Organ Sharing (UNOS): http://www.unos.org

University of Pennsylvania: http://bioethics.net

University of Washington School of Medicine, Ethics in Medicine: http://eduserv.hscer.washington.edu/bioethics

US Commission on Civil Rights: http://www.usccr.gov

Updates can be found at **www.kellysnursing.com**

PART III

Professional Components and Career Development

Nursing Organizations

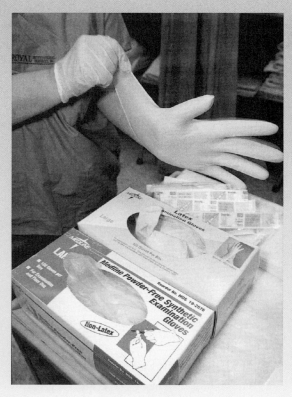
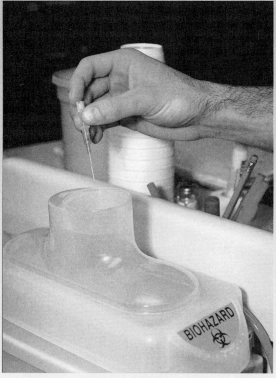

The work of organized nursing has frequently been to protect nurses.
(Courtesy of the American Nurses Association, Washington, DC)

Organizational Procedures and Issues

The more complex and highly organized society becomes, the harder it is for an individual to exert any significant influence or power. There are exceptions to this rule, of course. There will always be pioneers and crusaders—individuals who, through sheer force of personality, conviction, and determination, succeed in making an impact. However, by and large, the concerted effort of a group of people working in an organized manner is necessary today to accomplish a given purpose, to effect a change in the status quo.

This is as true in nursing as in any other field on both student and graduate levels. One student alone, for instance, can do little to change what may seem to be the out-of-date or autocratic practices of the nursing school administration, but working through the student association in the school or through a unit of the National Student Nurses' Association (NSNA), she or he may very well bring about improvements. Similarly, one nurse, no matter how dedicated or determined, would never have been able to make it easier and less expensive for older citizens to get needed hospital and medical care. Yet the strong voice of the American Nurses Association (ANA), speaking out in favor of health insurance coverage for the aging under the Social Security system, was one of the forces that brought about Medicare. ANA took this stand because the majority of its members indicated that this was what they wanted. So, working through the professional organization, the individual was heard, did have influence, and did help to bring about change.

There are many persons who are inclined to do nothing more than grumble to themselves and others about what they do not like or what they would like to see accomplished. But so long as they do no more than complain, and unless they join with their colleagues to act in an organized, effective way, they will probably continue to be powerless and dissatisfied.

That does not mean that a person should simply become a *joiner*—someone who seems to become a member of almost any organization. Such a process only scatters the person's interests and energies in many directions and provides no focus. There are many organizations concerned with health and nursing that a nursing student or registered nurse (RN) will want to join, support, or at least be familiar with. By joining some of them, individuals will be able to work with colleagues in advancing not only their own interests, but also those of nursing as a whole; through others, they will find the companionship of those with more specific practice interests.

The nature and purpose of these nursing and health organizations will be discussed in the following chapters. Of concern in this chapter is the nurse's role—or anyone's role, for that matter—as an organization member. Presumably, people join an organization because its concerns and goals are the same as their own. Joining is not enough. An association's success depends on intelligent, industrious, and conscientious leadership; a willing, enthusiastic, and well-informed membership; adequate financial support; and sound business organization and administration. It is the responsibility of each member to help make all of these things realities.

■ MEMBERSHIP RESPONSIBILITIES

Members of any organization should feel responsible for learning as much as possible about the organization—its history, purposes, the number and composition of its membership, and its principal activities. They should study the constitution and bylaws, the code of ethics (if there is one), and subscribe to its official publication. They should learn the names of the organization's principal current officers and preferably their background. When attending meetings, they should listen carefully to the discussion and become familiar with the most important issues under consideration and the conditions and facts that influence the decisions to be taken. This will take time, but spending just a few hours can prepare new members for rewarding participation in the organization's work.

As soon as a person is ready to take a more active part in the meetings, he or she can enter into discussions, ask relevant questions, help clarify issues by presenting a fresh and knowledgeable point of view, accept appointments to committees, and volunteer to help as time and ability dictate. Restraint, diplomacy, and a sense of good timing should guide new members as they find their place in any group.

Individuals who hold or want to hold office should have a copy of authoritative rules of order for organizing and conducting an organization's business and should become familiar enough with the publication so that they can readily find the information needed. Whoever presides over formal business meetings in any other capacity must know how to do so efficiently, without referring to the book of rules, except for an answer to unusually difficult questions. The rules of order used by a particular association are usually named in its bylaws.

Most members do not need to be as familiar as an officer with the minute details of parliamentary procedure, but should know how to address the presiding officer; formulate, present, and vote on a motion; and be familiar with other basic procedures that facilitate the progress of the meeting. This knowledge will enhance their ability to express views and contribute to the discussion without embarrassment or lack of confidence.

On the other hand, it would be naive not to recognize that parliamentary procedure can be used as a manipulative tool to bring about certain action or lack of action. For instance, if an item is not placed on the agenda by the president, other officers, or members, it is not likely to be discussed and certainly not acted on. If the item is placed in an unfavorable position—at the end of a long session when people are less alert, at a point when a certain voting constituency is present for a short time (some bylaws allow any member present to vote), or at a point when certain information is not yet available, or after a controversial,

emotional, related item—the action taken might be quite different than it would be if the topic were discussed at another time. There are also those who misuse the intricacies of parliamentary procedure by complex motions to amend or substitute a motion repeatedly so that the members may be totally confused about the real issue in the motion on which to be voted. Those speaking to a motion may also be deliberately or inadvertently obscure, incorrect, or inappropriate in their statements, which, if the usual procedure of speaking from the floor is observed, may make the point difficult to correct and clarify. (Then there are always those who like to be heard whether or not what they say is pertinent.) Therefore, the average member should be alert to these machinations and learn how to combat them. If a motion seems to have been railroaded through, it is particularly useful to know how that action can be reversed before the final adjournment. Because any organization has its political aspects, those who are interested in seeing that a certain action is taken seldom take a chance on this simply occurring during a business meeting. An effort is made to sell individuals or subgroups within the organization on the idea before formal action is taken—that is, lobbying. The formal action can be orchestrated: Who makes the motion, who speaks to it, what supporting information must be introduced, is it best referred to a taskforce or committee, and, most important of all, are the votes there? A politically astute member tries to estimate at what point the issue is more likely to be voted in the desired direction, delaying the vote by some form of postponement, if necessary.

■ WHO DOES THE WORK?

Even the most careful plans and the finest constitution and bylaws do not ensure a healthy, productive organization. The plans and directions must be put into action. Who does this? Every officer, every committee member, and every member at large shares the responsibility for knowing what that person as an individual can do for the good of the entire membership and for doing it—unless health or some other serious problem is a deterrent.

An incapacitated officer or committee chair should resign promptly and give the organization the opportunity of deciding whether or not to choose another. Members who accept an appointment to a committee and later find themselves unable to assist with its work should withdraw, leaving the chairman or other authorized person free to appoint another, more productive member.

Members in today's organizations can be categorized as owners, potential owners, the unambitious, or dissidents. The owners of an organization know the system and how to work it; are adept at organizational politics; are the leaders or the supporters of leaders; and make decisions and dispense rewards. The owners are satisfied members, highly involved, and make up about 10 percent of an organization's membership. Potential owners comprise about 50 percent of the membership and are usually too busy to participate in leadership, although they might like to have some kind of organizational power. Potential owners pay dues and may be an untapped bounty for an organization because they have opinions and views that are not sought out but might be important for the organization to have. Dissidents are those who are generally very involved in organizations but are dissatisfied—dissatisfied with leadership, policy, programs, or positions. The dissident often enjoys the role of the contrarian, seeking recognition through opposition. Dissidents comprise about 10 percent of an organization's membership. The fourth category of member is the unambitious. Approximately 30 percent of an organization's members are satisfied with the organization's work but have little involvement in the organization. They would rather "pay than do," shun power, and enjoy watching from afar. They are invaluable to the health of any association, and should know that when, and if, they are ever more disposed toward active involvement, the opportunities will be there for them.

President, Chairperson, Moderator

Although the elected or appointed head of an association does a great deal of work behind the scenes during a term of office, the membership thinks of this person most frequently as the one who presides at meetings. This is one of the most important responsibilities for which a leader needs particular skills, talents, and personality assets.

The individual should be in complete control of emotions; avoid distracting mannerisms; speak clearly; be discreet, impartial, and courteous; have considerable stamina; and be businesslike. However, a good sense of humor is a decided asset. A good leader should be able to sense the atmosphere of a meeting and prevent it from becoming explosive or detrimental to progress. It is even important to be sensitive to the physical comfort of the assembly and to do what is possible to improve ventilation, lighting, seating arrangements, or whatever else is indicated to keep everyone alert and interested. The presiding officer should be prompt for every meeting, ready to function at the appointed time, and, as soon as a quorum is present, call the meeting to order. This encourages habitual latecomers to be on time and helps to ensure prompt adjournment.

The president must have a thorough knowledge of the history of the organization, what it has done in the past, and what it plans to do in the future. Rarely should a question find this person completely unprepared; if the president does not know the answer, he or she should know who does or where it can be found. Sometimes the questions are referred to someone else even if the chair knows the answer. This might happen when a question is asked about the organization's finances and the president asks the treasurer to answer. Any officer must know when it is appropriate to withhold information as well as when to disclose it. It is important always to be in control of the situation and to keep the audience informed about the discussion before the group to avoid the confusion that results when members do not understand the issue.

Generally, the presiding officer should not express a personal opinion on an issue. This is because of the need to maintain a neutral attitude and because one of the chief duties of a leader is to encourage others to participate. It is a good policy to subtly encourage the less assertive member to speak up and discourage the individuals who always want to express their views at length. In doing this, the presiding head must be eminently fair and unbiased, allowing all the right to air their views.

The chair (whoever is presiding, and not necessarily the president) must be thoroughly familiar with the agenda of every meeting over which she or he presides and know how to complete it expeditiously and in accordance with the rules of procedure adopted by the organization. This is learned by studying the rules, observing other presiding officers in action, and experience. Every meeting will bring confidence and learning from successes and failures.

A president may have exhibited considerable ability to lead discussions, but may not have had extensive practice in handling motions, one of the major responsibilities of a presiding officer. Sometimes this is a simple procedure, but it can become involved. The chair who understands the intricacies guides the action deftly and gains the respect of the group; the one who gets confused about what step takes precedence over another, for example, may create a chaotic situation that will leave the members dissatisfied and possibly highly critical. Many organizations have a parliamentarian in attendance to avoid problems, and some others even have a parliamentarian preside at meetings that will have a large volume of formal business.

It is vital to be acquainted with as many members of the organization as possible and to become familiar with their interests and abilities. This will help in making appointments to committees and selecting members for other assignments. If the organization is widespread, visits to several different areas or constituent associations each year are helpful; giving necessary help often stimulates the members in their work. On social occasions the president should mingle with members; this will establish rapport with the various groups and will tend to promote interest and enthusiasm.

The president must keep in touch with the work and progress of other officers and the committees in the organization and cooperate amicably and constructively with them. Democratic principles must be observed, allowing each person to use the initiative and authority necessary to discharge assigned duties and responsibilities without interference while demanding first-rate performance. If the organization has a paid chief staff officer or director and a headquarters staff, the officers must observe the same principles, carrying the appropriate responsibilities but never usurping prerogatives that are rightfully those of the staff.

The head of any organization needs leadership qualities in large measure. Although every individual elected to such an office probably will not possess all of them, there will be many opportunities to develop them.

Vice President

Although, theoretically, a vice president—particularly a first vice president—is as capable as the president, because she or he must be prepared to function in the president's absence or in an emergency, the qualifications tend to be less exacting. Many persons with outstanding leadership ability are unwilling to accept the relatively inactive post of the vice presidency. This happens in organizations of all sizes and types, from a local volunteer group to the federal government.

To make the office more challenging, some associations declare in their bylaws that the vice presidents shall also be heads of committees or assume other responsibilities. Among the most common are chairperson of the program, policy development, or bylaws committees. Vice presidents may also represent the organization in meetings, inter-organizational committees, or taskforces. This gives the vice president an opportunity to make a specific contribution to the organization and also gives visibility. Sometimes large organizations have more than one vice president, all with specific responsibilities.

It is common practice for many organizations to include a president-elect on the board, preparing that person for assumption of the presidential office with minimal orientation. There are some disadvantages: a double-term commitment on the part of that individual and probable inability to prevent that person from succeeding to the presidency if she or he proves to be ineffectual at the board level.

Secretary

The secretary often takes the minutes and may deal with correspondence. If the organization is large enough to have a professional staff, staff does the actual taking of detailed minutes and handling of correspondence, but both are checked and sometimes signed by the secretary, president, or other appropriate person. Nevertheless, the functions of the secretary are spelled out in the bylaws and may be the responsibility of an elected person or duly authorized staff.

In a smaller organization, the secretary who thinks and writes clearly, is well informed about the association's business, and has the necessary knowledge and skill to write appropriate minutes is invaluable. The secretary must be able to keep alert throughout meetings that can be both tedious and frustrating, and maintain an outward attitude of equanimity, neutrality, and cooperation regardless of inner conflicts. The secretary must be objective and impartial in all reports in spite of the fact that at times it is necessary to interpret the interpretations of others when transcribing the notes taken at a meeting. It is important to be methodical, reliable, and prompt in getting out all reports and memoranda. The corresponding secretary needs to be a master of the courteous and appropriate phrase, because these responsibilities have important public relations connotations. Neatness and promptness in correspondence are highly desirable.

Treasurer

It is not unusual for the treasurer of an organization to be selected more carefully than the president, and almost as much is expected. The principal qualifications should be honesty, accuracy, and conscientiousness in keeping records, and knowledge of bookkeeping procedures, budgeting, and financial reporting. Business experience is a decided asset. The membership, even when it knows better, often judges the treasurer's ability by the balance on hand in the treasury.

The treasurer of any organization is often chair of its committee on finance. This post requires the usual skills necessary to conduct a committee meeting plus additional ability to discuss facts and figures intelligently, often before board members who may not be well versed in financial matters but are vitally interested in the organization's purse strings. The president's work is also made easier by a competent treasurer because so many of the organization's activities depend on its financial status. Even if skilled employees carry out the details of the financial management of the organization, the board has fiduciary responsibility for the association. Budgets cannot be properly developed or adhered to and intelligent financial decisions cannot be made, nor a myriad of state and federal reports filed, if accurate information is not available. Therefore, board members and especially the treasurer must have at least a basic understanding of financial management.

Committees

An organization's bylaws usually call for standing committees, with the number depending more on the scope of the activities than on the volume. The bylaws also indicate whether committee members are appointed or elected.

The quantity and quality of work done by each special group greatly influence the status and progress of the organization, although sometimes so indirectly that the general membership is unaware of their extent. For example, the nominating committee is responsible for finding persons who are willing and eligible to fill elected offices and who have the qualifications for them. This requires diligence and excellent salesmanship, especially if the prospective candidate is initially reluctant to serve. In large or widely scattered organizations, many members do not know the candidates personally. They must depend on the nominating committee to select the best available people; they then base their voting decisions on whatever information about them is released through official channels.

Members of the nominating committee, therefore, must always seek the best person or persons regardless of friendships, school ties, personal obligations, or any other influencing factor. And it follows logically that the persons responsible for appointing or electing members of this committee must consider integrity to be one of their most important personal qualifications. Their influence on the future of the organization is considerable: A ballot can be set up in such a way that a certain individual or someone representing a particular constituency is sure to win that

election. This is especially true with a mail ballot, where a strong write-in vote is almost impossible to achieve unless it is highly organized.

The work of other committees often is equally important. Some aspects may be obvious; others may need definition and delineation of responsibilities.

■ PARLIAMENTARY PROCEDURES

The purpose of the business meetings of any organization is to transact business efficiently while recognizing the rights of individual members and giving minority and opposing groups ample opportunity to air their views, yet ensuring that the wishes of the majority prevail. To achieve this purpose, a methodical order of conducting the meetings is essential.

When early American congresses first organized, they borrowed from the British Parliament many practices that they adapted for their own use. Further changes were made from time to time until a distinctive American system evolved. The terms *parliamentary procedure* and (incorrectly) *parliamentary law* are used, however, in referring to both the American and British systems, which still have a good deal in common.

The procedures that have been used for many years by the US Senate and House of Representatives developed from four sources:

1. The Constitution of the United States
2. Jefferson's *Manual of Parliamentary Procedure*, which he prepared while he was vice president and presided over the Senate
3. Rules that have been adopted by the House since its beginning and that may be changed with each Congress; these rules are sometimes called the *legislative manual*
4. Decisions rendered by the presiding officer and the chairman of the Committee of the Whole House

The transactions of less imposing bodies than the US Congress are governed similarly. Each usually has a constitution and bylaws citing the officers and their duties in general, the order of business, voting regulations, and other matters related to the conduct of business meetings. The presiding officer makes decisions consistent with his or her authority, often with the advice of a parliamentarian employed by the organization. Each major meeting of the membership or House of Delegates may produce changes in rules or the formulation of new ones needed to expedite its own activities, and each organization adopts a manual of parliamentary procedure to guide the business transactions.

The most popular guide for formal business procedure is *Robert's Rules of Order, Newly Revised*. This reference work, written by General Henry M. Robert of the US Army and published originally in 1876, is based on the rules and practices of Congress. It is generally considered the most authoritative book of its kind, and some organizations attempt to follow it to the letter. Others use it only as a final authority to settle a controversial point. Still others select simpler but equally reliable rules of order to guide their transactions, such as *Sturgis' Standard Code of Parliamentary Procedure* by Alice F. Sturgis or *Parliamentary Law* by F. M. Gregg. As stated in *Robert's Rules of Order, Newly Revised*,

> The application of parliamentary law is the best method yet devised to enable assemblies of any size, with due regard for every member's opinion, to arrive at the general will on the maximum number of questions of varying complexity in a minimum amount of time and under all kinds of internal climate ranging from total harmony to hardened or impassioned division of opinion.[1]

Although *Robert's Rules of Order* and other such publications include duties of officers and committees and other information, the discussion here will be concerned with the conduct of a business meeting because duties of officers and other details are defined in an organization's constitution and bylaws, which supersede any other rules.

Some of the principles and techniques of parliamentary procedure can perhaps be best presented by following an imaginary annual meeting of the National Student Nurses' Association (NSNA) from beginning to end. This organization, described in Chapter 24 , is the membership organization for nursing students. When the NSNA bylaws do not specify a procedure, *Robert's Rules of Order, Newly Revised* is used as a guide.

Most formal meetings have an order of business. A classic example follows:

1. Call to order
2. Minutes of previous meetings
3. Reports of executive staff, officers, board, and standing committees
   a. Executive reports (executive director/chief-of-staff)
   b. Executive announcements
   c. Order of reports
      i. President
      ii. Vice president
      iii. Secretary
      iv. Treasurer
      v. Board of directors
      vi. Standing committees
4. Reports of special committees
5. Announcements
6. Unfinished business
7. New business
8. Adjournment

In this meeting, these steps will be considered one at a time and others that are often included in the order of business may be added.

Although the following discussion implies that the NSNA's business is completed in one session, it generally takes several sessions to finish. This is usual at business (convention) meetings and may be required in the bylaws by certain wording, such as the need for the nominating committee to report the ticket at a certain time.

An order of business must be flexible enough to be realistic. For example, if there is good reason for having the reports of special committees given ahead of the standing committees, the *president is privileged* to make that change simply by announcing it from the chair. The president is also privileged to make announcements or have others make them and to invite the headquarters staff members and guests to address the assembly whenever it appears appropriate and helpful. A major reordering of the agenda by the presiding officer or another member may require approval of the total group.

Call to Order

The president calls the meeting to order by rapping a gavel for attention if necessary and saying, "Will the meeting please come to order?" or words to that effect. The secretary then presents the agenda for the meeting and the parliamentarian explains the basic rules of parliamentary procedure that will be followed.

To make sure that a *quorum* (as defined in the NSNA bylaws) is present, the president asks the secretary to call a roll of delegates. If a quorum is present, the president so states, or the president may declare a recess or fill in the time with matters of a nonbusiness nature until enough members arrive.

Minutes of the Preceding Meeting

Although the NSNA's secretary keeps accurate and complete files on all business transacted at every meeting of the association, it is highly improbable that minutes of the association's last meeting will be read, because these would be long, detailed, and time-consuming. So, in lieu of reading the minutes, most large membership organizations distribute mimeographed copies of the previous meeting's minutes or make them available on request.

However, in meetings of smaller groups within the NSNA, such as the executive board or one of the committees, the second step in the order of business could be the reading of the minutes of the preceding meeting. This is done by the secretary at the request of the chairman or silently by the members. It is also possible that minutes will have been distributed and read before the meeting. When this is finished, the chair asks the members if they wish to make any additions or corrections. A member wishing to make a change rises (or remains seated as may be the custom) and after being recognized makes a statement that might be something like this: "Madame Chair, my name is Helen Gibson [or simply 'Helen Gibson'], Kentucky. The secretary reported that the president of the New Jersey association moved that the executive board investigate the feasibility of promoting a national student nurse week. The motion was actually made by the president of the New York State association."

Small groups in which members know each other may not need to identify themselves. Nonetheless, it is correct parliamentary procedure. The chairman and the recording secretary must know who is speaking and other members like to know.

The president says "thank you" to the member and asks the secretary to change the record, unless someone contradicts the correction. When all requests for corrections, additions, or deletions have been made, the president states, "The minutes will be (or are) accepted as corrected." If no changes are indicated, she says, "The minutes will be (or are) accepted as read."

Report of the President

The president usually presents her/his own report but has the privilege of asking the secretary or someone else to read it. If presenting it personally, she or he will ask the first vice president to take the chair until the report is completed. This is because correct parliamentary procedure requires that a meeting must always have a presiding officer and the president cannot preside and present a report at the same time.

Although the president's report may contain some facts and figures, it is not usually a business report. Rather, it is of a general nature and greatly influenced by the president's personality. Included will be an account of the progress made by the association during the past year, the satisfactions and perhaps the disappointments; some of the things done while president, such as visiting state nurses' associations and speaking at meetings; plans and ambitions for the future with implied and possibly formulated recommendations based on needs as the president sees them; and expressions of appreciation to others for their support and assistance.

No formal acceptance procedure of the president's report is indicated. If reports are not captured electronically, a copy is given to the secretary for the record and the president resumes the chair.

Report of the Secretary

The secretary's report includes information about his or her personal activities in the office, stressing the broad scope of official duties. When the report has been completed, the president accepts it as presented without asking for a vote by the delegates.

Report of the Treasurer

The treasurer's report is a statement showing the income and expenses of the association during the past year and its financial status at the end of the fiscal year. When the treasurer has finished presenting the report, the president says, "The treasurer's report is accepted as presented," and may add, "and it is filed for audit."

Any questions about the treasurer's report should be asked at this time. The president may reply or may ask the treasurer to do so. General discussion is permitted at the president's discretion.

Report of the Committee on Nominations

Much of the work of the nominating committee—deciding on appropriate candidates for office, securing their permission to be nominated, and compiling their biographies—is done prior to the annual meeting. At the meeting, the chairperson (sometimes simply called *chair*) of the nominating committee, when called on by the president, reads the slate of officers to the assembly. When finished, she or he says, "Madame President, I move the adoption of this slate of officers." The president then asks the house if there are other nominations. If there are none, a delegate will move that the nominations be closed. This motion will be seconded and voted on promptly.

Any delegate can make a nomination from the floor by addressing the chair, naming the proposed candidate, and giving briefly the proposed nominee's qualifications for the post. A special form supplied by the nominating committee, containing detailed information about the candidate, is submitted to the nominating committee if the nomination is seconded. Nominations from the floor are closed by house vote.

Following the meeting, the nominating committee reviews the information about candidates who were nominated from the floor and may post their names and offices for which they are candidates near the voting place where balloting is done. It is also possible that a convention paper or other form of written communication will be distributed to members with election information and the nominees' names and qualifications. It may or may not be possible to have the new names printed on the ballot in time for the election. If not, the delegates wishing to vote for them may write in the names.

Voting is done at a time and place designated by the executive board. Delegates must present credentials before they are allowed to vote. When voting is completed—usually within a few hours—the tellers who were appointed by the president at the first meeting count the ballots and prepare a report to be given at the NSNA's closing business session. A plurality vote (more votes than any other candidate for the same office) is required for election by the NSNA. If a majority vote were required, a candidate would need at least one more than half the votes cast to be elected.

Reports of Other Committees

As the NSNA president calls for reports of the association's other committees, the chairperson of each goes to the platform—if invited by the president—or to a microphone or other place where she or he can be seen and heard easily by the entire assembly, addresses the chair, and presents the report. If any action is to be taken (usually recommendations), the committee chair or someone else says, "Madame President, I move the acceptance of this report" or "adoption of the recommendation." A delegate may second the motion, and the motion is handled like any other. If no action is required on any sections of the report, the preceding step may be omitted and the president will

thank the reporting person. At times, reports are presented in a book of reports and are not read if the business of the committee does not appear controversial or call for action. They can still be discussed, however, if members desire.

Unfinished Business

At this point the president makes sure that any items of business left incomplete because of time limitations, absent persons, and so on, are satisfactorily completed.

New Business

New business is often the most interesting and exciting part of the agenda. If the issues are controversial, debate may be heated and lengthy. Even if they are not, the topics discussed indicate the course the association will take during the months ahead.

Resolutions

Resolutions may be one of the most important parts of a major meeting, because they are indications of the organization's position on key issues. Resolutions are submitted by individual members, groups, or committees within the organization to a resolutions committee or the board of directors. A resolutions committee may, usually with the permission of the originators, combine similar resolutions or change some aspect of a resolution.

The board has the privilege of supporting or not supporting the resolution, and in some organizations it can withhold it from the voting body. Some organizations hold preliminary hearings to expedite action or agreement without the formality of strict parliamentary procedure. This often clarifies misunderstandings and saves time during the business meeting. Generally, a member whose resolution has been rejected for presentation has the right to introduce it from the floor.

Resolutions, except courtesy resolutions, are often meant to be acted on by the organization after the meeting. For instance, a resolution may call for a letter to the President of the United States requesting better federal funding of nursing education, or it could direct long-term activities of the organization. Although the wording is often formal, with one or more whereas clauses giving the reasons for the resolution preceding the resolution, there is no reason why the wording cannot be clear and concise, so that the message is understood by all. Reviewing the past resolutions of an organization gives an excellent picture of its philosophy and goals and is one means of judging its quality.

Therefore, although resolutions frequently come toward the end of a meeting, they should be given thought before voting.

Adjournment

After the amenities have been observed, such as the passing of other resolutions expressing appreciation for services and courtesies, and perhaps introduction of the new officers, the meeting is adjourned by motion and vote.

■ MANAGING MOTIONS

The work of a business session goes much better if officers and members know and practice the proper methods of handling motions according to parliamentary procedure. A motion is a proposal or suggestion intended to initiate action, effect progress, or allow the assembly to express itself as holding certain views. It is through these motions—made, seconded, discussed, and approved by a majority of the delegates—that the association is enabled to transact its business, make decisions, and move forward.

Uncomplicated motions may be passed very quickly by silent assent, such as accepting the secretary's report as read or by *viva voce*, which means a voice vote or responding *aye* or *no* (*yea* or *nay*) in response to a request from the presiding officer; *viva voce* may also be used in voting on involved issues. However, if the vote is or is likely to be close, the chair will ask for a show of hands or a standing vote, because they permit an actual count. Some organizations now use electronic systems to give an instant count, which saves time and arguments about accuracy. A written vote, or ballot, may be indicated and is usually required for elections.

To Make a Motion

A member who wishes to make a motion always

1. Stands and goes to the microphone when indicated.
2. Waits, if necessary, until the speaker ahead has stopped talking. In general, it is advisable to remain seated until the previous speaker has finished, but if several members have motions to present, it is better to get in line.
3. Waits for the chair's signal to go ahead. This may be done with a nod of the head or verbally.
4. Addresses the presiding officer as Madame (or Mister) Chairman, Chairperson, President, or Speaker.

5. Identifies oneself by name and state or other designation as indicated. Sometimes stating the name of the office held, the committee, or some other affiliation is appropriate.
6. States the motion clearly and succinctly. When time permits, it is a good idea to write out a motion before rising to make it. This helps the individual say what is intended and also to repeat it verbatim, if requested. Frequently, it is required that the motion be written and forwarded to the secretary before it is read by the chair; this provides more assurance that the motion will be recorded accurately, and that it is correctly presented to the membership.

Most motions require seconding before action. The chair will call for a second, if indicated. The member who does the seconding rises (if custom), addresses the chair, and after identification, says, "I second the motion." If no one seconds a motion calling for seconding, the motion is automatically lost and the president so states. No mention of it is made in the official records.

Discussion

Assuming that a motion is seconded, the chair next says, "It has been moved and seconded that . . . Is there any discussion?" If there is none, she or he asks for a vote by one of the methods previously mentioned. A member wishing to ask a question or make a comment follows the usual procedure for recognition.

Sometimes discussion is prolonged, heated, and confused, involving proposed amendments to the original motion and perhaps even amendments to the amendment, known as subsidiary amendments. The presiding officer must be fair and skillful to permit all persons to express their views and yet not seriously impede the progress of the meeting. The action must then be guided back to the original motion, disposing of the last mentioned items first.

Discussion of a motion may be terminated if a member calls for "the question." This means that the member feels that the matter has been discussed sufficiently for the members to vote intelligently on it. Because terminating the discussion without the approval of the assembly would infringe on the privilege of unlimited debate, the chair then asks, "Are you ready for the question?" If a sufficient number, as predetermined by the association's rules of order, vote in the affirmative, the motion is put to a vote. Otherwise, debate must be reopened or some other method must be used to handle the motion before the house.

Decision

The ultimate disposition of a motion depends on the majority decision of the delegates. If more than half of them vote *yes*, it is passed; if the majority vote *no*, the motion is, of course, defeated. Sometimes a motion is passed "as amended," that is, not in its original form, but with one or more changes in it, or additions to it, as proposed from the floor during the discussion. Some organizations require a two-thirds vote for passage of a motion or of motions in certain areas. These requirements are spelled out in the association's bylaws.

When there is obvious conflict or confusion about a particular motion, especially when it may have become complicated or unclear as a result of several proposed amendments, a motion to refer it to a committee may be made. This motion in itself may be debated. If it is passed, then the original motion goes to an appropriate committee for further study and possible presentation at some later date.

It is also possible to vote to table a motion; this means that it is set aside temporarily, permitting the chair to move on with the agenda, but will be taken up again later in the same session or meeting. A vote to postpone action on the motion until some other time may also be taken. Decisions to table or postpone action on a motion are most likely to be made when the matter at hand is a complicated or hotly debated issue.

Any of these actions gives the members more time to clarify their thinking about the motion. It also permits more time to marshal arguments pro and con and, finally, permits the president, possibly aided by the parliamentarian, to study the motion so that at some later date it may be reviewed clearly for the delegates. Sometimes a tabled motion never comes for action again, because everyone agrees that it is better not acted on (or it is forgotten).

Occasionally, members pass a motion that they later regret, either because the decision was made hastily, with incomplete information, or in a state of confusion. To bring that same motion before the assembly again, an individual voting on the prevailing side may move to reconsider. Anyone can second. The motion to reconsider takes precedence over other motions, and therefore is acted on at once, regardless of what else is being discussed. It is debatable, and if passed, the entire issue of the previously passed motion is open for discussion, with the opportunity to clarify or to introduce needed information. It is then handled in the usual manner.

The responsible member and, especially, the officer of any organization will not want to depend on this necessarily brief presentation of parliamentary procedure as the sole guide to informed action. If a meeting is not run efficiently and fairly, members become rapidly disenchanted with the entire organization. Meetings may be the only way in which members participate in the decision-making process of the organization, and if they see it as disorganized or a setup, many will withdraw completely. The knowledge and skill of both officers and members are required to ensure that meetings are conducted as they should be, so that the voice of the members prevails.

■ MEMBER–STAFF RELATIONSHIPS

As nursing organizations grow larger, many acquire professional staff, supported by clerical and sometimes technical assistants. In the past, an executive secretary was a retired member of a nursing association, untutored in association management, who learned on the job. Today, the professional executive is seen as essential because she or he deals with complex issues, policies, structure, and human and financial resources, and, frequently, thousands of volunteers.

Although the professional staff of nursing associations may consist of nurses, members of the same organization, with voting and office holding rights, the role is different. The members make policy through the volunteer board and officers; the staff carries out policy. Because volunteers are transient—a board of directors inevitably changes after each election—it is often only the staff that provides continuity. Yet, should their opinions as to a certain action be in direct opposition to the board or committee's, unless they can sell their point of view, it is the staff's responsibility to do what the volunteers decide. Staff may try very hard, directly or indirectly, to influence the key members of the organization.

Many members do not have a clear concept of the careful balance needed between board and staff lines of authority and responsibility. Just as volunteers should expect to devote an adequate amount of time to the association and bring to it the same amount of intellectual commitment and judgment used in their professional pursuits, staff members are expected to provide not just services but leadership, and must create confidence in their judgment and in the program. Staff is expected to synthesize and analyze issues and prepare materials and options for decision making so that volunteers' time is not wasted and they can react to specifics, not generalities. Staff and volunteers should regard each other as valuable colleagues with whom bad news as well as good news is shared. Staff must learn to identify the special abilities of volunteers so that they are put to use.

It is also important that staff identify their roles, responsibilities, and activities, so that expectations are real. Volunteers should not get involved in what is not their responsibility. An executive director (ED) manages the office and personnel. When volunteers attempt to interfere in personnel matters, problems inevitably result. If the ED is incompetent, the board should terminate her or him.

The ED is an employee of the board, the only employee of the board. Often a search committee reviews and selects candidates to recommend to the board. Criteria for selection should be carefully thought through to meet the needs of that organization. A study done by the Foundation of the American Society of Association Executives noted that the qualities considered most important for a successful association executive for the twenty-first century are sevenfold. First, the association executive must have a desire to serve others manifested through a commitment to board, staff, members, and external publics. A vision of the future and the ability to succeed through change, forge partnerships, and manage information and technology are also key ingredients for success. Dealing with diversity and maintaining a personal and professional life balance are necessary qualities of the association executive. The most significant point to remember in staff–volunteer relationships is that it is a partnership; both are supposed to be working toward the same goals, and when there are unusual tensions between the two, it is often the result of misunderstanding or disagreement on how these goals are to be achieved. As in any other professional and human relationship, good communication is essential.

Issues and Concerns

Probably because of the proliferation of professional associations, there are many more concerns about them. At one time, organizations were run by volunteers in their spare time, typing notices with two fingers or with the help of somebody's sister; now they are a form of big business, including powerful unions and well-funded professional organizations. All seek economic and other advantages for their members, as well as the power necessary to succeed. However, members and the spirit of volunteerism continue to be the ingredients that make power possible. Volunteers look for different roles in organizations and different rewards than they did a generation ago.[2]

Politicians do not want a strong, organized group against them, and there is no doubt that an organized lobby gets action, especially if associations cooperate with each other. Still, there is concern that the power of such organizations is not good for the public, and trade associations and professional organizations have been found subject to the Sherman Anti-trust Act and the Federal Trade Commission Act, which relate to price fixing and restraint of trade. There have also been questions about certification and accreditation by the professional organizations. Nursing has responded to maintain its credibility, reorganizing and restructuring our systems to comply with both the letter and spirit of the law. In addition, the tax-exempt status of many associations is under scrutiny and challenge.

Because of this growth and power, or potential power, the concerns of voluntary organizations have become more and more similar to those of their for-profit counterparts. Recently, for instance, attention has been given to ethical dilemmas of staff and management, whereas previously this was considered more of a theoretical topic relating to a profession or business in general. An important factor is good management; a voluntary organization, like any business, must be solvent. Few, if any, can expect an automatic increase in members or can retain members without considerable effort. Today's members expect an association to be sensitive to their needs and to be instantly responsive in meeting those needs. Members expect quality products and services. Such products or services might take the form of liability insurance, professional and technical publications, and videos or computerized information systems.

Most members look to organizations for two basic things—information and networks. Prospective members should query association members about the quality and speed of service, information and networks provided, and how often the association assesses member needs. The answers to these questions will determine the value of joining and the viability of an organization. The organization that survives in the twenty-first century will be fast, friendly, flexible, and focused.

Most critical is the issue the president of one professional organization called the *internal crisis of identity and mission*. The key question asked about this professional organization for university professors is also pertinent to nursing's professional organization. The heterogeneity of professionals generates threatening tensions and divisions within the organization; is there a sufficient residue of common concern to justify the creation of one body to bring together all who call themselves professional nurses?

One problem in nursing is that so many nurses do not understand what the functions of a professional association are and therefore have inappropriate expectations. Sociologist Robert Merton in his classic article has delineated the functions in three categories: functions for individual practitioners, the profession, and society. For individuals, the association (1) gives social and moral support to help them perform their roles, especially in terms of economic and general welfare (salary, conditions of work, opportunities for advancement), continuing education, and working toward legally enforced standards of competence, and (2) develops social and moral ties among its members so that each becomes his or her brother's keeper. For the profession, the organization must set rigorous standards and help enforce them (quality of those recruited and of education, practice, and research). The profession must always press for higher standards. For society, the organization helps furnish the social bonds through which society coheres, providing unity in action.

> The association mediates between the practitioner and profession on the one hand, and on the other, their social environment, of which the most important parts are allied occupations and professions, the universities, the local community, and the government.[3]

The membership of most organizations is and probably always will be made up of people with varying degrees of commitment. No association can please them all. Yet, it is widely agreed that unless there is one voice for a profession, no one will listen. Adequate numbers of participating members are crucial. Nevertheless, although ANA is the largest generalist nursing organization in the United States, the lack of internal agreement on issues is often evident; however, we are a pluralistic society and why should nursing be different? The best testimony to this statement are the differences that often divided ANA and a growing number of nursing specialty associations. By bringing all of these associations together in a coalition of and for the profession, nursing has come together to speak with "one strong voice" on the issues that are most important.

In the following chapters, it will be seen how the increasing numbers of organizations that nurses can and do join come together around a common cause when it counts.

KEY POINTS

1. Being licensed as individuals, nurses need their professional organizations to provide peer support in their practice.

2. The level of organizational participation varies through a professional lifetime from just paying your dues, to ad hoc involvement, to committee membership, to accepting leadership positions.

3. Organizational leaders need particular skills, talents, and personality assets to preside at meetings, and these can be developed.

4. The vice president should be as qualified and adept as the president, and take an active role in governance.

5. The treasurer should be well versed in the financial operations of the association.

6. Recording of precise, yet not overly lengthy, minutes is essential to a meeting.

7. Parliamentary procedure during meetings allows both minority and majority opinions to be heard, and business to be transacted efficiently.

8. Formal meetings have an order of business that is predetermined and most commonly guided by *Robert's Rules of Order* or some similar guide.

9. The proper handling of motions according to parliamentary procedures is meant to facilitate business, not confuse the membership.

10. The staff of an association is often the only source of continuity.

REFERENCES

1. Robert's Rules of Order, Newly Revised, 10th ed. Introduction, p. xlviii. http://www.rulesonline.com. Retrieved Jun 5, 2010.

2. Rotolo T, Wilson J. What happened to the "long civic generation"? Explaining cohort differences in volunteerism. *Social Forces* 82(3):1091–1121, March 2004.

3. Merton R. The functions of the professional association. *Am J Nurs* 58:50–54, January 1958.

Updates can be found at **www.kellysnursing.com**

National Student Nurses' Association

The National Student Nurses' Association (NSNA), established in 1952, is the national organization for nursing students in the United States and its territories, possessions, and dependencies. NSNA's mission is to

1. Bring together and mentor students preparing for initial licensure as registered nurses (RNs), as well as those nurses enrolled in baccalaureate (BSN) completion programs.
2. Promote the development of the skills that students will need as responsible and accountable members of the nursing profession.
3. Advocate for high-quality, evidence-based, affordable, and accessible health care.
4. Advocate for and contribute to advances in nursing education.
5. Develop nursing students who are prepared to lead the profession in the future.[1]

The functions of the organization, as listed in the bylaws, are as follows:

1. To have direct input into the standards of nursing education and influence the educational process
2. To influence health care, nursing education, and practice through legislative activities, as appropriate
3. To promote and encourage participation in community affairs and activities toward improved health care and the resolution of related social issues
4. To represent nursing students to the consumer, to institutions, and to other organizations
5. To promote and encourage students' participation in interdisciplinary activities
6. To promote and encourage recruitment efforts, participation in student activities, and educational opportunities regardless of a person's race, color, creed, sex, age, lifestyle, national origin, or economic status
7. To promote and encourage collaborative relationships with the American Nurses Association (ANA), the National League for Nursing (NLN), and the International Council of Nurses (ICN), as well as the other nursing and related health organizations[2]

The NSNA is autonomous, student financed, and student run. It is the voice of all nursing students speaking out on issues of concern to nursing students and nursing.

■ MEMBERSHIP

Students are eligible for active membership in NSNA if they are enrolled in state-approved programs leading to licensure as an RN or are RNs enrolled in programs leading to a baccalaureate degree in nursing. Students are eligible for associate membership if they are prenursing students enrolled in college or university programs designed to prepare them for programs leading to a degree in nursing. Associate members have all of the privileges of membership except the right to hold office as president and vice president at state and national levels.

Application for membership is made directly to NSNA. Dues paid to NSNA are a combination of national and state association dues; the latter vary from state to state. The dues structure is decided by a vote of the membership.

NSNA also has two categories of membership not open to students. *Sustaining membership* is open at the national level to any individual or organization interested in furthering the development and growth of NSNA. Sustaining members receive literature and other information from the NSNA office. Dues vary for sustaining members, which may include NSNA alumni, other individuals, local organizations, and national organizations. Honorary membership is conferred by a two-thirds vote of the House of Delegates on recommendation by the board of directors on persons who have rendered distinguished service or valuable assistance to NSNA. This is the highest honor NSNA can bestow on an individual.

History

Just when or where the idea of a national association of nursing students originated will probably never be known. But for many years and in increasing numbers, students had been attending the national conventions of ANA and NLN, eager to learn of the activities of these two associations that would soon be affecting them as graduate nurses. Special sessions were arranged at these conventions so that students could meet and discuss mutual problems. At the same time, some student nurses' organizations had been formed on the state level, giving students an awareness of both the strength and values of group association and action. It was inevitable, of course, that sooner or later the idea of a national association would arise. Once it did, nursing students throughout the United States began to work enthusiastically in that direction.

In June 1952, approximately 1000 students attending a national nursing convention in Atlantic City, New Jersey, voted to form an organization under the sponsorship of the Coordinating Council of the ANA and NLN. A committee of nursing students and representatives of ANA and NLN worked on organization plans, and in June 1953 the National Student Nurses' Association was officially launched. Bylaws were adopted and NSNA's officers were elected.

In its first few years, NSNA had little money, a small membership, no real headquarters of its own, and no headquarters staff. Its main assets at the time were the persistence, determination, and dedication of its members, plus financial and moral support from ANA and NLN. A year after NSNA's founding, these two organizations appointed (and paid) a coordinator to help NSNA function; many of the association's activities were transacted through correspondence. Each organization also provided a staff consultant to NSNA and helped finance the association's necessary expenses and publications. Among the latter were the bylaws and a newspaper. The next step was a headquarters office. Today, NSNA leases its own office at 45 Main Street, Suite 606, Brooklyn, New York 11201.

Even in its early years, NSNA was able to help finance itself. Year after year, NSNA's share of the costs increased. Membership grew, and annual dues, which had originally been 15 cents per year, were raised to 50 cents in 1957. Finally, in 1958, only 5 years after its inception, NSNA became financially independent. Frances Tompkins, the original coordinator appointed in 1954, became the executive secretary (the title was later changed to executive director) and headed a staff of two. In 1959, NSNA became legally incorporated as the National Student Nurses' Association, Inc., a nonprofit association.

Today, the association pays for headquarters offices, a staff, and all the other expenses incidental to running the business of a large association. It holds and finances its own annual convention. At the same time, it has initiated and financed several important projects in the interests not only of its members, but also of the nursing profession as a whole.

General Plan of Organization

Its House of Delegates, whose membership consists of elected representatives from the school and state associations, determines the policies and programs of NSNA. The delegates at each annual convention elect NSNA's three officers; six non-officer directors, one of who serves as editor of *Imprint*, the official journal of NSNA; and a four-member nominating committee. Officers serve for 1 year or until their respective successors are elected.

Two consultants are appointed, one each by the ANA and NLN, in consultation with the NSNA board of directors. They serve for a 2-year period or until their respective successors are appointed. According to the bylaws, these consultants are charged with providing an interchange of information between their boards and NSNA. All consultants are expected to serve only as resource persons, consulting with officers, members, and staff and attending the meetings of the association. Consultants and advisers serve several major purposes.

1. To assist elected and appointed officers to identify issues, problems, and alternatives as they carry out their legal, fiduciary, and organizational responsibilities

2. To provide students in leadership positions with information about professional issues and positions taken by the appointing organization

3. To strengthen organizational ties between the student association and the appointing organization by serving as a liaison with these organizations

4. To provide continuity to the organization where the student leadership is short term and changes composition from year to year

5. To act as a professional role model and mentor[3]

The board of directors manages the affairs of the association between the annual meetings of the membership, and an executive committee, consisting of the president, vice president, and secretary/treasurer, transacts emergency business between board meetings. There are two standing committees: the nominating and elections committee, and the resolutions committee. The board has the authority to establish other committees as needed. State and constituent organizations may or may not function in a similar manner; their bylaws must be in conformity with NSNA's bylaws.

In 1976, the NSNA House of Delegates mandated a change in the structure of the association, giving school chapters the eligibility for constituency status and delegate representation. Under this system, school chapters must verify that their bylaws conform with NSNA's bylaws and must have 10 members. If a school has fewer than 10 students enrolled, membership by 100 percent of the students entitles the school to constituency status. Delegate representation is based on the number of students in the school who are members. State associations that have two recognized school chapters and their own bylaws in conformity are recognized as NSNA constituents and are entitled to one voting delegate.

Projects, Activities, and Services

NSNA has a wide variety of activities, services, and projects to carry out its purpose and functions. Even in its early years, the association sought participation in ANA and NLN committees and sent representatives to ICN.

Early projects were the Minority Group Recruitment Project (which has developed into Breakthrough to Nursing) and the Taiwan Project. The latter project, carried out in cooperation with the American Bureau for Medical Aid to China, grew out of NSNA members' interest in nursing students in other countries, coupled with a desire to assist whenever possible. After a firsthand report about the inadequate, overcrowded living conditions for nursing students at the National Defense Medical Center in Taiwan, delegates to the 1961 NSNA convention voted to raise $25,000 to build and equip a new dormitory for this group. By 1965, through vigorous fundraising drives carried out at all levels of NSNA, the larger sum of $37,000 had been accumulated. The completed 50-student residence, named the *NSNA Dormitory*, was officially dedicated in March 1966, with American government officials cutting the traditional ribbon at the ceremony and representing both NSNA and the US government.

Today, NSNA collaborates with several nursing and other health organizations. NSNA is a member of the Nursing Organizations Alliance (the Alliance). The Alliance is composed of national nursing organizations and serves as a forum for networking and addressing nursing issues. NSNA is also a leading participant in the student assembly of the ICN, and the NSNA president served as its chairperson during the 1977 ICN in Tokyo. NSNA served as host for the 1981 student assembly. Through a special program funded by the Helene Fuld Health Trust, in 1997 NSNA sent a delegation of 52 nursing students to the ICN Quadrennial Congress in Vancouver, British Columbia, Canada. The 1996/1997 NSNA president led the delegation and served as chair of the student assembly.

NSNA members are involved in community health activities such as hypertension screening, health fairs, child abuse, teenage pregnancy, education on death and dying, and disaster preparedness. Some of these activities are carried out in cooperation with other student health groups. In addition to health- and nursing-related issues, NSNA supports social, women's, and human rights issues.

Community health and disaster preparedness activities receive major emphasis by NSNA, and projects planned and implemented by NSNA members cover a wide variety of community health needs, such as heart attack risk reduction education programs, aid to homeless families, disaster relief efforts, and health fairs for all age groups.

Breakthrough to Nursing

NSNA has always been involved in recruiting qualified men and women into nursing. In 1965, however, NSNA launched a nationwide project directed toward the recruitment of blacks, Native Americans, Hispanics, and members of other underrepresented groups into the nursing profession. Known as the *National Recruitment Project*, this long-term effort grew out of an increasing awareness on the part of nursing students of their collective responsibility for supporting the civil rights movement, for recruiting for nursing, for alerting young men and women in minority groups to the opportunities in a nursing career, and in recognition of the value of such nurses in improving the care of their own ethnic groups.[4]

The national project was proposed at the 1965 NSNA convention by the 1964–1965 NSNA Nursing Recruitment Committee, whose recommendations were based on results of pilot projects conducted in Colorado, Minnesota, and Washington, DC. The delegates voted to undertake the project on a national scale.

By early 1967, the project was well under way in many different areas of the country, with the state associations tackling the problem in various ways. In collaboration with other appropriate community groups—the Urban League, those associated with Head Start or other anti-poverty programs, and civil rights groups—nursing students throughout the United States worked diligently not only to interest minority group members in nursing, but also to help them financially, morally, and educationally to undertake such a career.

In 1971, NSNA set the Breakthrough to Nursing Project, as it is now called, as a priority and sought funds to strengthen and expand the existing program. Later that year, NSNA was awarded a contract for $100,000 by the Division of Nursing. In 1974, a 3-year grant expanded Breakthrough to 40 funded target areas. The grant ended in June 1977, but NSNA continues to support the project, and the chair of the Breakthrough to Nursing Committee holds a director position on the NSNA Board of Directors.

The objectives of the project are to (1) develop and implement a publicity campaign to inform and interest potential nursing candidates in a nursing career; (2) coordinate nursing student recruitment efforts with community organizations and schools of nursing in support of the program to reach more minority students; (3) participate in recruitment program activities such as conferences, workshops, and career days focused on increasing the number of minority students recruited into nursing; (4) work with public school counselors, teachers, school nurses, and other secondary school personnel to assist with the identification, motivation, and encouragement of disadvantaged or minority group students interested in a career in nursing; and (5) inform the public and the nursing community of the goals of the project.

To carry out these objectives, the involvement and support of nursing student volunteers, faculty, and heads of schools of nursing is essential. Student volunteers carry out such activities as career fairs, education of school counselors, working with schools and community groups to provide tutorial and counseling services, the development and distribution of brochures, help with the application and registration procedures in colleges, and the provision of information about financial resources.

Breakthrough to Nursing guidelines and materials are available for distribution nationally. In addition to the *Nursing—The Ultimate Adventure* DVD, the *Nursing—The Career of a Lifetime* DVD was produced to provide information and career-planning guidance to prospective nursing students as well as to nursing students and RNs.

Although there are still problems, such as racial polarization and retention of students after recruitment, there is no doubt that the Breakthrough has had an impact on nursing, NSNA members, and the community. In 2010, the project celebrated its 45th anniversary. Over the years, the project has evolved to reflect the needs of contemporary society. For example, in addition to those groups already cited, the Breakthrough to Nursing project also focuses on nontraditional students (second-degree students) and encourages all qualified people to enter the profession.

Legislation

One of the most impressive NSNA developments in recent years is the active and knowledgeable participation of NSNA members in legislation. Excellent resources on legislative activities and political education on a national level and assistance and support in legislation provided by NSNA to constituent associations resulted in legislative committees in most states. During the various crises of federal funding for health, students have testified before congressional committees and supported the passage of the Nurse Education Act by their active participation in the political process. They have also urged the passage of social and health care reform legislation. Students are also encouraged to work with state nurses' associations (SNAs), state political action committees (PACs), and other groups on health legislation on the local and state levels, and to educate members in such areas as state nurse practice acts and political activism.

NSNA is a member of Americans for Nursing Shortage Relief (ANSR). This alliance of nursing and health care organizations played a key role in assisting legislators to create the Nurse Reinvestment Act, which supports funding for nursing education, faculty preparation, and the retention of nurses in the workplace.

Interdisciplinary Activities

NSNA has shown a forward-looking interest in the health and social problems, often combined with like interest in interdisciplinary cooperation. With the American Medical Student Association (AMSA), Student American

Pharmaceutical Association (SAPhA), and American Student Dental Association (ASDA), individual nursing students have participated in Head Start, Appalachian and Indian health, migrant health, and Job Corps projects. Recently reinstated as the Coalition of Health and Professional Students, students from various health-related disciplines meet routinely to discuss mutual interests and concerns.

One major interdisciplinary activity in which NSNA participated was Concern for Dying's *Interdisciplinary Collaboration on Death and Dying.* This student program recruited representatives from the AMSA, the Law Student Division of the American Bar Association, and students from social work and theology schools. The Collaboration, begun in 1977, introduced students to a variety of professional perspectives on death and dying and created a dialogue among future professionals.

Other Professional Activities

Almost since the inception of NSNA, members have been invited to participate in the committees of ANA and NLN. Such participation has increased as NSNA has sought to take an active part in the debates, discussions, and decisions concerning nursing. Usually the resolutions of NSNA support the goals of the ANA and NLN and, at times, they move ahead of the others in their acceptance of change. The support of both organizations is often asked on issues that require the support of nurse executives, educators, or others. Some of the issues involved have been in relation to curriculum change, clinical experience opportunities, education for practice, career mobility, and accreditation.

Scholarship Funds

The Foundation of the National Student Nurses' Association (FNSNA) administers its own scholarship program. The Foundation was established in 1969 as the Frances Tompkins Educational Opportunity Fund to enable individuals and organizations to contribute funds for undergraduate nursing education scholarships. The fund is incorporated and has obtained federal tax exemption. Scholarship monies are obtained from corporations, individuals, and professional organizations. Scholarship applications become available in the fall of each year and can be easily downloaded from NSNA's website (click on Foundation). The NSNA has established the Forever Nursing endowed scholarship campaign for undergraduate nursing education. This fund ensures that money is always available to support students seeking RN licensure as well as those in BSN completion programs.

The NSNA supports the Laura D. Smith Scholarship Fund through Nurses Educational Fund, Inc. Each year this fund awards a scholarship for graduate study. The recipient must have been a member of NSNA while in nursing school. This scholarship was established in 1962 in honor of Laura D. Smith, former senior editor of the *American Journal of Nursing* and NSNA adviser, who died in 1961.

NSNA Projects and Activities

Imprint, the official NSNA magazine, came into existence in 1968, and a subscription is given to members. Subscriptions are also available to other interested groups, schools, and individuals. *Imprint,* published five times during the academic year, is the only publication of its kind specifically for students. It is the only nursing magazine written by and for nursing students, and students are encouraged to contribute articles and letters. The January issue of *Imprint* focuses on career planning and offers students guidance to explore different nursing roles and plan their nursing careers.

Other publications include the *NSNA News,* an online newsletter that keeps NSNA members informed of pertinent issues and activities; *The Dean's Notes,* a newsletter for deans and directors of schools of nursing; the *Business Book,* which serves as an annual report and is printed for the annual convention; *Getting the Pieces to Fit,* a yearly handbook for state and school chapters; and informational, supportive materials on students' rights. Most states and some schools also publish newsletters. NSNA's two websites, www.nsna.org and www.nsnaleadershipu.org, offer resources and opportunities for students to receive academic recognition for their participation in NSNA's many leadership activities.

At the 10th anniversary of its founding, NSNA had accomplished a great deal.[5] Before its 30th, it had become an involved group whose activities demonstrated committed professionalism.[6] Gone were the talent shows and uniform nights of the early days. "Students learned to conduct meetings and to use parliamentary procedure, they showed concern about their education and their future practice, and they showed concern for others."[7] It was involved in many of the same issues as ANA and NLN and often seemed to show more foresight. With its 40th anniversary, NSNA had reason to celebrate its history and its future.[8]

In 2002, NSNA celebrated its 50th anniversary in Philadelphia, Pennsylvania. Four thousand students, faculty, NSNA alumni, and invited guests packed the Pennsylvania Convention Center to learn about NSNA's past, be involved in the present, and plan the future. A book entitled *50 Years of the National Student Nurses' Association* was distributed to all convention attendees and is available from NSNA. A documentary videotape with interviews of past NSNA leaders tells the story of NSNA history and the role the association played in advocating for the rights of nursing students and advancing nursing education.

Education is of prime interest to NSNA members. Among the many issues discussed in the NSNA House of Delegates are curriculum planning, accreditation, entry into practice, career mobility, and student rights. NSNA recognizes and values the contributions of associate, baccalaureate, diploma, generic master's, and doctoral programs that prepare students for RN licensure. As early as 1969, NSNA delegates encouraged the development and demonstration of nursing education programs that would recognize an individual's previously acquired knowledge and skill. NSNA encourages articulation agreements for the easy transition of associate degree and diploma graduates into RN to BSN programs. In 1976, the NSNA House of Delegates recognized the need for baccalaureate education in nursing and encouraged the increased availability of baccalaureate programs in nursing and increased enrollment of RNs in baccalaureate programs.

As in other fields, nursing students have also fought for their own rights, and NSNA has maintained a commitment to student rights. In 1970, a guideline for a student bill of rights was distributed to all constituents, a mandate of the 1969 delegates. In 1975, a comprehensive bill of rights, responsibilities, and grievance procedures was accepted and published. The statement was adopted in schools throughout the country. The document was revised by the 1991 House of Delegates. The NSNA has also developed a *Code of Ethics* to address professional, academic, and clinical conduct. The *Code of Professional Conduct*, the *Code of Academic and Clinical Conduct*, and the *Student Bill of Rights* are available from www.nsna.org.

In the area of practice, students have taken positions on the prevention of violence in the workplace, increasing awareness of child abuse identification, increased primary care access for older adults, increased education in self-care awareness for nursing students and nurses, and increasing awareness and advocacy for homeless youth, to name a few.

Finally, NSNA members have been involved in issues affecting the public's health—for instance, by participating in projects to educate children and young people about the dangers of drugs. NSNA has taken numerous positions on contemporary issues such as women's health, pregnancy, infant and child health, sexually transmitted diseases, AIDS/HIV prevention and education, smoking and health, drug and alcohol abuse, infection control, and promotion of a positive image of nursing.

NSNA offers the opportunity for the voice of nursing students to be heard and the association provides a forum for debate on health and social issues as well as nursing issues; provides opportunities for interdisciplinary contacts; and is a training ground for learning and practicing shared governance. Participation and involvement can be a meaningful and valuable part of the nursing student's education.[9] Many involved NSNA members go on to leadership positions in nursing organizations and continue their lifelong commitment to advancing the profession of nursing.

In 1999, NSNA developed a new program, the *NSNA Leadership University*, to help nursing students earn academic credit for their involvement in NSNA. The NSNA Leadership University provides an opportunity for nursing students to be recognized for the leadership and management skills they develop through participation in the Association's programs and governance activities. From the school chapter level to the state and national levels, nursing students learn how to work in cooperative relationships with peers, faculty, and students in other disciplines, community service organizations, and the public. NSNA's Leadership University is not a brick and mortar structure. It is a university being built by the students who want to participate. There is no tuition. All NSNA members may participate in the Leadership University. All they have to do is become active in NSNA's many shared-governance leadership opportunities. Complete details can be found at www.nsnaleadershipu.org.

Nursing students in all programs leading to RN licensure are invited to learn more about NSNA. Contact NSNA at www.nsna.org or at 45 Main Street, Brooklyn, New York 11201, (718) 210-0705.

KEY POINTS

1. The NSNA develops leaders whose future membership in their state associations will strengthen the profession.
2. Student leaders are very transient in NSNA, so they are highly dependent on capable staff.
3. Appointees from the ANA and NLN are advisory to the board of NSNA.
4. The Breakthrough to Nursing Project has been highly successful in attracting diverse students to nursing.
5. Students have been visible and effective in working with nursing and interdisciplinary organizations around legislative issues.
6. *Imprint*, as the official magazine of NSNA, encourages articles and letters by students.
7. NSNA has spoken out loudly through its House of Delegates on all dimensions of proper conduct: student's rights and professional, academic, and clinical conduct.
8. NSNA encourages enrollment in all basic RN programs: associate, diploma, baccalaureate, and generic master's programs.
9. NSNA views basic registered nursing education as a pathway to academic progression and supports articulation between educational programs as well as recognition of previously acquired knowledge and skills.

REFERENCES

1. *Getting the Pieces to Fit.* New York: National Student Nurses' Association, 2010.
2. NSNA. *Bylaws.* New York: The Author, 2010.
3. NSNA. *Guidelines for Planning for School Advisors and State Consultants.* New York: The Author, 2010.
4. Johnson N. Recruitment of minority groups: A priority for NSNA. *Nurs Outlook* 14:29–30, April 1966.
5. NSNA. *NSNA's Ten Tall Years.* New York: The Author, 1963.
6. NSNA today. *Am J Nurs* 77:624–626, April 1977.
7. NSNA. *NSNA '77: A Retrospective.* New York: The Author, 1977.
8. NSNA's 40th Anniversary Issue. *Imprint* 30, April–May 1992.
9. Fitzpatrick M. NSNA: Path to professional identity. *Imprint* 34:63–66, April–May 1987.

Updates can be found at **www.kellysnursing.com**

American Nurses Association

The American Nurses Association (ANA) is composed of organizations and individuals who have member or affiliate status. Member status is available to organizations meeting the criteria for constituent member associations (often called state nurses' associations [SNAs]). Affiliate status is available for organizations meeting the criteria for organizational affiliates; in 2010, there were 24 specialty nursing and workforce advocacy organizations that connected to ANA as affiliates. Both member and affiliate status are available for individuals (Individual Member Division [IMD]). The constituent member associations (CMAs) are state and territorial nurses' associations, US nurses overseas associations, and a federal nurses' association (whose employers are members of the Federal Nursing Services Council) consisting of active duty military. As of 2010, there is a CMA in every state and territory with the exception of Alaska, the District of Columbia, Hawaii, Michigan, and Minnesota. The organizational affiliates are freestanding national organizations and labor and workplace advocacy entities who support ANA in its work. Individual members can choose to join ANA directly. Direct ANA individual members receive full ANA member benefits but no benefits at the state level. Individual Affiliate Status is a virtual ANA membership for RNs who want to support their profession and access the Members Only section of nursingworld.org. It does not include benefits in the state nurses' association. ANA membership totaled over 180,000 registered nurses (RNs) in 2010.

The ANA was established in 1897 by a group of nurses who, even then, recognized the need for a membership association within which nurses could work together in concerted action. Its original name was the Nurses' Associated Alumnae of the United States and Canada, but to incorporate under the laws of the state of New York, it was necessary to drop the reference to another country in the organization's title. This was done in 1901; however, the name remained Nurses' Associated Alumnae of the United States until 1911, when it became the American Nurses Association. Canadian nurses also formed their own membership association.

History shows that ANA's primary concern has always been individual nurses and the public they serve. Thus, in its early years ANA worked diligently for improved and uniform standards of nursing education, registration, and licensure of all nurses educated according to these standards, and improvement of the welfare of nurses. The need for such actions and the difficulties involved become apparent if one remembers that in the early 1900s many hospitals opened schools for economic reasons only, with no real interest in the education or employment of nurses after graduation, and the public had no guarantee that any nurse gave safe care. ANA's efforts served to protect the public from unsafe nursing care provided by those who might call themselves nurses but who had little or no preparation. In recent years, ANA has continued to give major attention to setting standards of practice. The ANA subsidiary, the American Nursing Credentialing Center (ANCC), accredits continuing education providers as well as offering certification in specialty areas for individual nurses and designating institutional systems of nursing for excellence (Magnet and Pathway status). The National League for Nursing Accrediting Commission (NLNAC) and the Commission on Collegiate Nursing Education (CCNE) address the accreditation function for nursing education programs.

■ PURPOSES AND FUNCTIONS

Throughout its existence, ANA's functions and activities have been adapted or expanded in accordance with the changing needs of the profession and the public. As a changed or changing major function becomes crystallized, it is incorporated in the bylaws by vote of the ANA House of Delegates. Thus, the purposes of ANA, as stated in the current bylaws, are to

- Work for the improvement of health standards and the availability of health care services for all people.
- Foster high standards of nursing.
- Stimulate and promote the professional development of nurses and advance their economic and general welfare.

ANA's current functions, also as outlined in the bylaws, are to

- Establish standards of nursing practice, nursing education, and nursing services.
- Establish a code of ethical conduct for nurses.
- Ensure a system of credentialing in nursing.
- Initiate and influence legislation, governmental programs, national health policy, and international health policy.
- Support systematic study, evaluation, and research in nursing.
- Serve as the central agency for the collection, analysis, and dissemination of information relevant to nursing.
- Promote and protect the economic and general welfare of nurses.
- Provide leadership in national nursing and, through appropriate channels, in international nursing.
- Provide for the professional development of nurses.
- Conduct an affirmative action program.
- Ensure a collective bargaining program for nurses.
- Ensure a workplace advocacy program for nurses.
- Provide services to CMAs and the IMD.
- Maintain communication with CMAs and the IMD through official publications.
- Assume an active role as consumer advocate.
- Represent and speak for the nursing profession with allied health groups, national and international organizations, governmental bodies, and the public.
- Protect and promote the advancement of human rights related to health care and nursing.[1]

■ GENERAL PLAN OF ORGANIZATION

From time to time, ANA's organizational structure undergoes some minor or major changes to enable the association to function more efficiently in the light of changing circumstances or needs. The major changes are included in the following description of how ANA is organized and how it functions. An organizational chart is presented in Exhibit 25–1.

House of Delegates, Officers, and Board

The business of the association is carried on by its House of Delegates and Board of Directors. The House of Delegates (HOD), consisting of up to a total of 675 delegates, is apportioned at 600 delegate seats for the CMAs, 15 delegate seats for the elected ANA Board of Directors, and up to 60 delegate seats for the IMD and representatives of organizational, labor, and workforce advocacy affiliates. The ANA HOD also includes the following, which have courtesy seats without vote:

1. The past presidents of ANA
2. The chairperson or designee of the ANA congress
3. Presidents/chairpersons or designees of the American Academy of Nursing (AAN), American Nurses Association-Political Action Committee (ANA-PAC), American Nurses Credentialing Center (ANCC), and the American Nurses' Foundation (ANF), if the unit does not have representation through its president serving on the ANA Board of Directors
4. One representative each of the Federal Nursing Services Council and the National Student Nurses' Association

The HOD is the highest authority in the association. The number from each CMA is based on the overall size of the CMA membership. The HOD meets biennially. The members of the House elect ANA's Board of Directors and officers, the majority of the members of its Nominating Committee, and some members of its congress (to be described later). Thus, control of the association remains always in the hands of its membership.

Throughout the years, ANA's HOD has made many important decisions related to nursing and nurses. At many successive conventions, for instance, it went on

ANA Members' and Affiliates

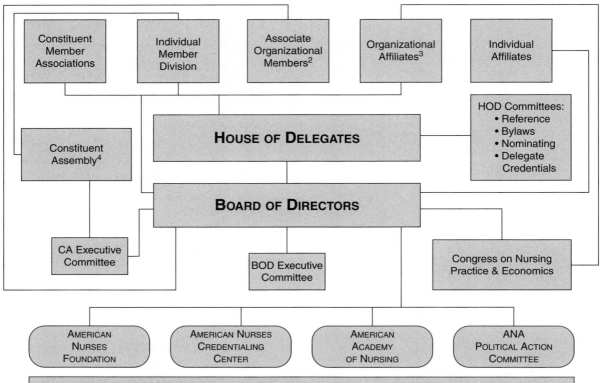

EXHIBIT 25-1. ANA: organizational structure.

record as supporting the principle underlying the legislation that eventually brought Medicare into being. As early as 1946, it began to support bold statements designed to discourage discriminatory policies in regard to nationality, race, religion, or color within the nursing profession. In 1964, it voted to revise the bylaws so that ANA's responsibility for nursing education and nursing services might be more explicitly stated. In 1966, it adopted a national salary goal with a differential for nurses with a baccalaureate degree. In 1968, the *Congress on Practice* was created,

reemphasizing ANA's concern with practice. In 1970, even with the news that ANA was in a financial crisis because of mismanagement of funds and a consequent cutback of programs, the delegates resolved to recruit more of the disadvantaged into nursing, help to reduce the many threats to the environment, become more deeply involved in health planning, and develop closer working relationships with consumers of health care.

In 1972, it became a priority to define the requirements for high-quality nursing services, clarify the scope of nursing

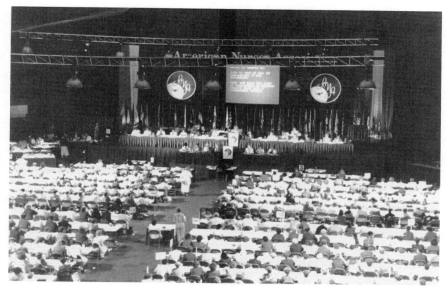

The ANA House of Delegates meets yearly to set policy for nursing in this country. (Courtesy of the American Nurses Association)

practice, provide for continuing peer review, recognize excellence and continued competence among practitioners of nursing, expand and improve all aspects of nursing education, and assist SNAs with their economic security activities. An affirmative action program was also established that called for the appointment of an ombudsman to the ANA staff.

In 1974, convention action gave major emphasis to national health insurance, nurses' participation in Professional Standards Review Organizations (PRSOs), implementation of standards for nursing practice, certification for excellence in practice, reaffirmation of support of individual licensure (as opposed to institutional licensure), support of continuing education (CE) programs, and a mandate to the ANA Board of Directors to establish a system of accreditation of CE programs, commit the association to pursue direct fee-for-service reimbursement for nurse practitioners (NPs), establish the role of ANA in collective bargaining, and eradicate the exploitation of foreign nurses and assist in their becoming qualified to practice.

In 1976, the bicentennial convention year, the House passed resolutions on nurse advocacy for the elderly, the responsibilities of nurses in nursing homes, alternatives to hospitalization for the mentally disabled and retarded, and the involvement of nurses in health planning.

The 1978 and 1980 Houses set as priorities for the next biennium improving the quality of care provided to the public; advancing the profession so that the health care needs of people are met; enlarging the influence of the nursing profession in the determination and execution of public policy; and strengthening ANA so that it may better serve the needs and interests of the profession. Also approved were major resolutions on national health insurance, quality assurance, human rights, career mobility, and identifying, titling, and developing competency statements for two categories of nursing practice.

In 1982 and 1984, the House adopted the following statement of association priorities for the biennium: "To promote and protect the economic worth, the education and the practice of nurses." Specific goals were related to better communication with the public, standard setting for nursing, influencing health policy, and strengthening ANA's role in credentialing. The action taken in the House and the actions taken by the association throughout the year focused on these efforts. For instance, proposals accepted by the House in 1984 were related to smoking and other hazards of the workplace; the role of nurses within the prospective payment system, in home care, and in long-term care; implementing the goal of entry into practice at the baccalaureate level; supporting the Equal Rights

Amendment (ERA); action to improve the economic status of women and children; nurse accountability and ethics; and the protection of collective bargaining rights.

In 1986, the ANA adopted a long-range strategic and business plan for the organization, with the HOD retaining the right to identify funding priorities. The 1988 House directed the association to move its headquarters' location to Washington, DC; that was accomplished by 1992. The years between 1982 and 1989 were particularly volatile, with heated discussions around who should be the individual member of the SNA. Tensions were fueled by the lingering debate over educational preparation for entry into practice and the uncertainty of transition to the federation model. It became evident that the radical changes in the association demanded careful study of all aspects of organizational life: structure, function, membership, and interorganizational relationships. Out of this turmoil, the Commission on Organizational Assessment and Renewal (COAR) was born. In 1989, after 3 years of study and consensus building, the recommendations of COAR were adopted and cast into bylaws, creating the stability that allowed ANA to move on to issues other than internal maintenance.

By 1990, the HOD had turned its attention outward to the most provocative social problems of the period, including the need for national health care reform. The association's authorship of *Nursing's Agenda for Health Care Reform* provided the credibility for ANA to become a major presence in the health policy debate.[2] By the 1992 House, *Nursing's Agenda* was supported by over 70 nursing and non-nursing organizations.

In 1994, the ANA HOD continued to discuss health policy and the impact of the nation's concern over cost on the employment of RNs and the quality of their work environment. Delegates reaffirmed the commitment to universal coverage and a basic benefit package that includes health promotion and restoration, disease prevention, and long-term care.

The 1995 House continued to focus attention on health care reform and showed significant support for a single-payer mechanism as the best model for financing, but incorporated enough latitude in its phrasing to allow ANA to support other options. Concern about the slow progress toward establishing the baccalaureate as the educational requirement for entry into practice resurfaced in the form of an appeal to facilitate the career mobility of RNs pursuing the bachelor's degree. In response to the Pew Health Professions Commission, delegates supported the maintenance of individual licenses for nurses, with authority vested in boards of nursing.[3]

The 1996 delegates expressed opposition to the practice of linking pay increases to dollars saved by withholding health care services from beneficiaries. The House further opposed the idea of a second license for advanced practice and the Pew Commission's call for giving institutions more discretion in defining nurses' scope of practice. Here was the specter of institutional licensure. The issue of the regulation of unlicensed assistive personnel (UAPs) prompted heated debate among those who supported regulation and others who vehemently objected to any formal regulatory recognition of UAPs, seeing this as the first step toward autonomy.

The year 1997 brought additional licensure concerns, this time the multistate license and the association's apprehension that this model would seriously weaken nursing regulation. Bylaw changes ensured a staff nurse's presence on the ANA Board of Directors. A surplus of nurses brought concerns over immigration issues, the *North American Free Trade Agreement* (NAFTA), and the *General Agreement on Tariffs and Trade* (GATT). There was an expression of concern over whether all members of the American Academy of Nursing actually maintained their membership in the SNA.

In 1998, the delegates spoke against government policies that reduced payments to home care. They further responded to the prospective payment system instituted for nursing homes. Other issues were the confidentiality of electronic systems for health care information, continuing concern over multistate licensing, and the revision of the *Code of Ethics*. Delegates declined to support revisions in the code, seeing more wisdom in its current broad statements.

The year 1999 brought about major restructuring within the association. The proposal was approved by the House to consolidate various structural units into one congress, the *Congress on Nursing Practice and Economics*, and create a new labor entity, the *United American Nurses* (UAN). This new congress replaced the Congress on Nursing Economics, the Congress of Nursing Practice and its various councils, the Commission on Economic and Professional Security, and the Institute of Constituent Members on Nursing Practice. The Institute of Constituent Member Collective Bargaining Programs was incorporated into the UAN. When and where necessary, additional organizational work was to be accomplished through "adhocracy." It should be noted that historically congresses participated widely in policy development and program evaluation, made appointments, assigned work, monitored trends, and recommended to the Board, but essentially had no clear authority except for the adoption of standards. The reader is referred to the eighth edition of *Dimensions* for a discussion of the structural units that were dissolved through bylaws revision.

At this same time, the onset of another nursing shortage demanded new solutions. The aging of the nurse workforce, withdrawal of many experienced nurses from practice, a serious shortfall of qualified faculty, decreased admissions to entry-level educational programs, and multidisciplinary shortages all complicated the situation. The House rejected looking to the immigration of nurses as a solution. Instead, they called to create an environment that would retain experienced nurses and encourage the development of models and programs to improve the attraction of academic life for potential faculty. They were outspoken in their demands for equitable pensions for women and workplace safety.

In 2000, it became obvious that ensuring an adequate nurse workforce for the public would be a slow, painstaking process. Five Core Issues were identified to guide the agenda of the association: nursing shortage, appropriate staffing, workplace rights, workplace health and safety, and patient safety/advocacy. A National Center for Patient Safety was established to foster consumer education and a state-based error reporting system. These strategies created a consumer outcry for nurses to participate in their care and made the connection between short staffing and errors in treatment. Through the bylaws process a *Commission on Workplace Advocacy* (CWPA) was formed to service states that did not look to collective bargaining as a strategy for workplace improvement. While ANA sought productive solutions to the nursing shortage, the industry turned to mandatory overtime.

The years 2001 and 2002 still found ANA coping with the problems of workforce shortage and holding firm to the conviction that there are enough domestic nurses if the environment were enriched for their practice. "Nurses love their work, but hate their job." The Magnet facilities are offered as an exemplar of a quality practice environment. A revised Code of Ethics was approved in 2001 (see Chapter 10).

In 2002, delegates again made the appeal for workplaces conducive to the more mature worker and expressed the desire to help nurses afflicted with addictions or psychiatric illness to be rehabilitated and restored to their practice.

The ANA House of Delegates, after much deliberation, took no action on a proposed bylaws revision. As a result, ANA maintained its current bylaws, at least temporarily. The bylaws revision included adding both organizational and individual membership options and creating new relationships with ANA's current programs that deal with workplace rights, the UAN, and CWPA. The goal was to strengthen these programs and provide them with greater autonomy as associate organizational members that would be connected to ANA through formal agreements.

The 2003 HOD approved resolutions requiring ANA to work with other nursing organizations to develop policies that will ensure equitable practice guidelines for HIV-positive nurses, without undue limitations on their practice. Other resolutions sought to protect the workplace rights of nurses infected with other bloodborne diseases, such as hepatitis, and to support the dissemination of the CDC's *Plan to Prevent Emerging Infectious Diseases*. Further, ongoing education of RNs regarding appropriate mechanisms to protect themselves and their patients from infectious diseases was identified as a priority. The role of the public health nurse and the infrastructure for public health was also the source of controversy. The number of RNs identified as "public health nurse" in the *National Sample Survey of Registered Nurses* decreased from 39 percent in 1980 to 17.6 percent in 2000. Meanwhile, demands on these nurses and the entire public health structure have continued to increase, particularly in relation to preparedness requirements for anthrax, smallpox, and other biological threats. Delegates directed the ANA to advocate for public awareness of the critical nature of the public health nurse's role in promoting and protecting the health of individuals, families, and communities. As nurses protect our communities, delegates sought protection for nurses who become ill or injured as the result of terrorist attacks by advocating that insurance carriers offer policy coverage for such eventualities. Delegates took upon themselves some emotionally charged issues with resolutions on the use of marijuana for medical purposes, and therapeutic and reproductive applications in genetics science.

Discussion on health care reform focused on ensuring universal coverage. There was much suspicion over demands for cost containment and what effect this would have on the nursing workforce. Concern was expressed over accepting advertising or exhibitors who have policies that conflict with ANA's policy of anti-discrimination. Along these same lines, the HOD demanded intervention with members of Congress, the President, and Joint Chiefs of Staff urging the military to abandon discrimination against lesbians and gays. ANA continues its opposition to the military's discriminatory "don't ask, don't tell" policy, while maintaining its support for nurses in the military.

In one of its first actions, the 2004 HOD approved a measure that builds on the Institute of Medicine's (IOM's) recommendations outlined in a report called *Keeping Patients Safe: Transforming the Work Environment of Nurses*, which addresses needed workplace changes, including maintaining appropriate staffing to prevent medical errors and ensure quality patient care. In another action, delegates agreed with a plan to ensure APRNs' rights to provide care as defined in their scope of practice. This action was spurred by policies in some health care facilities in which medical staff determines who can have clinical privileges and oversee patient care—essentially preventing some APRNs from practicing fully. Delegates also discussed the valuable role that technology can play in preventing medical errors. However, they want to ensure that technology does not replace or interfere with RNs' clinical judgment. Therefore, the HOD passed a resolution asking ANA to support the essential role of the individual RN in maintaining responsibility and accountability for independent decision making. The HOD also approved two resolutions addressing environmental issues. One centers on the need for ANA to define how nurses and the profession can assume leadership in reducing the burden of environmentally associated disease now and in the future. The other environmental caution centered on the agricultural use of antibiotics leading to antibiotic resistance in humans. Delegates urged Congress and the meat and poultry industry to phase out the non-therapeutic use of medically important antibiotics and fluoroquinolones (a class of drugs that includes ciprofloxacin) in poultry. Delegates voiced their concerns about the need to protect the integrity of the scientific peer-review process from political and ideological forces. Delegates further addressed the need for patient safety measures in light of medication cost-savings efforts, such as the movement to purchase drugs from other countries. And there was international business. Delegates condemned the death sentences handed down to five Bulgarian nurses and a Palestinian physician in Libya. The six health professionals were falsely accused of spreading HIV in a children's hospital in Benghazi, Libya. Delegates also supported the US ratification of two United Nations treaties: the "Convention on the Rights of the Child" and the "Convention on Elimination of All Forms of Discrimination Against Women."

In internal politics, delegates approved periodic increases in the dues paid to ANA by CMAs, called a "dues escalator," that will be tied to the Consumer Price Index-Urban (CPI-U). The increased funding will be used to assure that ANA remains the singular, national voice of nurses.

The 2005 HOD directed ANA to work with other health care organizations and citizen action groups to support the goals outlined in the association's updated blueprint for health care reform, called *ANA's Health Care Agenda 2005*. In that document, ANA states that health care is a basic human right and calls for an emphasis on preventive, community-based care and universal health coverage. In a related action, the HOD protected RNs' vital role in providing care in community-based and ambulatory care settings. This included reconsidering position statements that condoned replacement of RNs in these settings, as well as accepting UAPs to administer medications. Another resolution requests the dissemination of information showing the impact of nurses' fatigue, rotating shifts, long work hours, and insufficient break time on patient safety, quality of care, and the personal safety of RNs. Recent world events prompted delegates to advocate for prisoners' and detainees' right to health care and humane treatment, and to ensure that RNs do not voluntarily participate in any deliberate physical or mental suffering. Further, delegates held the *Code of Ethics for Nurses* as a set of precepts that encompass all nursing activities and supersede policies of institutions or employers. To prevent the deaths of an estimated 85 abandoned newborns each year, the HOD approved a resolution that promotes public awareness of "safe haven" laws. Forty-five states currently have programs that allow parents to take unwanted infants to a safe place without fear of exposing their identities or being charged with child abandonment. ANA delegates also called for collaboration with other national nursing and child advocacy organizations toward a nationwide Ad Council campaign educating parents and others about the dangers of leaving children unattended in and around motor vehicles.

The 2006 HOD acknowledged nurses who responded to Hurricane Katrina and other disasters and emergencies. The HOD reaffirmed the RN's unencumbered authority to practice with the rights, responsibilities, and accountability as defined in the profession's fundamental documents: the ANA *Social Policy Statement*, *Code of Ethics for Nurses with Interpretive Statements*, and *Nursing Scope and Standards of Practice*. The ANA HOD strongly urged all RNs involved in direct patient care, particularly those caring for vulnerable patient populations, to receive the seasonal influenza vaccine annually (though ANA opposes mandatory vaccination policies). Also reaffirmed was the right of the RN to be represented for collective bargaining.

With one-half of all new graduate nurses leaving their first professional assignment in less than 1 year, the 2008 HOD resolved to support the integration of new nurses into the work environment through varied educational and practice strategies, such as residency programs, and to support nursing research efforts that demonstrate effective plans for the successful integration of new nurses into the work environment. Delegates also resolved to increase awareness among nurses about the effects of intimate partner violence on the health, safety, and welfare of families, children, and communities, and advocate for the use of evidence-based clinical guidelines in caring and treating victims of violence. Delegates approved a resolution that recognizes the impact global climate change has on the health of the world's population and encourages nurses to advocate for change on both individual and policy levels. Also resolved was the need to advocate for research to identify real or perceived gaps and barriers to health care for veterans and their families. Recognizing concerns over the adverse effects linked to food additives and contaminants, ANA has resolved to work collectively with CMAs, affiliates, and health care organizations to eliminate purchasing milk and dairy products that contain hormones for use in the health care industry. Attention was also focused on the impact human trafficking has on public health and the profession of nursing. There is a need to ensure that nurses have the skill set to properly identify and refer victims of human trafficking. The HOD also resolved to advocate for public policy that decreases the incidence of human trafficking. ANA, as one of the original supporters of the Social Security program, resolved to work with Congress and the President to strengthen Social Security and ensure its solvency beyond 2042. The HOD also advocated for the expansion of Medicare from the traditional "medical model" to include a focus on prevention, wellness, and primary care services. There was support for increasing the level of education required for continued registration as an RN by requiring RNs to attain a baccalaureate degree in nursing within 10 years after initial licensure, while maintaining the multiple entry points into

the profession. It was further resolved to advocate for legislation that increases access to oral health care for older adults, and support efforts to raise awareness of the importance of oral health. ANA resolved to begin a dialogue with the American Red Cross over the elimination of its Chief Nurse Officer position, and to urge the Red Cross to reinstate a Chief Nurse Officer at its national headquarters.

The 2010 biennial HOD revisited many items from ANA's past. Hostility, abuse, and bullying have continued to escalate since 2006 when they were originally considered. Implementation policies were discussed which are proactive and look to institutional and public policy for protection. The need for an "escalator clause" in dues assessment was reaffirmed, and discussion followed on the apportionment of delegates and dues when IMD and CMA members without ANA governance rights are considered. These points were never clarified as new membership options have been added, and more are proposed for the future. A resolution questioned the health literacy of the general population. Health care reform is a monumental paradigm shift from a reactive to a preventive/predictive model. Success will demand that the population have a strong role in health decisions and actions. Nurses have to be prepared to address health literacy concerns. More research is needed in this area. Cost containment has prompted a need to study the safety and effectiveness of reprocessed single-use devices. Another obstacle to cost containment and quality is the exclusion of all qualified health care providers from authorizing home care services and supplies needed by patients, with the exception of physicians. Delegates supported providing health care services to undocumented immigrants. There was discussion on the usefulness of Internet social networking sites to nursing. The HOD reaffirmed its support of initiatives to facilitate the integration of novice nurses into the work environment, and urged dissemination of information about successful models.

In the intervals between the HOD's meetings, the Board of Directors transacts the business of the association. This is a 15-member voting body, consisting of five officers: president, first vice president, second vice president, secretary, and treasurer; 10 directors elected at large, four of whom are staff nurses and one a recent graduate of an RN licensure program. Additionally, non-voting seats are provided to the chair of the Constituent Assembly, an RN representative of the organizational affiliates and of the labor and workforce advocacy affiliates, each of who shall be a CMA/ANA or an IMD member. Terms of office are staggered to prevent a complete turnover at any one time and to provide for the continuity of programs and action.

Serving to implement ANA policies and programs is the headquarters staff, made up of RNs, economists, attorneys, lobbyists, statisticians, writers, and other professionals, as well as support staff. They carry out the day-to-day activities of the association in accordance with the policies adopted by the HOD and ANA's general functions. ANA headquarters is located at 8515 Georgia Avenue, Suite 400, Silver Spring, MD 20910.

Other Organizational Entities

Like other large organizations, ANA has its *standing committees*, those that are written into the bylaws and that continue from year to year to assist with specific, continuing programs and functions of the association. There are four such committees of the HOD: bylaws, nominating, reference, and delegate credentialing to verify and report on the credentials of delegates at meetings of the House. These standing committees differ from what are called *special committees*, which are appointed on an ad hoc basis to accomplish special purposes. Special committees may be board committees or HOD committees.

Except for the nominating committee and committees of the congress, the board appoints committee members. The standing committees are accountable to the house and submit reports to the board. The board also appoints its own committees to carry out its work.

The *Constituent Assembly* consists of the president and chief administrative officer of each SNA or their designees. They meet periodically to discuss nursing affairs of concern to ANA, SNAs, and the profession.

■ MAJOR ANA PROGRAMS AND SERVICES

The programs and services of ANA represent the total results of the efforts of members and staff, elected officers, and structural units. These include meeting with members of other groups and disciplines; planning or attending institutes, workshops, conventions, or committee meetings; developing and writing brochures, manuals, position papers, standards, or testimony to be presented to Congress; and implementing ongoing programs, planning new ones, or trying to solve the problem of how to serve the members best within the limitations of the budget. Every issue of the *American Nurse Today* carries reports of these many and varied activities. Presented here are brief descriptions of some (but not all) of the major ANA programs and services.

Nursing Practice

ANA works continually and in many ways to improve the quality of nursing care available to the public. In its role as the professional association for RNs, it defines and interprets principles and standards of nursing practice and education. These publications are available from ANA.

ANA's concern for quality nursing care is clearly demonstrated by the development of practice standards, with their implications for peer review, and the consequent action of ANA and many state associations to assist nurses to implement the standards. ANA's *Nursing: Scope and Standards of Practice* provides a framework for the constantly growing numbers of specialty standards, nursing performance, and public assurance as a measure of competence (see Chapter 9). Most specialty standards were developed jointly with ANA within the context of its framework, or were later endorsed by ANA. There are many publications available through NursesBooks.org, the publishing program of ANA that provide guidance in using standards for peer review, understanding their legal aspects, and applying them to practice.

For over 100 years, ANA has been working to improve patient safety by promoting nursing quality. The National Center for Nursing Quality (NCNQ®) was created by ANA to address patient safety and quality in nursing care and nurses' work lives. The center advocates for nursing quality through quality measurement, novel research, and collaborative learning. Issues such as the nursing workforce and impact on patient outcomes are tackled through innovative initiatives, which include the National Database for Nursing Quality Indicators (NDNQI®) and *Safe Staffing Saves Lives*, ANA's national campaign to solve the nurse staffing crisis, among others.

The association's programs are interrelated and overlapping. In March 1994, the ANA Board launched Nursing's Safety and Quality Initiative. This was a direct response to the suspicion that organizational restructuring in health care was compromising safety and quality for both patients and nurses themselves. During the course of this project, 10 initial quality indicators were identified (*Nursing's Report Card*) to test the relationship between nursing actions and patient outcomes. Today, over 1500 hospitals participate in NDNQI®.

ANA's concern for quality is also manifested through its *Center for Ethics and Human Rights* and *Code for Nurses*.

One of the center's purposes is to develop and disseminate information on ethical and human rights issues facing the profession of nursing. The center provides consultation and resources for addressing practice dilemmas and controversies. For example, the center helps nurses and SNAs with the application of the *Code for Nurses* and prepares documents such as the *Position Statements on the Nurse's Role in End-of-Life Decisions*. This is only one example of a variety of position papers that ANA has authored and approved to provide guidance for the practice of nursing. A list of current position statements is presented in Exhibit 25–2.

Professional Nursing Policy

The ANA HOD and the ANA Board of Directors are charged with setting policy in health care, the workplace, patient care, and many other areas where nurses are engaged. When a hot topic arises or there are various views and opinions about current events, the HOD and/or the Board of Directors may address these concerns by way of a position statement. Position statements are an explanation, a justification or a recommendation for a course of action that reflects ANA's stance regarding the concern. The development process for position statements initially involves internal deliberation by the Congress on Nursing Practice and Economics. A draft of the proposed position statement is then posted on ANA's website for public comment. Following public comment, the statement is revised if necessary and approved by the ANA Board of Directors. This process allows each and every nurse to voice his or her views and opinions on the various dimensions of the issue at hand. Position statements expire or are retired by the organization when appropriate.

Nursing Education

According to ANA's 1917 Certificate of Incorporation, two of the purposes of the organization are ". . . to promote the professional and educational advancement of nurses in every proper way; to elevate the standard of nursing education . . ." However, as noted in the *Compendium of ANA Education Positions, Position Statements and Documents,*[4] the association did not take any significant action in this area until the 1960s when the association made a definitive statement on nursing education, *A Position Paper on Educational Preparation for Nurse Practitioners and Assistants to Nurses.*

In 1959, the association established the Study Committee on the Functions of ANA, which was charged with developing "criteria to aid in a determination of the functions which ANA as the professional association must carry if it is to discharge its responsibilities to the public and to the nursing profession." One area of exploration was nursing education and the roles and responsibilities of both the ANA and the NLN. After extensive study, the committee proposed the establishment of a permanent ANA structure to deal with matters related to nursing education, and in 1960, the HOD agreed to continue to elevate standards on nursing education by formulating principles of education essential to effective practice. In 1961, the Board of Directors established a Committee on Education. To this day, nursing education remains a priority of the association, and a variety of structural units within the association address this issue.

In 1963, the Consultant Group on Nursing, appointed by the Surgeon General of the Public Health Service, published a report entitled *Toward Quality in Nursing: Needs and Goals.* The consultant group made the following observations:

> The present educational structure for the training of nurses lacks system, order, and coherence. There is no clear differentiation as to the levels of responsibility for which the graduates of each type of program are prepared. The consultant group is convinced that the baccalaureate program should be the minimal requirement for nurses who will assume leadership positions.

ANA's Committee on Education proposed the establishment of an autonomous commission that would design and spearhead a comprehensive study regarding the results of the consultant group. Both the ANA and the NLN appropriated funds to establish a joint committee to investigate ways to conduct and finance the study. The ANA Board of Directors believed that an association position paper on nursing education would serve as useful resource material to the proposed commission.

In 1964, the Nurse Training Act of 1964 was signed into law, the first federal law to give comprehensive assistance for nursing education. The passage of the nurse training act and the establishment of federal programs providing funds for training various categories of health workers made it imperative that ANA provide sound guidelines regarding the preparation needed for nursing practice and for the work of ancillary nursing personnel.

The 1964 ANA HOD adopted a motion that "ANA continue to work toward baccalaureate education as the educational foundation for professional nursing practice."

■ **EXHIBIT 25–2. Select ANA Position Statements and Date of Approval**

Abuse of Prescription Drugs – 4/5/91	Drug and Alcohol Abuse
Active Euthanasia – 12/8/94	Ethics and Human Rights
Adolescent Health – 9/30/00	Social Causes and Health Care
Adolescent Immunization – 12/12/02	Social Causes and Health Care
Adult Immunization – 12/12/02	Social Causes and Health Care
Additional Access to Care: Supporting Nurse Practitioners in Retail-Based Health Clinics – 12/11/09	Nursing Practice
AIDS/HIV Disease and Socio-Culturally Diverse Populations – 4/2/93	Bloodborne and Airborne Diseases
ANA Response to Pew Commission Report – 12/5/96	Nursing Practice
Assisted Suicide – 12/8/94	Ethics and Human Rights
Association of Operating Room Nurses Official Statement on RN First Assistants – 4/1994	Nursing Practice
Assuring Patient Safety: Registered Nurses' Responsibility in All Roles and Settings to Guard Against Working When Fatigued – 12/8/06	Workplace Advocacy
Assuring Patient Safety: The Employers' Role in Promoting Healthy Nursing Work Hours for Registered Nurses in All Roles and Settings – 12/8/06	Workplace Advocacy
Assuring Safe, High Quality Health Care in Pre-K Through 12 Educational Settings – 3/16/07	Nursing Practice
Childhood Immunizations – 3/30/95	Social Causes and Health Care
Credentialing and Privileging of Advanced Practice Registered Nurses – 10/11/06	Nursing Practice
Credentials for the Professional Nurse: Determining a Standard Order of Credentials for the Professional Nurse – 12/11/09	Nursing Practice
Cultural Diversity in Nursing Practice – 10/22/91	Ethics and Human Rights
Discrimination and Racism in Health Care – 3/26/98	Ethics and Human Rights
Drug Testing for Health Care Workers – 12/8/94	Drug and Alcohol Abuse
Education and Barrier Use for Sexually Transmitted Diseases and HIV Infection – 9/6/91	Bloodborne and Airborne Diseases
Electronic Health Record – 12/11/09	Nursing Practice
Elimination of Manual Patient Handling to Prevent Work-Related Musculoskeletal Disorders – 3/14/08	Nursing Practice
Elimination of Violence in Advertising Directed Toward Children, Adolescents, and Families – 7/13/07	Social Causes and Health Care
Equipment/Safety Procedures to Prevent Transmission of Bloodborne Diseases – 9/6/91	Bloodborne and Airborne Diseases
Ethics and Human Rights – 9/5/91	Ethics and Human Rights
Forgoing Nutrition and Hydration – 4/2/92	Ethics and Human Rights
HIV Disease and Correctional Inmates – 9/11/92	Bloodborne and Airborne Diseases
HIV Disease and Women – 9/11/92	Bloodborne and Airborne Diseases
HIV Exposure from Rape/Sexual Assault – 4/2/93	Bloodborne and Airborne Diseases
HIV Infection and Nursing Students – 4/3/92	Bloodborne and Airborne Diseases
HIV Infection and US Teenagers – 12/13/91	Bloodborne and Airborne Diseases
HIV Testing – 9/6/91	Bloodborne and Airborne Diseases

■ EXHIBIT 25–2. Select ANA Position Statements and Date of Approval

Human Cloning by Means of Blastomere Splitting and Nuclear Transplantation – 6/21/00	Ethics and Human Rights
In Support of Patients' Safe Access to Therapeutic Marijuana – 12/12/08	Ethics and Human Rights
Joint Statement on Delegation American Nurses Association (ANA) and National Council of State Boards of Nursing	Unlicensed Assistive Personnel
Just Culture – 12/28/10	Workplace Advocacy
Lead Poisoning and Screening – 4/8/94	Social Causes and Health Care
The Mayday Fund Report: A Call to Revolutionize Chronic Pain Care in America: An Opportunity in Health Care Reform – 11/04/09	Nursing Practice
Mechanisms Through Which SNAs Consider Ethical/Human Rights Issues – 12/8/94	Ethics and Human Rights
Mercury in Vaccines – 6/21/06	Consumer Advocacy
Needle Exchange and HIV – 4/2/93	Bloodborne and Airborne Diseases
Nurse-Midwifery – 4/2/93	Nursing Practice
Nurses' Participation in Capital Punishment – 12/8/94	Ethics and Human Rights
Nursing and the Patient Self-Determination Acts – 11/18/91	Ethics and Human Rights
Nursing Care and Do-Not-Resuscitate Decisions – 12/20/03	Ethics and Human Rights
Pain Management and Control of Distressing Symptoms in Dying Patients – 12/5/03	Ethics and Human Rights
Patient Safety: Rights of Registered Nurses When Considering a Patient Assignment – 3/12/09	Workplace Advocacy
Personnel Policies and HIV in the Workplace – 9/6/91	Bloodborne and Airborne Diseases
Polygraph Testing of Healthcare Workers – 12/8/94	Workplace Advocacy
Polypharmacy and the Older Adult – 12/15/90	Drug and Alcohol Abuse
Post-Exposure Programs in the Event of Occupational Exposure to HIV/HBV – 9/6/91	Bloodborne and Airborne Diseases
Privacy and Confidentiality – 12/8/06	Ethics and Human Rights
Professional Role Competence – 5/28/08	Nursing Practice
Promoting Safe Medication Use in the Older Adult – 3/12/09	Nursing Practice
Promotion and Disease Prevention – 7/2/95	Social Causes and Health Care
Reduction of Patient Restraint and Seclusion in Health Care Settings – 10/17/01	Ethics and Human Rights
Registered Nurse Education Relating to the Utilization of Unlicensed Assistive Personnel – 4/13/92	Unlicensed Assistive Personnel
Registered Nurses' Rights and Responsibilities Related to Work Release During a Disaster – 6/24/02	Workplace Advocacy
Registered Nurses Utilization of Nursing Assistive Personnel in All Settings – 7/13/07	Unlicensed Assistive Personnel
Reproductive Health – 3/27/89	Social Causes and Health Care
Risk and Responsibility in Providing Nursing Care – 6/21/06	Ethics and Human Rights
Role of the Registered Nurse in the Management of Analgesia by Catheter Techniques – 9/1991	Nursing Practice
Safety Issues Related to Tubing and Catheter Misconnections – 10/10/07	Nursing Practice
Sexual Harassment – 4/2/93	Workplace Advocacy
Stem Cell Research – 1/10/07	Ethics and Human Rights

■ **EXHIBIT 25–2. Select ANA Position Statements and Date of Approval**

The Nonnegotiable Nature of the ANA Code for Nurses with Interpretive Statements – 12/8/94	Ethics and Human Rights
Travel Restrictions for Persons with HIV/AIDS – 9/6/91	Bloodborne and Airborne Diseases
Tuberculosis and HIV – 4/2/93	Bloodborne and Airborne Diseases
Tuberculosis and Public Health Nursing – 4/2/93	Bloodborne and Airborne Diseases
Use of Placebos for Pain Management in Patients with Cancer – 12/1996	Social Causes and Health Care
Violence Against Women – 3/24/00	Social Causes and Health Care
Work Release During a Disaster: Guidelines for Employers – 6/24/02	Workplace Advocacy

The above are a sample of current position statements. The reader is referred to http://www.nursingworld.org for the full narratives of these statements and others not included here.

The house requested that the Committee on Education work with "all deliberate speed to enunciate a precise definition of preparation for nursing at all levels." This request resulted in the development and ANA Board of Directors endorsement in 1965 of *A Position Paper on Educational Preparation for Nurse Practitioners and Assistants to Nurses.*

The major assumption underlying the development of the position paper was that "education for those in the health professions must increase in depth and breadth as scientific knowledge expands." According to members of the Committee on Education, the purpose of the position paper was to describe a system of education rather than to label practitioners. The following principles were set forth in the position paper:

• The education for all those who are licensed to practice nursing should take place in institutions of higher education.

• Minimum preparation for beginning professional nursing practice at the present time should be a baccalaureate-degree education in nursing.

• Minimum preparation for beginning technical nursing practice at the present time should be an associate-degree education in nursing.

• Education for assistants in the health care occupations should be short, intensive preservice programs in vocational education institutions rather than on-the-job training programs.

As approximately 78 percent of the nurses in practice in 1965 were graduates of hospital-based diploma programs, concern was expressed regarding the impact of the document on the status of these nurses. Therefore, in 1966, the ANA Board of Directors approved the publication of a brochure, *A Date With the Future*, which interpreted the meaning of the position paper for graduates of hospital schools of nursing. The brochure stated,

> The position paper addresses itself to the future of the nursing profession to insure that nursing will exercise its rightful voice and influence in the health care complex of tomorrow. As ANA plans for the future, ANA members are assured that: 1) There is no change in legal status for the diploma nurse. Nurses graduated from and now enrolled in state approved diploma programs are eligible upon graduation to become licensed as registered nurses. 2) The position paper does not in any way affect what nurses have already achieved, but rather it focuses on the impending and long overdue changes in the system of nursing education.

Also in 1966, the ANA Board of Directors adopted a motion that "appropriate groups within ANA be encouraged to develop statements on qualifications, utilization, distribution, and enumeration of nursing personnel needed to provide nursing care in health care facilities." In addition, the board endorsed an ANA-NLN Joint Statement on Community Planning for Nursing Education. A second joint statement on the same topic was endorsed in 1967.

This all led to the board adopting a statement in 1967 on continuing education for nurses. The brochure, *Avenues for Continued Learning*, was described as a companion document to the 1965 position paper to encourage continuing professional education of all practicing nurses without regard to their previous preparation.

In 1968, the ANA HOD adopted three platform planks relative to nursing education including support for community planning for "the sound and orderly transition of nursing education into institutions of higher learning."

During the 1968–1970 biennium, the Commission on Nursing Education spelled out criteria for all new nursing programs in a communication to state boards of nursing and SNAs. The commission outlined the following minimum requirements: control by an educational institution (college or university), adequate numbers of competent faculty with graduate preparation in nursing and education, adequate financial support, and provision of clinical learning laboratories for the projected number of students.

In 1969, the ANA Board of Directors approved a statement on graduate education in nursing. This statement was considered one statement in a continuing series to comprise a comprehensive philosophy of nursing education. On the basis of an examination of the traditional goals and values of graduate education and an analysis of the expanding responsibilities of nurses, the association declared, "The major purpose of graduate education in nursing should be the preparation of nurse clinicians capable of improving nursing care through the advancement of nursing theory and science." Also in 1969 and 1970, the board endorsed various statements aimed at ending discrimination in education for nursing practice.

Upon completing its 2-$\frac{1}{2}$ years of investigation in 1970, the National Commission for the Study of Nursing and Nursing Education stated that nursing's educational system should be centered in collegiate institutions to insure enlarged social, economic, and educational opportunities. The report, *An Abstract for Action*, contained four recommendations (more on this report is presented in Chapter 5):

1. Federal agencies and private foundations should appropriate grant funds and research contracts to investigate the impact of nursing practice on the effectiveness of the health care.

2. Each state should create a planning committee to recommend specific guidelines to insure the inclusion of nursing education within collegiate institutions.

3. A national joint practice commission composed of representatives of physicians and nurses should be established to discuss the congruent roles of the two professions.

4. Federal, regional, state, and local governments should adopt measures for the increased support of nursing research as well as nursing education.

In meetings in 1970 and 1971, the Board of Directors reviewed the commission's report and endorsed its principal recommendations, pointing out that these recommendations were closely allied to ANA's long-held objectives for nursing education. The board urged SNAs to study the report and to intensify their efforts to advance implementation. The HOD endorsed the report of the commission in 1970, and for the next biennium the association worked to implement the commission's recommendations. Special attention was placed on the securing of federal aid for nursing education. Also in 1970, the house agreed that ANA should seek the development of remedial programs that will prepare minorities to enter schools of nursing; seek increased funds to provide schools of nursing with low cost loans and scholarship aid; and urge schools of nursing to develop programs of cultural studies.

In 1971, the Board of Directors took steps to establish a permanent structural unit (Council on Continuing Education) to deal with continuing education matters. Also in 1971, the National Student Nurses' Association (NSNA) passed a resolution requesting that ANA submit in writing to NSNA its definition of the role and the status of the diploma programs and graduates before the 1972 NSNA convention. The board approved a response that contained the following statements:

> The belief of ANA is that the education of all future licensed practitioners of nursing should be in institutions of higher education . . . where a student earns an associate or baccalaureate degree. The ANA Position Paper (1965) addressed itself to the future to insure that nursing would exercise its rightful voice and influence in the health care complex of tomorrow. The position paper did not in any way affect what nurses had already achieved. . . . There is no change in the legal status of graduates of diploma programs. Nurses graduated from and now enrolled in state-approved programs are eligible upon graduation to become licensed as registered nurses, subject to individual state laws.

NSNA expressed dissatisfaction with ANA's response and requested that ANA write a new position paper and include student participation in the rewriting.

In 1973, the Board of Directors approved a *Statement on Graduates of Diploma Schools of Nursing* developed by an ad hoc committee composed of representatives from ANA's membership and specialty nursing organization membership. This statement contained the following observations:

> The ANA Board of Directors wants to reaffirm its recognition that graduates of diploma schools of nursing are giving the bulk of the professional nursing care in the country. . . . The primary purpose of the 1965 Position Paper was twofold: to declare that general education should assume its full responsibility for the preparation of nursing, as it does for the preparation of other professionals; and to assure the youth of nursing the kind of education that can be equated academically with that of others. . . . Nurses have reacted primarily against the attempt to distinguish between preparation for 'professional' or 'technical' practice. These references were intended as goals for future educational programs, and were not to be used to describe nurses as individuals.

In conjunction with the adoption of the *Statement on Graduates of Diploma Schools of Nursing*, the board took the following action:

1. That every program unit of ANA take into account the special needs and interests of diploma school graduates when developing their plans for each biennium.

2. That the Commission on Nursing Education identify means by which diploma school graduates can continue their education and that the commission use its knowledge and influence to make educational opportunities available, and to promote the standardization and use of challenge mechanisms which would permit diploma graduates to have their skills and knowledge recognized and credited.

3. That all structural units and particularly the Commission on Economic and General Welfare in its concern with classification systems explore mechanisms that can be adopted to allow for horizontal and vertical mobility, and thus recognize an individual's experience, competency, and demonstrated abilities.

4. That the Commission on Nursing Education be asked to examine and determine the relevancy of the use of the terms 'professional' and 'technical' to distinguish basic preparation for nursing practice and to recognize all RNs as professionals.

(The commission presented a report to the board in 1974, prepared by its Task Force on Technical Terms, examining the terms "professional" and "technical." However, the board voted to take no action on the report as presented and referred it again to the commission. In 1975, the commission present a revised statement to the board and the board tabled a motion that "the Board of Directors accept the commission statement on the terms 'professional' and 'technical' for use within and by ANA structural units.")

In 1975, the Commission on Nursing Education issued *Standards for Nursing Education*.

The HOD, in 1976, requested that the Board convene a national conference of appropriate representatives for the purpose of developing a statement on entry into nursing practice. The House also urged the Board and staff to continue energies to counteract efforts to subjugate nursing education and nurse educators to the supervision, direction, and control by any discipline other than professional nurses. Also in 1976, the House referred to the Board a motion to reaffirm the position taken by the 1966 House that the baccalaureate degree in nursing be established as a requirement for entry into the profession of nursing. Later in 1978, the Board reported that this motion was incorporated into the discussion during the national conference on entry into practice held in 1978.

During the 1976–1978 biennium, the Commission on Nursing Education completed for publication three statements: "New Directions for Graduate Education in Nursing," "Policy for Public Funding of Nursing Education," and "Flexible Patterns in Nursing Education."

The conference mandated by the HOD in 1976 to develop a statement on entry into nursing practice occurred in 1978. The purpose of the conference was to provide the opportunity for selected representatives of the nursing profession to (1) debate the issues related to entry into nursing practice; (2) explore and discuss methods that can be utilized to implement ANA's 1965 statement on educational preparation; and (3) propose recommendations for further plans and activities regarding entry into the practice of nursing. The National Conference on Entry Into Nursing Practice was a working conference planned for 400 participants, which included nurse legislators, representatives from the Division of Nursing, educators from each type of nursing program, representatives from a variety of other nursing organizations, and three representatives for each state nurses' association. Resolutions presented to the 1978 HOD from this conference brought about agreement of the House to ensure that two categories of nursing practice be clearly identified and titled by 1980 and that by 1985 the minimum preparation for entry into professional nursing practice be the baccalaureate in nursing, and to support increased accessibility to high-quality career mobility programs that utilize flexible approaches for individuals seeking academic degrees in nursing.

The 1980 HOD agreed to consider the effects the proposed changes in educational requirements for nurses might have on minority representation in nursing. The House also agreed to endorse, publish, and disseminate educational mobility guidelines to be utilized as a mechanism to promote increased accessibility to nursing education programs for individuals seeking academic degrees in nursing. ANA agreed to advocate that nurses interested in pursuing a baccalaureate in nursing seek enrollment in colleges and schools that give consideration to the ANA standards for nursing education.

The year 1982 brought about an agreement for ANA to move forward to expedite implementation of the baccalaureate in nursing as the minimal educational qualification for entry into professional nursing practice. And in 1984, ANA agreed to establish the goal that the baccalaureate for professional nursing practice be implemented in 5 percent of the states by 1986, 15 percent of the states by 1988, 50 percent of the states by 1992, and 100 percent of the states by 1995. The ultimate goal would be congruence of professional nurse licensure with the educational base of the baccalaureate in nursing.

Titling for licensure initiated major discussion at the 1985 HOD as the House agreed to urge SNAs to establish the baccalaureate with a major in nursing as the minimum educational requirement for licensure and to retain the legal title, Registered Nurse, for that license and to establish the associate degree with a major in nursing as the educational requirement for licensure to practice technical nursing. ANA also went on record as supporting the legal title of Associate Nurse (AN) for the technical level of nursing. The House that year also supported the National Federation of Licensed Practical Nurses to increase the educational preparation of the Licensed Practical Nurse/Licensed Vocational Nurse to the associate degree level and to work with this group and the National Association for Practical Nurse Education and Service to achieve their support for ANA's position on the title Associate Nurse for the technical level.

Grandfathering of Licensed Practical Nurse/Licensed Vocational Nurse to the Associate Nurse was an issue in

1986 as the House agreed that whenever a given state implements the title "associate nurse," currently licensed LPNs/LVNs be grandfathered into technical nursing practice with that title. The educational requirement of the associate degree in nursing for those individuals would be waived.

The 1995 HOD entertained *Report NDNA: Educational Requirement for Professional Nursing Practice*, submitted by the North Dakota Nurses Association, which asserted that action must be taken to implement the baccalaureate in nursing degree as the minimum requirement for RN licensure. It further contended that ensuring that future nurses will be prepared at the appropriate level would strengthen the position of nursing in the health care debate. Following much discussion both in the Reference Hearing and on the floor of the House, the report, declaring the baccalaureate degree in nursing as the educational requirement for the beginning RN, as amended, was adopted. Thereby, the 1995 HOD agreed to (1) declare the baccalaureate degree in nursing as the educational requirement for the beginning registered or "basic" nurse in the final edition of *Nursing: A Social Policy Statement*, now renamed *Nursing's Social Policy Statement*; and (2) collaborate with selected major nursing organizations and other affected groups to identify factors impeding baccalaureate education as the entry level for professional nursing practice. In addition, the HOD voted to develop alternatives to achieve ANA's 1965 position on education for professional nursing with intent for state specific grandparenting provisions.

In 2006, the Board of Directors adopted *Education for Nurse Managers Promoting Positive Outcomes for Patients and Nurses* to promote quality patient outcomes, nurse satisfaction, and nurse retention by clarifying the education needed to develop nurse managers with the knowledge, skills, and competencies to perform their roles well. In 2008, the HOD affirmed that increased numbers of RNs with a baccalaureate degree are needed to address the ongoing challenges of an increasingly complex health care delivery system and a critical nursing faculty shortage and supported initiatives to require RNs to obtain the BSN within 10 years of initial licensure and activities to attain the degree. In addition, the 2008 HOD supported new nurse orientation programs and research efforts to demonstrate their effectiveness.

Continuing education (CE) has also been given considerable attention by ANA, gaining impetus in 1971 with the establishment of the Council on Continuing Education and the awarding of a grant for a project entitled "Identification of Need for Continuing Education for Nurses by the National Professional Organization." See Chapters 12, 13, and 20 for discussion of issues in CE, as well as information on CE units and accreditation.

ANA endorsed the concept of CE for all nurses as one of the means by which they can maintain competence. ANA believes that maintaining competence is primarily the responsibility of the practitioner. Because of a practical and philosophical reluctance to transfer this responsibility to government, the Association, by a vote of its 1972 HOD, opposed mandatory CE as a condition for renewal of a license to practice. The ANA House reversed this position in 1974, but particular emphasis was put on SNA control rather than government control. The House directed ANA to provide support to those states that choose to establish CE as one prerequisite for re-licensure, as well as to those states that choose to encourage CE through a voluntary program. By 1979, most SNAs had some sort of approved CE programs. Further, during the era when NP programs proliferated on a CE basis, some type of accreditation of these educational programs was seen as essential. ANA provided, and still provides, accreditation services for such programs that continue to exist. Since 1975, the association has provided a mechanism for the voluntary national accreditation of continuing education in nursing (now carried out by the ANCC).

Legislative, Regulatory, and Legal Advocacy

ANA's legislative and regulatory programs are focused on matters affecting nurses, nursing, and health, but in today's society these matters represent an extremely broad area of activity, ranging from child care to gun control.

ANA's governmental affairs consist of three dimensions: (1) to help SNAs promote effective nursing practice acts in their states to protect the public and the nursing profession from unqualified practitioners; (2) to offer consultation on other legislative and regulatory measures that affect nurses; and (3) to speak for nursing in relation to federal legislation for health, education, labor, and welfare, and for social programs such as civil rights.

The first ANA Committee on Legislation was established in 1923, with the responsibility of watching federal legislation affecting nursing and representing ANA in such matters. The ANA Board also determined at that time to confine the Association's legislative and regulatory work to matters of health, nurses, and nursing. ANA now has a Board-appointed Legislative Committee that recommends

legislative priorities to the Board annually. Legislative advocacy is based on ANA policy statements, House resolutions, and, of course, the ANA goals and priorities.

The major responsibility for coordinating legislative information and action lies with the ANA governmental affairs arm. It was not until late 1951 that ANA opened an office in Washington, with one staff person to act as full-time lobbyist, and direction for the legislative program emanated from ANA headquarters (then in New York). From those modest beginnings, the Washington staff and its work has grown exponentially as has its influence, including lobbying (through its registered lobbyists); development of relationships with congressional members and their staffs and committee staffs; contacts with key figures in the executive branch of government; maintaining relations with other national organizations; preparing most of the statements and information presented to congressional committees; drafting letters to government officials; presenting testimony; acting as backup for members presenting testimony; and representing ANA in many capacities. Over the years, ANA has represented nursing in the Capitol on many major issues: funds for nursing education, pension reform, national health insurance, quality of care in nursing homes, collective bargaining rights, pay equity, health hazards, civil rights, Federal Trade Commission authority and regulations, problems of nurses in the federal service, tax revision, higher education, problems of health manpower, direct reimbursement to nurses, health care reform, and more.

Major newspapers and journals have commented on nursing's influence on Capitol Hill. It is important to note that as invaluable as the ANA Washington staff is, with its behind-the-scenes and visible lobbying activities, there would be no success without the active backup of nurses, as well as consumers, labor, and other health groups. ANA has often cooperated and coordinated with other health disciplines, but has also faced areas of disagreement (such as early opposition of AMA and other groups to funding for nurse education). Such philosophical differences still occur, but there has been increasing cooperation with other groups to achieve mutual legislative goals.

Communication about legislative matters is particularly important to help members keep abreast of key legislative issues. Beginning in 1955, *Capital Commentary*, first called *Legislation News*, was sent to state associations, schools of nursing, state boards of nursing, state boards of health, chief nurses in federal services, and selected individuals. The demand and the need became so great that news of a legislative and regulatory nature is now regularly incorporated in *The American Nurse*. *Capitol Update* is now available on-line: http://nursingworld.org/gova/federal/gfederal.htm#update.

ANA is noted for its grassroots network, the Nurses Strategic Action Team (N-STAT). *N-STAT* is a program coordinated by ANA in partnership with the SNAs. It consists of the N-STAT Rapid Response Team and a legislative network that links a knowledgeable, articulate, and politically astute member of the SNA with almost every member of the US Congress. N-STAT is the power behind ANA's success on Capitol Hill. Tens of thousands of nurses in this country are formally involved in the N-STAT network.

In addition to specific legislative action, ANA becomes involved in various legal matters that affect the welfare of nurses. In some cases, ANA acts as a friend of the court, providing information about the issues involved. Since 1973, ANA has filed charges of discrimination in various district offices of the *Equal Employment Opportunities Commission* (EEOC), some of which it won and some of which are still unsettled. ANA has also presented oral arguments and briefs on various matters before the *National Labor Relations Board* (NLRB) and the US Supreme Court. The number of such services that ANA offers expands yearly.

Economic and General Welfare

The ways in which ANA has worked to promote the welfare of its membership have varied with the times. When it was first incorporated, it gave as one of its purposes, "To distribute relief among such nurses as may become ill, disabled, or destitute." Until 2009, ANA, thanks to an economic security program established in 1946, steadily expanded and strengthened that purpose, and worked actively to ensure that nurses have a voice in determining their employment conditions that nursing salaries are appropriate to nursing responsibilities, and that employment conditions are of the kind to enable nurses to give high-quality care. In 2009, the Association's economic security program (United American Nurses) disaffiliated to join in forming a rival union: National Nurses United (NNU). The following section is offered to provide a glimpse of ANA's rich history in economic and general welfare, which continues in forms other than collective bargaining.

ANA's economic security philosophy promotes the concept that nurses have a right to form a group to choose a representative to negotiate for them with their employer, and to have the mutually agreed-on provisions put in

writing. It endorses the constructive use of collective bargaining techniques in nurses' negotiations with their employers. Although ANA never served as bargaining agent for groups of nurses, many SNAs do so. ANA helped to develop the principles and techniques for such employer–employee negotiations and advised and assisted the SNAs with their economic security activities as much as possible. In addition, a major role of the ANA on the national level was to develop policy positions on economic and general welfare. Because of this role, ANA held the status of a collective bargaining organization.

Overall, ANA was concerned not only with improving salaries, fringe benefits, and working conditions, but it has also expanded its activities to improve the quality of nursing care, to assure the public of the individual and collective accountability of qualified professional nurses, and to increase the accessibility of health care services for the public. These concerns remain and are addressed through professional policy, the Magnet and Pathway Programs, and the Center for American Nurses, to name a few of the programs of ANA and its subsidiaries. Remember job action by nurses has often been in protest of inadequate patient care, which has not been improved by the employer.

Members, nonmembers, and others often misunderstand the ANA economic and general welfare program. Seeing that the economic security of its members is maintained is one of the classic roles of a professional association, and, especially in recent years, economic security has been seen as extending beyond purely monetary matters and conditions of employment to involvement of nurses in the decision-making aspects of nursing care. An example might be that, through an agreed-on process, perhaps including a formal committee structure, nurses' objections to inadequate staffing or illegal or inappropriate job assignments would be instrumental in bringing about changes that would provide improved care.

In the last few years, the nurse's right to adequate monetary compensation has been recognized almost universally, although in many places, salaries and benefits are still abysmal, and there is still a struggle involved for improvement, with or without SNA representation as a bargaining agent. There is still significant employer resistance to allowing nurses a voice in policy making, both because of the possible financial impact and because of fear of loss of control, as well as on the basis of general philosophical disagreement.

Over the years, the ANA House has made many major decisions in relation to economic security issues. In 1968, ANA's 18-year-old no-strike policy was rescinded, and in

1970, the 20-year-old neutrality policy (that nurses maintain a neutral position in labor–management disputes between their employers and non-nurse employees) was also rescinded.

The 1974 passage of a *National Labor Relations Act* (NLRA) amendment to include employees of nonprofit health care institutions created a flurry of activity. In 1975, as the result of a legal brief presented by ANA, NLRA ruled that a separate collective bargaining unit of RNs is appropriate under the normal local unit determination criteria, and by early 1980, the professional organization was the largest collective bargaining representative for RNs. Also in 1975, the ANA board of directors established the Shirley Titus Award in recognition of individual nurses' contributions to the association's economic and general welfare program. Finally, the formation of the *Commission of Economic and General Welfare* in 1976 was a further indication of increased ANA membership interest and commitment to economic and general welfare issues.

In the years following the 1974 NLRA amendments, ANA and SNAs were frequently involved in legal actions regarding various aspects of collective bargaining that are unique to nursing: whether nurses could be in separate units, the status of head nurses and supervisors as management, and whether the fact that supervisors and directors of nursing may sit on the board of directors of an SNA means that the collective bargaining agent (the SNA) is controlled by management. Decisions favoring unions have been less frequent in the last few years as unions have lost ground. Such cases are not settled with one ruling, and frequently further action is taken through appeal mechanisms or legislation. One major victory was a 1990 decision by the US Court of Appeals for the Seventh Circuit to allow nurses to organize in separate (all-RN) bargaining units. (The US Supreme Court ultimately upheld the decision.) The NLRB had made such a ruling, but a suit by the American Hospital Association (AHA) had enjoined the NLRB from implementing it. In a more negative decision of May 1994, the US Supreme Court ruled that an LPN who directed less-prepared personnel in a nursing home was considered a supervisor and therefore exempt from any legal employee protections. This could potentially challenge the right for nurses to organize and bargain collectively and to join in any concerted activity about patient care or employment conditions, whether or not a union represents them. In other words, the majority of the justices said that the direction of assistive workers was a responsibility the nurse assumed as an agent of the employer, rather than as an agent of the patient, because the consumer looked to the employer to guarantee service and safety. The decision holds implications far beyond nursing and may have to be addressed through legislation. In a minority opinion, one justice noted that every professional's work involves to some degree directing the work of others. There have since been other organizing activities that have tested this same principle and been found to support the fact that nurses supervise UAPs as part of their personal advocacy for their patients, not on behalf of their employers, and thus have a right to organize.[5] The issue is far from resolved. Further discussion on labor and collective bargaining is included in Chapters 19 and 30.

Unions, which have been successful in organizing nonprofessional health workers and a number of professionals, have been giving priority to organizing nurses. There is serious concern that large unions with strong economic backing and single-purpose goals to increase monetary and working benefits may prove competitive, for nurses frequently do not see the professional organization as a strong or even appropriate bargaining agent. Because past experience has shown that unions have taken little action to negotiate contracts involving nurses in decisions that could improve patient care and because many nurses are not even aware that such participation is possible, one of the most worthwhile purposes of collective bargaining could be lost. In 2001, SNAs represented over 100,000 RNs in 23 states, the District of Columbia, and the US Virgin Islands. The relevance of the SNAs in collective bargaining is affirmed in a 1997 study conducted by the AFL-CIO. Potential union members surveyed find association characteristics more appealing than those of the traditional union image.[6] This definitely placed the SNAs at an advantage as an amalgam of associations providing workplace representation as an optional membership benefit.

To add visibility and strength to the collective bargaining program, in 1999 a new labor entity, the United American Nurses (UAN), was established within ANA. In 2000, the HOD created the *Center for Work Place Advocacy* to service those states without collective bargaining programs. In June of 2001, registered nurse delegates to the UAN's National Labor Assembly (decision-making body) voted to affiliate with the AFL-CIO, forming a historic partnership with the federation's 64 unions. In 2009, leaders of the California Nurses Association/National Nurses Organizing Committee, United American Nurses, and Massachusetts Nurses Association came together to form National Nurses United, a competitive union. The UAN thereby disaffiliated from ANA.

In 2003, the *Center for American Nurses* became a separately incorporated organization independent of ANA. It retained this status until 2010 when the services offered by the Center were formally integrated into ANA. The Center collaborated and partnered with individuals and groups to create healthy work environments. Evidence-based solutions and powerful tools to navigate workplace challenges, optimize patient outcomes, and maximize career benefits were its forte. These services continue to be available to the nursing community through ANA. The Center never offered collective bargaining services.

It should be noted that concern for the economic security of nurses is not limited to the American scene. In 1973, the World Health Organization and the International Labor Organization jointly held an unprecedented committee meeting to discuss urgent and radical measures to alleviate international problems of the shortage, maldistribution, and poor utilization of nurses. A major objective of the meeting of health care experts from 19 nations was to set viable recommendations covering factors influencing the conditions of life and work in the nursing profession. Among the proposals presented were the right of collective bargaining, a 40-hour basic week, payment for overtime, 2 consecutive days of rest, and 4 weeks' compulsory paid leave per year. The meeting, initiated by the International Council of Nurses (ICN), of which ANA is a member, may have had positive effects on nursing around the world.

However, the issues are not easily resolved. At ICN meetings, economic issues are discussed extensively, and in meetings of the Council of National Representatives, the subject of social and economic welfare affecting nurses is a top priority. Reports indicate that unions in many countries are attempting to represent nursing and control the profession. Although the economic benefits gained through collective bargaining are obvious, the test of nurses' commitment to patient care will come as they acquire the right to become joint decision makers about conditions to improve patient care.

Human Rights Activities

ANA works toward integrating qualified members of all racial and ethnic groups into the nursing profession and tries to achieve sound human rights practices. From the time of its founding, ANA as a national organization has never had any discriminatory policies for membership in the association. Until 1964, however, a few of its constituent associations denied membership to black nurses. In these instances, ANA made provision for black nurses to bypass district and state associations and become members of ANA directly. In 1950, the *National Association of Colored Graduate Nurses* (NACGN) voluntarily went out of existence on the basis that there was no longer a need for such a specialized membership association. At the same time, strong pressure from ANA and the other state associations was exerted until now when all state and district associations have discontinued such discriminatory practices, and minority group nurses are appointed and elected to committees and offices at district, state, and national levels. ANA has also strongly supported every major civil rights bill affecting health, education, public accommodations, nursing, and equal employment opportunities. In 1956, long before most health and professional associations had taken a positive stance on civil rights, ANA's Board of Directors adopted a statement supporting the principle that health and education should not be supported by tax funds if there are any discriminatory practices. Testimony along these lines was presented at federal hearings.

Even so, there was some feeling that a greater effort was necessary, and in 1972, the HOD passed the Affirmative Action Resolution, calling for a taskforce to develop and implement a program to correct inequities. The program was defined as "a positive ongoing effort that is results-oriented and specifically designed to transcend neutrality." It was aimed at not only nondiscriminatory programming, but also at action to correct past deficiencies at all levels and in all segments of an organization. An ombudsman was also provided for and appointed.

The program went into action in 1973, and a taskforce of minority and non-minority members met with ANA units to identify problems and make plans. A minority position statement was developed, recommending methodology for change on such issues as recruitment and retention of minority students, lack of data on career patterns of minority group RNs, and the need to include information in nursing education about the health needs of minority groups. In the years that followed, several regional conferences were held on quality care for ethnic minority clients, and the papers were published. The taskforce also published a bibliography, *Minority Groups in Nursing*, in 1973; an updated bibliography was published in 1976 after the establishment of the Commission on

Human Rights. Both were a compilation of the literature on ethnic people of color, men, and those with different lifestyles who are in nursing, as well as other pertinent topics relating to minorities and the provision of health care to minorities.

In 1974, ANA was awarded a 6-year grant by the Center for Minority Group Mental Health Programs of the National Institutes of Mental Health to establish and administer the *Registered Nurse Fellowship Program for Ethnic/Racial Minorities*. The program continues today and supports minority nurses in doctoral study in psychiatric mental health nursing or a related behavioral or social science. Over half of the fellows have earned doctorates. Most are teaching or doing research on the health needs of minorities.

ANA has taken positive legal action on minority rights and women's rights (salary and pension discrepancies). With the support of most members, ANA also made a major statement on reproductive health and took action in the *Cruzan* case to uphold patients' rights (see Chapter 22).

Since 1974, ANA has taken a position in support of the ERA and participates in various women's rights programs and activities. There is no doubt that activities related to human rights will continue. It is important that the valuable services of all nurses be fully utilized and the nursing needs of the pluralistic American society be met.

Communication and Information Services

ANA is a veritable gold mine of information. The association publishes *The American Nurse*, which reports recent activities and happenings important to the nursing community. ANA is also a clearinghouse for information on the state-specific statutory requirements for nursing, language in collective bargaining contracts, and the prevailing demographics of practicing nurses, as some examples. ANA's website nursingworld.org is a comprehensive on-line source of current information about ANA and its affiliate structures, and is also the home of the *On-line Journal of Issues in Nursing*.

NursesBooks.org, the publishing arm of ANA, publishes standards of practice, the *Code for Nurses*, major reports, monographs, papers presented at meetings, and certain publications of the AAN and ANCC. The association also publishes position statements, guidelines for practice, bulletins, manuals, and brochures for specialized groups within the organization and sends out news releases and announcements concerning activities of interest to the public. Available from NursesBooks.org on request is its periodically revised *Catalogue*, and a list of publications is also available on-line.

■ THE AMERICAN ACADEMY OF NURSING

A significant action taken by the 1966 HOD was the creation of the American Academy of Nursing (AAN) to provide for the recognition of professional achievement and excellence. Because of the financial problems of ANA in the late 1960s, the Academy was not established until early 1973. At that time, 36 nationally prominent nurses were selected as charter fellows of the Academy by the ANA Board of Directors. Included were practitioners, researchers, academicians, and administrators from 34 states. The vision of the AAN is to transform health care so as to optimize the well-being of the American people and the world in general. The mission of the Academy is to

- Provide visionary leadership to the nursing profession.
- Potentiate the contributions of nursing leaders.
- Advance the development and synthesis of knowledge.
- Shape the formulation of effective health care policies and practices.

The AAN's goals are to

- Anticipate national and international trends in health care and address resulting issues of health care knowledge and policy.
- Inform public and professional constituencies of the state of health care knowledge and policy issues.
- Elect and sustain a distinguished, diverse, and active membership.
- Augment the senior-level leadership skills of distinguished nurses and encourage the deployment of these nurse leaders in a wide array of policy forums.
- Communicate effectively the accomplishments and values of the AAN to ensure public and private funding for articulated priorities.
- Develop an effective and efficient organizational structure to achieve the aforementioned goals.

The Academy was constituted as a self-governing affiliate of ANA to insulate its work from the inevitable politics of membership associations. The Academy has its own dues structure, bylaws, and elected officials. Using AAN as the vehicle, the leadership corps for the profession provides thinking on the critical issues confronting nursing. Their ability to create and disseminate intellectual products must be unencumbered by political pressure. The AAN has responded well to the challenge of shaping the future. *The Magnet Hospital Study of 1983* set the stage for the current Magnet Hospital and Nursing Home Programs instituted by ANCC to pay tribute to departments of nursing service that are exemplars. *The Teaching Nursing Home Program* contributed significantly to the nursing home reforms of 1987.[7] *The AAN Clinical Scholars Program* accorded advanced practice nursing intellectual respect and moved the practice toward the level of distinction it currently enjoys. The faculty practice initiative of the 1980s gave credibility to service-education unification efforts that have since become the standard to bring the best of nursing to both students and patients. The AAN has accomplished its work through demonstration projects, annual meetings, expert panels that are a major mechanism for continuing problem solving and discussion around issues, dissemination of ideas through *Nursing Outlook* (the Academy's official journal), and the wide reach of its influential members.

For the Academy, knowledge is power. And the establishment of three scholar-in-residence programs, each cosponsored with a major governmental or quasi-governmental entity, has augmented this image. *The Scholar with the National Institute of Nursing Research* (NINR) is challenged to develop a nursing research initiative that complements the NINR priorities. *The Agency for Health Care Research and Quality (AHCRQ)/AAN Scholar* focuses on areas of investigation that integrate clinical nursing with cost, quality, and accessibility concerns. *The Institute of Medicine (IOM)/AAN Scholar* is concerned with health policy issues.[8]

Two current Fellows in good standing must sponsor nurses who wish to become Fellows. The Academy's *Fellow Selection Committee* reviews the applications according to established procedures and determines those applicants who meet the criteria for fellowship. Criteria for selection of Fellows are as follows:

- Member in good standing of ANA
- Evidence of outstanding contributions to nursing, such as
  - Pioneering efforts that contribute information that is useful in surmounting barriers to effective nursing practice or facilitating excellence in nursing practice
  - Successful implementation of creative approaches to curriculum development, the definition of specialized areas for practice, or the development of specialized training programs
  - Research or demonstration projects that contribute to improvement in nursing and health service delivery
  - Creative development, utilization, or evaluation of specific concepts or principles in nursing education, nursing practice, nursing management, or health services
  - Authorship of books, papers, or other communication media that have had significant implications for nursing practice, health policy, or health planning
  - Successful development of health policy or health planning
  - Leadership in nursing organizations at the local, state, or national level
- Evidence of potential to continue contributions to nursing and to the academy, such as the following:
  - Efforts, projects, or other activities that relate to contemporary problems
  - Efforts, projects, or other activities that reflect a broad perspective on nursing including social, cultural, and political considerations
  - An expressed willingness to actively participate in and support academy activities

Members designated as Fellows of the American Academy of Nursing are entitled to use the initials FAAN following their names.

■ THE AMERICAN NURSES CREDENTIALING CENTER

The ANA established a certification program in 1973 to recognize professional achievement and excellence in practice. The impetus for the establishment of the certification program is found in the adoption by the 1958 HOD of the following goal: "To establish ways within the ANA to provide formal recognition of personal achievement and superior performance in nursing."[9] In 1968, interim certification boards began to work with the Congress for Nursing Practice to establish criteria for certification. By 1973, ANA was completing arrangements for its certification program. Included was an arrangement with the Educational Testing Service (ETS) of Princeton, New Jersey, to provide technical support in the development of systems for certification, including appropriate examinations.

(ANA-appointed expert panels provided the content for these tests, and ETS the test development expertise.) By 1974, criteria had been fully delineated for geriatric nursing, psychiatric and mental health nursing, pediatric NPs, and community health nursing. Any licensed RN who could demonstrate current knowledge and excellence in practice, regardless of the basic program from which the nurse graduated, was eligible to take the examination.

More than 5000 applications were received for the first examination given in May 1973. Until then, nurses had rarely been recognized or rewarded for excellent patient care. Monetary rewards, prestige, and promotion had been via the administrative route or through educational achievement.

ANA became one organizational entity among several who certified nurses. ANA's program was predated by successful certification offerings from the American Association of Nurse Anesthetists and the American College of Nurse Midwives. Other specialty societies also expressed the intent to begin to certify in their areas of practice.

In 1976, the ANA announced that it would certify at two levels: (1) certification for competence in specialized areas of practice with distinctive eligibility requirements, and (2) certification for excellence in practice, with the potential for diplomate status in a proposed American College of Nursing Practice for certified nurses who met additional criteria. The proposal was given a hostile reception, primarily because the diplomate status called for a master's degree, and many of those certified for excellence had no degree at all. In other words, the model provided for three levels of practice distinction: competence, excellence, and diplomate. In rethinking the program, two levels of certification were identified: competence in specialized areas of practice (generalist) and acknowledged achievement as a specialist. The former required a bachelor's degree by the end of 1998, and the latter called for the master's degree. Each was based on the assessment of knowledge, demonstration of current practice ability, and endorsement of colleagues.

During its 1989 review of ANA's organizational structure and functions, COAR recommended that the ANA Board of Directors establish a separately incorporated center through which ANA would serve its credentialing programs. At the HOD meeting in June 1989 it was voted to adopt this recommendation of COAR. As a result, in 1991 the ANA certification program became a separately incorporated entity called the American Nurses Credentialing Center (ANCC). The ANCC philosophy of credentialing *is based on, and is consistent with, the adopted ethical codes of ANA and its policies*, standards, and positions on nursing practice, education, and service.

ANCC offers certification, accreditation, and recognition programs that reflect a commitment to professionalism in nursing and provide consumer safeguards. Certification by ANCC provides tangible recognition of professional achievement. The ANCC Accreditation Program administers a national system for the evaluation and recognition of continuing education in nursing. *The Magnet Recognition Program and Pathway to Excellence Designation* recognizes excellence in nursing services. Together these programs contribute to ANCC's position of national leadership.

The Pathway to Excellence has a lot of the qualities of Magnet status, but it focuses on the professional work environment and whether the organization values nurses. Focus is on the workplace, balanced lifestyle, the collaborative atmosphere, positive nurse job satisfaction and retention, as examples. Pathway differs from Magnet in that Magnet also recognizes excellence in patient care, with standards that encompass leadership, professional practice and development, innovation and research, and outcomes. Magnet builds on research and evidence-based practice. Pathway is suitable to all sized facilities, but it is ideal for small and medium health care organizations, and it is well suited to rural hospitals that may not have the resources of a large, urban center. Facilities can hold both Magnet and Pathway designations, but many organizations use Pathway as a bridge or first step toward Magnet.

Its Board of Directors is the governing body of ANCC. ANA appoints all Board members, and six ANCC members are sitting members of the ANA Board of Directors. The ANCC Commission on Certification is responsible for implementing the certification program. Among its functions, the commission sets certification program policy; establishes boards on certification; serves as the final appellate body for certification candidate appeals; receives, reviews, and comments on proposals from the ANA Congress on Nursing Practice and Economics for new certification programs; and provides a mechanism for the systematic evaluation of the certification program. There is a Test Development Committee (TDC) responsible for each certification exam. Each TDC is composed of certified nurses who are content experts in their specialty field. TDC members typically represent a variety of practice settings and educational backgrounds.

In 2002, ANCC certified in 40 specialty and advanced practice areas. ANCC certification exams are administered by authorized testing agencies at locations across the country. The exams are given in either computer-based or written format. Twenty certification examinations were being offered at the generalist level and 20 at the advanced practice level for nurses, including certifications for dieticians and pharmacists in diabetes management (see Exhibit 25–3).

In 2000, ANCC approved an additional certification for diploma and associate degree nursing practice. This policy change was called *Open Door 2000* and created the implementation of two levels of specialty credentialing: Clinical Nurse Specialists are to use the title CNS-BC after their name; NPs, on the other hand, use the corresponding specialty certification followed by the letters NP-BC, that is, ANP-BC, FNP-BC, ACNP-BC, and so on. The BC stands for Board Certified. Since its inception in 1991, ANCC has certified over 150,000 nurses.

The eligibility criteria for each certification vary according to the specialty area. Applicants submit proof of their eligibility in the form of documentation of CE, educational transcripts, and nurse colleague endorsement forms. Some of the specialty areas require both past and present practice, whereas all require current licensure as an RN in the United States or its territories. Once awarded, the certification is valid for 5 years and may be renewed by either completing a stipulated amount of CE or by reexamination. Specific information on eligibility criteria for each specialty area and the cost of the exam may be obtained by contacting ANCC through its website at http://www.nursingworld.org/ancc.

The accreditation program, which is also administered by ANCC, was established in 1974 by ANA as a voluntary system for accreditation of CE in nursing. The essential purpose of this system is to provide professional nursing judgment on the quality of the CE offered. Accreditation is a peer review system based on designated standards and criteria for CE in nursing. *The ANCC Commission on Accreditation*, utilizing the ANA's *Standards for Continuing Education in Nursing*, is responsible for developing and monitoring the operational policies, procedures, and criteria that govern the accreditation and approval processes. The commission defines *accreditation* as a voluntary process for appraising and granting recognition to an organization or institution that meets established standards based on predetermined criteria. The two categories of accreditation available in the ANCC system are (1) accreditation as an approver of CE in nursing and (2) accreditation as a provider of CE in nursing.

■ **EXHIBIT 25–3. American Nurses Credentialing Center Board Certifications**

Nurse Practitioners
Acute Care NP
Adult NP
Adult Psychiatric and Mental Health NP
Diabetes Management – Advanced
Family NP
Family Psych and Mental Health NP
Gerontological NP
Pediatric NP
School NP

Clinical Nurse Specialists
Adult Health CNS
Adult Psychiatric and Mental Health CNS
Child/Adolescent Psych and Mental Health CNS
CNS Core Exam
Diabetes Management – Advanced
Gerontological CNS
Home Health CNS
Pediatric CNS
Public/Community Health CNS

Other Advanced Level
Diabetes Management – Advanced
Forensic Nursing – Advanced
Nurse Executive – Advanced
Public Health Nursing – Advanced

Specialties
Ambulatory Care Nursing
Cardiac Rehabilitation Nursing
Cardiac Vascular Nursing
Case Management Nursing
College Health Nursing
Community Health Nursing
General Nursing Practice
Gerontological Nursing
High-Risk Perinatal Nursing
Home Health Nursing
Informatics Nursing
Maternal-Child Nursing
Medical-Surgical Nursing
Nurse Executive
Nursing Professional Development
Pain Management
Pediatric Nursing
Perinatal Nursing
Psychiatric and Mental Health Nursing
School Nursing

Source: ANCC. http://www.nursecredentialing.org/certification. aspx. Retrieved March 10, 2010.

The ANCC introduced the Magnet Recognition Program in 1994. It is built on the 1983 Magnet Hospital Study conducted by the AAN. The baseline for its development is the ANA *Standards for Organized Nursing Services and Responsibilities of Nurse Administrators Across All Settings* (1991). The program is a joint endeavor of ANA and ANCC. The goal of the Magnet Recognition Program is to recognize excellence in nursing services and to identify health care facilities that act as a "magnet," creating a work environment that attracts and retains professional nurses. The *Commission on Magnet Program* currently recognizes 55 health care organizations for their excellence in nursing service.

■ THE AMERICAN NURSES ASSOCIATION POLITICAL ACTION COMMITTEE

Important components of nursing lobbying efforts are the nursing political action groups. Most professional organizations have such groups, which are independent of the organization but related to it. This is because a tax-exempt, incorporated professional organization such as ANA (or AMA) is under definite legal constraints as far as partisan political action is concerned. In 1971, a small group of nurses in New York formed the Nurses for Political Action (NPA) to serve as a political arm for ANA by providing financial support for candidates and engaging in other political activities, as well as providing political education to nurses. In 1973, ANA directed an ad hoc committee to explore the possibility of a political action committee (PAC). For various reasons, a new organization evolved: *Nurses' Coalition for Action in Politics* (N-CAP), which was officially organized in 1974 with a $50,000 ANA grant, as a voluntary, unincorporated, nonpartisan political action group. This is now called the *American Nurses Association Political Action Committee* (ANA-PAC). ANA does not give money to ANA-PAC to give to candidates, but it does provide funds for ANA-PAC administrative support. ANA-PAC has a single purpose: to promote the improvement of health care through political action. Its two major functions are education and support. Education is directed toward encouraging nurses and others to take a more active part in governmental affairs, educating them on the political process and political issues relevant to health care, and assisting them in organizing themselves for effective political action. For this purpose, ANA-PAC has sponsored workshops and prepared educational materials. It has also encouraged and assisted PACs on the state level. Many states now have active PACs that primarily give attention to state issues, but are also able to coordinate collective action on national legislation.

Support is offered to political candidates (regardless of political party affiliation) whose acts demonstrate dedication to constructive health care legislation. This support may be in the form of endorsement or include monetary contributions. Endorsements are made in consultation with state PACs whenever possible. State political action coalitions endorse state candidates. The fact that nurses, or at least SNA members, are perhaps more politically active than other citizens was shown by one survey: 91 percent are registered to vote, 75 percent have written a letter to an officeholder expressing an opinion, 58 percent have attended a political meeting or rally, and about 58 percent have contributed money to a candidate.

To support these activities, ANA-PAC accepts donations from nurses and others. It is headquartered at 8515 Georgia Avenue, Suite 400, Silver Spring, MD 20910.

■ THE AMERICAN NURSES' FOUNDATION

The American Nurses' Foundation (ANF) was created by ANA to meet the need for an independent, permanent, nonprofit organization devoted to nursing research. It was an outgrowth of the ANA's expanding research activities, particularly the 5-year *Studies of Nursing Function*, which was undertaken by ANA after the 1950 convention, both because of a mandate by membership and as an assumption of the profession's responsibility to determine its own functions.

Initial financing of this project was provided by the SNAs, but by the third year the ANA Board of Directors decided to finance the program from the Association's budget. Between 1950 and 1955, 27 studies were funded. *Nurses Invest in Patient Care*, a preliminary report, was prepared and published by ANA in 1956. Written by Everett C. Hughes, Helen MacGill Hughes, and Irwin Deutscher, *20,000 Nurses Tell Their Story* was published in 1958; it was a synthesis of the findings of ANF-funded studies.

So that such research could be continued and expanded, the ANA Board recommended that the 1954 HOD "authorize the incoming board of directors to secure information and to develop a foundation or trust for receiving tax-free funds for desirable charitable, scientific, literary or educational projects in line with the aims and purposes of the American Nurses Association." After 6 months of committee study, the establishment of the ANF was approved by the new Board. It was incorporated in

1955, and its tax-exempt status was approved in 1956. The foundation was organized exclusively for charitable, scientific, literary, and educational purposes.

Between 1955 and 1973, the major objectives of ANF were to provide financial support for research and to disseminate and promote the dissemination of research findings through publications, conferences, and other communications media.

In 1979, the ANF Board established major new objectives focusing on the analysis of health policy issues of priority to nursing, support for the career development of nurses, and assistance to the educational and research activities of ANA.

ANF has continued its *Nursing Research Grants Program*, funded through the contributions of corporations, nursing organizations, and individuals. In 1983, the ANF *Distinguished Scholar Program* was established. The purpose of the program, jointly sponsored by the IOM, is to permit nurse health policy analysts and scholars to analyze selected policy issues related to economics, the delivery of nursing services, nursing practice, and nursing education as identified by the nursing profession. In 1980, in collaboration with the American Nurses Association Council of Nurse Researchers, ANF also established a *Distinguished Contribution to Nursing Science Award* to recognize nurse researchers who have made significant contributions to the nursing profession.

The Professional Practice for Nurse Administrators in Long-Term Care Facilities Project (NA/LTC) was cosponsored by ANF and the Foundation of the American College of Health Care Administrators, Inc. (FACHCA) and was supported by a grant from the W. K. Kellogg Foundation. The primary goal of this 3-year project (completed in April 1984 and then refunded) was the continued professional development of nurse administrators and directors of nursing in long-term care. A health education project involving Missouri elementary schools was another early ANF project. ANF also partners with ANA in the *Quality and Safety Initiative*, which has resulted in the Nursing Report Card implementation through the SNAs. This is only representative of some of the work accomplished directly through the Foundation over the years. The ANF solicits, receives, and/or administers funds.

Obviously, funding is of vital concern to ANF. In 1992, ANF concluded a successful *Nursing on the Move* campaign, raising $1.5 million toward the relocation of its headquarters to Washington, DC. In 1993, ANF received a $2 million bequest from the estate of Julia Ondo Hardy,

RN, the largest bequest in the history of nursing in the United States.

ANF is governed by its bylaws and directed by a nine-member board of trustees; six of the trustees are RNs. A finance committee and a research advisory committee report to the board of trustees. The finance committee monitors budget preparation, the investment portfolio, and fundraising activities. The research advisory committee establishes guidelines for administering the small grant program and recommends recipients to the board for final approval. A Corporate Advisory Council lends the strength of big business. The executive director of ANA is the executive director of ANF. There is also a professional headquarters staff involved in fundraising and managing grant-funded projects.

Requests for information about completed ANF research projects or applications for grants (which should include an outline of the research question and the proposed design) may be sent to ANF headquarters at 8515 Georgia Avenue, Suite 400, Silver Spring, MD 20910.

ANA Participation with Other Groups

In the conduct of business, the ANA staff, officials, and members meet with some 300 organizations and groups. Much of this participation is in the form of official liaisons and coalitions. There are also many occasions for cosponsorship of conferences, educational programs, and projects.

One formal liaison that warrants mentioning is the *Tri-Council*, composed of ANA, NLN, the American Organization of Nurse Executives (AONE), and AACN. The Tri-Council is discussed in Chapter 26.

ANA is a member of the National Quality Forum (NQF), a private, not-for-profit membership organization created to develop and implement a national strategy for health care quality measurement and reporting. The mission of the NQF is to improve American health care through the endorsement of consensus-based national standards for measurement and public reporting of health care performance. This data must provide meaningful information about whether care is safe, timely, beneficial, patient centered, equitable, and efficient. In a report issued in 1998, the President's Advisory Commission on Consumer Protection and Quality in the Health Care Industry proposed the creation of the Forum as part of an integrated national quality improvement agenda. Leaders from consumer, purchaser, provider, health plan, and health service research organizations met as the Quality Forum Planning Committee throughout 1998 and early 1999 to define the mission, structure, and financing of the Forum. The Forum was incorporated as a new organization in May 1999. There are approximately 400 members currently and ANA, joining in 2000, was the first and is one of only 19 nursing organizations that are members.

ANA and NQF convened a group of interprofessional health experts for a day and a half workshop. The workshop focused on the role of nursing within the National Priorities Partners (NPPs) priorities and goals. The ANA, one of the 32 official NPPs, hosted the event at their headquarters in Silver Spring, Maryland.

The purpose of this workshop was to provide an intensive interprofessional forum for the timely ongoing discussion of the ways in which the field of nursing is contributing to moving the National Priorities agenda forward and how this work can be further leveraged toward the attainment of the national priorities and goals. Participants were asked to highlight current work in respect to the efforts of nursing around the six NPP priorities and goals.

The framework for discussions centered on the drivers of transformation in health care, including

- Performance measurement
- Public reporting
- Payment systems
- Research and knowledge dissemination
- Professional development: education and certification
- System capacity

Particular emphasis was placed on professional development, research and knowledge dissemination, system capacity, and professional development.

A small planning group from ANA, AAN, and NQF staff worked within a tight time frame to organize a robust agenda to set a framework and goals for the discussion. The need for transforming the health care system is urgent and the ability to demonstrate value and continuous improvement is essential. Nurses and nursing are vital to these endeavors. Nursing joins many other private and public organizations and professional groups mobilized to create a coherent and accountable system for assuring the quality of health care.

A diverse group of experts joined the NQF Nursing Organizational Members and ANA Organizational Affiliates in actively strategizing how nursing will advance the priorities. Day two of the conference focused on the development of an overall nursing strategy and action plan to advance the National Priorities and Goals developed by the NPPs. The voices of nursing's many constituencies, including consumers, quality organizations, policy makers, and colleagues in other health disciplines, contributed to the development of the action plan. This action plan will provide guidance to nursing in developing and implementing activities to improve patient care centered on the NPP priorities. Workshop materials, including participant and observer biosketches, are posted on nursingworld.org. ANA continues to monitor ongoing NQF projects and spearheads the nomination of highly qualified nurses to Steering Committees, Technical Advisory Panels, workgroups, and the Board of Directors on behalf of the 19 NQF Nursing Organizational Members. Since that process began, over 55 RNs have been appointed to a host of NQF Steering Committees and Technical Advisory Panels.

In addition, ANA participates as a Principal in the Hospital Quality Alliance's (HQA's) *Improving Care through Information*, a public–private collaboration to improve the quality of care provided by the nation's hospitals through measuring and publicly reporting on that care. This collaboration includes the Centers for Medicare and Medicaid Services (CMS), the American Hospital Association, the Federation of American Hospitals, and the Association of American Medical Colleges, and is supported by other organizations such as the Agency for Healthcare Research Quality, National Quality Forum, Joint Commission on Accreditation of Healthcare Organizations, American Medical Association, American Nurses Association, National Association of Children's Hospitals and Related Institutions, Consumer-Purchaser Disclosure Project, AFL-CIO, and American Association for Retired Persons. The goal of the program is to identify a robust set of standardized and easy-to-understand hospital quality measures. An important element of the collaboration, *Hospital Compare*, is a website/web-tool developed to publicly report credible and user-friendly information about the quality of care delivered in the nation's hospitals.

ANA also serves on the National Priorities Partnership, the right people coming together at the right time. The Partners are committed to real action that will transform the nation's health care system. The 32 Partner organizations have significant influence over health care, uniquely positioning them to improve America's health and health care system. The Partnership has a vision for world-class, affordable health care and is transforming health care from the inside out. Throughout the process, ANA seeks input from the greater nursing community that is shared with NQF staff. A number of suggested examples of nursing actions were included in the NPP document that is available at http://www.nationalprioritiespartnership.org/.

Mapping of the work of NPP to health reform legislation takes place on an ongoing basis. The Care Coordination Workgroup is focusing on the period immediately following hospital discharge to promote the timeliness of patient follow-up with the goal that all health care organizations and their staff will work collaboratively with patients to reduce 30-day readmission rates. This will be accomplished by convening key stakeholder groups to develop a strategy for measuring and improving the timeliness of post-acute follow-up to prevent hospital readmissions, considering the appropriate window of time (e.g., 0 to 14 days); data to be captured, data sources and tools (e.g., EHR, PHR), and alignment with "meaningful use" requirements; and types of visits (office, phone, or e-visits). Stakeholders include, among others, providers (hospitals, home health, nursing home, etc.), health care practitioners (primary care, APN, etc.), and purchasers.

Other Activities and Services

Among other ANA benefits for nurses is insurance of various kinds at favorable group rates. Many educational programs, seminars, workshops, clinical conferences, scientific sessions, and so on are also available at reduced rates for members. The state or national association may offer these benefits.

Nurses are also increasingly interested in international nursing. ANA was one of the three charter members of the ICN and is an active participant in the work of this organization. Essentially, ICN is a federation of national associations of professional nurses (one from each of the countries), and ANA is the member association for the United States (see Chapter 27).

ANA established the *International Nursing Center* in 1992. The Center sponsors an international talent bank composed of nurses with expertise in international work and foreign language capability. The Center was awarded a grant by the World AIDS Foundation in 1993 to train nurses in Sri Lanka and India in HIV/AIDS prevention and care.

■ THE INDIVIDUAL NURSE AND ANA

A classic article by sociologist Robert Merton cites the functions of any professional organization as including social and moral support to help the individual practitioner perform the professional role, to set rigorous standards for the profession and help enforce them, to advance and disseminate research and professional knowledge, to help furnish the social bonds through which society coheres, and to speak for the profession. In carrying out some of these functions, the association is seen as a "kind of organizational gadfly, stinging the profession into new and more demanding formulations of purpose."[10] Not all members agree with their organization's goals, and the difficult task of achieving a flexible consensus of values and policies must be accomplished with full two-way communication between the constituencies and the organizational top. However, the key to the success of any organization is the participation of its members. This review of the ANA and its activities is at best an overview. As the needs of members and the demands of society require, changes occur rapidly, inevitably, and, it is hoped, appropriately— but not always easily. The best way for a nurse to keep up with and share in the changes taking place is through active membership. ANA speaks for nurses; nonmembers have no part in that voice and have no right to complain if it is not representing them. The strength in the organization and in nursing lies in thinking, communicating nurses committed to the goal of improving nursing care for the public and working together in an organized fashion to achieve this goal.

KEY POINTS

1. The rapid increase in specialty associations resulted in some initial lack of coordination in advancing nursing goals.

2. The National Federation of Specialty Nursing Organizations (NFSNO), the Tri-Council, and the Alliance are examples, past and current, of the way that nursing organizations have established relationships that allow them to communicate and collaborate in areas of mutual interest.

3. ANA focuses considerable attention on nursing practice, education, human rights, economic and general welfare, and standard setting. ANA sees itself as speaking for America's nurses.

4. ANA has been sensitive to changing times, reorganizing and speaking out on unpopular subjects when it was necessary for the public good.

KEY POINTS

5. Many programs started internal to the association and then became independent organizations or affiliates as they matured.

6. The American Academy of Nursing was established to recognize leadership in the profession; it is insulated from the politics of the association so that its members may safely provide their best thinking on issues critical to nursing.

7. ANCC is an internationally renowned credentialing center that certifies nurses in specialty practice; recognizes health care organizations for excellence through the Magnet and Pathway Programs; and accredits providers of continuing nursing education.

8. The ANA-PAC's major strength is its grassroots organization.

9. ANA has always been committed to the welfare of nurses, and established its economic security program in 1946.

REFERENCES

1. ANA. *Bylaws*. Silver Spring, MD: The Author, 2008.

2. *Nursing's Agenda for Health Care Reform*. Washington, DC: ANA, 1991.

3. ANA. http://www.nursingworld.org. Retrieved September 26, 1998.

4. Gallagher RM, Sullivan K. *Compendium of ANA Education Positions, Position Statements and Documents*. Silver Spring, MD: Author, 2009.

5. Time line: The evolution of the NLRB decision. *Am Nurse* 28:32, March 1996.

6. *AFL-CIO: 1997 Communications Survey*. Internal document. ANA, August 20, 1997.

7. Mezey M, Lynaugh J, Cartier M. The teaching nursing home program. *Nurs Outlook* 23:146–150, May–June 1984.

8. American Academy of Nursing. http://www.nursingworld.org/aan. Retrieved September 24, 1998.

9. ANA. *Summary of the 1958 House Action*. Kansas City, MO: The Author, 1958.

10. Merton R. The functions of the professional association. *Am J Nurs* 58:50–54, January 1958.

Updates can be found at **www.kellysnursing.com**

CHAPTER 26

The Tri-Council for Nursing

The Origins of the Tri-Council for Nursing are in the American Nurses Association/National League for Nursing (ANA/NLN) Joint Coordinating Committee, which dates back to 1952. In 1952, a major reorganization of nursing associations resulted in a strengthened and expanded ANA, the establishment of the NLN, and the need for a coordinating mechanism. The Tri-Council became this mechanism. In time, the American Association of Colleges of Nursing (AACN) and the American Organization of Nurse Executives (AONE) were added to this coalition. Despite the addition of AONE as a fourth member in 1986, the name *Tri-Council* was retained. Business is carried out through the presidents and executive directors of these organizations, who meet regularly.

The Tri-Council positions nursing strongly by bringing to one table those organizations that have the broadest perspective on the affairs of the profession, representing practice, education, and nursing services in organized health care systems. The actions of any one of these associations have implications far beyond its own constituency. The Tri-Council's common agenda focuses on the management of issues that touch every nurse either directly or indirectly, and action has taken the form of grantsmanship or pooled resources such as federal lobbying or consolidation of staff in a number of different arrangements. Each association maintains its autonomy but is to some degree accountable to each of the others. Examples of Tri-Council areas of concern in the past are nursing's public image, the nursing shortage, recruitment to the field, federal funding for nursing research and education, and a host of other legislative and regulatory concerns. In the past, the National Commission on Nursing Implementation Project (NCNIP), the Ad Council Campaign, Nurses of America (nurses in the media), and more were created by the Tri-Council, funded through their efforts, and executed by one, several, or all of the members assuming a leadership role.

This chapter presents each of the Tri-Council organizations in more detail and also identifies other coalitions that have been created to speak with one strong voice in more specialized areas. ANA, as the membership organization for every nurse through his or her state or constituent nurses' association (SNA), has already been discussed. NLN, AACN, and AONE are included here.

■ NATIONAL LEAGUE FOR NURSING

It is easier to understand the origins of the Tri-Council and the uniqueness of NLN if the events surrounding the restructuring of nursing organizations in 1952 are reviewed. In many ways, NLN is older than the date suggests, because it grew out of several preexisting nursing organizations and absorbed many of the functions they had performed (see Chapters 3 and 4). In the mid-1940s, the nursing profession decided to take a long, hard look at its entire organizational structure. At this time there were six national nursing organizations and a host of jointly sponsored committees, activities, and services. This somewhat cumbersome arrangement resulted not only in an overlapping expenditure of time, effort, and resources but also in confusion in the minds of both nurses and the public as to the purpose and functions of each organization.

Starting in 1944, nurses, under the leadership of the Committee on Structure of National Nursing Organizations, began to study the way in which their profession was organized. The culmination of this long and painstaking self-examination came in 1952 in Atlantic City, New Jersey. At that time, nurses voted in favor of having two major organizations: a strengthened and reorganized ANA, which would continue to serve as the membership association for registered nurses (RNs), and the NLN, through which nurses and others interested in nursing, along with institutions (both educational and service), could work together to strengthen nursing education and nursing services.

The six organizations prior to the 1952 decision were ANA, the National League of Nursing Education (NLNE), the National Organization for Public Health Nursing (NOPHN), the Association of Collegiate Schools of Nursing (ACSN), the National Association of Colored Graduate Nurses (NACGN), and the American Association of Industrial Nurses (AAIN). NACGN voluntarily went out of existence in 1951, because ANA required all its constituents to admit to membership RNs without discrimination on the basis of color. AAIN decided to continue as a separate organization. The newly created NLN, however, inherited the major functions of the other three organizations—excluding, of course, ANA. So education and public health/community health practice became the NLN's domain.

NLNE was the first nursing organization in the United States. Established in 1893 under the formidable title of the American Society of Superintendents of Training Schools for Nurses of the United States and Canada (it became NLNE in 1912), its purpose was to standardize and improve the education of nurses. Originally for nurses only, it broadened its membership policies in 1943 to admit lay members.

NOPHN was established in 1912. As its title implies, it was an organization concerned not only with public health nurses but also with the development of public health nursing services. It provided for both agency and individual membership—the latter, except in NOPHN's very early years, open to non-nurses as well as nurses.

The prime objective of ACSN, started in 1933 when baccalaureate degree education for nurses was just beginning to make headway, was to develop nursing education on a professional and collegiate basis. Membership was open principally to accredited programs offering college degrees in nursing.

Mission and Goals

"The National League for Nursing promotes excellence in nursing education to build a strong and diverse nursing workforce."[1] This is the NLN's mission statement. The following goals support the mission statement and are organized around four major themes—leadership in nursing education, commitment to members, champions for nurse educators, and advancement of the science of nursing education:

- Enhance the NLN's national and international impact as the recognized leader in nursing education.
- Build a diverse, sustainable, member-led organization with the capacity to deliver NLN's mission effectively, efficiently, and in accordance with its values
- Be the voice of nurse educators and champion their interests in political, academic, and professional arenas.
- Promote evidence-based nursing education and the scholarship of teaching.

Membership and Structure

The NLN is unique in that it provides the opportunity for both organizational and individual membership. Additionally, its membership is not exclusive to nurses, but allows the participation of consumers and friends of nursing. Membership currently includes

- More than 1200 institutions
- Approximately 30,000 individual nurse educators, graduate students, and consumers
- 23 constituent leagues

The NLN is governed by an 18-member Board of Governors that consists of four elected officers (president, president-elect, secretary, and treasurer) and 14 members at large. The chief executive officer of NLN reports to the board. Members of the board of governors serve staggered 3-year terms, and one-third of the board turns over yearly. Balloting is done by proxy or in person, with both individuals and agency members entitled to vote. All of these offices and elected positions are open to both nurse and non-nurse NLN members.

In 2001, the Board of Governors approved a new member involvement structure. That structure provided for four Advisory Councils, each of which focuses on broad issues that affect all types of educational programs. The five-member Executive Committee of each Advisory Council is elected by the member to serve staggered 3-year terms, and a member of the Board of Governors serves as a liaison to each Advisory Council.

The four Advisory Councils are the Nursing Education Advisory Council (NEAC); Nursing Education Research, Technology, and Information Management Advisory Council (NERTIMAC); Nurse Educator Workforce Development Advisory Council (NEWDAC); and Constituent Advisory Council (COAC). Individual members are involved in the work of the Advisory Councils through Task Groups that are appointed. In 2002, each of the 10 Task Groups was focusing on an issue that is significant to nursing education and relevant to the mission of the NLN: educational standards, recruitment and retention of students, articulation and mobility, the development of a nursing education minimum data set, gaps in the science of nursing education, faculty competencies, faculty development needs, and the recruitment and retention of faculty. In addition to the 20 members who serve on the Advisory Council Executive Committees, more than 100 NLN members contribute to the viability of the organization by serving on Task Groups.

In addition to the Executive Committees of the Advisory Councils, the only other elected committee is Nominations. There also are appointed committees on bylaws, finance, program planning, awards, and public policy. The Board serves as the strategic planning committee for the NLN.

NLN members also participate locally through their constituent leagues. The constituent league is a state or regionally based unit that offers programs, engages in public policy work, and promotes innovations that are consistent with the NLN mission and goals.

Accreditation

The NLN was the first and remains the only accrediting body that services all types of nursing education programs. NLN accrediting activities began in 1949. Presently, this service is offered through the *National League for Nursing Accrediting Commission* (NLNAC). NLNAC is a wholly owned subsidiary of the NLN. It is separate and independent with sole authority over its finances and administration. NLNAC has its own governing board with a consumer presence. In 2010, more than 1191 educational programs held NLNAC accreditation. This included one DNP, 102 master's, 259 baccalaureate, 617 associate degree, 59 diploma, and 153 LPN/LVN programs.[2]

Between 1965 and 2001, the NLN also was involved in the accreditation of community-based care programs. In 1987, the Community Health Accreditation Program (CHAP) became a fully independent subsidiary of NLN. In 2001, the NLN terminated its membership in CHAP.

Data Collection and Dissemination

For over 60 years, the NLN has been a focal point for formulating data bases, conducting research, and publishing results of survey studies. It has been and remains a major supplier of data about nursing education to the federal government and other policy-making bodies, and it is a leading resource for information about faculty, students, and workforce supply. Since 1953, the NLN has maintained a comprehensive data bank on all state-approved nursing education programs. Every year, NLN surveys all state boards of nursing and all 2500 schools of nursing (that "house" approximately 3500 nursing programs) in the United States and its territories.

Educational Supports: Testing, Publications, and Programming

NLN offers more than 70 different tests for both nursing students and practicing nurses. In addition, the organization reaches out to its membership and its public through several means: its official journal, *Nursing Education Perspectives*, is published every other month and available online; a quarterly newsletter, *Shaping the Future*, is a biweekly electronic newsletter from the CEO; *Update*; Position Statements; and numerous books and monographs. The annual NLN Education Summit is a conference for nurse educators where topics of discussion include innovations in teaching/learning, curriculum development, outcomes assessment, distance learning, faculty issues, graduate education, and other significant issues. The NLN also assists faculty in their lifelong learning by offering online courses, regional workshops, and an educational programming bureau.

National League for Nursing, 61 Broadway,
33rd Floor, New York, NY 10006
http://www.nln.org

◼ AMERICAN ASSOCIATION OF COLLEGES OF NURSING

The AACN was established in 1969 to answer the need for a national organization dedicated exclusively to furthering nursing education in America's universities and 4-year colleges.

For approximately 2 years prior to that date, a group of deans of NLN-accredited graduate programs in nursing had been meeting informally to discuss the kind of organization needed to focus on nursing higher education and to provide a forum for deans and directors to meet and take rapid and concerted action on significant issues. In May 1969, deans of nursing, 44 in all, gathered in Detroit and voted to establish an independent Conference of Deans of College and University Schools of Nursing composed of the deans and directors of NLN-accredited baccalaureate and graduate programs in the United States.

The first general meeting of the newly organized group was held in Chicago in October 1969. In February 1972, the name of the organization was changed to the American Association of Colleges of Nursing.

Mission

The American Association of Colleges of Nursing is the national voice for baccalaureate and graduate-degree nursing education. A unique asset for the nation, AACN serves the public interest by providing standards and resources, and by fostering innovation to advance professional nursing education, research, and practice. Its strategic goals are to

- Provide strategic leadership that advances professional nursing education, research, and practice.
- Develop faculty and other academic leaders to meet the challenges of changing health care and higher education environments.
- Leverage AACN's policy and programmatic leadership on behalf of the profession and discipline.[3]

Membership, Structure, and Governance

Membership in the association is institutional, represented by the dean or other highest administrative officer of a baccalaureate or graduate program leading to a degree in nursing. From an original 121 member institutions in 1969, AACN today represents 645 schools of nursing at public and private universities and senior colleges nationwide.[4]

An 11-member Board of Directors, each of whom represents a member institution, governs AACN. The Association has standing committees on nominating, finance, government affairs, membership, and program; maintains taskforces on such areas as faculty development; and sponsors interest groups on nursing education, practice, and scholarship.

Membership Services

It is AACN's objective to provide nursing educators and the health care community with a consistently responsive level of programming, assistance, and policy guidance. To this end, in 1986, AACN directed the national panel that defined the knowledge, clinical skills, values, and other essential abilities that must be possessed by graduates of America's bachelor's degree nursing education programs. AACN publishes and disseminates these *Essentials of Baccalaureate Education for Professional Nursing Practice* to nursing schools and policy makers throughout the nation, and revises the teaching components to stay current with changing conditions in nursing and health care. In 1996, the AACN members approved a document entitled *The Essentials of Master's Education for Advanced Practice Nursing*. Care was taken to ensure that policies on graduate education were in harmony with the work of the National Organization of Nurse Practitioner Faculty, who brought clinical acumen to the topic of education for advanced practice. This consensus seeking did much to establish the profession's credibility in ensuring the quality of nurse practitioner (NP) education and practice. It additionally opened the door for negotiation with the NCSBN over requiring a governmental credential for advanced practice as opposed to professional certification. This issue is discussed in Chapter 20.

Through its government relations and other advocacy programs and as a member of the Tri-Council for Nursing, AACN works to advance public policy on nursing education and research. AACN has been a vigorous leader in securing federal support for nursing education and research; influencing legislative and regulatory policy affecting nursing education, practice, and health care delivery; and obtaining continuing financial assistance for nursing students.

Accreditation

In 1997, AACN responded to what it saw as concern over specialty accreditation in higher education and assumed leadership in developing a new alliance of multiple organizations to the end of accrediting nursing higher education in a more streamlined, coordinated process. This happened after the full support of its membership (246 to 59) in October 1996. As part of this proposal, AACN members also authorized the creation of a new entity that would have the sole purpose of providing accreditation services to baccalaureate and higher degree nursing programs. The Commission on Collegiate Nursing Education (CCNE), which was established as an autonomous accrediting arm of AACN, participates in the alliance and work for consensus on standard setting within this larger group.

The members of the alliance again bring the credibility of clinical experts to the accreditation process.

CCNE's draft accreditation standards and procedures were refined through a series of regional meetings in cities across the nation during 1997. CCNE began offering accreditation services to baccalaureate and graduate nursing programs during 1998.

CCNE states its mission as follows:

> CCNE is an autonomous accrediting agency contributing to the improvement of the public's health. CCNE assures the quality and integrity of baccalaureate and graduate education programs preparing effective nurses. CCNE serves the public interest by assessing and identifying programs that engage in effective educational practices. As a voluntary, self-regulatory process, CCNE accreditation supports and encourages continuing self-assessment by nursing education programs and the continuing growth and improvement of collegiate professional education.

This mission and its complementary purposes emphasize any nursing education program's accountability to its community of interest, the process of continual self-assessment, and a respect for the variable ways in which a program may choose to respond to its mission, goals, and anticipated outcomes.

Other Membership Services

AACN also operates the Institutional Data System, a central data source publishing current reports on enrollment, graduations, and other trends in baccalaureate and graduate nursing education. Other AACN publications provide policy makers with critical information and guidance on key issues facing the profession.

The government has already looked to AACN on at least two occasions to ensure the adequacy of its data bases for policy decisions. In 1992, AACN facilitated a Survey of Certified Nurse Practitioners and Clinical Nurse Specialists on behalf of the Division of Nursing to determine whether there were adequate numbers of advanced practice nurses to assume the roles that were created for them in proposed legislation. In 1997, AACN responded to a call from the Health Resources and Services Administration (HRSA) for a formula to determine how NPs, certified nurse-midwives (CNMs), and physician assistants (PAs) should be used to meet health care needs in underserved areas. AACN does not necessarily do the hands-on work, but subcontracts and maintains responsibility for the finished product.

Published in 1994 in cooperation with AACN, *Peterson's Guide to Nursing Programs* is the only comprehensive guide to accredited baccalaureate and graduate nursing education programs nationwide. In addition, AACN conferences provide deans and other education administrators with enhanced skills in areas such as student recruitment and retention, legal issues, and master's and doctoral program development.

AACN's publications include *Syllabus*, the bimonthly AACN newsletter; the bimonthly *Journal of Professional Nursing*; and a variety of books and reference directories for nursing educators, administrators, researchers, and students. AACN maintains a website rich with information.

American Association of Colleges of Nursing, 1 Dupont Circle, Suite 530, Washington, DC 20036
http://www.aacn.nche.edu

■ AMERICAN ORGANIZATION OF NURSE EXECUTIVES

Founded in 1967, AONE is a national organization of nearly 7000 nurses who design, facilitate, and manage care. It is a corporate subsidiary of the American Hospital Association (AHA). It has been so since 1988, when the boards of AONE and AHA approved a restructuring proposal to enhance the role of nursing at the AHA.[5]

Mission

As the national organization representing nurse executives and managers, AONE provides direction and leadership for the advancement of nursing practice and patient care in organized health care systems, for the achievement of excellence in nurse executive practice, and for shaping policy affecting health care delivery from the perspective of the nurse manager.

Membership and Structure

The members of AONE are nurse executives as individuals. AONE conducts its business operations through an elected governing board and board committees. National initiatives are reinforced through chapters at the state and regional levels, which in some cases include nurse managers in their membership.

As part of the AHA, AONE participates directly in policy development through involvement on AHA committees and the AHA board of trustees. Additionally, AONE holds ex officio membership on AHA regional policy boards, observer status in the AHA House of Delegates, and appointment to the AHA committee of commissioners to the Joint Commission.

Membership Services

AONE publishes a monthly newsletter, *The Nurse Executive*, as well as other monographs and publications. In 1989, it collaborated with the ANA in issuing six monographs on strategies for the nursing shortage. AONE sponsors annual meetings, educational conferences, and teleconferences that address issues central to nursing management, administration, and leadership.

American Organization of Nurse Executives, 155 N. Wacker Drive, Suite 40D, Chicago, IL 60606
http://www.aone.iorg

■ COALITIONS

The proliferation of nursing organizations, although meeting the special needs of some nurses, has also caused confusion among nurses, other health workers, and the public. Do these organizations speak for nursing in addition to ANA? In place of ANA? Members of these nursing organizations were also concerned. A perceived or real lack of unity can frustrate the achievement of desired goals. Therefore, in November 1972, ANA hosted a meeting of 10 specialty groups and NSNA to "explore how the organizations can work toward more coordination in areas of common interest." It was found that concerns were similar and that such a meeting was generally considered long overdue.

In a second meeting, hosted by the American Association of Critical Care Nurses and held at the Western White House in San Clemente, California, in January 1973, federal nurses and representatives from the National Commission on Nursing and Nursing Education were also invited, and the group was asked to consider forming a National Nurses Congress. Although this suggestion was rejected, participants came away with great respect for the role of specialty associations and for the unique contribution of ANA to the organizational life of the profession.

In June 1973, at a third meeting of presidents and executive directors of the specialty nursing organizations, this group adopted the name of the Federation of Specialty Nursing Organizations and the American Nurses Association. They identified a specialty nursing organization as a "national organization of registered nurses governed by

an elected body with bylaws defining purpose and functions for improvement of health care; and a body of knowledge and skill in a defined area of clinical practice." Those attending expressed mutual support and agreed on some of the issues of the times. Meetings of the group began to be held on a semiannual basis.

In 1981, the title of the organization was changed to National Federation for Specialty Nursing Organizations (NFSNO), which more clearly defined the membership. The mission of the NFSNO was to promote specialty nursing practice and its contributions to the health of the nation through the collaborative and educational efforts of member organizations and provide a forum for networking and addressing areas of mutual concern. NFSNO also established the Nurse in Washington Internship (NIWI) program to enhance the ability of registered nurses to influence the legislative and regulatory processes. As of 2000, NFSNO consisted of 34 regular and 5 affiliate members. ANA participated as an auditor, because all the NFSNO members also belong to the Nursing Organization Liaison Forum (NOLF).

NOLF was an organizational unit of ANA, formed in 1982 to promote the unified action of allied nursing organizations under the auspices of ANA. In December 1983, ANA invited 45 nursing organizations to Kansas City to explore the possibilities of coming together in such a forum. The meeting was cordial, but the results were somewhat noncommittal. There was a question as to whether NOLF and NFSNO would be duplicative efforts. Over time, NOLF grew and unified over 80 nursing organizations by 2001. Its members were regularly updated on the work of ANA, their opinions sought, and they frequently spoke for both ANA and their specialty organization to the media, Congress, and in a variety of other instances. NOLF organizations also voluntarily shared their resources with ANA to help fund political and professional issues of mutual concern. In the 1990s, *Nursing's Agenda for Health Care Reform prompted particular solidarity among nursing.*

In 2001, these two coalitions, NFSNO and NOLF, merged into the Nursing Organizations Alliance (the Alliance). The Alliance is a freestanding organizational entity and held its first meeting in the fall of 2002. NOLF will continue, pending the necessary revision of the ANA bylaws. NIWI will be continued by the Alliance. Membership in the Alliance is open to any nursing organization whose focus is to address current and emerging nursing and health care issues. Structural nursing components of a multidisciplinary organization are also welcome to join. Nursing leaders see this new alliance as a broader opportunity for specialty organizations to discuss best practices, as well as advocate for legislation and other measures that advance the profession.[4] It also replicates the egress from ANA of other organizational units as they grew to maturity.

National Alliance of Nurse Practitioners

In 1986, in response to the need for a united voice among NP groups, the National Alliance of Nurse Practitioners (NANP) was formed. The alliance evolved out of several earlier meetings of NP leaders, including an attempt in 1984 to center NP issues within the ANA Council of Primary Health Care NPs. However, the consensus among NPs was to build a national consortium that would encompass the ANA council of the time as well as other NP groups. For those interested, the NANP has a fact sheet summarizing its history.

The purpose of the alliance is to address the health care of the nation by promoting the visibility, viability, and unity of NPs. The organization is committed to achieving cost-effectiveness in health care, improving the organization and delivery of health care services, and supporting the education of health professionals. Its focus is on legislative and political action, public relations and marketing of NPs, and communication among its members and with other health professions, other nurses, and the public. All national, state, regional, or local NP organizations qualify for membership based on the four NANP categories:

1. National organization
2. Freestanding organization with more than 500 members
3. Freestanding organization with fewer than 500 members
4. State organization with a national parent body

Currently, the NANP represents 30,000 NPs through its organizational members, which make up its governing body:

American Academy of Nurse Practitioners
American College Health Association (Nurse/NP sections)
ANA, Council of Nurses in Advanced Practice
National Association of NPs in Reproductive Health
National Association of Pediatric Nurse Associates and Practitioners
National Conference of Gerontological Nurse Practitioners

Such collaborative activities among nursing organizations as described here show a new maturity in nursing that not only recognizes the importance of joining together on major health issues, but also fosters continual positive cooperative action. This action will enable nurses to be a stronger force in the planning and delivery of health care services.

KEY POINTS

1. The Tri-Council organizations have expanded judiciously and worked together effectively for over 60 years.
2. NLNAC and CCNE are the subsidiaries of NLN and AACN that provide accreditation services to nursing education.
3. AACN directs its efforts to baccalaureate and higher degree education programs, and their administration.
4. NLN services the full range of nursing education programs and its faculty, additionally offering testing services and accreditation through a subsidiary.
5. AONE, as a subsidiary of AHA, serves the needs of nurse executives and nurse managers.
6. The merger, disbanding, and egress of coalitions from parent organizations have a deeper meaning than proposed, but this is also a necessary adjustment to changing times.

REFERENCES

1. NLN. Mission and Goals. http://www.nln.org. Retrieved June 5, 2010.
2. Ibid.
3. AACN. Mission, Values, and Goals. March 2010. http://www.aacn.nche.edu/ContactUs/strtplan_mission.htm. Retrieved June 6, 2010.
4. Ibid.
5. AONE. http://www.aone.org/aone/about/home.html. Retrieved June 6, 2010.

Updates can be found at **www.kellysnursing.com**

27 CHAPTER

Other Nursing and Related Organizations in the United States

Within the last 10 years, an increasing number of specialty organizations for nurses have been added to those already well established. Although all nurses can find a place for themselves within the American Nurses Association (ANA), some have elected to join one of the other nursing organizations instead of or in addition to ANA. This is not unrealistic today, with the expectation for continued competence and the rapidly changing scientific base for practice. Once that initial employment decision is made on graduation, the nurse becomes specialized and needs reliable sources of information for state-of-the-art practice in that specialty area.

Each nurse has a need for at least two organizations, one that protects his or her broad professional interests and a second to maintain a cutting edge on practice. Many specialty associations are presented here. Some are totally independent; others are part of other organizations. Some restrict membership to nurses; others include medical-technical personnel as well as consumer members. Occasionally there is no provision for individual membership, but you should know about these organizations too; their publications are valuable resources.

It would be impossible to describe all the organizations in nursing today. This chapter lists primarily those that were part of the ANA's Nursing Organization Liaison Forum (NOLF) or the National Federation for Specialty Nursing Organizations (NFSNO). These coalitions merged in 2001, forming the Nursing Organizations Alliance (the Alliance).

The first of the specialty organizations, which still exists, was the American Association of Nurse Anesthetists (1931). In the 1940s and 1950s, the American Association of Industrial Nurses (AAIN), now the American Association of Occupational Health Nurses (AAOHN); the Association of Operating Room Nurses (AORN); and the American College of Nurse-Midwives (ACNM) followed. Beginning in 1968, however, literally dozens of others were organized. They were either splinter groups that broke off from ANA and formed their own association, or others that evolved as the profession became more specialized.

Special interest groups seem to have several things in common, such as providing a forum of peers for sharing experiences and problems related to a particular specialty or interest, continuing education (CE), standard setting, and leadership development. Some certify for specialty practice, but in time establish a separate corporate entity for credentialing. The separation of standard setting or the peer group from the certifier is necessary for credibility.

The nursing organizations noted in this chapter are not all clinical specialty groups; some exist to serve other needs of nurses educationally, socially, or spiritually. Still others focus on nurses' practice settings as opposed to the populations they serve. It is predictable that more organizations will evolve as nurses assume new and diverse roles. Those discussed here appear to be the most firmly established and active at this time. All are national organizations and a few have or aspire to an international constituency. The exceptions are the four regional associations presented later in the chapter.

As a group and individually, these organizations are impressive. Each has a passion for its specialized area and the expertise to speak with credibility. And more important, nurses identify with their practice. Readers are urged to use these rich resources. Websites are also noted.

■ MEMBERSHIP ORGANIZATIONS

The Academy of Medical-Surgical Nurses

The Academy of Medical-Surgical Nurses (AMSN) was established in 1991 to advance the practice of medical-surgical nursing through CE, standard setting, providing peer support, and creating a forum for the management of issues related to this area of specialty practice.

The association has about 5000 members and 20 local chapters, and has published standards of practice and a core curriculum. The AMSN sponsors an annual meeting. Official publications are *Med-Surg Nursing, MedSurg Matters!* (newsletter), and *MedSurg Nursing Connection* (e-newsletter).

Academy of Medical-Surgical Nurses, Box 56, East Holly Avenue, Pitman, NJ 08071 **http://www.amsn.org**

Alpha Tau Delta

The Alpha Tau Delta (ATD) Nursing Fraternity, Inc., is a national fraternity for professional nurses founded on February 15, 1921, at the University of California, Berkeley. Chapters are established only in schools of nursing where baccalaureate or higher degree programs are fully accredited by NLN. ATD has many active collegiate and alumnae chapters. Membership is based on scholarship, personality, and character and has no restriction as to race, color, creed, or sex. Members must be enrolled in a baccalaureate or higher degree program. Because ATD is a professional fraternity, its membership is limited to those in the nursing profession, and it organizes its group life to promote professional competence and achievement within the field of nursing.

The purposes of ATD are to further raise professional and educational standards, develop character and leadership, encourage excellence of individual performance, and organize and maintain an interfraternity spirit of cooperation.

Besides the chapter scholarships, financial aid is given annually through the Miriam Fay Furlong National Grant Awards and the PRN Alumni Awards. Other awards are the National Chapter Members of the Year and award keys and merit awards to individuals for outstanding accomplishments.

The governing body of ATD is its biennial national convention. It is composed of elected delegates from each college and alumnae chapter and the national council officers. ATD reports 6000 individual members.

The national paper *Captions of Alpha Tau Delta* and the *President's Letter* are published in the spring and fall of each year. ATD is a member of the Professional Fraternity Association and, through this organization, is represented in the Interfraternity Research and Advisory Council.

Alpha Tau Delta, 1904 Poinsettia Avenue, Manhattan Beach, CA 90266 **http://www.atdnursing.org**

American Academy of Ambulatory Care Nursing

The American Academy of Ambulatory Care Nursing (AAACN) was formally chartered in 1978. Its purpose is to promote high standards of ambulatory care nursing administration and practice through education, the exchange of information, and scientific investigation. In 1993, AAACN revised its standards for nursing administration and practice in the ambulatory care setting. The association has since authored *Telephone Nursing Practice Administration and Practice Standards* and contributes a regular monthly column to *Nursing Economic$.*

AAACN provides the bimonthly newsletter, *Viewpoint*, as a benefit of membership. It also sponsors an annual convention. Membership is about 2100.

American Academy of Ambulatory Care Nursing, Box 56, East Holly Avenue, Pitman, NJ 08071 **http://www.aaacn.org**

American Association of Critical-Care Nurses

The American Association of Critical-Care Nurses was founded in 1969 as the American Association of Cardiovascular Nurses. The Association was reincorporated in California in 1972 under its present name, which more accurately reflects the professional practice of its members. The American Association of Critical-Care Nurses is the world's largest specialty organization, with over 80,000 members and 250 chapters nationwide in 50 states and 2 foreign countries. The Association's growth has directly paralleled the increasing importance of nursing specialties that deal with human responses to life-threatening health problems. The major function of the American Association of Critical-Care Nurses is to provide education directed at advancing the art and science of critical care nursing and promoting environments that facilitate comprehensive professional nursing practice for people experiencing critical illness or injury. The American Association of Critical-Care Nurses' vision is one of a health care system driven by the needs of patients, in which critical care nurses make their optimal contribution.

The Association prepares critical care nurses for the continuing challenges and demands of the profession by offering a series of programs throughout the year. The largest and most widely attended program is the National Teaching Institute and Critical Care Exposition held annually in May.

Membership benefits currently include subscriptions to four AACN publications: *Critical Care Nurse*, the *American Journal of Critical Care*, AACN *Bold Voices*, and AACN's e-newsletter *Critical Care Newsline*. Other official American Association of Critical-Care Nurses publications include *AACN Clinical Issues*, a quarterly peer-reviewed hard-bound journal available by subscription; *AACN Nursing Scan in Critical Care*; and *Technology for Critical Care Nurses*. The American Association of Critical-Care Nurses encourages professional accountability and has established its *Standards for Nursing Care of the Critically Ill*, *Outcome Standards for Nursing Care of the Critically Ill*, and *Education Standards for Critical Care Nursing* to define and frame nursing care of the critically ill and injured.

Through its affiliate, the American Association of Critical-Care Nurses Certification Corporation, CCRN certification in adult, pediatric, and neonatal critical care nursing is offered to nurses who meet eligibility requirements. Certification examinations are offered by computer-based testing at hundreds of sites, and certification is valid for a 3-year period, after which time recertification is available through CE or retesting. Currently almost 60,000 nurses hold certification in one of six specialty areas. An agreement was finalized in 1994 between the Certification Corporation and the American Nurses Credentialing Center (ANCC) to jointly offer a certification for NPs in acute care.

Other membership benefits include reduced registration fees at AACN programs, professional liability and other group insurance programs, and professional discounts on American Association of Critical-Care Nurses publications. Membership and program information is available from the following address, as well as certification information from the Certification Corporation.

American Association of Critical-Care Nurses, 101 Columbia, Aliso Viejo, CA 92656 **http://www.aacn.org**

American Association for the History of Nursing

The American Association for the History of Nursing (AAHN), formerly the International History of Nursing Society, was incorporated in October 1982. Its purpose is to educate the public regarding the history and heritage of the nursing profession by stimulating interest and national and international collaboration in promoting the history of nursing; supporting research in the history of nursing; promoting the development of centers for the preservation and use of materials of historical importance to nursing; serving as a resource for information related to nursing history; and producing and distributing to the public educational materials regarding the history and heritage of the nursing profession. Membership is open to individuals interested in the purpose and work of the association.

The AAHN's *Bulletin* is published quarterly. AAHN sponsors two awards that recognize exemplary historical research and writing: the Lavinia A. Dock Award for established historians of nursing and the Teresa E. Christy Award for work conducted in a student status.

American Association for the History of Nursing, 10200 W. 44th Avenue, Suite 304, Wheat Ridge, CO 80033 **http://www.aahn.org**

American Association of Neuroscience Nurses

The American Association of Neuroscience Nurses (AANN) was founded in 1968 as the American Association of Neurosurgical Nurses. Its purpose is to foster the health, education, and welfare of the general public through promoting education, research, and high standards of care of the patient with neurologic dysfunction and to promote the growth of nursing as a profession. Criteria for membership include

- Active involvement or primary interest in neurosurgical nursing
- A license to practice as an RN in the United States or Canada

AANN currently has a membership of over 3400, and all members are also members of the World Federation of Neuroscience Nurses.

Major publications of AANN include the *Journal of Neuroscience Nursing* (six issues a year); *Synapse E-News*, the membership newsletter, published bimonthly electronically; and the *Core Curriculum for Neuroscience Nursing*,

3rd ed. Other materials include a research directory, which lists nurses involved in neuroscience research; a speaker's bureau; and *Neuroscience Nursing Practice: Process and Outcome Criteria for Selected Diagnoses* (published with ANA). CE programs are offered nationally and through a series of regional chapters (over 60) throughout the country.

Certification is provided through the American Board of Neurosurgical Nursing, which offers examinations twice a year. Information may be obtained from AANN. The Association holds its annual meeting each spring and another meeting in the fall.

American Association of Neuroscience Nurses, 4700 W. Lake Avenue, Glenview, IL 60025 **http://www.aann.org**

American Association of Nurse Anesthetists

Organized in 1931, the American Association of Nurse Anesthetists (AANA) is the professional organization for nurses who have specialized in anesthesia. Certified Registered Nurse Anesthetists (CRNAs) and student nurse anesthetists are eligible for AANA membership. AANA represents 96 percent of the nation's CRNAs, and its members automatically become members of their state associations. There are over 28,000 members nationwide.

To become a CRNA, a registered nurse must be a graduate of an accredited program of nurse anesthesia and have passed the national certification examination administered by the AANA's Council on Certification of Nurse Anesthetists.

In 1952, the AANA developed an accreditation program for schools for nurse anesthetists, currently administered by the AANA's Council on Accreditation of Nurse Anesthesia Educational Programs. A third credentialing council, the AANA's Council on Recertification of Nurse Anesthetists, oversees the recertification process.

Ongoing activities of the AANA include developing standards that ensure high-quality anesthesia care to safeguard patients; offering a continuous quality and risk management program for anesthesia departments, group practices, and individual practitioners; facilitating the nurse anesthesia education process and research; taking a leadership role in efforts to ease the CRNA shortage; seeking private and public sector funding sources for educational advancement and research; providing educational opportunities and professional recognition; and monitoring, assessing, and working with legislative and regulatory bodies regarding governmental initiatives.

AANA also promotes a professional and equitable work environment by addressing legal and ethical issues facing CRNAs; facilitates effective cooperation between nurse anesthetists and other health care groups; works with state nurse anesthetist associations on projects of mutual interest; disseminates information about nurse anesthesia by publishing a scientific journal, a newsletter, and miscellaneous monographs; and conducts an annual membership survey regarding the practice of anesthesia by CRNAs.

Continuing tension is associated with the relationship between CRNAs and anesthesiologists. AANA recognizes an anesthesia specialty in both nursing and medicine and supports a collaborative model when these professionals practice together. AANA's *Quality of Care in Anesthesia*, published in 1998, summarizes the relevant research in anesthesia practice, building the case that a supervisory/ subordinate relationship between the CRNA and anesthesiologist is unjustified based on demonstrations of quality and safety. Among CRNAs, 80 percent practice with anesthesiologists and the remaining 20 percent function as sole anesthesia providers.

The association holds an annual convention. Sessions are open to AANA members as well as others in the health care field. The *AANA Journal*, the official publication of the American Association of Nurse Anesthetists, is published bimonthly, and the AANA *Newsletter* is published monthly for members only. The headquarters building is located at the following address; there is also an office in Washington, DC.

American Association of Nurse Anesthetists, 222 South Prospect Avenue, Park Ridge, IL 60068-4001 **http://www.aana.com**

The American Association of Nurse Attorneys

The idea of organizing nurses who are attorneys was proposed in 1977, when it became apparent that no national association addressed the needs and interests of this growing group of professionals. Meetings were held in areas where nurse attorneys were clustered. The American Association of Nurse Attorneys (TAANA) was incorporated in 1982.

The aims and purposes of the Association are to assist the professional development of nurse attorneys and to educate the public on matters of nursing, health care, and law. Specific goals are to educate the membership on relevant issues; facilitate information sharing among nurse attorneys and with related professional groups; establish an employment network; provide mutual support among nurse attorneys; develop the nurse attorney profession; become well-known experts, consultants, and authors in nursing and law; educate nurses about legal aspects of the profession; and offer educational seminars and workshops for nurse attorneys.

An annual meeting whose educational component addresses issues of national concern to nurse attorneys occurs every fall in a different area of the country. Educational and social gatherings are held at regular intervals in approximately 25 metropolitan areas. *Inside TAANA*, the official newsletter of TAANA, is published four times a year.

Current membership is over 600. Membership is open to any nurse attorney, nurse in law school, or attorney in nursing school. Information regarding TAANA or its activities may be obtained from the national office at the following address.

The American Association of Nurse Attorneys, PO Box 14218, Lenexa, KS 66285-4218 **http://www.taana.org**

American Association of Occupational Health Nurses

The AAOHN was organized in 1942 as the American Association of Industrial Nurses and in 1977 changed its name to reflect the broadened scope of practice and its settings.

The professional association for registered nurses who provide on-the-job health care for the nation's workers, AAOHN has about 8000 members with 125 local, state, and regional constituent associations. Its mission is to advance the profession of occupational health nurses by promoting professional excellence in achieving workers' health and safety through education and research; establishing professional standards of practice and a code of ethics; influencing legislative and regulatory issues that have an impact on health and safety; and fostering internal and external communications to facilitate AAOHN's goals and objectives.

AAOHN has developed a comprehensive professional affairs program covering academic education, CE, professional practice, research, and association leadership training. Specific projects include assisting constituent associations with program planning, offering CE opportunities, and publishing resource documents.

The association maintains a strong governmental affairs program, which publishes the *Governmental Affairs Program Guide for Constituent Associations*. It represents occupational health nurses in public policy discussions that affect their day-to-day practice. It also studies and attempts to influence legislative actions.

AAOHN believes that increased professional competency is the method for the occupational health nurse to achieve economic opportunity and security. Its goal is to promote the occupational health nurse as a professional worker.

AAOHN's annual meeting is held in conjunction with that of the American College of Occupational and Environmental Medicine; the combined meeting is called the *American Occupational Health Conference*. Symposia and workshops are also held on other occasions. In addition to its official monthly magazine, *AAOHN Journal*, AAOHN provides a comprehensive communications program, including a monthly newsletter, *AAOHN News*. The organization's headquarters is located at the following address.

American Association of Occupational Health Nurses, 7794 Grow Drive, Pensacola, FL 32514 **http://www.aaohn.org**

The American Association of Office Nurses

The American Association of Office Nurses (AAON) was founded and incorporated in 1988. It has a membership of approximately 2000, with local chapters in most states. AAON views the office practitioner as one of the physician's most important professional assistants and allies, helping to facilitate the delivery of quality care to patients, and to manage the daily operation of the office. It is committed to the continuing education and long-term welfare of all professional personnel working in the physician's office, ambulatory nursing, and clinic settings. Because AAON believes that comprehensive quality care depends on the medical office team, it offers various levels of membership and invites RNs, nurse educators, NPs, licensed practical nurses (LPNs), nursing assistants, and office managers to avail themselves of educational opportunities.

The mission of AAON is to enhance the delivery of effective patient care by providing CE specific to the field of office nursing, patient education, leadership, and office management. It is dedicated to promoting the professionalism of the office nurse and recognition of this specialized field of nursing among its peers. AAON also provides a networking forum for office professionals to share ideas and knowledge to help in delivering comprehensive, safe, and effective patient care.

AAON offers a quarterly newsletter, *Nurses Exchange Office News (NEON)*, as a benefit of membership. It also sponsors an annual convention each fall and regional meetings each spring that highlight office nursing care, nursing assessment, patient education, interpersonal communications, organizational management, and leadership classes. In addition to the annual and regional meetings, CE programs include local seminars and monthly meetings as well as home study programs offered in *Office Nurse*. Standards of office nursing practice are available.

The American Association of Office Nurses, 52 Park Avenue, Park Ridge, NJ 07656-1277 **http://www.aaon.org**

American Association of Spinal Cord Injury Nurses

The American Association of Spinal Cord Injury Nurses (AASCIN) is a national specialty nursing organization formed in 1983 to promote excellence in meeting the health care needs of individuals with spinal cord injury. It is a unit of the Academy of Spinal Cord Injury Professionals, a multidisciplinary association committed to the advancement and improvement of care of spinal cord–injured individuals, promotion of education and research, and dissemination of information. There are about 1500 members.

The official publication of the Association is the *Journal of Spinal Cord Medicine*, published online four times a year for spinal cord injury professionals including physicians, scientists, psychologists, social workers, researchers, nurses, and therapists. AASCIN also publishes the *SCI Nursing: Educational Guidelines for Professional Nursing Practice, Standards of Spinal Cord Injury Nursing Practice*, and *SCI Patient/Family Education Manual for Nurses.*

AASCIN also sponsors a research program, prepares position papers on key issues on spinal cord injury, and convenes an annual education conference.

American Association of Spinal Cord Injury Nurses, The Academy of Spinal Cord Injury Professionals, 801 18th Street NW, Washington, DC 20006 **http://nurses.ascipro.org/sci-nursing.html**

American College of Nurse-Midwives

The philosophy of the ACNM is based on the beliefs that every childbearing family has a right to a safe, satisfying experience with respect for human dignity and worth, for variety in cultural forms, and for the parents' right to self-determination. ACNM defines a *certified nurse-midwife (CNM)* as an individual educated in the two disciplines of nursing and midwifery who possesses evidence of certification according to the requirements of the organization.

The mission of the ACNM is to develop and support the profession of nurse-midwifery to promote the health and well-being of women and infants within their families and communities. In pursuit of its goals and working frequently in cooperation with other groups, ACNM identifies areas of appropriate nurse-midwifery practice, studies the activities of the nurse-midwife, establishes qualifications for those activities, approves educational programs in nurse-midwifery, sponsors research and develops literature in this field, and serves as a channel for communication and interpretation about nurse-midwifery on regional, national, and international levels.

The American College of Nurse-Midwifery was established in 1955; it merged in 1969 with the American Association of Nurse-Midwives, founded in 1929, to become the American College of Nurse-Midwives. Membership is limited to ACNM-certified nurse-midwives, although they do not have to live in the United States.

Accreditation is done by the ACNM's Division of Accreditation, which functions autonomously. The ACNM Division of Competency Assessment has handled certification activities. In 1990, the ACNM membership voted to separately incorporate the Division of Competency Assessment as the ACNM Certification Council, Inc. This sister organization provides certification for professional nurse-midwives for entry into practice. ACNM and its 4800 members conduct or take part in conferences, institutes, and workshops concerned with the practice of nurse midwifery and with the improvement of services in the maternal and child health fields. A national meeting is held annually. The official newsletter is the bimonthly *Quickening*; the official publication is *The Journal of Nurse-Midwifery and Women's Health*. Additionally, the *Advocate* and *Quick eNews* is provided periodically to members online.

American College of Nurse-Midwives, 8403 Colesville Rd, Suite 1550, Silver Spring, MD 20910 **http://www.midwife.org**

American Holistic Nurses' Association

The American Holistic Nurses' Association (AHNA) was organized in 1980 by a group of nurses and others dedicated to the principles and practice of holistic nursing. Its purposes are to promote the education of nurses in the concepts and practice of the health of the whole person and to serve as an advocate of wellness. AHNA strives to support the education of nurses, allied health practitioners, and the general public on health-related issues; to examine, anticipate, and influence new directions and dimensions of the practice and delivery of health care; and to improve the quality of patient care through research on holistic concepts and practice in nursing.

Local, area, regional, and national educational programs, workshops, seminars, and conferences are presented. AHNA is over 2000 members strong. *Beginnings*, the official newsletter of AHNA, is published quarterly, and the *Journal of Holistic Nursing*, a peer-reviewed publication, is also published quarterly. News from AHNA is sent electronically to all members monthly.

Membership is open to nurses and others interested in holistically oriented health care practices.

American Holistic Nurses' Association, 323 N. San Francisco Suite, Suite 201, Flagstaff, AZ 86001
http://www.ahna.org

American Nephrology Nurses' Association

The American Nephrology Nurses' Association (ANNA) is the professional organization for registered nurses practicing in nephrology, transplantation, and related therapies. It was founded in 1969 as the American Association of Nephrology Nurses and Technicians. In 1984, it was reorganized and retitled. Its purpose is primarily educational with numerous national, regional, and local programs, seminars, and conferences given. Other major activities include a registry for CE credit and the provision of standards of nursing practice in the hemodialysis and transplantation areas. The objectives of ANNA are to develop and update standards for the practice of nephrology nursing, provide the mechanisms to promote individual growth, and promote the research, development, and demonstration of advances in nephrology nursing.

There are over 12,000 members of the national organization. ANNA provides membership services through an organizational structure that includes a national board of directors, four membership regions, and more than 112 local chapters. Any RN interested in the care of patients with renal disease is eligible for full membership. Dietitians, social workers, LPNs, and technicians may participate as associate members. Major publications are the *Nephrology Nursing Journal*, ANNA's peer-reviewed publication, *ANNA Update*, *Standards of Clinical Practice*, *Core Curriculum for Nephrology Nursing*, *Nephrology Nursing—A Guide to Professional Development*, and a number of clinical monographs and other publications on topics such as scope of practice, core curriculum, careers, and nephrology nursing research.

American Nephrology Nurses' Association, East Holly Avenue, Box 56, Pitman, NJ 08071-0056
http://www.annanurse.org

American Psychiatric Nurses Association

The American Psychiatric Nurses Association (APNA) is committed to the vision that all people will have accessible, effective, and efficient psychiatric–mental health care in delivery systems that fully utilize the skills and expertise of psychiatric nurses. The mission of APNA is to provide leadership to advance psychiatric–mental health nursing practice; improve mental health care for individuals, families, groups, and communities; and shape health policy for the delivery of mental health services. In pursuit of its mission, APNA is extensively involved in interdisciplinary and consumer liaisons related to its specialty, notably the Mental Health Association and the National Alliance for the Mentally Ill. APNA has developed a psychopharmacology curriculum and an aggression management program for the geriatric population.

Educational resources include the print and online *Journal of the American Psychiatric Nurses Association (JAPNA)*, published six times a year, and the monthly newsletter, *APNANews: The Psychiatric Nursing Voice*.

APNA reports over 6500 members in 40 state and regional chapters. The vast majority of these members are over age 40 with significant experience in the field. In addition, about 655 members hold master's or doctoral degrees. The membership is evenly divided between inpatient and outpatient venues of care.

American Psychiatric Nurses Association, Colonial Place Three, 1555 Wilson Boulevard, Suite 515, Arlington, VA 22209 http://www.apna.org

The American Public Health Association–Public Health Nursing Section

The American Public Health Association (APHA), established in 1872, is the largest organization of its kind in the world, with a membership of some 32,000 in addition to the approximately 25,000 members of its affiliates. As a professional organization, it represents over 75 disciplines in public health concerned with shaping national and local public health policies; as a communications network, it disseminates new knowledge through the internationally respected *American Journal of Public Health* and a publishing house operation of major proportions. *Nation's Health* is the official newspaper of the association, published 10 times a year.

Of the 24 specialized sections that make up APHA, the Public Health Nursing Section is one of the largest, with approximately 1700, and also one of the oldest, having been established in 1923. Highly active and influential, the Public Health Nursing Section provides a voice for nursing interests within the APHA structure and nationally through that structure. Section members participate on APHA's program development board, on taskforces and committees, and with other sections of the association. Through cooperative relationships with other nursing groups—such as ANA, the Association of Community Health Nursing Educators, the Association of State and Territorial Directors of Nursing, and NLN—its mission is to enhance the health of population groups through the application of nursing knowledge to communities. This section has been instrumental in establishing the Quad Council (ANA, ACNE, ASTDN, and APHA) to promote a strong, coordinated voice for public health nursing.

Over the eight decades of its existence, the Public Health Nursing Section has studied numerous aspects and issues of public health nursing, including the definition and roles of public health nursing, relationships between hospitals and public health agencies, planning services to certain high-risk populations, salaries, educational and professional qualifications, quality assurance, staffing issues, research priorities, and the role of public health nursing in health care reform.

In its investigation of these issues, the Public Health Nursing Section has continuously been in the organizational forefront of the APHA structure. Over the years, numerous nurses have been elected members of APHA's governing council, including the executive board. Nurses Marion Sheahan, Margaret Dolan, and Iris Shannon served as president of the APHA in 1960, 1973, and 1988, respectively, and several nurses have held the office of vice president. In addition, Marion Sheahan, Margaret Arnstein, and Doris Roberts have won the Sedgwick Memorial Medal, one of APHA's highest citations; the Albert Lasker and Martha May Eliot Awards have been won by nurses several times; and the prestigious Bronfman Prize was given to Ruth B. Freeman in 1971.

The APHA annual meeting provides an excellent forum for the Public Health Nurses' scientific and business exchanges and social events, but meetings of the various section councils and committees are also held throughout the year. The Ruth B. Freeman and creative achievement awards are given by the section at each annual meeting to recognize nurses who have made outstanding contributions to public health nursing.

A fascinating and detailed *History of the Public Health Nursing Section, 1922–1972*, by Ella E. McNeil, is now out of print but is on file in the APHA archives. In 1977, the Public Health Nursing Section established the Margaret B. Dolan Lectureship Fund. At the 1978 APHA Convention, the first Dolan lecture was presented as the keynote address. The lectures have continued as an annual keynote convention event.

The first century of public health nursing came to a close at the 1993 annual APHA meeting, following a year focusing on the history, accomplishments, and future role of public health nursing. Archives of the PHN Section of APHA are located at Mugar Library, Boston University.

American Public Health Association (PHN Section), 800-I Street, NW, Washington, DC 20001-3710 **http://www.apha.org/membergroups/sections/aphasections/phn**

American Radiological Nurses Association

The American Radiological Nurses Association (ARNA) was founded in 1981 as the professional organization representing nurses who practice in diagnostic and therapeutic imaging environments. These nurses provide, promote, and maintain the continuity of quality patient care in imaging environments such as general diagnostic, neuro/cardiovascular, interventional, ultrasonography, computed tomography, nuclear medicine, magnetic resonance imaging, and radiation oncology. ARNA accomplishes its purpose by defining the functions, qualifications, and educational criteria of radiology nurses; promoting the practice; assessing, recommending, and evaluating radiologic nursing standards; facilitating efficient networking among radiologic nurses and allied health care professionals; and promoting scholarly activity and education in all areas of radiologic nursing.

An elected board of directors governs ARNA, and there are various standing committees to do its work. The association has 1393 members. ARNA holds an annual business meeting and sponsors educational programs.

American Radiological Nurses Association, 7794 Grove Drive, Pensacola, FL 32514

American Society for Parenteral and Enteral Nutrition

Founded in 1975, the American Society for Parenteral and Enteral Nutrition (ASPEN) is the nation's only multidisciplinary group of health professionals chiefly concerned with the nutritional support of patients. ASPEN's staff manages the daily operations of the society for a membership of more than 5000 individuals comprising physicians, dietitians, pharmacists, and nurses. Student membership and membership for individuals not included in one of the above disciplines is available under an affiliate status category. They receive all benefits of membership except voting rights and the right to hold a position on committees or the board of directors.

ASPEN is committed to promoting quality patient care, education, and research in the field of nutrition and metabolic support in all health care settings. Its specific objectives are to promote communication among professional disciplines in the field, proper applications of clinical and research experience in the practice of nutritionally sound medicine, and professional competence in the field. ASPEN publishes two bimonthly journals, the *Journal of Parenteral and Enteral Nutrition (JPEN)*, and *Nutrition in Clinical Practice (NCP)*. JPEN contains original research, reviews, and editorials, whereas NCP provides reliable, practical, "hands-on" information for health professionals concerned about nutrition. They are available in both print and online forms. In addition, the society publishes bibliographies, textbooks on core curriculum, course syllabi, standards of practice, and guidelines for the proper administration of parenteral and enteral nutrition (PEN).

The society holds an annual educational convention, its Clinical Congress, which attracts over 3500 attendees. It gives six research awards at this event. In 1993, the ASPEN Rhodes Research Foundation was established to promote further and fund new research in the field of parenteral and enteral nutrition.

ASPEN provides certification examinations for both nurses and dietitians that are administered twice a year. In addition, its board of directors has approved offering a certification program in parenteral and enteral nutrition for physicians. These examinations are carefully designed and administered under the auspices of ASPEN's National Board of Nutrition Support Certification (NBNSC). Although the NBNSC is legally a part of the society, it functions as an independent credentialing agency.

American Society for Parenteral and Enteral Nutrition, Fenton Street, Suite 412, Silver Spring, MD 20910-3805
http://www.nutritioncare.org

American Society of Ophthalmic Registered Nurses

Organized in 1976, the American Society of Ophthalmic Registered Nurses, Inc. (ASORN) is open to all professional RNs engaged in ophthalmic nursing. ASORN's purpose is to unite professional ophthalmic RNs to promote excellence in ophthalmic nursing for the better and safer care of the patient with an eye disorder or injury. Specific objectives are to study, discuss, and exchange knowledge, experience, and ideas related to ophthalmic nursing to provide CE to its members; hold regular meetings to advance the purpose of the society; and cooperate with other professional associations, hospitals, universities, industries, technical societies, research organizations, and government agencies in matters affecting the purposes of the society. There are 1800 members.

A national meeting is held annually in conjunction with the American Academy of Ophthalmology meeting. *Insight*, the official journal, is published quarterly; two electronic newsletters, *Blink* and *Connection*, are provided to members monthly. Local chapters, which are independent of the national organization, meet at regular intervals in 14 regional areas.

American Society of Ophthalmic Registered Nurses, PO Box 193030, San Francisco, CA 94119
http://www.asorn.org

American Society of PeriAnesthesia Nurses

Established as the American Society of Post Anesthesia Nurses (ASPAN) in 1980, the organization's name was changed in 1996 to the American Society of PeriAnesthesia Nurses. This change was made to accommodate the expansion and natural growth of the nursing role in preanesthesia screening and ambulatory surgery care. However, the acronym, ASPAN, remains the same.

ASPAN is the national association representing nurses practicing in the perianesthesia environment. The purposes for which ASPAN was organized are educational, scientific, and charitable. Founded in 1980, ASPAN has over 11,000 members representing 40 state and regional associations and international constituencies. The Conference Center accessed through the ASPAN website allows nurses to ask questions, make comments, and communicate with their colleagues about perianesthesia nursing practice.

The association provides members with a bimonthly newsletter published online and called the *Breathline*, and a scientific journal also published bimonthly, the *Journal of Post Anesthesia Nursing*. Other reference publications offered include the *Standards of Nursing Practice*, the *Review Text*, *Redi-Ref*, and numerous videotapes on postanesthesia nursing. An annual conference is held in April. ASPAN also offers both perianesthesia and ambulatory postanesthesia certifications.

The first week in February is recognized as National Post Anesthesia Nurses Week and is celebrated throughout the country. ASPAN's national office is located at the following address.

American Society of PeriAnesthesia Nurses, 90 Frontage Road, Cherry Hill, NJ 08034-1424 **http://www.aspan.org**

American Society of Plastic Surgical Nurses

Incorporated as a nonprofit organization in 1975, the American Society of Plastic Surgical Nurses (ASPSN) has a growing membership of more than 1700 plastic and reconstructive surgical nurses. ASPSN serves its members through a national structure of four regions and a network of local chapters in the United States and Canada. The mission of ASPSN is to promote high standards of plastic and reconstructive surgical nursing practice and patient care through education, the exchange of information, and scientific inquiry. RNs, LPNs, and licensed vocational nurses (LVNs) who support the philosophy, mission, and objectives of the Society are eligible to become Regular Members. LPNs and LVNs are also eligible to become Associate Members along with technicians and medical assistants.

An annual convention is held each fall. Local and regional chapters provide supplementary seminars throughout the year. ASPSN publishes *Plastic Surgical Nursing*, a quarterly, and a bimonthly newsletter, *ASPSN News*. ASPSN's *Core Curriculum* is available from the national office, at the following address.

American Society of Plastic Surgical Nurses, 7794 Grow Drive, Pensacola, FL 32514 **http://www.aspsn.org**

Association of Nurses in AIDS Care

The Association of Nurses in AIDS Care (ANAC) is a nonprofit professional nursing organization committed to fostering the individual and collective professional development of nurses involved in the delivery of health care to persons infected or affected by the human immunodeficiency virus (HIV) and to promoting the health, welfare, and rights of all infected persons. Founded in 1987, ANAC has grown to a membership of over 2200 nurses and 45 local chapters.

ANAC's active members include RNs, associate members, LPNs or LVNs, and student nurses. Services to members include publication of *JANAC* (the *Journal of ANAC*) and *ANACdotes*, ANAC's official newsletter; the Annual National Conference; local meetings, conferences, support groups; and publication of other educational materials. ANAC's *Core Curriculum for HIV/AIDS Nursing* was published in 1995. Two ANAC fellowship awards are given annually to nurses pursuing graduate education in the field of HIV/AIDS.

The organization has 11 active committees, including a government relations committee addressing health care policy issues, an education committee producing educational programs and materials, and a clinical issues committee to address new research and clinical information of interest and importance to the members.

Association of Nurses in AIDS Care, 3538 Ridgewood Road, Akron, OH 44333-3122 **http://www.nursesinaidscare.org**

Association of periOperative Registered Nurses

The Association of periOperative Registered Nurses (AORN) is a voluntary organization of professional RNs with a national and international membership and a universal interest in the care of the surgical patient. Founded in 1954, AORN has about 41,000 members in 335 chapters and 23 specialty assemblies in the United States and abroad who manage, teach, and practice perioperative nursing; who are enrolled in nursing education; and who are engaged in perioperative research. The chapters meet the needs of geographic regions, and specialty assemblies address issues of specialty perioperative practice. Specialty assemblies include advanced technology, ambulatory surgery, cardiothoracic surgery, management, nurse educator/clinical specialist, orthopedics, RN first assistant, pediatric and rural, nurses in business, industry, and consulting.

AORN's mission states that it is the professional organization of perioperative nurses that unites its members by providing education, representation, and standards for quality patient care. AORN believes that the OR nurse must be responsible for patients undergoing surgery. Its philosophy recognizes its responsibility to health care and the operating room by setting standards of practice, contributing to essential nursing education, and providing the opportunity for continuous learning through a broad program of educational activities.

AORN sponsors activities to meet the educational needs of its members. CE offerings are sponsored throughout the United States and in foreign countries. These include the national AORN Congress, the biennial World Conference, national seminars, week-long courses, and self-directed study materials. The AORN Foundation is vital to this work and has raised about $1 million yearly in support of its educational, research, and scholarly agenda. Research and consumerism have become major AORN commitments. A director of perioperative research has been added to the headquarters staff, and local chapters are recognized for their projects to educate the consumer about the perioperative specialty.

An extensive list of publications is available to its members including the *AORN Standards and Recommended Practices in Perioperative Nursing*, which is widely recognized in the field, the *AORN Journal* (online or in print for a small additional fee), which is published monthly, and *AORN Connections* also published monthly.

A registered professional nurse who currently manages, teaches, or practices perioperative nursing either full or part time is eligible for active membership. A registered professional nurse enrolled in formal nursing education or engaged in perioperative research may retain active status. Associate membership is available to registered professional nurses who are engaged in an allied field of nursing.

Association of periOperative Registered Nurses, 2170 S. Parker Rd., Suite 300, Denver, CO 80231
http://www.aorn.org

Association of Pediatric Oncology Nurses

The Association of Pediatric Oncology Nurses (APON) is an organization of RNs who are either interested in or engaged in pediatrics, oncology, and/or pediatric oncology nursing. The group was formally begun in 1973 in Atlanta as a result of increasing demands for education and support for nurses who care for and about children with cancer and their families. The overall objective of APON is to promote an optimal level of nursing care for pediatric oncology patients and their families. This is achieved

through an annual national educational conference, the quarterly electronic *Journal of Pediatric Oncology Nursing*, and the quarterly *APHON Newsletter*. In addition, APON promotes the implementation of standards of pediatric oncology nursing practice and encourages research in nursing care of children with cancer.

Membership is open to all RNs in the United States, Canada, and foreign countries and currently has 3200 members and 40 local chapters in the United States and Canada. Members receive a newsletter, a chapter directory, an official journal, and other publications.

The most frequently expressed benefit of APON membership is the opportunity to network with nurses with common goals, interests, and values, as there is an ongoing improvement in the quality of life and life expectations for children with cancer.

Association of Pediatric Oncology Nurses, 4700 W. Lake Avenue, Glenview, IL 60025-1485
http://www.aphon.org

Association of Rehabilitation Nurses

The Association of Rehabilitation Nurses (ARN) is the membership organization for professional nurses who work with individuals with physical disabilities or chronic illness. Formed in 1974, ARN has over 5600 members who practice in a variety of settings. There are 47 local chapters throughout the country and 10 special interest groups. ARN's mission is to promote and advance professional rehabilitation nursing practice through education, advocacy, and research to enhance the quality of life for those affected by disability. Rehabilitation nurses work in general hospitals, rehabilitation and long-term care facilities, insurance companies, home health care operations, educational institutions, and private consulting firms.

ARN offers a certification program through its Rehabilitation Nursing Certification Board (RNCB). Over 10,000 rehabilitation nurses have met the qualifications to be certified rehabilitation registered nurses (CRRNs). The CRRN program is a member of the American Board of Nursing Specialties.

Over the years, ARN has focused much of its energies on education programming for rehabilitation nurses. In 1975, it established an education and research foundation, the Rehabilitation Nursing Foundation (RNF), and prepared a comprehensive educational plan in 1993. ARN and RNF have developed many educational and communications resources, including annual educational conferences, regional seminars, a rehabilitation nursing management seminar, an intermediate-level seminar that concentrates on current rehabilitation concepts and skills applicable to various rehabilitation nursing courses, standards and scope of practice, and a core curriculum. ARN has increased its visibility in subacute care, long-term care, and home care. Two significant ARN publications are *Rehabilitation and Restorative Nursing in the Subacute Setting* and *Rehabilitation Nursing in the Home Health Setting*. Annual conferences feature tracks in subacute care, home care, disease management, and case management.

The organization publishes the *ARN News* 10 times a year; *Rehabilitation Nursing*, a bimonthly journal; and the electronic *Health Policy Digest*. The Rehabilitation Nursing Foundation continues to develop educational resources and has strengthened its role as the research and development resource for rehabilitation nursing.

The organization funds annual grants for rehabilitation nursing research, and a novice researcher grant was initiated in 1995. ARN conducts its own research on rehabilitation nursing diagnoses. A biennial research symposium has been instituted. External activities include working with other organizations and participating in national health care improvement efforts. ARN provides testimony to government bodies—such as the National Institute for Nursing Research, the National Center for Medical Rehabilitation Research, and the National Institute for Disability and Rehabilitation Research—to share rehabilitation nursing's perspective where appropriate.

Association of Rehabilitation Nurses, 4700 W. Lake Avenue, Glenview, IL 60025-1485 http://www.rehabnurse.org

Association of State and Territorial Directors of Nursing

The Association of State and Territorial Directors of Nursing (ASTDN) was established in 1935 as the public health nursing leadership affiliate of the Association of State and Territorial Health Officials. Its primary purposes were to encourage state and local health authorities to improve the quality and extend the volume and scope of their public health nursing services, to encourage the development of nursing leadership for all public health nursing within the respective states, to participate in joint efforts with federal and national nursing groups in the promotion of a unified approach to existing public health nursing problems, and to promote the establishment of sound educational facilities

for the preparation of additional public health nurses. Public health nursing directors for the official state or territorial health department make up the membership, in addition to over 300 associate members from academia, professional organizations, and governmental agencies as well as alumni members who previously served as state PHN directors.

Members of ASTDN hold an annual meeting and CE session for members and guests, which include nurses in leadership positions within the federal government and current presidents of the affiliating organizations of the Quad Council (the Association of Community Health Nursing Educators, the Public Health Nursing Section of the American Public Health Association, the Community Health Nursing Council of the American Nurses Association, and ASTDN). Additionally, the executive committee meets in conjunction with the fall meeting of APHA. Membership services include these meetings, a quarterly newsletter, assorted committee assignments, and networking opportunities with colleagues across the country.

Research activities have focused on public health nursing staffing and career ladders, leadership positions with state health departments, utilization of NPs in local health departments, and other similar work. The association has an active research committee, with research disseminated at the annual meeting. Legislative activities concern funding for nursing education and public health's structure, function, and financing under health care reform. For mailing purposes, the address of ASTDN's president can be obtained through the following office.

The Association of State and Territorial Health Officials, PO Box 4166, Halfmoon Station, Clifton Park, NY 12065 http://www.astdn.org

The Association of Women's Health, Obstetric and Neonatal Nurses

The Association of Women's Health, Obstetric and Neonatal Nurses (AWHONN) was originally established in 1969 within the American College of Obstetricians and Gynecologists as the Nurses' Association of the American College of Obstetricians and Gynecologists (NAACOG). In 1993, the organization became an independent, nonprofit association as AWHONN. Its purpose is to promote excellence in nursing practice with women and newborns. AWHONN's 22,282 members represent a rich diversity of skills and experience, and demonstrate why the association is considered the voice for women's health as well as obstetric and neonatal nursing.

AWHONN is divided into 11 geographic districts in the United States, its territories, and Canada, plus one district to include members of the armed forces wherever stationed. Districts further divide into sections, which subdivide into chapters. Members interact at these grassroots levels to coordinate workshops, educational outreach, and other programs that improve career skills, help provide better service to the community, and set a course for future professional success.

The organization concentrates on nursing education, research, and practice. Through video and audiotapes, computer-assisted instruction, video satellite seminars, and a fetal heart-monitoring program offered nationwide, it offers many CE opportunities. It also encourages individual members' research projects through grants presented annually. Additionally, the department of research coordinates national research utilization projects. In everyday practice, AWHONN has consistently been known for its standards, guidelines, and position statements that specifically address women's health and obstetric and neonatal nursing practice issues. In the present era of health care reform, it contributes as a resource to legislators and participates in many nursing coalitions.

AWHONN's newsletters, *Legislative News & Views* (quarterly), *AWHONN Vitals* (monthly), and *AWHONN News* (quarterly), inform members about the association's activities and reports on new developments that affect perinatal and women's health nursing. The *Journal of Obstetric, Gynecologic, and Neonatal Nursing* (JOGNN) is a refereed publication that includes the latest in practice and research in these nursing specialties. *Nursing for Women's Health* is a refereed clinical practice journal that delivers health care trends and everyday issues. *Healthy Mom & Baby* is a new AWHONN consumer magazine and website that guides women through all trimesters of a healthy pregnancy to give newborns the best start possible. *Health4Women.org* is an online resource that delivers the latest evidence-based and trusted information to promote healthy living for women, their families, and aging relatives.

The Association of Women's Health, Obstetric and Neonatal Nurses, 2000 L Street NW, Suite 740, Washington, DC 20036 **http://www.awhonn.org**

Chi Eta Phi Sorority

Chi Eta Phi Sorority, Inc., is an international sorority of registered and student nurses. Founded in 1932, its purposes are to encourage the pursuit of CE among members of the nursing profession, to have a continuous recruitment program for nursing and the health professions, and to constantly identify a corps of nursing leaders within the membership who will function as agents of social change on national, regional, and local levels. There are over 8000 registered and student nurses who hold membership in Chi Eta Phi Sorority. There are over 78 graduate chapters and 38 undergraduate chapters located in 26 states, the District of Columbia, St. Thomas, the US Virgin Islands, and Monrovia Liberia, West Africa. Membership is by invitation and is both active and honorary.

The sorority's national projects include those designed to stimulate interest in nursing; facilitate recruitment and educational preparation for nursing and the health professions; increase retention of students in nursing programs; and provide scholarship funding for educational advancement. Service programs involve health screening, health education, and tutorial programs. Benefits of membership include the *Journal of Chi Eta Phi Sorority* (JOCEPS), a scholarly nursing journal published annually, and additionally *Chi Line*, the national newsletter (semiannual publication).

Chi Eta Phi Sorority, 3029 13th Street NW, Washington, DC 20009 **http://www.chietaphi.com**

Dermatology Nurses Association

The Dermatology Nurses Association was established in 1982. Its mission is to provide quality education, foster high standards of nursing, and promote wellness.

An annual convention and business meeting are held each December in conjunction with the annual meeting of the American Academy of Dermatology. A total of 25 local Dermatology Nurses Association chapters have been formed. Membership numbers over 3000 with 26 local chapters, and is open to nurses, medical assistants, and technicians involved in dermatology. Special interest groups exist for advanced practice nurses (NPs, CS, MSN): Laser, Human Resources Management/Administration, Photopheresis, Phototherapy/Psoriasis, Skin Cancer and Surgery, University/Research Coordinator, VA Nurses, Wound Care, and Cosmetic Surgery.

The Dermatology Nurses Association publishes *Dermatology Nursing* as its official journal as well as a bimonthly newsletter, *Focus*.

Dermatology Nurses Association, 15000 Commerce Parkway, Suite C, Mount Laurel, NJ 08054 **http://www.dnanurse.org**

The Emergency Nurses Association

The Emergency Nurses Association (ENA) was incorporated in December 1970; since that time ENA has grown to an active membership in excess of 30,000 members in 32 countries. It is the world's largest emergency organization. ENA was founded to represent nurses faced with all the problems of providing emergency care, so that these nurses could pool their knowledge and seek solutions to these problems, set standards, and develop improved methods for practicing efficient emergency care. Eligible for membership are RNs engaged in emergency care who have special skills or knowledge related to emergency nursing. Any other health professional may join the Association as an affiliate member.

The major objective of ENA is to provide optimum emergency care to patients in emergency departments. Members are urged to promote a positive attitude toward education on all levels within the emergency department by continuing study through the ENA organization; to support formal programs of instruction for emergency techniques and for postgraduate courses on the professional level; and to participate in the community planning of total emergency care.

The Board of Certification of Emergency Nursing was established in 1979 by the ENA. Since 1980, it has been a not-for-profit, autonomous organization delivering evaluation and certification services to emergency nurses. Four certifications are offered: emergency nurses (CEN), flight nurses (CFRN), critical care ground transport nurses (CTRN), and pediatric emergency nurses (CPEN). Over 21,000 nurses in the United States and Canada hold either the CEN or CFRN credential alone.

ENA publishes *ENA Connection* 10 times a year and the *Journal of Emergency Nursing*. The Association also publishes an emergency nursing core curriculum, a trauma nursing core course, a pediatric emergency guide, and several new resource materials to assist members. During the annual ENA Scientific Assembly, business and clinical programs are presented.

Emergency Nurses Association, 915 Lee Street, Des Plaines, IL 60016-6569 **http://ena.org**

Home Healthcare Nurses Association

Founded in 1993, the Home Healthcare Nurses Association (HHNA) is a nursing organization of more than 3000 individual members involved in home health care practice, education, administration, or research. Its goals are to develop the specialty of home health care nursing, foster excellence in practice, influence public policy as it affects home health care nursing practice, and enhance communication among members and other publics with the outcome of quality health care services for home health care clients.

Membership is made up of RNs engaged in any aspect of home health care. At present, no provision exists for institutional, student, associate, or non-nurse membership. Membership dues include a subscription to *Home Healthcare Nurse* and the bimonthly *HHNA News*.

HHNA is the first and only organization specifically targeted toward nurses in home health care. It is an organization of, for, and by the nurses caring for clients and their families in the home.

Home Healthcare Nurses Association, 228 7th Street, SE, Washington, DC 20003 **http://www.hhna.org**

Hospice and Palliative Nurses Association

The Hospice and Palliative Nurses Association (HPNA) was established in 1986 for the purpose of exchanging information, experiences, and ideas among hospice nurses and promoting understanding of the specialty of hospice nursing within the wider health community and the general public.

The Association's mission is to foster excellence in hospice nursing by promoting the highest professional standards; studying, researching, and exchanging information, experiences, and ideas leading to improved nursing care for terminally ill patients and their families; encouraging nurses to specialize in the practice of hospice nursing; fostering the professional development of nurses; responding to the changing needs of HPNA members and the population they represent; and promoting the recognition of hospice care as an essential component of the health care system.

Although primarily a professional membership association for practicing hospice RNs, HPNA offers categories for associate members and students. Membership currently numbers almost 8000. Benefits include the *Journal of Hospice and Palliative Nursing* (JHPN), which is the official journal of the Hospice and Palliative Nurses Association. It is published bimonthly and is a membership benefit. The *Journal of Palliative Medicine* (JPM) is a leading peer-reviewed journal covering medical, psychosocial, policy, and legal issues in end-of-life care and the relief of suffering for patients with intractable pain. It is a second journal of the Hospice and Palliative Nurses Association and all HPNA members have access to the current and archived *JPM* in the Members Only area of the HPNA website. The Journal presents essential information for professionals in hospice/palliative medicine, focusing on improving the quality of life for patients and their families, and the latest developments in drug and non-drug treatments. Current HPNA members are also entitled to an e-subscription to the innovative weekly online *JPM* newsletter, *Briefings in Palliative, Hospice, and Pain Medicine & Management.*

The National Board for Certification of Hospice and Palliative Nurses (NBCHPN®) offers credentialing in this specialty for all levels of nursing (APN, Generalist Nurse, LP/VN, Nursing Assistant) and the Administrator. The Board maintains an arm's-length relationship with HPNA. The organization funds research on hospice nursing, including a spiritual care perspectives study to determine the attitudes and practices of hospice nurses in this area.

Hospice and Palliative Nurses Association, Penn Center West One, Suite 229, Pittsburgh, PA 15276
http://www.hpna.org

International Association of Forensic Nurses

The International Association of Forensic Nurses (IAFN) is the only international professional organization of registered nurses formed exclusively to develop, promote, and disseminate information about the science of forensic nursing.

Forensic nursing is a clinical subspecialty. It focuses on the areas in which medicine, nursing, and human behavior interface with the law. Forensic nurses apply the nursing process to public or legal proceedings; they engage in the scientific investigation of trauma involving both living and deceased individuals. They are concerned with the impact of victimization, offender motivations, crime scene analysis, self-destructive behavior, and the exploitation of the vulnerable. Forensic nurses provide services to individual clients and consultation services to nursing, medical, and law-related agencies. They give expert court testimony in areas dealing with trauma and/or questioned death investigative processes, adequacy of services delivery, and specialized diagnoses of specific conditions as related to nursing.

Several groups of nurses in various specialties are eligible to join IAFN, ranging from sexual assault nurse examiners to nurses in clinical or community-based nursing practice involving victims of injuries. Categories are regular members, associate members (for non-RNs), and students and retired members. There are currently 2852 active paid members in the United States.

IAFN publishes the *Journal of Forensic Nursing* twice a year and its newsletter *On the Edge* four times a year, an annual directory of membership, and protocols and guidelines for identifying crime victims and proceeding with evidence collection. The organization sponsors an annual scientific assembly, which features the papers and research of renowned scientists.

IAFN, through the Forensic Nursing Certification Board, offers the only international certification examination for adult/adolescent and pediatric Sexual Assault Nurse Examiners. The Forensic Nursing Certification Board (FNCB) began offering a certification exam for Sexual Assault Nurse Examiners–Adult/Adolescent (SANE-A®) in 2002. The examination is based on an analysis of adult and adolescent SANE practice. Certification as a SANE-A demonstrates the SANE's high level of knowledge, expertise, and professional commitment. In addition, the certification validates the status and experience of sexual assault nurses who often testify as expert witnesses in court trials. As of December 2009, there were 1106 nurses with the SANE-A credential. The FNCB completed the development of the Sexual Assault Nurse Examiners—Pediatric (SANE-P®) credential with the first examination offered throughout North America in the spring of 2007. There are now 214 nurses who hold the SANE-P credential.

International Association of Forensic Nurses, 1517 Ritchie Hwy, Suite 208, Arnold, MD 21012-2323
http://www.iafn.org

International Society of Psychiatric–Mental Health Nurses

The mission of the International Society of Psychiatric–Mental Health Nurses (ISPN) is to unite and strengthen the presence and the voice of specialty psychiatric–mental health nursing while influencing health care policy to promote equitable, evidence-based, and effective treatment and care for individuals, families, and communities.

ISPN is composed of three founding divisions, which had existed as separate organizations before coming together under ISPN:

- Association of Child and Adolescent Psychiatric Nurses (ACAPN)
- International Society of Psychiatric Consultation Liaison Nurses (ISPCLN)
- Society of Education and Research in Psychiatric–Mental Health Nursing (SERPN)

The three divisions maintain their specialized identity. ISPN invites other psychiatric–mental health nursing groups to join as other divisions. Additionally, there are four councils: Practice, Education, Research, and Legislative.

Membership is open to nurses practicing in or having an interest in psychiatric nursing. ISPN members enjoy networking opportunities with others in the specialty; an annual conference; a bimonthly newsletter; free listing in the membership directory; participation on committees such as core curriculum, bylaws, and research; a peer consultation program; team building; and access to publications that are state-of-the-art tools prepared for novices to experts practicing in the field. A triannual newsletter, *Connections*, and one of three division journal(s)—*Archives of Psychiatric Nursing, Journal of Child and Adolescent Psychiatric Nursing*, or *Perspectives in Psychiatric Care*—are benefits of membership.

International Society of Psychiatric Nursing, 2424 American Lane, Madison, WI 53704-3102 http://www.ispn-psych.org

Infusion Nurses Society

The Infusion Nurses Society, formerly the Intravenous Nurses Society, is a nonprofit professional nursing association established in 1973 that represents nurses involved in the practice of intravenous (IV) therapies both in hospitals and at alternative clinical practice settings. The Infusion Nurses Society's mission is to enhance the practice of IV nursing through education, standards, and research to achieve the highest level of patient care.

The Infusion Nurses Society has developed its *Intravenous Nursing Standards of Practice*, which relate to all the major areas of the IV nursing specialty (e.g., blood and blood component therapy, total parenteral nutrition, and oncology). The Infusion Nurses Society Certification Corporation was established in 1983 and annually provides a national certification exam to credential the practicing IV nurse.

Membership is offered on an active or an associate basis to all health care professionals from any practice setting who are involved in or interested in the specialty practice of infusion therapy. Membership currently numbers about 6000 US members dispersed among 44 chapters. The Infusion Nurses Society publishes a professional journal, the *Journal of Intravenous Nursing*, and a newsletter, *INS Newsline*, both of which are bimonthly. An annual 4-day meeting and three 2-day advanced study programs provide, on an annual basis, CE and professional networking opportunities. The Infusion Nurses Society has more than 50 chapters nationwide that hold bimonthly meetings and annual seminars.

Infusion Nurses Society, 220 Norwood Park South, Norwood, MA 02062 http://www.ins1.org

National Association for Health Care Recruitment

The National Association for Health Care Recruitment (NAHCR), formerly the National Association of Nurse Recruiters, was founded in 1975. It seeks to promote and exchange principles of professional health care recruitment. The association maintains appropriate but separate relationships with voluntary and government hospitals, leading community health care organizations, educational institutions, nursing organizations, and advertising media. NAHCR serves its members by strengthening the recruitment and management skills needed to be effective in the profession and gives health care recruiters an opportunity to meet with their peers to exchange ideas and discuss mutual concerns.

An annual conference featuring speakers, exhibits, workshops, and a new recruiter orientation is held. Problem solving is the emphasis of free, informal discussions held frequently in each of NAHCR's nine regions. There are 28 NAHCR regional chapters. NAHCR also holds fall, spring, and regional 1-day workshops.

Recruitment Directions, NAHCR's newsletter, is published 10 times per year. This publication reports on industry trends, events, and association happenings. An annual recruitment survey provides up-to-date data of importance to health care recruiters. A membership directory and resource guide is published annually. A recruitment and retention manual is also available.

Membership, currently numbering over 850, is open to those working in a hospital or health care agency that is actively involved in nurse and allied health recruitment. Nonvoting associate membership is available to individuals interested in supporting NAHCR activities. Subscriptions are available to *Recruitment Directions*. Institutional membership is open to organizations interested in promoting and supporting the Association's development.

National Association for Health Care Recruitment, 2501 Aerial Center Parkway, Morrisville, NC 27560 http://www.nahcr.com

National Association of Clinical Nurse Specialists

The National Association of Clinical Nurse Specialists (NACNS) was established in 1995 by a geographically diverse group of over 60 CNSs. NACNS is currently composed of more than 2500 individual members representing a broad scope of specializations across the continuum of care. The Association's purpose is to enhance and promote the unique contribution of the advanced practice work of the CNS. NACNS is committed to providing members with an arena for educational, networking, and mentoring opportunities and will work to increase the visibility of the CNS's impact on cost, quality, and access to nursing care. NACNS will serve as a forum for the identification and discussion of issues and trends that affect and shape CNS practice, and will promote unity in the CNS community. A prime benefit to membership is the publication, *CNS: The Journal for Advanced Nursing Practice*.

National Association of Clinical Nurse Specialists, 100 North 20th Street, 4th Floor, Philadelphia, PA 19103
http://www.nacns.org

The National Association of Hispanic Nurses

The National Association of Hispanic Nurses (NAHN) was formed in June 1976 in Atlantic City, New Jersey, under the name National Association of Spanish Speaking/Spanish Surnamed Nurses. Evolving from an ad hoc committee of the Spanish Speaking/Spanish Surnamed Caucus formed at the 1974 ANA convention, it brought together for the first time Hispanic nurses from all Hispanic subgroups—Mexican American, Puerto Rican, Cuban, and Latin American—to provide a forum for exchange of information and experiences about health care services to the Hispanic community. Its name was changed in 1979.

The objectives of NAHN include providing a forum in which Hispanic nurses can analyze, research, and evaluate the health care needs of the Hispanic community; disseminate research findings and policy perspectives dealing with Hispanic health care needs to local, state, and federal agencies to influence policy making and the allocation of resources; identify Hispanic nurses throughout the nation to ascertain the size of this group of health care professionals available to provide culturally sensitive nursing care to Hispanic consumers; identify barriers to the delivery of health services for Hispanic consumers and recommend appropriate solutions to local, state, and federal agencies; identify barriers to quality education for Hispanic nursing students and recommend appropriate solutions to local, state, and federal agencies; assess the safety and quality of health care delivery services for the Hispanic community; work for the recruitment and retention of Hispanic students in nursing educational programs, so as to increase the number of bilingual and bicultural nurses who can provide culturally sensitive nursing care to Hispanic consumers; and provide an opportunity for Hispanic nurses from all over the United States and Puerto Rico to share information dealing with their professional concerns, experiences, and research.

Membership is open to any Hispanic nurse in the United States, the Commonwealth of Puerto Rico, or other jurisdiction of the United States. Non-Hispanic nurses and nursing students interested and concerned about the health delivery needs of the Hispanic community as well as the professional needs of Hispanic nurses are welcome to become members. There are currently 2300 members dispersed among 37 chapters.

The NAHN publishes the *International Journal of Hispanic Health Care*, which is peer reviewed. The organization holds biennial national conferences (even years) and national conventions (odd years).

National Association of Hispanic Nurses, 1455 Pennsylvania Ave., NW, Suite 400, Washington, DC 20004 **http://www.thehispanicnurses.org**

National Association of Nurse Practitioners in Women's Health

The National Association of Nurse Practitioners in Women's Health (NPWH; formerly the National Association of Nurse Practitioners in Reproductive Health) was founded in 1980. NPWH's mission is to ensure the provision of quality health care to women of all ages by NPs. NPWH defines quality health care to be inclusive of an individual's physical, emotional, and spiritual needs.

NPWH recognizes and respects women as decision makers for their health care. NPWH's mission includes protecting and promoting a woman's right to make her own choices regarding her health within the context of her personal, religious, cultural, and family beliefs.

NPWH represents NPs who provide care to women in the primary care setting as well as in women's health specialty practices. NPWH members can be found in state- and federally funded family planning and maternal–child health programs, sexually transmitted disease clinics, health maintenance organizations (HMOs), the armed forces, private practices, and a variety of other settings. The Association's work includes advocating for the NP role, educating the public about the value and cost-effectiveness of NPs in reproductive health, functioning as a clearing-house for information and consultation on current issues, accrediting women's health NP programs, and monitoring state and national legislation. Programs and publications produced and sponsored by NPWH offer special expertise in reproductive health as well as primary care women's health issues. Programs and offerings include but are not limited to contraception, menopause, sexually transmitted diseases, pregnancy, women's sexuality, female urinary problems, cancer detection and prevention, colposcopy and the management of cervical disease, and women's wellness.

There are nearly 2000 members in five membership categories: active membership for RNs who have completed an NP program or are certified (or eligible for certification); associate membership for nurses and other clinicians who support the purpose of NPWH; student membership; corporate membership; and supporting membership for executives, employers, physicians, and other individuals who uphold the purpose of NPWH. Membership benefits include a newsletter, the *Monthly Cycle*, and *Women's Health Care Journal*.

National Association of Nurse Practitioners in Women's Health, 505 C Street, NE, Washington, DC 20002 **http://www.npwh.org**

National Association of Orthopaedic Nurses

The National Association of Orthopaedic Nurses (NAON) was established in 1980 to promote education and research related to the nursing care of persons with orthopaedic conditions.

Today, NAON is one of the premiere national nursing associations with 6000 members dispersed among 91 chapters and 15 special interest groups. NAON's major purpose is to promote, in cooperation with all members of the health care team, the highest standards of nursing practice; to promote research; and to maintain effective communication between orthopaedic nurses and other external interested persons and groups.

The association offers certification examinations for orthopaedic nurses through the associated Orthopaedic Nurses Certification Board, the *Orthopaedic Nursing* journal, a newsletter, a bibliography on orthopaedics, a core curriculum, patient education videos, and other monographs and videos.

In addition to awards for excellence in orthopaedic nursing practice, writing, and research, NAON also offers its active members competitive scholarships for continuing education.

National Association of Orthopaedic Nurses, 401 N. Michigan Avenue, Suite 2200, Chicago, IL 60611 **http://www.orthonurse.org**

National Association of Pediatric Nurse Associates and Practitioners

The National Association of Pediatric Nurse Associates and Practitioners (NAPNAP) was founded in 1973 as a nonprofit specialty nursing organization devoted to improving the quality of infant and child health care. Today, NAPNAP represents practitioners working with populations across the pediatric spectrum, including infants, children, adolescents, and young adults. The pediatric NP provides an advanced level of care to children and their families, including counseling on normal development and behavioral problems, the prevention of illness and preventable injuries, and the care of children with acute or chronic conditions. NAPNAP promotes high standards of child health care through education, research, and legislative action involving over 7000 members in 48 chapters across the country.

NAPNAP publishes the *Journal of Pediatric Health Care*, a bimonthly pediatric journal containing articles about research and current developments in pediatric care, and the *Pediatric Nurse Practitioner*, a bimonthly newsletter that reports on NAPNAP's activities as an association. NAPNAP sponsors an annual convention and CE opportunities. NAPNAP has had an active role in influencing legislation relevant to pediatric NP practice, especially in the areas of child abuse, childcare and safety, and reimbursement of pediatric NPs.

National Association of Pediatric Nurse Associates and Practitioners, 20 Brace Road, Suite 200, Cherry Hill, NJ 08034-2634 **http://www.napnap.org**

National Association of School Nurses

The National Association of School Nurses (NASN) was formed in 1969 as a department of the National Education Association. In 1977, the name was changed to its current one. In 1979, the NASN incorporated and became an affiliate of the National Education Association, a status that still exists. The mission of NASN is to advance the practice of school nursing and provide leadership in the delivery of quality health programs to the school community.

To become an active member, a registered professional nurse must meet the requirements for school nursing in the member's state and fulfill other qualifications or requirements set forth in the bylaws. Other membership categories are associate, student, retired, corporate, and institutional. Currently there are over 10,000 members with 51 school nurse organization affiliates in 49 states, one overseas, and one in the District of Columbia.

NASN is producing a series of self-study modules on *Nursing Assessment of School-Age Youth* with funding from the Robert Wood Johnson Foundation and offers an Internet program called *Asthma Education for School Nurses.* NASN established an Academy of Fellows to recognize excellence in school nursing in 1997.

Besides initiating a variety of projects aimed at educating school nurses, NASN sponsors a newsletter, the *Journal of School Nursing,* an annual conference, and two regional conferences. It has developed several publications including *School Nursing Practice: Roles and Standards* and *Guidelines for School Nursing Documentation: Standards, Issues, and Models.* NASN also offers a certification examination for school nurses.

NASN sponsors School Nurse Day each year on the fourth Wednesday in January and monitors federal legislation that pertains to school health, testifying on important health issues.

National Association of School Nurses, 8484 Georgia Avenue, Suite 420, Silver Spring, MD 20910
http://www.nasn.org

National Black Nurses' Association

The National Black Nurses' Association (NBNA) was formed at the end of 1971 as an outgrowth of the Black Nurses' Caucus held during the 1970 ANA convention. These nurses believed that black Americans and other minority groups "are by design or neglect excluded from the means to achieve access to the health mainstream of America" and that black nurses have the "understanding, knowledge, interest, concern, and experience to make a significant difference in the health care status of the black community."

Membership is open to all RNs, LPNs, and nursing students regardless of race, creed, color, national origin, age, or sex. The NBNA represents 150,000 African American registered nurses, licensed vocational/practical nurses, nursing students, and retired nurses from the United States, Eastern Caribbean, and Africa, with 79 chartered chapters in 34 states. The first national conference was held in 1972, and annual conferences have continued to be held.

The NBNA's mission is to "provide a forum for the collective action by black nurses to investigate, define and advocate for the health needs of African Americans." The NBNA has established several avenues for the dissemination of knowledge about critical issues in nursing practice, research, education, and other health care issues relevant to African Americans. Publications are the *NBNA News* and the *Journal of the National Black Nurses Association.*

National Black Nurses' Association, Inc., 8630 Fenton Street, Suite 330, Silver Spring, MD 20910-3803
http://www.nbna.org

National Council of State Boards of Nursing

The National Council of State Boards of Nursing (NCSBN) was created in 1978 by boards of nursing throughout the United States and its territories that are its members. It is an organization through which the boards act and counsel together on matters of common interest and concern affecting the public health, safety, and welfare, including the development of licensing examinations in nursing. To accomplish its mission of promoting public policy related to the safe and effective practice of nursing, NCSBN provides services and guidance to its members in performing functions that regulate entry to nursing practice, continuing safe practice, and nursing education programs.

Under the direction of its member boards, NCSBN develops the National Council Licensure Examinations for Registered Nurses (NCLEX-RN) and Practical Nurses (NCLEX-PN). Each member board uses the examinations to test the entry-level competency of candidates for nursing licensure. More details are included in Chapter 20.

NCSBN provides support for boards of nursing through collecting and analyzing information pertaining to the licensure and discipline of nurses (including a disciplinary data bank), developing model nursing legislation and administrative rules, and sponsoring educational programs.

The organization publishes a quarterly newsletter, *Issues,* and offers a series of videotapes on the NCLEX as well as numerous other resource materials. Its members consist of 61 boards of nursing. A delegate assembly meets annually to determine policies and provide future direction.

National Council of State Boards of Nursing, 111 E. Wacker Drive, Suite 2900, Chicago, IL, 60601
http://www.ncsbn.org

National Gerontological Nursing Association

Established in 1984, the National Gerontological Nursing Association (NGNA) aims to provide a forum in which gerontological nursing issues are identified and explored; to develop and support educational programs for nurses, health providers, and the general public; and to educate and inform the general public on health issues, particularly those affecting elders.

NGNA's mission also supports innovative approaches in gerontological health care, disseminating information and research related to gerontological nursing and enhancing the professionalism of gerontological nurses.

Among membership benefits are a subscription to *Geriatric Nursing*, which has a special NGNA section; *Supporting Innovations in Gerontological Nursing* (SIGN), an informative newsletter designed to keep members aware of current issues and NGNA activities; CE programs; networking at local chapters; and *New Horizons*, the official bimonthly newsletter.

Membership is open to RNs, nursing students, nursing assistants, and non-nurses in the associate member category. There are about 1500 members.

National Gerontological Nursing Association, 1020 Monarch Street, Lexington, KY 40513
http://www.ngna.org

National Nursing Staff Development Organization

Established in 1989, the National Nursing Staff Development Organization (NNSDO) exists to foster the art and science of nursing staff development; promote the image and professional status of nursing staff development educators; encourage and support nursing research and its application of findings in practice; and provide a platform for nurses engaged in staff development practice to discuss issues related to the continuing evolution of the field of nursing staff development. NNSDO also provides a forum for members to further define staff development practice.

In addition, it offers staff development services for members through its publications, meetings, conferences, consultations, mentoring activities, and so on. Members include individual nurses engaged in any aspect of nursing staff development.

The organization holds an annual convention, and members receive a bimonthly newsletter, *Trend-Lines*, and the bimonthly *Journal for Nurses in Staff Development*. NNSDO conducts workshops on various topics relating to staff development.

NNSDO collaborates in developing the certification examination for continuing education and staff development through the ANCC. It offers certification preparation courses under contract with its affiliates (local groups of nursing staff development educators). The organization recently initiated a research fund to stimulate projects.

National Nursing Staff Development Organization, 7794 Grow Drive, Pensacola, FL 32514-1350
http://www.nnsdo.org

North American Nursing Diagnosis Association–International

The North American Nursing Diagnosis Association (NANDA)–International was formally organized in 1982 for the purpose of developing, refining, disseminating, and promoting nursing diagnostic terminology as well as taxonomic structure for use by professional nurses. NANDA was begun by a small group of nurses at St. Louis University concerned about the unavailability of specific patient data that could be computerized and used for providing patient care in a team approach. In 1973, they organized the first invitational conference of the National Conference Group for the Classification of Nursing Diagnoses to identify, develop, and classify nursing diagnoses. At the fifth conference (1982), formal bylaws were adopted, and the name *North American Nursing Diagnosis Association* was adopted to recognize the significant contribution made by Canadian nurses.

NANDA has assumed responsibility for developing and maintaining a diagnosis classification system or taxonomy for professional nursing. The NANDA database is included in the *Meta-thesaurus* of the Unified Medical Language System of the National Library of Medicine. The NANDA classification, titled *NANDA Nursing Diagnoses: Definitions and Classification*, has been translated into numerous foreign languages.

It is updated and published every 2 years. The organization has a process for the review and inclusion of new nursing diagnoses into the taxonomy, and it encourages interested individuals and groups to submit new diagnoses.

Membership is organized into seven geographic districts of the United States and Canada, each of which may consist of smaller regional or local groups. Affiliate membership is available for regional groups, along with individual and institutional membership. Membership numbers about 900, including many international members. Registered professional nurses are eligible to be members, as are students and those with associate status.

The national organization holds a biennial conference; regional and smaller groups may hold more frequent meetings. NANDA has liaisons with many similar nursing diagnosis groups internationally, which are also developing nursing language systems. *The International Journal of Nursing Terminologies and Classifications* (IJNTC) is published quarterly and distributed internationally. The NANDA-I Newsletter is distributed to all members.

North Atlantic Nursing Diagnosis Association International, PO Box 157, Kaukauna, WI 54130-0157
http://www.nanda.org

Nurses Christian Fellowship

Established in 1948, Nurses Christian Fellowship (NCF) is both a professional organization and a ministry by and for Christian nurses and nursing students. It is a division of Inter-Varsity Christian Fellowship and aims to bring the good news of Jesus Christ to nursing education and practice. NCF is concerned for the nurse as a whole person and advocate of quality nursing care. The goals are to (1) develop a network of nurses who listen to God and pray with expectation; (2) equip nurses with a biblical world view that prepares them to represent Jesus Christ in nursing education and practice; (3) proclaim the gospel of Jesus Christ so that others will hear the good news of Christ's relevancy to people and issues in nursing; (4) demonstrate Christ's righteousness and justice through teaching biblical ethical standards and advocating health care for the poor and underserved; (5) develop leadership qualities and skills in Christian nurses who will communicate the gospel of Jesus Christ in nursing locally, nationally, and internationally.

NCF provides a local, regional, national, and international network for Christian nursing. Local groups meet for prayer, bible study, mutual encouragement, and outreach. NCF staff and volunteers provide mentoring, vision for ministry, and help to establish campus and area-wide groups. Area, national, and international CE programs and conferences provide spiritual and professional growth opportunities. Topics include Christian growth, spiritual care, suffering, death, healing, stress and conflict management, ethics, and values.

Written materials include guidelines for starting groups, textbooks on spiritual care and Christian ethics, bible study guides, and the quarterly *Journal of Christian Nursing*. Some workshops are available on videotape. Members receive regular newsletters and prayer updates. Specific resources are available for students, faculty, and graduate students, including the student newsletter *Campus Vitals* and listings of theses and dissertations that include the spiritual dimension from a Christian perspective.

Membership is open to nurses and nursing students who affirm NCF's vision and faith and are committed to involvement in some aspect of the ministry, both financially and practically.

Nurses Christian Fellowship, PO Box 7895, Madison, WI 53707-7895 **http://ncf-jcn.org**

Oncology Nursing Society

The Oncology Nursing Society (ONS) was founded in 1975. The purposes of the society include promoting the highest professional standards of oncology nursing; studying, researching, and exchanging information, experiences, and ideas leading to improved oncology nursing; encouraging nurses to specialize in oncology nursing; and fostering the professional development of oncology nurses individually and collectively. Registered nurses practicing in or interested in oncology are eligible to apply for membership. Today, ONS is the largest professional membership oncology association in the world.

A primary goal of ONS is to provide a network of peer support and exchange for oncology nurses on both the national and local levels. Currently there are more than 36,000 RNs and other health care professionals dedicated to excellence in patient care, teaching, research, administration, and education in the field of oncology. At the community level, ONS offers members the opportunity to join a chapter, where they can have access to education, information, peer support, and leadership opportunities. ONS currently has nearly 206 local chapters.

ONS invests heavily in the education of its members through position statements to guide practice, conferences, and publications. Major educational initiatives have focused on fatigue, cancer in black Americans, bone marrow transplantation, and pain and symptom management. Position papers give clinical direction for assisted suicide, cancer and genetics testing, short-stay surgery for cancer, medical oncology in the nonacute setting, clinical trials, and the use of placebos in pain management. The magnitude and importance of this work is obvious, and only limited examples have been included.

Members receive a subscription to the Society's official journal, the *Oncology Nursing Forum,* and to the newsletter, the *ONS News.* They can also receive a reduced rate on a variety of publications developed by ONS and benefit from a reduced registration fee at the ONS Congress and Fall Institute.

In 1981, the Oncology Nursing Foundation, an affiliate organization of ONS, was established to provide research grants, research fellowships, scholarships, cancer public education projects, and career development awards to oncology nurses.

A second affiliate organization, the Oncology Nursing Certification Corporation, was established in 1984 to develop, administer, and evaluate a program for the certification of oncology nurses.

Oncology Nursing Society, 125 Enterprise Drive, RIDC Park West, Pittsburgh, PA 15275-1214
http://www.ons.org

Respiratory Nursing Society

The Respiratory Nursing Society (RNS) is the professional association for nurses who care for clients with pulmonary dysfunction and who are interested in promoting pulmonary health. RNS was created in 1990 to promote coordinated, comprehensive, high-level nursing care for these clients by fostering respiratory nurses' personal and professional development. To accomplish this, the organization provides educational opportunities that help nurses enhance their knowledge and skills, has created standards of care in collaboration with the ANA, promotes and disseminates research, and serves as a formal network for communications in the field of respiratory nursing.

The purpose of RNS is twofold: to promote the specialty practice of respiratory nursing through the professional development of its members, and to promote safe and effective respiratory health care for society through activities related to health promotion, disease prevention, and care through all phases of illness and across all age spans and cultures.

RNS publishes a quarterly newsletter, *Perspectives in Respiratory Nursing,* which provides information on clinical practice issues, current research, and a calendar of events. The quarterly *RNS Bulletin* provides up-to-date information on organizational and member news. An annual educational conference offers programs covering basic pulmonary assessment, strategies for intervention, concepts in managed care, advanced techniques and skills, and new product information.

Respiratory Nursing Society, 309 E. Lee Avenue, Vinton, VA 24179
http://www.respiratorynursingsociety.org

Society for Vascular Nursing

Founded in 1982, the Society for Vascular Nursing (SVN) is an international association dedicated to promoting excellence in the compassionate and comprehensive management of persons with vascular disease. The Society aims to assume the leadership role in defining the vascular component of fundamental nursing education, establish and implement research-based standards of practice for vascular nursing, collaborate with other professions to address the unique needs of the patient with vascular disease, and enhance public awareness of vascular disease.

SVN offers active membership to licensed nurses as well as associate membership to non-nurse health professionals and corporate membership to related industry. Benefits include subscriptions to the quarterly *Journal of Vascular Nursing* and the bimonthly newsletter, *SVN . . . prn.* SVN features an annual national symposium each spring. A vascular nursing fellowship grant program provides funding for approved research projects by SVN members. A taskforce is currently exploring a specialty certification program.

SVN also sponsors a nationwide health education and screening campaign for peripheral arterial disease, "A Step Ahead," and assists in the coordination of screening programs across the country and in Canada. Currently there are approximately 900 members.

Society for Vascular Nursing, 100 Cummings Center, Suite 124 A, Beverly, MA 01915 http://svnnet.org/

Society of Gastroenterology Nurses and Associates

Formed in 1974, the Society of Gastroenterology Nurses and Associates (SGNA) works to advance the science and practice of gastroenterology and endoscopy nursing through education, research, advocacy, and collaboration. By the end of 2010, membership in the Society numbered more than 8000.

Members receive *Gastroenterology Nursing* bimonthly, and additionally a monthly newsletter. Certification is offered through the Certifying Board of Gastroenterology Nurses and Associates.

Society of Gastroenterology Nurses and Associates,
401 N. Michigan Avenue, Chicago, IL 60611
http://www.sgna.org

Society of Otorhinolaryngology and Head-Neck Nurses

The Society of Otorhinolaryngology and Head-Neck Nurses (SOHN) was chartered with 47 nurses in 1976 and has grown to a membership of 1100 nurses. The Society provides a nurturing environment to enhance the professional growth and development of nurses dedicated to the health of the otorhinolaryngology (ORL) patient population. SOHN's major vehicles to accomplish this are networking, education, and research. To this end, the Ear, Nose, and Throat Foundation was established in 1998. Additionally, special interest groups have been established in advanced practice, allergy/sinus, federal/military, head and neck, office based, otology, and pediatric.

Publications to members include SOHN's official journal, *Head and Neck Nursing*, and *Update*, a newsletter. A spring seminar and a congress are annual events.

Society of Otorhinolaryngology and Head-Neck Nurses,
207 Downing Street, New Smyrna Beach, FL 32168
http://www.sohnnurse.com

Society of Pediatric Nurses

Established in 1990, the Society of Pediatric Nurses (SPN) aims to improve the nursing care of children and their families and to further the development of pediatric nursing as a sub-specialty within the nursing profession. Members include staff nurses, school and outpatient nurses, clinical nurse specialists, practitioners, administrators, educators, and researchers.

The society offers a newsletter, membership directory, educational scholarships, and a small grants research program. Chapters are located throughout the nation, with 2000 members to date.

SPN holds an annual meeting each spring. An awards program recognizes outstanding contributions to pediatric nursing. SPN publishes the peer-reviewed research publication, *Journal of Pediatric Nursing*, six times a year, and *SPN News*, a bimonthly e-newsletter.

Society of Pediatric Nurses, 7794 Grow Drive, Pensacola, FL 32514-7072 http://www.pedsnurses.org

Society of Urologic Nurses and Associates

Organized in 1972, the Society of Urologic Nurses and Associates (SUNA) is dedicated to advancing the cause of professionalism and better patient care in the field of urology. The care of the urologic patient requires a high degree of education, skill, and dedication. Education is the key to achieving these objectives; thus, SUNA was organized to supplement and extend the urology curriculum provided by nursing schools. The purposes of SUNA are to serve as a vehicle for the distribution of all available information in the field of urology; to point the way to advanced nursing techniques and new equipment; and to help those who wish to become urology specialists.

The SUNA board of directors plans educational meetings on national, regional, and local levels. An annual conference is held in conjunction with that of the American Urological Association, the professional association for urologic surgeons.

SUNA provides certification and recertification for members and nonmembers through the American Board of Urologic Allied Health Professionals. Certification is based on assessment of knowledge, demonstration of current clinical practice, and colleagues' endorsement. SUNA currently has over 3000 members and 42 chapters located in four regions of the United States: Northeast, Southeast, North Central, and the West.

A bimonthly newsletter, *Urogram*, and a quarterly journal, *Urologic Nursing*, are provided to members. Active membership is open to persons in the health care professions who are engaged in the care of urology patients.

Society of Urologic Nurses and Associates, East Holly Avenue, Box 56, Pitman, NJ 08071-0056
http://www.suna.org

■ REGIONAL NURSING ASSOCIATIONS

Council on Collegiate Education for Nursing (SREB)

The Council on Collegiate Education for Nursing (CCEN), in affiliation with the Southern Regional Education Board (SREB), engages in cooperative planning and activities to strengthen nursing education in colleges and universities in the South. SREB, the nation's first interstate compact for higher education, appointed a committee on graduate education and research in nursing in 1948 to establish graduate programs in nursing. In 1963, CCEN was formed as the major mechanism for working toward strengthening and expanding nursing education programs at all levels. Two successive 5-year grants (1962–1972) from the W. K. Kellogg Foundation of Battle Creek, Michigan, supported a variety of activities addressing statewide planning, new instructional techniques, curriculum theory and development, and in-service programs for faculty and administrators. In 1972, SREB and the council, with funding from the Division of Nursing, US DHHS, developed plans for conducting regional activities on a more permanent basis.

The CCEN became a membership organization in 1975, maintaining an affiliation with SREB. Regionally accredited colleges and universities that provide nursing education programs leading to the associate degree, baccalaureate, and higher degrees are eligible for membership. Each member institution pays an annual fee that is established by the council.

CCEN functions as a forum where the chief administrator of college-based nursing programs can obtain information; discuss developments at national, state, and local levels; and conduct regional planning. This group generates ideas for and implements nursing-related projects administered by SREB.

Projects address relevant issues and concerns of nursing education in the 15 SREB member states (Alabama, Arkansas, Florida, Georgia, Kentucky, Louisiana, Maryland, Mississippi, North Carolina, Oklahoma, South Carolina, Tennessee, Texas, Virginia, West Virginia). Notable among the projects are Continuing Nursing Education in Computer Technology; Faculty Preparation for Teaching Gerontological Nursing; and Faculty Development for Graduate Nurse Educators.

Council on Collegiate Education for Nursing, 592 10th Street NW, Atlanta, GA 30318-5790
http://www.sreb.org

Western Institute of Nursing

The Western Institute of Nursing (WIN), a nonprofit organization, was established in 1986 and represents nurses in the following 13 states: Alaska, Arizona, California, Colorado, Hawaii, Idaho, Montana, Nevada, New Mexico, Oregon, Utah, Washington, and Wyoming. The institute expands on the 29-year heritage of the Western Council on Higher Education for Nursing (WCHEN) to provide leadership and representation for nursing in the West by joining practice and education in a full and active partnership. Over the years, WIN has developed into the western region's comprehensive, knowledgeable, and action-oriented organization involved with regional and national issues, concerns, and trends in nursing.

Recognizing the complex needs within the region, WIN has a proven track record of helping nurses address common interests as well as special problems. WIN has acquired the capacity and expertise to improve health care and advance the profession. Through the assistance of WIN, the efforts of individual and agency members are leveraged, creating diverse benefits for nurses. The mission of WIN is to influence positively the quality of health care for people in the West through monitoring relevant issues and trends and through designing, implementing, and evaluating regional action-oriented nursing strategies in nursing education, practice, and research.

There are six categories of membership in WIN—agency, associate, individual, student, retired, and honorary. *Agency memberships* are open to organized nursing education programs and organized nursing practices in the 13 western states. *Individual membership* is open to RNs who support the mission of WIN. *Student members* must be matriculated in a degree-granting program. *Associate memberships* are open to individual non-nurses and to organizations, agencies, and businesses outside the western region that support the mission of WIN. *Honorary memberships* include those designated for Emeritus status, and those who have made supporting contributions to WIN. An elected board of governors manages the affairs of the institute.

Membership in the institute's Western Society for Research in Nursing (WSRN) is open to all members of WIN. WSRN supports research efforts, providing a network for researchers and sponsoring an annual research conference.

WIN holds an annual assembly that provides a forum and networking for the discussion of relevant issues, trends, and activities related to the mission and goals of the institute and a business session for organizational matters. Through the annual Communicating Nursing Research Conference, nursing research is presented and discussed. Papers are selected for the quality of the research and the impact of the research on the discipline of nursing. Proceedings of the combined WIN/Assembly/Nursing Research Conference are published annually.

To recognize outstanding leadership and the promotion of excellence, WIN has established an awards program. Each year, the Carol A. Lindeman Award for a New Researcher is given.

Western Institute of Nursing, 3455 SW Veterans Road, Portland, OR 97239-2941 **http://www.ohsu.edu/son-win/**

■ NURSING-RELATED ORGANIZATIONS

There are a variety of organizations that allow for the participation of nurses through some form of exclusive or general membership. They are too varied to begin to list. The American Heart Association, the American Cancer Society, and the Catholic Hospital Association are just three examples.

In addition, there are those organizations that can either trace their roots to nursing or that serve a constituency closely involved with the registered nurse. The practical nurse organizations and the American Red Cross are of that nature and are presented here.

American Red Cross

Clara Barton, a volunteer who cared for soldiers during the Civil War, founded the American Red Cross in 1881. She became committed to ensuring that the US government ratified the Geneva Convention and established an organization in the United States that would alleviate human suffering. The American Red Cross is a humanitarian organization, led by volunteers, that provides relief to victims of disasters and helps people prevent, prepare for, and respond to emergencies. It does this through services consistent with the 1905 Congressional Charter and the fundamental principles of the international Red Cross movement. The 50-member, all-volunteer board of governors directs the American Red Cross and establishes the policies under which chapters and blood regions across the country operate. The Red Cross is a nongovernmental agency and relies primarily on the generosity of the American people for support.

The Division of Nursing was formally reestablished in the American Red Cross in July 1992. Its function is to provide support for nurse involvement throughout the organization. Nurses are recognized through nurse enrollment within the American Red Cross after providing a minimum number of hours of service.

Ever since it was founded, Nursing and Health Services has been one of the important units in many Red Cross societies. In the United States, a Division of Nursing Services was established in the American Red Cross in 1909, with Jane A. Delano as its first director. The maintenance of a reserve of qualified professional nurses who could be mobilized quickly in emergencies such as disaster or war was the initial purpose of the Red Cross Nursing and Health Services.

Red Cross Nursing and Health Services today are designed to extend community resources in helping to meet the health needs of people at home and in the community. Policies and standards for all Red Cross services are determined at the national level. At the local level, the chapter Nursing and Health Services committees are responsible for planning and implementing the nursing services. Not all chapters have identical services because community needs, resources, and interests vary. However, standardized educational courses are available throughout the nation. Although the services may vary, Nursing and Health Services maintains a reserve of volunteer nurses who become enrolled as Red Cross nurses for the following activities.

Disaster Relief, Education, and Preparedness

The Red Cross responds to more than 60,000 hurricanes, floods, earthquakes, tornadoes, fires, hazardous material spills, and transportation accidents each year. Trained Red Cross paid and volunteer staff members are ready to respond when a disaster threatens or strikes. Nurses are prepared through a series of training courses to adapt their nursing skills to meet needs brought about by disasters. Basic training is offered for emergency mass care, emergency assistance, and long-term recovery. Through advanced training and experience on disaster operations, nurses can be prepared to serve at the supervisory and director levels on national disasters.

Emergency Communications and Assistance to Members of the Armed Forces and Their Families

The Red Cross provides emergency communications, financial assistance, and counseling to members of the Armed Forces, their families, and veterans during both peacetime and conflict, on US military installations within the United States and around the world.

Biomedical Services: Blood and Tissue Services

Red Cross volunteers help to collect blood donations that amount to almost half of the nation's blood supply. Red Cross develops, tests, and implements training programs in areas such as the operations of blood testing laboratories and selection of donors. Red Cross tissue services collect, process, and distribute human tissue products.

Health and Safety Services

The Red Cross is a recognized provider of first aid, CPR, swimming and water safety, lifeguarding, and other health and safety programs. An average of 10 million people are trained each year. The Red Cross teaches people how to prevent HIV infection and works to increase understanding of the realities facing those who are living with HIV infection and AIDS.

International Services

As a major part of the international Red Cross movement, the American Red Cross supports humanitarian relief around the world in areas affected by natural disasters and war, and educates the public in international humanitarian law and the fundamental principles of the Red Cross. International tracing and location services are offered by every chapter of the American Red Cross to help locate, reunite, and exchange messages between people separated from their loved ones because of war, civil disturbance, or natural disaster.

National Association for Practical Nurse Education and Service

The National Association for Practical Nurse Education and Service (NAPNES) is the oldest organization for practical nurses (PNs) in the United States. It was founded in 1941 by a group of nurse educators for the purpose of improving and extending the education of the PN to meet the critical need for more nursing personnel. Founded as the Association of Practical Nurse Schools, the name was changed to the National Association for Practical Nurse Education in 1942; Service was added to the title in 1959.

Within a few years, after professionally planned curricula had been set up and duties of the PN defined, NAPNES expanded its activities to include a broad program of service to schools of practical nursing and the LPN/LVN. At one time this included accreditation of PN programs.

NAPNES serves as one of the spokesmen of the LPN on federal and state levels on such matters as licensing, laws governing LPN/LVN practice, educational opportunities for the LPN/LVN, and matters of general welfare. NAPNES publishes the *Journal of Practical Nursing* quarterly.

National Association for Practical Nurse Education and Service, 1940 Duke Street, Suite 200, Alexandria, VA 22314 **http://napnes.org**

National Federation of Licensed Practical Nurses

The membership of the National Federation of Licensed Practical Nurses (NFLPN), a federation of state associations organized in 1949, is made up entirely of LPNs and LVNs. In states with a PN association affiliated with the federation, members enroll through the state association. In other states, individual LPNs and LVNs may join NFLPN as members at large. Each member participates in formulating policies and programs through the election of a house of delegates, which meets during the annual convention. Students may attend meetings with voice but no vote.

Some of the major purposes of the NFLPN are to preserve and foster the ideal of comprehensive care for the ill and the aged; to bring together all LPNs or persons with equivalent titles; to secure recognition and effective utilization of the skills of LPNs; to promote the welfare and interests of LPNs; to improve standards of practice in practical nursing; to speak for LPNs and interpret their aims and objectives to other groups and the public; to cooperate with the other groups concerned with better patient care; to serve as a clearinghouse for information on practical nursing; and to continue improvement in the education of LPNs. A code of ethics for LPNs that stresses many of the same points as the ANA code has been developed by the NFLPN as a "motivation for establishing and elevating professional standards."

To help carry out its objectives, NFLPN maintains a government relations consultant in Washington, DC, and other consultants on labor relations. In 1962, NFLPN established the National Licensed Practical Nurses' Educational Foundation "for scientific, educational, and charitable purposes."

Seminars, workshops, and conferences are financed by the Federation, as are leadership-training conferences for persons engaged in PN association activities at the national, state, or local level.

Both ANA and NLN work with NFLPN on matters of mutual concern, principally through liaison committees. NFLPN supports NLN as the recognized agency for accreditation. NFLPN also supports NLN efforts in the development and improvement of PN programs.

National Federation of Licensed Practical Nurses, 605
Poole Drive, Garner, NC 27529
http://www.nflpn.com

KEY POINTS

1. The proliferation of specialty organizations is testimony that nurses identify with their practice.
2. With your first job as a registered nurse you become specialized, and it is impossible to make the transition to a new area of practice without updating your skills.
3. Most state and national associations have local chapters.
4. Most nursing organizations focus on education, leadership development, peer support, and standards of practice.
5. A specialty organization will not protect the broader professional interests, which are the raison d'être of your state nurses' association.

Updates can be found at **www.kellysnursing.com**

Major International Organizations

The organizations discussed in the preceding chapters are all national, although some have international members or affiliations. Included in this chapter are the major international organizations related to nursing and health.

■ INTERNATIONAL COUNCIL OF NURSES

The International Council of Nurses (ICN) antedated by many years the international hospital and medical associations. ICN is the largest international organization primarily made up of professional women in the world.[1] (There are, of course, men in ICN member organizations.)

The originator and prime mover of ICN was Ethel Gordon Manson (Mrs. Bedford Fenwick), a distinguished and energetic English nurse who first proposed the idea of an international nursing organization in July 1899.[2] Among the American nurses present in London at that time, attending a meeting of the International Council of Women was one whose name figures prominently in the nursing history of our own country, Lavinia Dock. She was quick to support Mrs. Fenwick's idea and, shortly thereafter, a committee of nurses from nine different countries began laying the groundwork and drawing up a constitution for the proposed new organization. When ICN was officially established in 1900, Mrs. Fenwick became its first president. Miss Dock became its first secretary, a position she held for the next 22 years. Annie Goodrich became the first ICN president from the United States.

The essential idea for which the ICN stands is, in Miss Dock's words, is

> . . . self government of nurses in their associations, with the aim of raising ever higher the standards of education and professional ethics, public usefulness, and civic spirit

of their members. The International Council of Nurses does not stand for a narrow professionalism, but for that full development of the human being and citizen in every nurse, which shall best enable her to bring her professional knowledge and skill to the many sided service that modern society demands of her.[3]

Today ICN is sometimes referred to as the *United Nations of Nurses*, an appropriate enough title. Although nonpolitical, and certainly less affluent than the UN, ICN does bring together persons from many countries who have a common interest in nursing and a common purpose—the development of nursing throughout the world.

Membership

From the beginning, ICN was intended to be a federation of national nursing organizations. The association was a little ahead of its time, however, because in 1900 very few countries had organized nursing associations. Until 1904, therefore, ICN had individual members. (These included male nurses, although the first time men were specifically mentioned as attending an ICN congress was in 1912 in Cologne, Germany, where greetings were given from the president of the association of male nurses in Berlin.) In 1904, three countries reported that their national nursing organizations were "ready and eager to affiliate with the International Council of Nurses," and thus Great Britain, the United States, and Germany became the three charter members of ICN.[4]

ICN today is a federation of national nurses' associations. The requirements for membership have been, essentially, that the national association be an autonomous, self-directing, and self-governing body—nonpolitical,

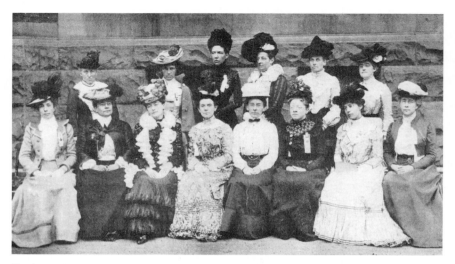

Foreign delegates and officers of the International Council of Nurses, Buffalo, New York, 1901. (Courtesy of Lucie Kelly, private collection)

nonsectarian, with no form of racial discrimination—whose voting membership is composed exclusively of nurses broadly representative of the nurses in its country, and that it be able to honor its financial obligation to ICN. Its objectives must be in harmony with ICN's stated objective: to provide a medium through which national nurses' associations may share their common interests, working together to develop the contribution of nursing to the promotion of the health of people and the care of the sick. A majority vote by the ICN's governing body determines the admission of national associations into membership.

At the 1973 meeting of ICN, a constitutional change was made to broaden the criteria for membership to include nurses who constitute a section or chapter of a national organization composed of other health workers as well as nurses. The ICN definition of *nurse* (the basis for national membership eligibility) was also broadened. In 1989, this definition (for membership purposes only) was as follows: "A nurse is a person who has completed a programme of basic nursing education and is qualified and authorized in his/her country to practice nursing."

A reiteration of the principle of nondiscrimination was also reinforced at this meeting through a resolution requiring the South African Nursing Association (SANA) to take action to enable nonwhite nurses to serve on SANA's board of directors or face the possibility of expulsion from ICN. (This discrimination apparently existed because of certain clauses in that country's nursing practice act, which had to be changed.) Later that year, SANA withdrew from ICN because of its inability to comply with the mandate. By 1995, South African nurses had established a new organization, the Democratic Nursing Organization of South Africa (DENOSA). DENOSA was admitted into ICN membership in 1997.

Each country may be represented in ICN by only one national nursing organization. For the United States, the ICN member is ANA, which allocates a small percentage of membership dues to the support of ICN. Thus, even though individual nurses are not ICN members, those who are ANA members can consider themselves part of this great international fellowship. In 2010, there were 132 geopolitical areas affiliated with ICN through their national nurses' associations (see Exhibit 28–1).

Organization

The governing body of ICN, according to a new constitution adopted in 1965 and revised in 1999, is the Council of National Representatives (CNR), consisting of the presidents of the member associations. This group meets at least every 2 years to establish ICN policies. It also has the responsibility of electing the members of the board of directors.

ICN's board of directors consists of 15 members: its four officers (president and three vice presidents), plus seven members elected on a regional basis and four members at

■ **EXHIBIT 28–1. ICN Member Associations as of 2011**

Andorra	Egypt	Lesotho	St. Lucia
Angola	Estonia	Liberia	St. Vincent and Grenadines
Argentina	Ethiopia	Lithuania	Samoa
Aruba	Fiji	Luxembourg	São Tomé and Principe
Australia	Finland	Macao	Serbia
Austria	France	Malawi	Seychelles
Bahamas	FYR Macedonia	Malaysia	Sierra Leone
Bahrain	Gambia	Malta	Singapore
Bangladesh	Georgia	Mauritius	Slovakia
Barbados	Germany	Mexico	Slovenia
Belgium	Ghana	Monaco	Solomon Islands
Belize	Greece	Mongolia	South Africa
Bermuda	Grenada	Morocco	Spain
Bolivia	Guatemala	Mozambique	Sri Lanka
Botswana	Guyana	Myanmar	Swaziland
Brazil	Haiti	Namibia	Sweden
British Virgin Islands	Honduras	Nepal	Switzerland
Brunei	Hong Kong	Netherlands	Taiwan
Bulgaria	Hungary	Netherlands Antilles	Tanzania
Burkina Faso	Iceland	New Zealand	Thailand
Canada	Indonesia	Nicaragua	Togo
Chile	Iran	Nigeria	Tonga
Colombia	Ireland	Norway	Trinidad and Tobago
Congo Dem. Rep.	Israel	Pakistan	Turkey
Cook Islands	Italy	Panama	Uganda
Croatia	Jamaica	Paraguay	United Arab Emirates
Cuba	Japan	Peru	United Kingdom
Cyprus	Jordan	Philippines	United States
Czech Republic	Kenya	Poland	Uruguay
Denmark	Korea	Portugal	Venezuela
Dominican Republic	Kuwait	Romania	Zambia
East Timor	Latvia	Russia	Zimbabwe
Ecuador	Lebanon	Salvador (El)	

large, all elected by the CNR. The board, which meets at least once a year, carries on the general business of ICN, reporting to the council. The ICN president and vice presidents constitute its executive and planning and finance committees, responsible for general administration of ICN affairs and advice in relation to investments. The ICN constitution does not call for any standing committees, but rather supports flexibility and adhocracy.

Carrying out ICN's day-to-day activities is its headquarters staff—a group of professional nurses, including ICN's executive director. These nurses represent ICN's executive staff, but in their relationships with and services to the member associations, they serve in an advisory and consultative capacity. Staff members are selected from various member countries. In 1996, a Canadian nurse became the executive director, and in 2009 a nurse from Scotland. Usually all executive staff speak more than one language and have special qualifications in one or more of ICN's areas of activity and service.

ICN headquarters is located at 3 Place Jean Marteau, 1201, Geneva, Switzerland. For many years, its headquarters had been in London. The move to Geneva, however, locates ICN close to the many other international bodies in that city.

ICN Congresses

Once every 4 years, the ICN holds what is always referred to as its Quadrennial Congress: a meeting of the members of the national nurses' associations in membership with ICN. Nursing students are usually eligible to attend ICN congresses too, if they are sponsored and their applications are processed by their national nurses' association. Students meet as a student assembly during the congresses, where they discuss issues of concern across national borders, such as students' rights.

ICN met less regularly in its early years, and the two world wars also caused the canceling of meetings during those periods. World War I disrupted the first meeting, which was to have been held in the United States in 1915. Instead, the business of ICN was carried on during the ANA convention in San Francisco that year, attended by American nurses and a few intrepid English nurses who braved the submarine-infested Atlantic Ocean. The 17th congress was held in the United States in 1981; the 1985 congress was in Israel; the 1989 congress was in Korea; the 1993 congress was in Spain; the 1997 congress in Vancouver, Canada; 2001 congress in Copenhagen, Denmark; 2005 in Taiwan; and 2009 in South Africa.

During the last several congresses, discussion and resolutions ranged from those focusing specifically on nursing issues to general social concerns. Included, for instance, were career ladders, socioeconomic welfare, educational and practice standards, research, autonomy, the nurse's role in safeguarding human rights, the nurse's role in the care of detainees and prisoners, and nurse participation in national health policy planning and decision making. Related to general health care were topics such as primary care, excision and circumcision of females, increased violence against patients and health personnel, the uncontrolled proliferation of ancillary nursing personnel, environmental quality, and care for the elderly. On an even broader scale were the concerns about refugees and displaced persons, poverty, and the status of women.

Functions and Activities

In the foreword to its 1981 constitution, ICN points out that the primary purpose of nurses the world over is "to provide and develop a service for the public," and that ICN, as a federation of national nursing associations, provides for sharing of knowledge so that "nursing practice throughout the world is strengthened and improved." In pursuit of this objective, ICN promotes the organization of national nurses' associations and advises them in developing and improving health service for the public, the practice of nursing, and the social and economic welfare of nurses; provides a means of communication, understanding, and cooperation among nurses throughout the world; establishes and

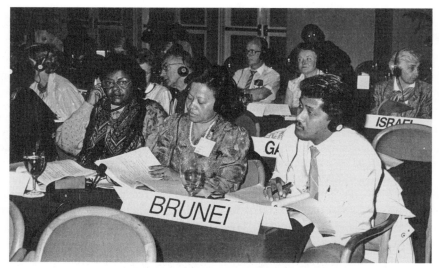

The biennial meeting of the ICN Council of Nurse Representatives (CNR) brings together the nursing leadership of over 132 countries. (Courtesy of the International Council of Nurses, Geneva)

maintains liaison and cooperation with other international organizations; and serves as a representative and spokesperson for nurses at an international level.

The work of ICN is focused on three main areas called the pillars of the association—professional practice, regulation, and socioeconomic welfare. Two of ICN's original goals were to provide for the registration of trained nurses to protect the public from practice by unqualified practitioners and to promote a standardized and upgraded system of nursing education. Important statements on basic beliefs about and principles of nursing education, practice, service, and social and economic welfare have been adopted. The nursing education statement indicates that nursing education should be conducted in institutions where education is the primary concern and that supervised practice related to theory should be provided with both healthy and sick populations. The nursing practice statement stresses health care as a basic human right, and the economic welfare statement calls for joint employer/employee consultation in determining conditions of employment and the right of nurses to participate in their national organization. These statements are simple and direct but ambitious, especially when we consider that they target the world of nurses and nursing.

Those who have attended any of the congresses will testify to the fact that they fully live up to the pomp and ceremony of their name. Held in various countries upon invitation of the national nurses' association of the host country, the congresses are inspiring demonstrations of international communication and fellowship in nursing. In conjunction with each congress, the CNR holds its meeting, with all those in attendance at the congress free to observe open sessions of the ICN council's deliberations. The official language of the congress is English, but facilitating communication is a system of simultaneous translation into the official congress languages: English, French, and Spanish. There is also a daily paper in all three languages, which is distributed during the congress.

One of the interesting traditions of the congress is that each outgoing president has left a watchword for the next 4 years. The first, left by Mrs. Fenwick in 1901, was *work*. That left by an American, Dorothy Cornelius, in 1977, was *accountability*. Establishing a new tradition, Margretta Madden Styles, an American and ICN president from 1993 to 1997, claimed the watchword *march* to begin her term of office. Kirsten Stallknecht, president from 1997 to 2001, chose the watchword *humanity* to guide ICN "in an age where technology is replacing caring." Each watchword is

engraved on a link of the silver chain of office of the ICN president and becomes a permanent part of ICN history.

At the congress, special program sessions are held, usually linked to one unifying theme. Among the most outstanding achievements of the CNR was the acceptance of a new *Code of Ethics* in 1999. The code makes explicit the nurse's responsibility and accountability for nursing care. Eliminated years ago, for instance, were statements that abrogated the nurse's judgment and personal responsibility and stressed a dependency on physicians, which nurses throughout the world saw as no longer appropriate.

Whenever possible, ICN has sought common denominators in education and practice throughout the world. One such common denominator, for instance, is the *International Code of Ethics* adopted by ICN and equally applicable to nurses in every country. Another example is the classic ICN publication authored by Virginia Henderson, *ICN Basic Principles of Nursing Care*, now available in 24 languages and useful to nurses throughout the world.[5] At the same time, ICN has always recognized the autonomy of its member associations and the principle that each country will develop the systems of education and practice best suited to its individual culture and needs.

Throughout the years, ICN has collected and disseminated data on patterns of nursing education and service throughout the world and provided information and advisory and consultative services in both areas to member associations requesting such service. In recent years, ICN has given special attention to primary care as a means of achieving health for all.

Some of ICN's activities in the educational field are financed, in whole or in part, by the Florence Nightingale International Foundation (FNIF), with which ICN is associated. FNIF was established in 1934 as an educational trust in honor of Nightingale. FNIF trust funds have also been used by ICN to encourage and stimulate research activities in nursing. One document developed by FNIF is *Ethics in Nursing Practice—A Guide to Ethical Decision-Making*, by Dr. Sara Fry, an American ethicist.

In recent years, ICN has been particularly active in the area of nurses' social and economic welfare, and its staff has carried out field work to assist national associations in this area. The economic and general welfare of nurses is still considered a concern of top priority.

Providing liaison for nurses with other international groups is one of ICN's most significant contributions to world nursing. Among the organizations, governmental and nongovernmental, with which ICN is associated in some way are the World Health Organization (WHO); the World Federation of Mental Health; the International Labor Organization; the World Medical Association; the International Hospital Federation; the International Federation of Red Cross and Red Crescent Societies; the International Committee of the Red Cross; the United Nations Educational, Scientific, and Cultural Organization (UNESCO); the Council of International Organizations of Medical Sciences (CIOMS); and the Union of International Associations.

Publications

Since 1929, ICN's official organ has been the *International Nursing Review* (INR), published quarterly by Blackwell Science, a prestigious publishing house located in Oxford, England. In addition to reports of ICN activities, the INR carries peer-reviewed nursing articles of international interest, usually written by nurses from the ICN member countries. Occasionally it reprints articles from publications of member countries. It is published in English, but some associations translate certain articles into their own languages.

Every year ICN celebrates International Nurses Day on a theme selected by the ICN Board of Directors by preparing a resource kit with a background paper, posters, and ideas for action and suggestions for planning and organizing International Nurses Day activities. Themes of the recent past have included the quality and cost-effectiveness of nursing, healthy aging, mental health, safe motherhood, school health, and nursing and the environment.

ICN has initiated a variety of activities to study issues and correct inequities critical to the development of nursing. Some have been the International Classification of Nursing Project,[6] the Regulation Project,[7] costing nursing services, nursing and AIDS, the international nursing research agenda, the use of assistive personnel, and mental health services, to name a few. Most of these initiatives produce publications that are available through headquarters, some free and others for a fee.

The Past and the Future

The preamble to ICN's original constitution stated, "We, nurses of all nations, sincerely believing that the best good of our profession will be advanced by greater unity of thought, sympathy and purpose, do hereby band ourselves in a confederation of workers to further the efficient care of the sick, and to secure the honour and interests of the nursing profession." From the beginning, ICN and its officers

were farsighted and pioneering. Included were members of every race and creed. The courageous Mrs. Fenwick stood firmly for her belief in women's suffrage and often spoke of the organization as a federation of women's organizations (for all its male members), with women's suffrage as one of its objectives. In 1901, she also stated a need for nursing education to be in colleges and universities and for nurses to be licensed. (Lavinia Dock missed one major ICN meeting because she was too busy lobbying for women's suffrage.)

In conservative 1900, at the ICN program meeting in London, one subject discussed was venereal disease. Nurses demanded early sex education for children and accessible treatment with no moral stigma attached. The members greeted this with a storm of applause. At other meetings, they tackled such subjects as criminal assault on young girls, the role of nurses in prisons, and many other taboo topics. They reached out to effect change and for over 110 years have been carrying on activities to meet their broadening objectives. It is impressive to see how an international group of nurses with such diverse backgrounds could agree on common goals on education, practice, and economic security when often nurses within an individual country, including the United States, cannot agree today.

The ICN's Strategic Plan identifies two major goals and a number of objectives and strategies related to each goal. The goals are as follows:

- To influence matters of health and social policy, and professional and socioeconomic standards worldwide
- To empower national nurses' associations (NNAs) to act on behalf of nurses, nursing, and the public well-being

Embodied in these goals are elements of strategic action that are as bold and risk taking as the history of international nursing. ICN offers the support to nurses in every country to come together as a critical mass and make their voices heard. For this, organizational structures need to be established and strengthened. High standards of education, practice, and management are the ultimate vision. For many countries, this requires slow steps toward a system of credentialing, with the necessary vigilance to protect autonomy. ICN pledges to work to make nursing prominent on the world stage and to work with nurses in their countries to achieve similar prominence in the best interest of the people they serve.

There are clear financial problems with which ICN must cope, reflecting perhaps the financial problems of each country's association, and there are disagreements about policy. However, the strategic plan is a good example of cooperative thinking and goal setting.

ICN realizes that it is only as strong as its NNA members. Building on that realization and the organization's responsibility of stewardship, ICN includes the following among its current priorities:

- *Development of the family nurse.* In this capacity, the nurse becomes a primary care provider and must embrace the concepts of community development, health promotion, and collaborative practice. One of ICN's current initiatives is a study of a variety of family nurse practice models that have demonstrated good outcomes. It will define the competencies of this role, comparing the effectiveness of each model internationally.

- *Implementation of the global study of the girl-child.* The United Nations' Fourth World Conference on Women held in 1995 in Beijing, China, focused international attention on the girl-child. ICN has identified the young urban girl-child as especially needy, and is currently involved in a study that will define the needs of young urban girls and position the nursing profession to intervene on their behalf.

- *Expansion of the ICN leadership program.* This program teaches nurses how to be more effective leaders by increasing their knowledge and developing their skills; this is achieved through classes, projects, and mentorship programs that are tailored to each site. The program is designed to ensure that nurses continue to shape policy as health care systems are reformed around the world. ICN plans to extend the program to new regions of the world and to expand offerings to currently and previously served areas.

- *Endowment of the Virginia Henderson Fellowship.* Virginia Henderson, a professor at Yale, helped shape worldwide nursing and is often called the *American Nightingale.* As a lasting tribute to her contributions to nursing and health care, ICN has established a fellowship in her name. Henderson fellows will address such issues as nursing outcomes, the application of research findings, new nursing practice patterns, family- and community-based care, and workplace issues.[8]

The World View

ICN has become a valued partner of international organizations, businesses, industries, and UN agencies, including WHO, UNESCO, the United Nations Children's Fund (UNICEF), and the International Labor Organization (ILO). In many countries, ICN's intervention on behalf of nurses is what spurs the government to action. Our presence at international forums is greeted with immediate recognition of the extent of our worldwide penetration.

Nurses are believed to have a strong influence on their patients; at the same time, nurses are not viewed as being motivated by personal gain. Several examples illustrate the influence of nurses on the people they serve. We have been recognized as the determining element in UNICEF's *Baby Friendly Hospital Initiative,* ensuring that breastfeeding is fairly presented to mothers as a feeding choice. And international advocacy of birth registration (and therefore provision of the rights of personhood to children) is seen as critically dependent on nurses. Recognizing that their members form the core of the team, the international organizations representing the nurses, physicians, and pharmacists unveiled the Health Professions Alliance in May 2000 at the 53rd World Health Assembly in Geneva. ICN represents nursing in this alliance.

ICN celebrated its centennial in 1999. ICN's history has indeed been illustrious; with its many member countries and close ties with WHO, it has helped to change the health care of the world.

■ SIGMA THETA TAU INTERNATIONAL

Sigma Theta Tau International (STTI), nursing's honor society, is one of the largest and most prestigious nursing organizations in the world. STTI is headquartered in the 33,000-square-foot International Center for Nursing Scholarship on the Indiana University/Purdue University Indianapolis campus. Membership is by invitation, conferred upon students in baccalaureate and graduate nursing programs who demonstrate excellence in scholarship and to community leaders who are qualified college graduates and have demonstrated exceptional achievement in nursing. The society's leaders were visionary when they added the word *international* to the name in 1985, making it one of the first nursing organizations with individual international members. By 2002, STTI had more than 120,000 members active in more than 90 countries. The membership profile of STTI today is as follows:

- More than 405,000 members have been inducted worldwide.
- The honor society has more than 130,000 active members.

- Members reside in 86 countries.
- Forty-six percent of active members hold master's and/or doctoral degrees; 26 percent are staff nurse/clinicians; 21 percent are nurse practitioners, nurse midwives, nurse anesthetists, or clinical specialists; 18 percent are administrators or supervisors; and 22 percent are educators or researchers.
- There are 469 chapters on college campuses in Australia, Botswana, Brazil, Canada, Colombia, Ghana, Hong Kong, Japan, Kenya, Malawi, Mexico, the Netherlands, Pakistan, Singapore, South Africa, South Korea, Swaziland, Sweden, Taiwan, Tanzania, Wales, the United Kingdom, and the United States.
- The honor society communicates regularly with more than 100 nurse leaders who have expressed interest in establishing a chapter in other countries and territories, including Chile, China, Costa Rica, Denmark, Finland, India, Ireland, Israel, Germany, Jamaica, Lebanon, Lithuania, New Zealand, Spain, and Thailand.[9]

STTI has a long history of innovation and dedication to the development of nurse leaders and scholars who influence the health of people globally through scholarship and practice excellence. In 1936, it became the first organization in the United States to underwrite nursing research. Since that time, STTI has provided more than 350 seed grants contributing to the advancement of many of the world's leading nurse scientists. Together with its chapters and grant partners (corporations, associations, and foundations), the society contributes more than $500,000 each year for nursing research. Additionally, more than 300 research-oriented educational programs are sponsored or cosponsored annually. Research congresses have been held in Spain; Israel; Scotland; Taiwan; Washington, DC; Australia; Vancouver, Canada; the Netherlands; and the United States.

In 1987, STTI launched the first national capital campaign in nursing's history, culminating in the acquisition of $5 million to erect the International Center for Nursing Scholarship and electronic Virginia Henderson International Nursing Library. Recognizing that some of the most valuable clinical research information may be so current that it has not yet been published, the Virginia Henderson International Nursing Library, unlike any other nursing library in the world, acquires peer-reviewed, unpublished literature. The library also offers the *Online Journal of Knowledge Synthesis for Nursing*, a peer-reviewed electronic journal affording nurses easy access to the latest reviews of research findings, and the *Registry of Nursing Research*, a unique collection of research data including researchers' demographic information, research studies, projects, findings, and abstracts.

The *International Leadership Institute* was formed in 1991 to help nurses be effective leaders in assuming responsibility for addressing germane health and social problems, establishing linkages among nurses and with interdisciplinary partners in health care, assisting nurses in assuming leadership external to the profession, supporting nurses in leadership roles, broadening knowledge about leadership, augmenting the resources and opportunities available to nursing leaders, and acknowledging and celebrating the leadership roles of nursing in health care and society.

The Leadership Institute has embraced numerous activities, including the Leadership Extern Program, Honorary Member Program, Career Pathway Model, Archon Awards for outstanding contributions to the health and well-being of others, and Arista think tank series designed to bring the vision, passion, and logic of nursing to bear on health problems of international significance.

The 75th Anniversary Campaign was inaugurated in 1992 with a goal of $7.5 million to advance the electronic library, leadership institute, nursing research funding, and other important society activities. This second international funding effort concluded in 1998, with more than $9.2 million registered in outright and planned gifts from members, chapters, foundations, corporations, and individual friends of nursing. By the end of 1998, STTI had welcomed approximately 200 Virginia Henderson Fellows registering exceptional philanthropic commitments.

Center Nursing Press, the society's publishing arm, produces *Image: Journal of Nursing Scholarship*, a peer-reviewed scholarly journal in nursing; *Reflections*, the organization's award-winning quarterly news magazine; *Chapter Leader Emphasis*, a quarterly newsletter sent to 3000 chapter officers; and peer-reviewed scholarly monographs on significant topics.

The Board of Directors, composed of Sigma Theta Tau's five elected international officers, six elected directors, and the executive officer, meets four times a year. The House of Delegates, the society's governing body, meets biennially and includes two representatives from each chapter in addition to the Board of Directors and standing committee chairs. During the academic year, chapters at colleges and universities conduct at least four meetings that are usually educational in nature. Regional conferences are conducted in each of the seven geographic areas in years alternate to the international convention.

The society and its affiliated chapters grant scholarships, research funds, and awards for excellence. Commendations are presented in recognition of creativity and excellence in practice, research, education, leadership, professional goals, and chapter programming. Other awards recognize superior programs or publications by nurses and others. The Baxter Allegiance Foundation Episteme Award, Mead Johnson Nutritionals Perinatal Nursing Research Award, Glaxo Wellcome Research Grant, and Audrey Hepburn/Sigma Theta Tau International Award for Contributions to the Health and Welfare of Children are also major honors.

Sigma Theta Tau International, 550 West North Street, Indianapolis IN 46202
Tel. (toll-free): 888-634-7575, fax: 317-634-8188
http://www.nursingsociety.org

■ WORLD HEALTH ORGANIZATION

WHO, established in 1948, is one of the largest of the specialized agencies of the United Nations. WHO's constitution states as one of its beliefs: "The enjoyment of the highest attainable standard of health is one of the fundamental rights of every human being without distinction of race, religion, political belief, economic, or social condition" and defines health as "a state of complete physical, mental, and social well-being and not merely the absence of disease or infirmity."

Membership in WHO is open to all countries, including those that do not belong to the United Nations. WHO is organized on a regional basis so that WHO and the nations within each region or zone can work together on matters of mutual concern.

The six regions are Southeast Asia, the Eastern Mediterranean, the Western Pacific, Africa, Europe, and the Americas. The Pan American Health Organization (PAHO) also serves the American region, whose Pan American Sanitary Bureau acts as the WHO regional organization.

An executive board directs the work of WHO, which is administered by a director general. Among its working force, known as the secretariat, are members of the health professions, including nurses. (However, at WHO headquarters, physicians outnumber nurses by far.) WHO's activities are largely financed by assessments on the member countries on the basis of a scale authorized by the World Health Assembly.

World Health Assembly

WHO's governing body is the *World Health Assembly.* It is made up of delegates from all member countries and meets once a year in May. The United States was the only country to include a nurse (Lucile Petry Leone) in its delegation to the first World Health Assembly. Twenty countries now include nurses in their delegations, among them the United States. The United Kingdom includes its chief nurse and several officers of the Royal College of Nursing in its delegation every year.

National and International Services

WHO's services are divided into three broad areas: (1) assisting governments, on request, with their health problems; (2) providing a number of worldwide health services; and (3) encouraging and coordinating international research on health problems. The trained staff of technical advisers, doctors, dentists, sanitary engineers, nurses, and others who are dispatched to help and advise any nation requesting aid work with the national ministry of health, the main emphasis being on making health care accessible to all persons.

Personnel are trained to initiate problem-solving programs and, when progress toward solution is assured, to teach people in the locality or country to carry on by themselves. WHO personnel recognize the influence of a people's social and economic status on health practices and attempt to effect improvement in those areas also.

Among WHO's major programs in individual countries are aid to strengthen local health services through better administration; the eradication or control of such communicable diseases as dengue fever, malaria, typhoid fever, tuberculosis, leprosy, AIDS, syphilis, trachoma, and yaws; the provision of better care for mothers and babies; the development of better sanitation facilities; and the improvement of mental health. WHO also provides fellowships, usually short term, to enable health workers to observe or study in other countries, with the goal of improving practice or services in their own country. US nurses are among those eligible for these fellowships.

WHO, in cooperation with member nations, collects and disseminates epidemiologic information, develops and administers international quarantine regulations, establishes a uniform system of health statistics, promotes standards of strength and purity for drugs and recommends names for pharmaceutical products, keeps countries advised of the possible dangers in the use of radioisotopes and helps train personnel in protection measures, and institutes international vaccination programs such as those against poliomyelitis.

Since the WHO/UNICEF Conference at Alma Ata (USSR) in 1978, WHO has emphasized primary care as the key approach to achieving an acceptable level of health throughout the world. ICN, which has always supported the primary care concept, was among the first to follow up on the Alma-Ata conference through a workshop that identified and recommended changes required in nursing education, practice, and legislation to prepare nurses for primary health care. When the executive director later reported to the WHO secretariat on these ICN activities and recommendations, many members from around the world noted the importance of nursing in primary health care.

In other actions, WHO has also intensified its promotion of the health systems used by the majority of people in any culture. In Third World countries, most people depend on traditional healers, who have often been quite effective in caring for them. Their integration into the general health system is considered essential at this point of development and health care delivery.

Nursing Within WHO

Delegates at the first World Health Assembly realized that more and better nurses were needed in every area of the world. In some countries in 1948, there was not a single fully qualified nurse. Health care was given entirely by aides, who often had little or no training. In other countries, as in the United States, there were adequate nursing services that could have been even better if more nurses were available. Between these two extremes were countries with widely varying numbers of nurses and vastly different educational patterns for preparing them. The largest part of WHO's nursing support has naturally been directed toward the relatively less developed, underprivileged countries with the most urgent health and nursing needs. In May 1992, the World Health Assembly passed a resolution in recognition of the central role nurses and midwives play in primary health care. In response to this action of the assembly, a Global Advisory Group (GAG) on nursing was constituted to give nursing more prominence and advocacy in international health affairs. The nursing GAG has eight or nine nurse members and four non-nurse participants.

WHO nurses work primarily in an advisory capacity, helping the nurses in a given country with their specific problems. Sometimes, however, WHO nurses must temporarily assume operational responsibilities until one of the country's own nurses has been prepared for the job. Thus, in establishing a postgraduate nursing program in a university, the WHO nurse may have to serve as director of the program in its early stages.

The areas in which WHO is called upon to provide assistance cover practically all of nursing—education, organization, and administration of hospital and public health nursing services, mental health, maternal and child health, clinical nursing specialties, and community health care planning. Improved midwifery services and education are vitally needed in many countries, and so are programs to upgrade the training of auxiliary nursing personnel. WHO helps in these areas by cooperating with health workforce planning. Assistance from WHO is also available to governments and their nursing divisions (if any) to plan for the development of nursing in those countries and promote nursing legislation in the interests of both nurses and the public.

Another WHO nursing activity is the sponsorship, sometimes in cooperation with other agencies, of regional conferences and seminars that focus on the changing role of the nurse in relation to current health policies. These enable nurses with similar backgrounds and problems to exchange information and work toward solutions under the guidance of expert nurses from WHO or other international health agencies. Many of these nurses have never before had an opportunity to meet with members of their profession from other countries, and they derive not only knowledge, but also encouragement and moral support from such conferences.

It is obvious that WHO's nursing activities call for highly qualified nurses, expert in at least one of the fields in which WHO offers advisory services. Language requirements depend on the country of assignment, but it is desirable for nurses to be proficient in at least one language other than their own. The official languages of WHO are Spanish, English, French, Russian, Chinese, and Arabic. In addition to its more or less regularly employed nursing staff, WHO engages nurses for limited periods of time to carry out special projects in various countries. WHO nurses often work in collaboration with nurses from other agencies who are also helping with nursing development in a given country.

In addition to its advisory services, WHO has published a variety of documents in relation to nursing, most of them basic and intended to be widely applicable in many countries. WHO also publishes *World Health*, a monthly magazine on world health intended for the lay public, and a variety of technical papers, journals, and reports.

WHO has played a significant part in many of the major developments in the international health field, such as an increase in the average life span, a decrease in infant mortality, the total eradication of smallpox, a major reduction in poliomyelitis and malaria, and an increase in medical and other health profession schools.

WHO's address is Avenue Appia, 1211 Geneva 27, Switzerland. The Pan American Health Organization's address is Pan American Sanitary Bureau, WHO Regional Office for the Americas, 525 23rd Street NW, Washington, DC 20037 **http://www.who.org**

■ AGENCY FOR INTERNATIONAL DEVELOPMENT

The Agency for International Development (USAID), administered by the US Department of State, is one of a succession of agencies through which the United States has assisted other countries in their social and economic development, with nursing as one of the areas in which assistance has been provided. USAID is a national rather than an international agency, but is included in this chapter because of the worldwide nature of its activities.

The distinguishing feature of the health and other technical assistance programs that have been carried out by USAID and its predecessor agencies is that they have been bilateral—that is, undertaken cooperatively with the government of the country being assisted, upon the request of that country and with both nations sharing in the determination of the programs to be carried out and the goals to be achieved. These joint health programs had their beginnings in 1942, with the establishment of the Institute of Inter-American Affairs to work cooperatively with Latin American countries in improving their health and welfare services. Since that time, US technical assistance in nursing has been provided under a variety of administrative auspices (e.g., the Economic Security Administration, Foreign Operations Administration, International Cooperation Administration, and others), culminating in the establishment of USAID in 1961.

The overall objective of USAID's health activities is to increase life expectancy, primarily through reductions in infant mortality and mortality in other high-risk groups, and to improve the quality of life through reductions in morbidity. The goal is to assist countries to become self-sufficient in providing broad access to cost-effective preventive and curative health services.

The Office of Health provides broad technical and research support for the agency's health program. Its program focuses on the development and promotion of health technologies to reduce child mortality and increase life expectancy, prevent the transmission of disease, and promote a healthier environment.

The early nursing assistance projects were highly concerned with the development and improvement of public health nursing services; this was the most pressing health need in Central and South America in the 1940s. The US nurses working in these programs, however, soon discovered that public health nursing services could not be permanently strengthened without a continuing supply of well-prepared nurses, which would, of course, require improved nursing school systems and facilities. In turn, if nursing students were to have their clinical experience in a true learning environment, hospital nursing services also needed improvement.

These three areas—public health nursing, nursing education, and hospital nursing services—have been the target of most nursing assistance projects carried out under USAID's auspices. Like WHO, however, USAID has also provided assistance in other nursing areas, such as midwifery services, the preparation of auxiliary personnel, and the establishment of postgraduate programs to prepare nurses for teaching and administrative responsibilities, among others. USAID also operates a participant training program whereby qualified individuals, nurses among them, in the assisted countries are given an opportunity to get the basic or advanced education they need in educational institutions in the United States or elsewhere.

USAID employs nurses on a short- or long-term basis to carry out its nursing assistance projects. Some USAID nurses have been with the agency or one of its predecessors for many years, assisting with projects in various countries. Others are recruited on a more limited basis or act as consultants.

USAID currently funds very few nursing projects. The trend is for bilateral, multidisciplinary partnership projects between medical centers in the United States and medical centers in countries throughout the world. Nurses are involved on a short- or long-term basis on many of these and other projects funded and managed by USAID. This work is often carried out by nongovernmental organizations. Nurses are recruited on a limited basis as consultants to the agency.

■ SUMMARY

The purpose of this chapter was to provide an overview of international health and nursing activities. Therefore, only the largest and most significant organizations and agencies operating in this area have been included. There are many other organized groups—religious and lay, private and governmental, societies and foundations—carrying on similar or related functions. For additional information, the heading *international* in any nursing, hospital, or medical literature index will provide information about the activities being carried on around the world on behalf of people's health and nursing needs.

KEY POINTS

1. The international presence of the ANA is guaranteed through its membership in ICN.

2. The quadrennial Congresses of ICN are truly experienced in international sisterhood and brotherhood, transcending cultural, political, and educational barriers.

3. The ICN predates by many years the international hospital and medical associations.

4. ICN has initiated many world-class projects, including the International Classification of Nursing Practice.

5. ICN's current priorities are the family nurse, the girl-child, and expansion of leadership experiences.

6. Sigma Theta Tau, the honor society in nursing, has inducted more than 405,000 members worldwide in 86 countries.

7. WHO has adopted primary care as the key to achieving an acceptable level of health throughout the world.

8. USAID is administered by the US Department of State, and aims to assist other countries in their social and economic development.

REFERENCES

1. Bridges D. Events in the history of the International Council of Nurses. *Am J Nurs* 49:594–595, September 1949.

2. Breay M, Fenwick E. *The History of the International Council of Nurses 1899–1925*. Geneva: ICN, 1931. This is a detailed, fascinating and informative account of ICN's founding and first 25 years, throwing considerable light on the nursing problems and personalities of this period.

3. According to ICN records, Miss Dock wrote these words as part of a foreword to the program of ICN's Second Quinquennial Meeting, held in London in 1909.

4. Roberts M. *American Nursing: History and Interpretation*. New York: Macmillan, 1954, pp 80–81.

5. Henderson V. *ICN Basic Principles of Nursing Care*. London: ICN, 1958.

6. Clark J, Lang N. *ICNP: Version 2, International Classification for Nursing Practice*. Geneva: ICN, 2009.

7. ICN. *Regulation 2020: Exploration of the Present; Vision for the Future*. Geneva: ICN, 2009.

8. Joel L, Stallknecht K. A global connection. *Am J Nurs* 100(10):109–111, October 2000.

9. STTI. Organizational Fact Sheet. April 2010. http://www.nursingsociety.org. Retrieved June 14, 2010.

Updates can be found at **www.kellysnursing.com**

HELPFUL WEBSITES FOR PART III, SECTION ONE

International Council of Nurses: http://icn.ch (see the networks for regulation, research, and advanced practice)

Public Service International (PSI): http://www.world-psi.org

Robert's Rules of Order Revised: http://www.constitution.org/rror/rror—00.htm

UNICEF: http://www.unicef.org/

World Bank: http://www.worldbank.org/

World Health Organization (WHO): http://www.who.int

Association websites included in Chapters 24, 25, 26, and 27

Transition Into Practice

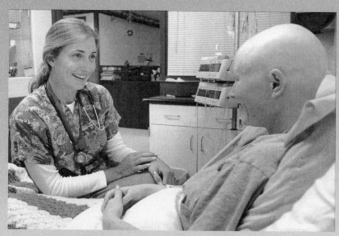

Your first job can set the tone of your nursing career. (Courtesy of Robert Wood Johnson University Hospital, New Brunswick, New Jersey)

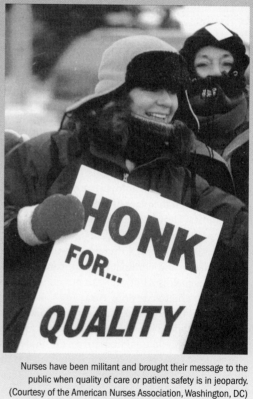

Nurses have been militant and brought their message to the public when quality of care or patient safety is in jeopardy. (Courtesy of the American Nurses Association, Washington, DC)

Making Choices: Job Selection

Graduation at last! And now what? For most nurses, "what" means it's now time to get a job. For some, the job is predetermined—commitment to the armed services, the Veterans Administration, or another agency that funded their education. Another group may have decided early on exactly the kind of nursing they prefer and the place where they want to do it. If all goes well and there are no problems, such as an oversupply of nurses for that specialty or geographic area, at least one major decision is made. But for all graduates, choosing that crucial first job and preparing for it are big considerations.

There are many employment opportunities for nurses today, although the place of employment preferred may not offer the exact hours, specialty, opportunities, or assistance a new graduate might want. Although nurses may be needed, some employers tend to retain less-qualified workers on lower salaries and eliminate patient care services. Another problem is maldistribution, with not enough nurses opting to work in ghettos or poor rural areas, although the need there is serious. Conversely, nursing graduates of a community college who wish to stay in that area may flood small communities. Still, qualified nurses are in demand almost everywhere. How, then, can you decide what is the best job for you? How do you maximize the chances of getting it?

◼ SOME BASIC CONSIDERATIONS

Personal and Occupational Assessment

It is a good idea to start thinking about career choices while you are still in your educational program. Because most schools have rotations through the various clinical specialty areas, this gives you a chance to compare as you learn. Generally, there is also access to someone who can advise you about the pros and cons of certain types of nursing—or at least there's a more experienced nurse, often a faculty member, to talk to.

More important than anything else, though, is to take a considered look at yourself—your own qualities and what you want out of life. There are a variety of approaches to this sort of self-assessment that are interesting to explore in depth, but there are certain commonalities. Some questions you might ask are as follows.

What are my personality characteristics? Do I like to do things with people or by myself? Am I patient? Do I like to do things quickly? Am I good at details, or do I like to take the broad view? Do I like a structured and quiet environment or one that is constantly changing? Am I relatively confident in what I undertake or do I look for support? Am I easily bored? Do I like to tackle problem situations or avoid them? Do I have a sense of humor? Am I emotional? Am I a risk taker? Do I care about the way I look? Do I care what others think of me?

What are my values? Do I believe in the responsibility to live or the right to die? Do I think everyone should have access to health care? Do I have a religious orientation? Do I think that too many people today are too rigid or too loose in their beliefs and behavior? Can I accept and work with those who have very different values? How do I feel about my responsibility to myself, my employer, my patient, the doctors, my profession, and society? Do I believe strongly that my way is the right way? Am I intolerant of others' beliefs?

What are my interests? In the broad field of nursing? In certain specialties? In the health field? In my private and social life? In the community? Do I like to travel?

What are my needs? Am I ambitious? Do I like to direct others? Is money important to me? Status? Do I need intellectual stimulation? Is academic success important? What about academic credentials? Am I willing to relocate? Does a city, suburb, or rural area fit my desired lifestyle? Is success in my field important? Am I willing to sacrifice personal and family time for success? Do I think that my first responsibility is to my family at this point? Is part-time work an option? Do I want plenty of time for family, friends, and leisure activities? Do I see nursing as a career or a way to earn a living as long as that is necessary? Do I really like nursing? If not, why not, and what can I do about it?

What kinds of abilities do I have? In manual skills? In communication? In intellectual/cognitive skills? In analyzing? In coordinating? In organizing? In supervising? In dealing with people? Do I have a great deal of energy and stamina? Are there certain times, situations, or climate conditions in which I have less stamina? Am I good at comforting people? Am I able to give some of myself to others?

It's good to prioritize some of these lists, because life and a job are usually full of compromises. What's most important? What would make you miserable? It might also be very helpful to share this list with others. Is this the way you are seen by them? Have you missed something? If some of your friends and peers are involved in their own decision making, get together with them and/or a trusted teacher or mentor to brainstorm about the possibilities in the field now or later to match your own profile most accurately with nursing opportunities. When compromises are necessary, you can decide ahead of time which ones are tenable or even perfectly acceptable at that point.

Because there will probably be economic constraints in the health care system for a long time, one way to look at the job market is in terms of future growth. For instance, you may choose a hospital for a first job to hone your new skills, but have you considered a long-term care facility, home care, or an ambulatory care outreach center? All are part of the trends in health care. You should examine those job prospects as carefully as any other. They may have components that do not fit in with your own self-assessment. But don't close doors because of preconceived notions.

It is also wise to be aware that there are both linear and nonlinear career routes. Historically the position of staff nurse led to charge nurse to assistant head nurse to head nurse to area coordinator or supervisor, and up you go. Or, in a more contemporary fashion, staff nurse to senior nurse to clinical coordinator to case manager to advanced practice, assuming the requisite academic preparation. These are the traditional routes and they imply sound planning. But there are other ways to conceptualize your career. Play to your passions and individual talents to create highly individualized career options.

If you are articulate and persuasive, with an insatiable interest in public policy, why should this be an avocation? How about work as a nurse lobbyist? You love to work with children, so you have chosen pediatrics. In your leisure you spend every minute outdoors. Why keep the two apart if you can choose to work in a children's camp or residential school? Be creative and explore every option, as crazy as it may seem. But know yourself first.[1]

Licensure

Regardless of the results of your self-study, a basic and essential step in your professional nursing career is to become licensed; you cannot practice in any state without an RN license. Information about how to apply to take the state board examination leading to licensure and other significant information is found in Chapter 20. The procedure for becoming licensed and getting the results is now very quick because of computer testing. State boards of nursing in most states permit nurses to practice temporarily, pending results of their examination. Theoretically, then, you can be employed as a graduate nurse until you pass the licensure exam. However, in reality, many, perhaps most, hospitals will interview you but not employ you until you become licensed. The administration generally feels that the cost of orientation is too great to take a chance that a nurse will fail. If a nurse fails after employment, he or she may be dismissed or must work as some type of nursing assistant.

What if you decide not to work right away? Stay home with your family? Take a long vacation? It's probably wise to study for the examination and take it anyway. Unused knowledge has a way of disappearing from the mind, and it might be much more difficult to pass later, without intervening learning and practice. Moreover, in most states, you are expected to take the examination within a certain time after graduation.

Should you take a nursing board review course? It depends on the confidence you have in your nursing knowledge and test-taking ability. The good courses can be very helpful and may provide backup materials as well as lectures. However, be careful to select a reputable company.

These are profit-making operations and expensive to you. Another way of preparing is to study with a group of peers, perhaps using board review workbooks or texts designed for that purpose.

■ PROFESSIONAL BIOGRAPHIES AND RÉSUMÉS

Now that you have done your self-assessment and thought about career alternatives, it's time to write your résumé.[2] No matter how you obtain a position in nursing, you will probably be asked to submit a résumé or summary of your qualifications for the job. This might include a personal history, education and experience, character and performance references, and professional credentials such as your license registration number.

Some universities and other educational programs still maintain files with updated information about your career provided by you and references that you have solicited. This has the advantage of eliminating the need to ask for repeated references from teachers who may scarcely remember you or to write again and again to a variety of places for records. However, this service is gradually fading away, and that may not be bad. As you and your career develop, a reference from your first teacher or your first staff position says little other than how you were perceived at that time. Newer references may be far more useful. Your academic record or simply evidence of your graduation may still be requested, and your school always provides that information, but today a well-prepared résumé is considered appropriate.

A résumé is a relatively short professional or business biography. In academia, a curriculum vitae (CV), which is somewhat lengthier and contains slightly different and more detailed information, is the appropriate form of professional biography. Résumés are usually shorter than CVs. However, *résumé* and *CV* are often used interchangeably.

The résumé should be businesslike, prepared with a word processor (with no insertion of hand-written comments) on one side of good-quality paper—plain white, off-white, or light gray—measuring $8\frac{1}{2}$ by 11 inches, with adequate margins all around and consistency of font and format. The envelope should match. Proofread for any spelling and grammatical errors. Typographical errors are guaranteed to turn off any employer. Have someone who has a critical eye read the document. No more than two pages are recommended; one is better. Some experts suggest that you have a professional printer duplicate your résumé on a photocopier that produces a sharp copy, absolutely free of dark areas or smudges. Quick-copy shops may specialize in making a résumé look good, doing layouts, typing, printing, and copying.

There are various ways to write a résumé; however, the content areas are generally the same. They start with name, mailing address, e-mail address, and telephone number, with the name written as you would sign it, but including appropriate degrees or credentials—for example, Mary Smith, RN, BSN or RN, MSN, CCRN. Periods are not necessary in these abbreviations as long as you are consistent in their use. Some nurses prefer to put the degree before the RN. Be sure your address and telephone number are complete. Include your business address only if you can accept calls there, although this is commonly omitted when you are seeking another job. An answering machine may be useful so that important calls from potential employers are not missed.

Résumés are organized in a chronological or functional—sometimes called *topical*—format. In a chronological format, you list your experience in reverse chronological order. The functional format calls for separate categories, such as clinical experience, teaching, education, and so on. The most common format is probably a combination in which the various areas of work experience, education, honors, publications, and other activities are presented in separate sections, but items are listed in reverse chronological order in each section. Remember that a résumé is a marketing tool that should show you to advantage. Therefore, although you must never be dishonest, the way you present your talents and credentials, especially after you have accumulated some work experience, may make the difference between whether you are interviewed or ignored, especially in a competitive situation. Although format is a matter of taste and style, a sample résumé that might be used by a new graduate is shown in Exhibit 29–1.

The following points may also be helpful. Stating a professional objective is not a must, especially if you are not sure exactly what you want to do. If you choose to write one, it should match the job for which you are applying and thus may need to be changed accordingly. For instance, someone with a master's degree in perinatal nursing may be interested in either a teaching or a clinical specialist position. Both the objective and the emphasis in the résumé must focus on the position for which the person is applying. Needless to say, if you are applying for your first or second staff nurse position in a hospital, the decision on what to write is less complex.

■ **EXHIBIT 29–1. Résumé**

LESLIE B. SMITH
120 Pine Street
Clearview, CA 91110

Home Phone 213-456-7890
Message Phone 213-482-6132

Professional Objective: Staff nursing in a community hospital

Experience:

2010–2011	University Hospital, Los Angeles, CA
	Nursing extern. Performed basic nursing activities under supervision on medical-surgical and pediatrics units.
2009–2010	Clearview General Hospital, Clearview, CA
	Unit clerk on medical-surgical units, evening shift. Assisted charge nurse in [list activities]; trained new clerks; developed end-of-shift report between clerks.
2007–2009 (Summers)	Williams General Hospital, Williams, CA
	Nurse's aide on medical-surgical units. Responsible for care of thirty patients under direction of RNs including [list major activities].

Education:

2009–2011	Blank University, School of Nursing Bachelor of Science (to be awarded May, 2011)
2007–2009	Clearview Community College, Associate in Science

Honors:

2009–2011	Dean's List
2010–2011	Member, Sigma Theta Tau, International Honor Society for Nursing
2010–2011	Honor Scholarship
2009	Outstanding Student Leader Award, Clearview Community College

Professional Activities:

2007–2011	Member, National Student Nurses' Association
2010–2011	Chair, Program Committee
May 5, 2010	Presented paper, "When Students Teach Patients," National Student Nurses Association (NSNA) Convention, Denver, CO
2009–2011	Member, Curriculum Committee, Blank University School of Nursing
May 4, 2011	Debate: "Be It Resolved: Everyone Has a Right to Health Care," NSNA Convention, New York, NY

Community Activities:

2010–2011	Art Club, Blank University
2009–2011	Volunteer for public television telethon, Blank University
2009–2011	Volunteer for March of Dimes
2005–2007	Candy-striper at Clearview General Hospital, Clearview, CA

All relevant work experiences should be included, with the most recent listed first. The usual format is to list the agency and date, followed by a brief description of duties performed, using "action" verbs—developed, initiated, supervised. Some experts suggest that if you have not had impressive positions, you should attempt to bury this fact in statements that focus on your personal qualities, such as "Leadership—demonstrated by ability to lead others—as night nurse on a pediatric unit at X hospital, such and such address." No one really knows whether this is more effective, but again, style is a matter of personal choice. Many nurses describe their nursing school clinical experiences in their résumé. This nonessential information can contribute substance to an otherwise thin résumé, but should only be used by new graduates. If the clinical experience section makes your résumé more than two pages in length, leave it out.

The education section should also begin with the most recent academic credential and should include the major and minor areas of study (if there is one) and such additions as research projects, special awards, academic honors, extracurricular activities, and offices held. Information on other honors, professional memberships and activities, and community activities might also be given in separate sections.

Under federal law, you cannot be required to include personal data such as your age, marital status, place of birth, religion, sex, race, color, national origin, or handicap. If you choose to do so, decide whether this makes you a more desirable candidate. For instance, a second language or extensive travel might be a plus in certain situations. It is usually best not to list specific references on your résumé, because this omission allows you to select the most appropriate reference for a particular position. If your school does maintain a file, you can state this, giving the correct address.

It is not necessary to say, "References available on request"; you would hardly refuse to give them. When you give the references, include the full names, titles, and business addresses of about three persons who are qualified to evaluate your professional ability, scholarship, character, and personality. Most suitable are teachers and former employers. New graduates should probably include a clinical instructor from the desired clinical practice area. Ask permission to use their names as references in advance. Choose carefully. If the individual, no matter how prestigious, really does not know you, your talents, and your abilities and the reference is noncommittal, it can do more harm than good. When you contact a reference, however, it is acceptable, even good sense, to offer to send a résumé to refresh that person's memory. For instance, almost everyone forgets the dates they knew you; you are not likely to be the only student or employee they know. If the individual is reluctant, do not push; the result can be a reference that says nothing much and the potential employer may read it as a negative. You might also keep in mind that employers frequently telephone the reference, either because they want a quick answer or because they want to ask questions that are not on a reference form or to explore some aspect of the written reference (particularly if it was noncommittal).

Therefore, if your reference is inclined to be abrupt, unpleasant, or irritated on the phone, choose another. As a rule, don't ask for a "To whom it may concern" letter and have it recopied. Most sophisticated employers see that as an uninterested response. Suppose you didn't get along with your last employer and, even though you left with appropriate notice, you fear a poor reference. Sometimes someone else who was your positional superior can be substituted or another person such as a clinical specialist who knows your work is suitable. (A peer's opinion may be discounted.) However, administrators often know each other, and your potential employer may know that you did not name the person who would be the usual reference and may check with him or her by phone. That could result in a really negative reference. Therefore, because lists of references are often not requested until after the interview, you could simply say then that you did not have a positive relationship. Be careful not to speak negatively of the former employer; try to be objective or neutral. Although references can be important, the impression you make in an interview can be much more important in the long run.

■ LOOKING OVER THE JOB MARKET

The potentials for a particular job are assessed both before and after applying for and/or being offered a nursing position. Chapter 15 should be helpful as an overview of the opportunities available in terms of both specialties and professional development (career ladder, internships), but reading the literature, talking to practitioners in the field, and, if possible, getting exposure to the actual practice at some time during your educational program will help answer some specific questions. Moreover, having written at least a basic résumé gives you a clearer picture of the position that will suit your talents and interests.

Today, even if an employer is actively recruiting for nurses, an application, a formal letter of interest, and often a résumé are necessary before a position is actually offered. There are those who feel that going through the entire process is worthwhile for the experience alone. However, unless you have at least some interest, it is rather unfair to take an employer's time to review an application and go through an interview for nothing. Therefore, after self-assessment, it is useful to do at least a potential job assessment in advance. The first logical consideration is a place with which you have already had experience.

Hospitals or other agencies affiliated with schools of nursing may offer new graduates staff positions. That has several advantages for the employer and usually for the student as well. Nurses who are familiar with the personnel, procedures, and physical facilities may require a shorter orientation period, which saves time and money.

In addition, the student has a track record; he or she is not an unknown entity. There are also benefits for new graduates. During these first months after graduation, you can gain valuable experience in familiar surroundings. There are opportunities to develop leadership and teaching skills and to practice clinical skills under less pressure because the people, places, and routines will not be totally strange. The potential trauma of relocating and readjusting your personal life is not combined with the tension of being both a new, untried graduate and a new employee. And it may be a wonderful place to work.

However, if the experiences offered do not help you to develop, if the milieu is one that eventually makes you resistant, resentful, indifferent, unhappy, or disinterested, the tone may be set for a lifetime of nursing jobs, not a professional career. Of course, that can also happen in other places, but if you're alert, you can often get a pretty good notion of how it would be to work at the agencies in which you have had student or work experience. This evaluation can be a little more difficult if you don't know a place at all, but the opinion of someone you respect, word-of-mouth information, the institution's newsletter and brochures, and even the way someone replies to your inquiry provides indirect as well as direct information.

On a more concrete level, you can give some thought to what you are willing to accept in terms of salary, shifts, benefits, and travel time. (Don't underestimate the value of the fringe benefits, which may not be taxable.) Balancing these with other advantages and disadvantages as determined by your self-assessment is important. And realistically, in times of a nursing shortage, you will have more choices than when the job market is tight.

Remember that in any health care organization there are critical indicators that send a message about how highly nursing is valued. Collect some telling information:

1. How is certification valued and rewarded?
2. How many staff nurses are certified in their practice areas?
3. How many advanced practice nurses are on staff?
4. What is their availability to the staff nurse?
5. What is the role of staff development—remedial, and responding to deficiencies, new procedures and policies, equipment and processes, or is enrichment also included?
6. Is there a career ladder?
7. How is education rewarded?
8. What is the quality of the nurse–physician relationship?
9. Are there integrated patient records; is there interdisciplinary care planning?
10. Do any nurses hold memberships on the medical staff organization, and what privileges do they have?
11. Is there an active presence of evidence-based practice and nursing research?
12. Where is the chief nurse executive in the organizational chart? (Nursing usually represents the single largest group of employees. If the nurse executive is buried somewhere down in the organizational hierarchy, this is a message about the respect given nursing.)

All of these factors must be considered seriously. You'll never have another first job in nursing, a job that could set the tone of your professional future. It's much better to move carefully and make sure that your choice is the best possible one for moving you toward your goal, whatever it may be.

■ SOURCES OF INFORMATION ABOUT POSITIONS

Three principal sources of information are available to nurses who are looking for a position: (1) personal contacts and inquiries, (2) advertisements, and (3) recruiters. At one time, employment agencies were also a common source, but over the years, hospitals and other health care agencies employed recruiters themselves and did not find it cost-effective to pay employment agencies. However, at another level of job seeking—executive positions—well-known agencies of good reputation (headhunters) are used by both employers and potential employees to match the best possible person to a suitable position.

Personal Contacts and Inquiries

The nursing service director or someone on the nursing staff of a student-affiliated agency, instructors, other nurses, friends, neighbors, and family may suggest available positions in health agencies or make other job suggestions. Hospitals not affiliated with schools of nursing sometimes ask the heads of nursing schools to refer graduates to them for possible placement on their staff. Often, letters or announcements of such positions are posted on the school bulletin board or are available in a file. Your own inquiries are likely to be equally productive in turning up the right position.

Never underestimate the value of personal contacts. People seldom suggest a position unless they know something about it. That gives you the opportunity to ask questions early on, and the information can help you decide as well as prepare you better for the interview. Moreover, if your contact knows the employer and is willing (better yet, pleased) to recommend you, your chances of getting the position are immediately improved. One business executive has said, "Eighty percent of all jobs are filled through a grapevine . . . a system of referrals that never see the light of day." When equally qualified people compete for the same position, the network recommendation could make the crucial difference. Asking for job-seeking help is neither pushy nor presumptuous, but you should be prepared to discuss your interests intelligently.

Most people like to be asked for advice and want to be helpful, but they have to be asked. On the other hand, you need to use some common sense in deciding how much and how often you ask for help from whom.

Advertisements and Recruiters

Local newspapers and official organs of district and state nurses' associations often carry advertisements of positions for professional nurses. National nursing magazines list positions in all categories of employment, usually classified into the various geographic areas of the country.

There are also regional nursing publications focused entirely on local nursing news and information, with major emphasis on nurse recruitment. National medical, public health, and hospital magazines carry advertisements for nurses, but they usually are for head nurse positions or higher, or for special personnel such as nurse anesthetists or nurse consultants. In times of shortage, employers also use billboards, radio and television announcements, and even letters.

Almost all publications carry classified advertisements. Rarely, if ever, does the publisher assume responsibility for the information in the advertisement beyond its conformity to such legal requirements as may apply. If you accept an advertised position that does not turn out to be what was expected, you cannot hold the publication responsible. Read the advertisement very carefully. Is the hospital or health agency well known and of good reputation? Is the information clear and inclusive? Does it sound effusive and overstress the advantages and delights of joining the staff? What can be read between the lines? How much more information will you need before you can decide whether the job is suitable? Some of these questions can be resolved through correspondence, telephone contact, or your network.

Career directories published periodically by some nursing journals or other commercial sources are free to job seekers. They have relatively extensive advertisements with much more detailed information than appears in the usual ad. The other advantage is instant comparison among geographic areas, and often preprinted, prepaid postcards that can be sent to the health agency of interest. Directories are frequently available in the exhibit section of student and other nursing conventions. Some carry reprints of articles on careers, licensure, job seeking, and other pertinent information. Some journals also do periodic surveys on job salaries and fringe benefits that can be useful when one is considering various geographic areas.

Recruiters are a major source of information and job opportunity. They represent hospitals and other agencies and are usually present at representative booths in the exhibit areas of conventions. Recruiters, who may or may not be nurses, also visit nursing schools or arrange for space in a hotel for preliminary interviews. Notices may be placed in newspapers or sent to schools. There are advantages to the personalized recruiter approach because your questions can be answered directly, and you can get "a feel" for the employer's attitude, especially if nurses accompany the recruiter. However, remember that recruiters are selected for their recruiting ability.

The so-called temporary nurse service is another option (see Chapter 15). These services function quite differently from agencies or registries, because they themselves usually employ the nurses and then, according to requests and a nurse's choices, send her or him to an institution or other agency for a specific period of time. In some situations, the nurse is an independent contractor as opposed to an employee. This arrangement would expect you to pay required taxes on your own. Nurses are usually placed in short-term situations in hospitals, but some services advertise home care. The single most important factor that seems to attract nurses to temporary nurse services is control over working conditions, including the time, place, type of assignment, and so on. New graduates may find this type of employment attractive as a temporary measure. Fringe benefits are not usually available, so this type of employment choice may be risky. There is also an opportunity to try out different types of nursing, but for the new nurse, the lack of individual support and supervision is a disadvantage.

■ PROFESSIONAL CORRESPONDENCE

New nursing graduates today have a wider variety of personal and educational backgrounds than they did a few years ago. Many have held responsible positions in other fields, and even more have worked part or full time before or during their educational programs.

Therefore, the suggested procedures for application and resignation presented are just that. They review generally accepted ways to handle certain inevitable professional matters in a sophisticated and businesslike way, and may serve as a refresher for those already familiar with these or other equally acceptable ways of relating and communication in professional business relationships. For the younger, less experienced nurse, this material provides a convenient reference and guide.

The first contact with a prospective employer is usually made by letter, followed by a personal interview, telephone conversation, and, occasionally, fax or e-mail. Every business letter makes an impression on its reader—an impression that may be favorable, unfavorable, or indifferent. To achieve the best effect, the stationery on which it is written should be in good taste; the message accurate and complete yet concise; the tone appropriate; and the form, grammar, and spelling correct.

Stationery and Format

Business letters should be neatly and legibly prepared using a word processor. Unlined white stationery that measures 8 ½ by 11 inches (standard business size) is the most suitable. Personal stationery is generally acceptable if it is of the right size; white, light gray, or off-white in color; and used with unlined envelopes. It should not look like social stationery. Notebook paper should never be used for business correspondence—neither should someone else's personal stationery or the stationery of a hospital, hotel, or place of business. Always keep copies of your correspondence.

Books on English composition and secretary's handbooks include correct forms for writing business letters. Two or more variations may be given; the choice is yours.

The block form is employed most widely in business correspondence and therefore is selected for illustration here (Exhibit 29–2). The left-hand words or margins are aligned throughout the letter, with extra space between paragraphs. Commas are used sparingly in this form, and a colon is used following the salutation. No abbreviations are used. If personal stationery on which the name and address are engraved or printed is used, this information

---

■ EXHIBIT 29–2. Cover Letter

Applicant's address
Applicant's phone number
Date of letter [3 blank lines to follow]
Employer's or recruiter's name and title [use complete title and address]
Employer's address [2 blank lines to follow]
Salutation:

Opening paragraph: State why you are writing. Name the position or type of work for which you are applying. Mention how you learned of the opening.

Middle paragraph: Explain your interest in working for this employer and specific reasons for desiring this type of work. Describe relevant work experience, pointing out any other job skills or abilities that relate to the position for which you are applying. If appropriate, state your academic preparation and how it relates to the job description. Be brief but specific; your résumé contains details. Refer the reader to your enclosed résumé.

Closing paragraph: Have an appropriate closing to pave the way for an interview and indicate dates and times of availability. Your e-mail address or a number is useful. If you cannot be reached during the day, designate a number for messages.

Sincerely,
Signature
Name typed
Enc. [probably your résumé]

---

should be omitted from the heading of the letter and only the date given.

In business correspondence, it is always advisable to address a person exactly as the name appears on her or his own letters. The full title and position should be used on the envelope as well as in the letter, no matter how long they may be. It is better to place the lengthy name of a position on the line below the addressee's name and to break up a long address in the interest of a neat appearance. Indent continuation lines as follows:

Selma T. Henderson, RN, PhD
Vice President for Patient Care Services
The Reddington J. Mason Memorial Hospital
1763 Avenue of the Twenty-first Century
Chesapeake-on-Hudson, OH 00000

People are sensitive about their names and titles; be accurate. If you do not know the name of the person to whom you are writing to inquire about a position, it might be a good idea to call and get the correct name and title from the person's secretary or other staff. (At the same time you could ask to be sent any information about the position and the institution.) The telephone number is usually in the ad, or you can find it on the Internet. Often the name of the person to whom an applicant should respond is also in the ad, and it may be a recruiter or someone from human resources. If no name is specified, make multiple phone calls, address the letter to the recruiter, and say, "Dear Recruiter."

It is correct to give a title before the name in an address in the heading of a letter and on the envelope—rather than using the form of initials after the name—for example, "Dr. Constance E. Wright" rather than "Constance E. Wright, Ed.D." In a signature, however, it is preferable to reverse this order and place the degree initials after the name of the signer of the letter. Never use both the title and the initials; "Dr. Constance E. Wright, Ed.D." is incorrect.

It is quite suitable, and even desirable, for a (licensed) nurse to use "RN" after his or her name, particularly in professional correspondence. Many nurses with doctorates sign their names with "RN, PhD" or "EdD, RN" to clarify that they are nurses as well as holders of a doctorate. They should be addressed as "Dear Doctor Whatever" (Doctor written out in the salutation).

A professional or business woman usually does not use her husband's name at all in connection with her work. Probably most business or professional women without a doctorate prefer to be addressed as "Ms." in correspondence. However, a woman can use the title "Mrs." to identify herself as a person who is or has been married if she desires. "Mrs." goes in parentheses before her typed name under her signature. "Ms." or "Mr." is not used at this point in a letter.

Cover Letter

The information included in any business letter should be presented with great care, giving all pertinent data but avoiding unnecessary details. It is often helpful to outline, draft, and edit a business letter, just as you would a term paper. This requires you to think it through from beginning to end to ensure completeness and accuracy. It is also helpful to tailor it to fit a well-spaced single page if possible.

Your writing style is your own, and how you word your message may be part of what you are judged on. The tone of a business letter has considerable influence on the impression it makes and the attention it receives. It is probably better to lean toward formality rather than informality. Friendliness without undue familiarity, cordiality without over enthusiasm, sincerity, frankness, and obvious respect for the person to whom the letter is addressed set the most appropriate tone for correspondence about a position in nursing. Although there are those who suggest very unusual, dramatic, or "different" formats, the reality is that they may backfire. A sample cover letter is shown in Exhibit 29–2.

If you feel that you need more information before you seriously consider a position (for instance, whether tuition reimbursement is a benefit or whether a particular specialty area has an opening), ask directly within the same application letter. The kind of response you get in terms of courtesy, promptness, and general tone will tell you a lot about the prospective employer. Be sure to mail, fax, or e-mail the cover letter with the résumé. A cover letter or résumé sent alone is not helpful for the recruiter or employer, and will most likely receive no response. If using e-mail, attach these documents; do not include them as the body of the e-mail. A letter included in the e-mail itself may lose its format in transmittal.

If you decide not to apply for the position after all or not to follow through with an interview, it is courteous to inform the person with whom you have corresponded. Specific reasons need to be given (briefly) only if you make such a decision after first accepting the position. This is not only courteous but also advisable, because you may wish to join that staff at another time or may have other contacts with the nurse executive or recruiter.

Applications

Applications are not just routine red tape. Whether or not a résumé is requested or submitted, the formal application, which is developed to give the employing agency the information it wants, can be critical in determining who is finally hired. Even if the information repeats information offered in the résumé, it should be entered. It is usually acceptable to attach the résumé or a separate sheet if there is not adequate space to give complete information. It's a good idea to read through the application first so that the information is put in the correct place. Neatness is essential. Erasures, misspellings, and wrinkled forms leave a poor impression. Abbreviations, except for state names and dates, should not be used as a rule.

If the form must be completed away from home, think ahead and bring anticipated data—social security and registration numbers, places, dates, and names. Although occupational counselors say that it is not necessary to give all the information requested (such as arrests, health, or race, some of which are illegal to request), it is probably not wise to leave big gaps in your work history without explanation.

■ THE JOB INTERVIEW

An interview may be the deciding factor in getting a job. Anyone who has an appointment for a personal interview should be prepared for it physically, mentally, emotionally, and psychologically. The degree of preparation will depend on the purpose of the interview and what has preceded it. Assuming that you have written and sent a résumé to a prospective employer and an interview has been arranged, preparation might include the following.[3]

Physical Preparation

Be rested, alert, and in good health. Dress suitably for the job, but wear something in which you feel at ease. It is important to be well groomed and as attractive as possible. First appearances are important and, given a choice, no one selects a sloppy or overdressed person in preference to someone who is neat and appropriately dressed. Have enough money with you to meet all anticipated expenses. If you are to be reimbursed by the employing agency, keep an itemized record of expenses for submission later. Get accurate directions to the interview site. Arrive at your destination well ahead of time, but do not go to your prospective employer, interviewer/recruiter's office more than 5 minutes before the designated time.

Mental Preparation

Review all information and previous communications about the position. You should also collect background information on the organization itself. Many health care organizations have their own Internet sites, and valuable information can be found there. Showing that you know about an employer is desirable and impressive. Make certain that you know the exact name or names of persons whom you expect to meet and can pronounce them properly. Decide what additional information you want to obtain during the interview. Consider how you will phrase your leading questions. Carry a small notebook or card on which you have listed the names of references and other data that you may need during the interview. If you bring an application form with you, place it in a fresh, unsealed envelope. Have it ready to hand to the interviewer when she or he asks for it; if it seems indicated, offer it at the appropriate time.

Emotional and Psychological Preparation

If you have any worries or fears in connection with the interview, try to overcome them by thinking calmly and objectively about what is likely to take place. (Role playing an interview with a colleague who may have been through the experience can be helpful.) Be ready to adjust to whatever situation may develop during the interview. For example, you may expect to have an extended conversation with the nurse executive or at least someone in nursing administration only to find, when you arrive, that a personnel officer or recruiter who is not a nurse will interview you; this is becoming more usual. She or he may interview you in a very few minutes and in what seems to be an impersonal way. Or you may have visualized the job setting as quite different.

Accept things as you find them, reserving the privilege of making a decision after thoughtful consideration of the total job situation. If the position offers both challenge and opportunity, you may sense it during the interview, or you may have reason to believe that it will develop after you assume your duties.

During the Interview

Usually, the interviewer will take the initiative in starting the conference and closing it. You should follow that lead courteously and attentively. Shake hands. Be prepared to give a brief overview of your experiences and interests if asked. At some point, you will be asked if you have any questions, and you should be prepared to ask for additional information if you would like to have it. Should the interviewer appear to be about to close the conference without giving you this opportunity, say, "May I ask a question, please?" Remember that the interview is a two-way process.

If you did not get this information in the handouts, you may wish to ask about the nursing delivery system, educational opportunities, advancement opportunities, staff participation in decision making, nurse–physician relationships, and the placement of the nursing department in the organization. It is perfectly acceptable to ask, before the interview is over, about salary, fringe benefits, and other conditions of employment if a contract or explanatory paper has not been given to you. In fact, it would be foolish to appear indifferent. A contract is desirable, but if that is not the accepted procedure, it is important to understand what is involved in the job. The job description should be accessible in writing, and it is best that you have a copy. Most interviewers agree that an outgoing candidate who volunteers appropriate information is likable. On the other hand, many use the technique of selective silence, which is anxiety provoking to most people, to see what the interviewee will say or do. A good interviewer will try to make you comfortable, in part to relax you into self-revelation; most do not favor aggressive methods. Good eye contact is fine, but don't stare. Be sensitive to the interviewer's reactions, such as disinterest in a certain response; maybe it's too lengthy. Don't interrupt. Don't mumble. Watch your body language (and observe that of the interviewer). It can denote indifference or irritation. Be enthusiastic but don't gush.

Some questions that are likely to be asked in an average 1-hour interview are

1. Why did you pick our organization instead of seeking a job somewhere else? (Be specific.)

2. What are your skills and achievements and how do they match our needs? (Know something positive.)

3. What kind of person are you? (Play up your strengths, and, although you should be honest, play down your weaknesses. Give examples—perhaps of what people say about you.)

4. What sets you apart from all the other people who can do the same thing? (Show your decision-making and judgment skills.)

5. What kind of people do you feel most comfortable working with? ("People who do their jobs well" is a good answer. Beware of falling into the trap of criticizing colleagues.)

6. Can we afford you? (Be realistic if this is your first job, and don't push.)

7. Tell me about yourself. (Keep it short; don't give more information than necessary to reassure the interviewer that you are suitable for the job, physically, mentally, and in terms of preparation. Stress your reliability. Don't be caught off guard, and get personal.)

8. What did you like most and least in school or on your last job? (Be honest, but don't list a series of gripes.)

9. How would you describe your ideal job? (Take the opportunity to do so, but let the interviewer know that you know that nothing's perfect.)

10. Where do you think you'll be 5 years from now? (If you say you don't know, you may come across as lacking initiative. Emphasize goals that show your interest in growing professionally.)

11. Do you have any questions? (Be prepared.)

In a survey of directors of nursing service in various settings, the characteristics valued most highly in rating a nursing job applicant were promptness to the interview, completion of the application prior to interview, neatness of the application, a well-groomed personal appearance, and questions asked. As other qualities that might be more important were bypassed, this list may show how important the external aspects of an interview can be.

When the interview is completed, thank the interviewer, shake hands, and leave promptly. A tour of the facility may be offered before or after the interview. This gives you a chance to observe working conditions and sometimes interpersonal relationships. You may or may not have been offered the position, or you might not have accepted it if it had been offered. If it was offered to you, it is usually well to delay your decision for at least a day or two until you have had time to think the matter over carefully from every practical point of view. Perhaps you will want more information, in which case you may write a letter, send a fax, use e-mail, or make a phone call to your prospective employer. It is always courteous and sometimes acts as a reminder to send a thank you letter.

Sometimes during the process of acquiring a position, you may have occasion to discuss some aspect of it over the telephone with the prospective employer. If you make the call, be brief, courteous, and to the point, with notes handy if needed. It may be helpful to take notes on the conversation. It is sensible to listen carefully and not interrupt. If you receive a call and are unprepared for it, be courteous but cautious and perhaps ask for time to think over the proposal—or whatever may have been the purpose of the call.

Agreements about a position made over the phone should be confirmed promptly in writing. If it is your place to do so, you might say, while speaking with the person, "I'll send you a confirming letter tomorrow." If it is the responsibility of the other party to confirm an agreement but she or he does not mention it, ask, "May I have a letter of confirmation, please?"

After any interview or conversation, it's useful to make notes about what happened for future use and reference.

If any business arrangements are made by fax, or e-mail, file this information with other related correspondence.

For positions sought through a registry or employment agency, the same courteous, thorough, and businesslike procedures used when dealing directly with a prospective employer are appropriate. A brief thank-you note for help received shows consideration of the agency's efforts on your behalf.

At the conclusion of this process of fact finding, interviewing, and the back and forth that characterizes the job-seeking and searching process, there are some very basic questions that you must be able to answer for yourself:

1. What does this job require?
2. Are my skills a "good match" for this job?
3. Are these the kind of people that I enjoy working with?
4. What sets me apart from all the others who can do this job, and how can I convey this to those who matter?
5. How can I persuade you to hire me, and pay me the salary I want?

Evaluation

What if you didn't get the job you wanted? There may simply have been someone better suited or better qualified in the recruiter's mind. Still, it is helpful to review the experience to refine your interviewing skills. Were you prepared? Did you present yourself as someone sensitive to the employer's goals? Did you articulate your personal strengths and objectives? Did you look your best? Sometimes discussing what happened with another person also gives you a different perspective. And there's no reason why you cannot reapply.

■ CHANGING POSITIONS

There seems to be an unwritten rule that new graduates should remain in their first permanent position for at least a year. Certainly, this is not too long—except in the most unusual circumstances—for you to adjust to the employment situation and find a place on the staff in which to use your ability and talents to their fullest. Furthermore, persons who change jobs frequently in any profession or occupation soon gain a reputation for this, and some employers are reluctant to hire them. However, should it be desirable or necessary to change positions, a number of points might be observed. Consider your employer and coworkers as well as yourself, and leave under amicable and constructive circumstances.

Depending on your reasons for leaving and how eager you are to make a change, some writers suggest that before you definitely accept a new position, the present employer should be informed about your desire to leave and why. It may be that, depending on the employer's concept of your value to the institution, a new, more desirable position might be offered. Other seasoned job hunters will caution you never to leverage or even attempt to "bluff." Once you have made a decision to leave, begin your search, but don't resign or reveal your intention to leave until you have a confirmed job offer.

It is important to give reasonable notice of your intention to resign. If there is a contract, the length of the notice will probably be stipulated. Two weeks to a month is the usual period, depending principally on the position held and the anticipated difficulty in hiring a replacement. Don't tell everyone else before you tell your immediate superior, privately and courteously.

Try to finish any major projects you have started; arrange in good order the equipment and materials your successor will inherit; and prepare memos and helpful guides to assist the nurse who will assume your duties. Check out employment policies about benefits, including accrued vacation or sick leave.

A letter of resignation should state simply and briefly, but in a professional manner, your intention of leaving, the date on which the resignation will become effective, and your reasons for making the change. A sincere comment or two about the satisfactions experienced in the position and regrets at leaving will close the letter graciously. There should be no hint of animosity or resentment, because this will serve no constructive purpose and may boomerang (see Exhibit 29–3). Don't burn your bridges. You may want to come back to that place at another time. At the least you may need a reference, and if you appear vindictive or childish, the employer is unlikely to give you an enthusiastic reference, even if you did your job satisfactorily. In these days of litigation, nothing may be written specifically, but employers are adept at reading between the lines of a bland reference. The administrative network (via a personal phone call) may paint you as someone with an "attitude problem," and you'll never know.

Terminal interviews are considered good administrative practice and are sometimes used for a final performance evaluation and/or a means to determine the reasons for resignation. There is some question of how open employees are about discussing their resignation (unless the reason is illness, necessary relocation, and so on), perhaps because

■ **EXHIBIT 29–3. Sample Letter of Resignation**

240 North Street
San Diego, California 00000
Date [3 blank lines to follow]
Ms. Ruth Green, RN, MSN
Vice President of Nursing
West Central Hospital
20 California Avenue
San Diego, California 00000 [2 blank lines to follow]
Dear Ms. Green:

I will be relocating to Phoenix, Arizona, in May and have accepted a position there at General Hospital as head nurse of the pediatric unit. Therefore, I wish to resign effective April 14, 1995.

Being at Central Hospital has been a very satisfying personal and professional experience. The atmosphere is one in which a nurse can grow, and I appreciate the support given by the staff of 4B and the head nurse, Melanie Rones. She has especially helped me to develop my managerial skills and encouraged me to take advantage of the hospital's tuition reimbursement. I expect to finish my degree in Phoenix. I am proud to have been a part of a group of practitioners and administrators who are committed to caring, competent patient care.

If there is anything I can do to help in the transition, I will be happy to do so.

Sincerely,

[Signature]

John Collins, RN

cc: Melanie Rones
Head Nurse 4B

of their fear of reprisal in references or even a simple desire to avoid unpleasantness. This is a decision you must make in each situation.

What if you're fired? Some common reasons for being fired are poor job performance, chronic tardiness, excessive absenteeism, or inappropriate behavior. Usually you are given a warning about any of these problems, and if you haven't done anything about correcting your problem (assuming that the charge is justified), you'd better take a good look at yourself. Those kinds of uncorrected problems may make your future prospects look dim. But more commonly today, you may be displaced from your job due to mergers, acquisitions, downsizing, or reorganization of the institution or agency. Be careful not to personalize the event or judge yourself too harshly. The health care industry is volatile and places all of us in permanent jeopardy.

Whether or not you're caught by surprise when you're told, try to maintain your composure. If you can't pull your thoughts together, request another interview to ask questions and find out about the termination procedure. If you are at fault, make a clean, fast break. If you are not at fault, try to clarify the situation to avoid negative references. You may choose to contest the action. This is discussed in Chapter 30. However, weigh whether it's worth it. You may need to clear your name, but it might be unpleasant or impossible to accomplish. If the dismissal is a layoff for economic reasons, it is a good idea to have a letter to this effect, both in terms of professional security and to get unemployment benefits if necessary.

When leaving a job is not your choice, it sometimes helps to talk with a supportive person, to ventilate and analyze what happened. Choose someone you can trust but who can help you see things as objectively as possible. Then it's time to get back to career planning. Perhaps you should look at the possibility of further education or training in a different kind of nursing. If not, be sensible about conserving your economic resources until you find another job. Try to select the next job, keeping in mind what made you unhappy in the last one and, of course, correcting those problems that got you fired. You need not volunteer to your prospective employer that you were fired, but if asked, don't lie. Just say that you were asked to leave and why. Don't criticize your previous employer and try to be as positive as possible about your last job. Your honesty and determination to do well could be a plus. It's doubtful that you will stay in the same institution throughout your career. This is a very mobile society, and there are many job opportunities for nurses throughout the country (and world). Without closing the doors to unexpected opportunities, beginning early to think in terms of a career will make nursing more satisfying and interesting to you in the long run.

KEY POINTS

1. Assessing yourself in terms of abilities, interests, characteristics, and values is a good idea before starting a job hunt.
2. A professional résumé and appropriate letters of application are factors in being selected for a job.

KEY POINTS

3. The résumé and any correspondence should be prepared meticulously.

4. Some of the best sources of information about the job market are advertisements in both electronic and print media, personal contacts, job fairs, and recruiters.

5. In interviewing for a job, it is important to be prepared physically and psychologically and to know, or get, as much information as possible about the position and environment.

6. In an interview be careful to look the part of a professional.

7. Consideration of a job's effect on future employment is an important factor in how the job should be terminated.

REFERENCES

1. Andersen C, Bednash G. Nursing as a launching pad for other options—A variety of nurses' paths to other roles. In Andersen C (Ed.): *Nursing Student to Nursing Leader.* Albany, NY: Delmar, 1999, pp 228–238.

2. College Grad. Resumes. http://www.collegegrad.com/resumes/. Retrieved June 9, 2010.

3. Nurse Jobs. Nursing Interview Tips. http://nursejobs.com/nursing-interview-questions.aspx. Retrieved June 9, 2010.

Updates can be found at **www.kellysnursing.com**

Career Management

■ SOCIALIZATION AND RESOCIALIZATION

Eventually, graduation does come, and for most nurses, the next step, with hardly a break, is that first nursing job. What can you expect?

Experts say that the transition from student to registered nurse (RN) is a psychological, sociological, and legal phenomenon. The student has spent 2 to 4 years being socialized into nursing in the educational setting; now resocialization into the work world is necessary. Socialization into a new role is not usually a conscious process, although both the individual being socialized and those doing the socializing consciously make certain efforts. These statements are accurate, but they trivialize the fact that the professions are set apart by their social position. Socialization should be anticipated and planned.

In reality, the expectations one experiences as a student in any field differ from those one encounters as an employee being compensated for professional services. For the most part, students are not integral to the systems of care; they look to faculty for their cues and rewards and are allowed to falter somewhat in their practice. Further, the socialization–resocialization phenomenon (student to full-fledged professional) is often presented as a one-time occurrence. In fact, given today's rapidly changing health care system—with the movement from hospitals into community practice, downsizing of hospital nursing staffs, and new markets for health services—nurses will be confronted with resocialization many times during their careers. All of these circumstances suggest that the only way to make a comfortable transition time after time after time is to know oneself and to understand the dynamics of a situation. There is nothing so unexpected or mystical about role transition and socialization. All of us have been

through the process at least once (but really many times) as we took on the attributes of participating members of society.

A role is a constellation of rights and responsibilities that characterize a social position. Because the individual role occupant is embedded in a social structure, the role behaviors are derived from the expectations of both the individual and the social systems with which that individual interfaces. *Socialization* is the process by which an individual acquires the behaviors necessary for acceptance by these interfacing groups or systems. This is accomplished through a reciprocal process of role shaping and role taking, with the eventual assimilation of the behaviors within one's repertoire as follows:

Step 1. Interaction with primary groups who mirror the expected behaviors (exposure)

Step 2. Development of an interpersonal attachment with significant others from that group (identification)

Step 3. Clarity on expectations; covert messages are made overt (empathy)

Step 4. Negotiation to resolve differences between the ideal and the real and determine how much freedom there is to modify the role to personal preference (role shaping)

Step 5. Continuing support to allow movement to behavioral synthesis; accommodated behavior becomes assimilated (role taking)[1]

Successful role transition is closely related to your personal desire to become part of the mainstream of nursing. The possibilities are greatly enhanced where there is a good feeling (*chemistry*) between you and your group of peers (staff nurses). This alerts you to the need to meet the people you will be working with on a day-to-day basis when applying for a position. The best of organizations go further, providing a preceptor or "buddy" arrangement with someone who is senior in the staff nurse role. Make sure you ask questions until you fully understand what is expected of you, and be cautious in bending the rules until you have established yourself. However, make inquiries that help predict how much personal role shaping will be possible. Some cues that may signify an organization allowing little flexibility in role development are

1. Highly precise and detailed job descriptions
2. Management by memo in situations where personal communication would have sufficed
3. Guarded interdisciplinary boundaries that hamper smooth operation
4. A hierarchy that is an obstacle to your work as opposed to facilitating it
5. Policies, procedures, and documentation systems that are cumbersome and even inconsistent with current practice
6. Absence of staff nurse autonomy in caring for patients
7. Verbalized discontent from staff but no evidence of any attempt to change things
8. High turnover rate

Individuals will enact roles based on their own knowledge, the modeling they have observed, and the social structure within which the role is situated. There is always some liberty or flexibility in role enactment, but this can vary quite dramatically from situation to situation. One ingredient of success will be how accurately you can estimate these degrees of freedom.

Successful role transition includes identifying with the right group, interpreting their expectations accurately, negotiating to the extent that is possible while maintaining your unique identity, and merging with the group on terms that are mutually acceptable. This is the best of all possible worlds. In less perfect situations, you have parties that refuse to tolerate any variance—individuals who are unable to read the expectations accurately or refuse to become fully involved. The latter situation has been labeled the *marginal man* syndrome.[2] This is the nurse who hangs on to the periphery of a system, never quite becoming part of it or bothering to know the personalities involved and refusing to assimilate nursing with the other aspects of life. This is particularly common in women who try to juggle multiple aspects of life, keeping each separate—obligations everywhere, multiple lists of things to do, each with a first-place priority, but a comprehensive plan nowhere. The wiser strategy is to integrate the dimensions of your life, with professional colleagues becoming personal friends, family participating in workplace and professional events, and so on (one list with one rank ordering of priorities).

For all but a few graduates, the first job is as an employee in some bureaucratic setting, which can often frustrate the best qualities of professionalism. For instance, a bureaucracy has specialized roles and tasks, and professionals have specialized competence with an intellectual component. The bureaucracy is organized into a hierarchical authority structure, but professionals expect extensive autonomy and collegiality in doing their work. The bureaucracy's orientation is toward rational, efficient implementation of specific goals and tends toward impersonality, yet professionals have influence and responsibility in the use of their specialized competence and make decisions governed by internalized standards.[3] On the basis of these differences alone—and there are others—professionals in a bureaucracy find themselves in conflict.

Kramer, in an extensive longitudinal study that is still relevant after over 30 years, has identified the problems of new graduates in establishing their roles in the midst of bureaucratic–professional conflict, and has termed it *reality shock*, "the specific shock-like reactions of new workers when they find themselves in a work situation for which they have spent several years preparing and for which they thought they were going to be prepared, and then suddenly find that they are not."[4] The phenomenon is seen as different from but related to both culture shock and future shock.

Thus, when the new nurse, who has been in the work setting but not of it, embarks on a first professional work experience, there is not an easy adaptation of previously learned attitudes and behaviors, but the necessity for an entirely new socialization to practice and simultaneous resolution of conflict with the bureaucracy. Kramer describes the steps as follows:

1. Skills and routine mastery: The expectations are those of the employment setting. A major value is competent, efficient delivery of procedures and techniques to clients, not necessarily including psychological support. New graduates immediately concentrate on skill and routine mastery.

2. Social integration: Getting along with the group; being taught by them how to work and behave; the "backstage" reality behaviors. If individuals stay at stage one, they may not be perceived as competent peers; if they try to incorporate some of the professional concepts brought over from the educational setting and adhere to those values, the group may be alienated.

3. Moral outrage: With the incongruence identified and labeled, new graduates feel angry and betrayed by both their teachers and employers. They weren't told how it would be and they aren't allowed to practice as they were taught.

4. Conflict resolution: The graduates may and do change their behavior, but maintain their values, or change both values and behaviors to match the work setting; or change neither values nor behavior; or work out a relationship that allows them to keep their values, but begin to integrate them into the new setting.[5]

The individuals who make the first choice have selected what is called *behavioral capitulation*. They may be the group with potential for making change, but they simply slide into the bureaucratic mold, or more likely they withdraw from nursing practice altogether. Those who choose bureaucracy (value capitulation) may either become "rutters" (staying in a rut), with an "it's a job" attitude, or they may eventually reject the values of both. Others become *organization men and women*, who move rapidly into the administrative ranks and totally absorb the bureaucratic values. Those who will change neither values nor behavior, what might be called *going it alone*, either seek to practice where professional values are accepted or try the "academic lateral arabesque" (also used by the first group), going on to advanced education with the hope of new horizons or escape. The most desirable choice, says Kramer, is *biculturalism*.

> In this approach the nurse has learned that she possesses a value orientation that is perhaps different from the dominant one in the work organization, but that she has the responsibility to listen to and seek out the ideas of others as resource material in effecting a viable integration of both value systems. She has learned that she is not just a target of influence and pressure from others, but that she is in a reciprocal relationship with others and has the right and responsibility to attempt to influence them and to direct their influence attempts on her. She has learned a basic posture of interdependence with respect to the conflicting value systems.[6]

Even though complicated by the bureaucratic–professional conflict, our original paradigm for socialization is visible in biculturalism.

New graduates do indeed go though variations of the reality shock experience. That there was little change in the adjustment process for decades can be seen by reviewing journals in the interim and by the nomadic patterns of nursing that must reflect deep-seated job dissatisfaction. Turnover may be a response to boredom, lack of involvement, and apathy, and traces its origin to incomplete socialization.

It is interesting that the shortage of the early 1990s and subsequent workplace enrichment programs greatly enhanced the recruitment and retention of nurses. In the intervening years many of those programs were lost, but they began to reappear with the next nursing shortage. These enrichments most commonly take the form of attempts to professionalize the workplace and decrease bureaucratic–professional conflict. They have been preserved in premier practice settings such as magnet facilities. Some of these strategies are summarized as follows:

1. Clinical ladders to recognize competence in direct care positions

2. Peer review

3. Shared governance and participatory management

4. Increased practice autonomy

5. Decentralization of operations

6. Interdisciplinary practice as evidenced in joint planning and integrated documentation systems

The realities of the workplace, albeit generally a bureaucracy, could certainly be softened if our nursing education programs and faculty brought more reality-based opportunities to students and provided more opportunities for "rehearsal." The following deserve consideration:

1. A synthesis semester at the end of the educational experience that incorporates, as far as legally possible, all the ingredients of full-time employment

2. Work-study programs that alternate semesters with work placements in your anticipated field

3. A curriculum that progresses toward more independence and personal accountability, with students and faculty moving to a collegial relationship as opposed to superiors and subordinates[7]

4. Service-education partnerships with faculty teaching students on their own panels of patients

5. Opportunity for any student to work with faculty on their personal research

6. Summer externships and new graduate internships or residencies

7. Patient areas with a primary commitment to the clinical learning needs of students

8. Assignment of each student to a staff nurse, who in fact should be his or her logical role model

9. Preceptor or "buddy" system involving agency staff

10. An experience with interdisciplinary or at the least multidisciplinary education[8]

Even with the most smoothly negotiated transition, reality finds most nurses as employees in large, complex bureaucracies; moreover, the role of nursing becomes more complex as the system of caring increases in size and sophistication and as nursing becomes more prominent. One should never lose sight of the fact that systems (large, small, simple, complex) exist to secure their goals and preserve their values. They accomplish this by responding to changing conditions, achieving solidarity among their parts, using a division of labor to accomplish work, controlling the environment, maintaining order, and using resources efficiently. *Efficiency* has caused a move to accomplish many things through adhocracy—systems established for a very limited goal and then disbanded. *Specialization* is another rational response to a highly complex world. Subcontracting as opposed to the creation of internal departments allows greater flexibility to adjust to change. In like manner, the nursing role has been forced to readjust or jeopardize organizational stability, so resocialization becomes a continuing process.

■ STRESS AND STRAIN: THE PERSISTING OCCUPATIONAL HAZARD

Stress and strain are synonymous with nursing, *stress* being the factors external to you and *strain* being those internal feelings of frustration and tension. Sometimes stress creates strain. Some individuals have the capacity to tolerate stressful conditions, putting them in perspective. In other instances strain is internally triggered and the search for external blame is fruitless. There are endless experts who can tell you how to deal with these frustrations and tensions. From Selye,[9] the father of the concept of stress, to Peplau,[10] the pioneer of psychiatric nursing, to Kobasa,[11] who introduced the descriptor of *hardiness* to explain why some people rise above it all. In summary, there is little predictability about who will respond negatively to stressful situations, but group cohesiveness or interpersonal

support seem to have a positive effect. This has been noticed in comparing nurses who work in high-stress environments with those where stress is less frequent and less intense. The only available responses to stress are to fight (and you never win), run, let the tension take its toll on you physically, or use the opportunity to learn more about yourself and cope productively.

Stress and strain are predictable in situations that include ambiguity, incongruity, conflict, under- and overload, and where the occupants see themselves as under- or overqualified for their role.[12] *Ambiguity* usually relates to a lack of structure and clarity. *Incongruity* stems from a poor fit between the person's abilities and their expectations or the expectations of the systems with which they interface. *Role conflict* indicates contradictions within the role behaviors themselves. The staff nurse feels an obligation to provide quality care, but then finds it impossible to achieve satisfactory outcomes within the limits of a predetermined length of stay. *Over- and underload* often require a more objective opinion. *Being over- or underqualified* moves us into areas of competence. Some individuals may consider themselves overqualified because they never strain to see the complexities of a situation. Peer discussion of such clinical situations is helpful to verify your opinion of yourself. Feelings of being underqualified must be talked through and validated, or they result in living the life of an imposter.[13]

The stress and strain that come with most of the service occupations are labeled *codependency* or *burnout* in the literature. In codependency, a person controls through the assurance that he or she is needed and works to keep things that way. "Unable to determine who owns a problem, they become angry and intolerant. The natural impulse to feel for their patients and occasionally bring home their frustrations is played out with exaggeration, and eventually rejected. Where once they felt too much, they now feel too little in defense of their ego. The result is poor judgment, insensitivity and burnout."[14] The codependent personality is at particularly high risk for burnout, which eventually results in negativism, and the severe loss of self-esteem as one's clinical competence is questioned.

There is no one prescription for coming to terms with an unmanageable personal or professional life. The problems are relative to the personality of the afflicted, and solutions must be individualized. The ultimate goal is to establish control and identity that is driven by internal strength, rather than being captive to the volatility of the environment. Given that your best investment is in self-care, consider the following:

1. Learn to use distance therapeutically. Allow people to fail and learn from their own mistakes. Find a comfortable and private place to retreat to when you are stressed. If you can't physically distance yourself, try meditation techniques.

2. Decide who owns a problem. If you don't own it, you have no obligation to fix it, especially if it requires self-sacrifice.

3. Examine the quality of the peer support you give and get, and correct the situation if needed. Sometimes support systems become habits as opposed to helps.

4. Invest in upgrading yourself. Expose yourself to new experiences; learn new skills. Plan your self-care as seriously as you plan your patient care.

5. Consciously schedule routine tasks and those requiring physical exertion as a break from complex and stressful activities.

6. Learn to trust your instincts. Every problem does not have a rational and logical solution.

7. Sometimes think in terms of what could be the worst consequence, then anything short of that is a bonus.

8. Identify one person who would be willing to serve as your objective sounding board. This may be one way to find out how you come across to people.

9. Make contact with your feelings about situations. Feelings are neither good nor bad; they just are.

10. Create options for yourself. Identify those circumstances that you need to personally control, those that are just as well controlled for you, and those that you choose to wait out.[15]

■ THE WORKPLACE: RIGHTS AND HAZARDS

The prevailing theme of this chapter has been successful career management through personal control. Aspects of that control were to understand how you move toward acceptable and satisfying role enactment and how you deal with stress and strain while protecting a personality that may be naturally vulnerable. An additional dimension of control is to know your rights and responsibilities as an employee—and to confront the hazardous conditions that will affect your work life as a nurse from start to finish. You have protections under the law, and other quasi-legal guarantees are included in personnel policies (employee handbooks, personnel policy manuals). Even though you may have nothing in writing, an expressed contract takes shape as you discuss the terms and conditions of your employment.

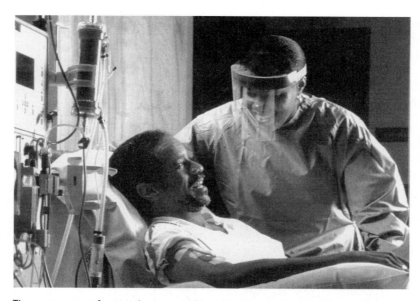

The proper use of protective gear makes a dangerous job much safer. (Courtesy of the US Department of Veterans Affairs)

A comprehensive overview of workplace rights would include issues of minimum wage, unemployment and disability, workmen's compensation, family leave, continuing health benefits after termination of employment, discrimination, job safety, pensions, unfair labor practices, and collective bargaining. The growing number of workplace concerns addressed through legislation and the courts is one circumstance that has contributed to the general decline in unionization. Unions appeared on the American scene when there were few legal workplace protections. Today's growing governmental involvement in professional practice, the workplace, and health care facilities makes it important to understand the interrelationships between administrative codes or regulations, employment law, and practice acts. When is the RN acting as an agent of the employer versus as an autonomous professional? If administrative codes allow nurses professional staff privileges in a hospital, can a specific facility deny this status? The degrees of complexity are endless, but you have the right to answers to any questions.

Given the broad range of issues and the degree to which they multiply once they are interrelated, the focus here will be on the most common questions:

1. Can I be fired without reason?
2. Is it possible to refuse an assignment?
3. Are there any protections for whistle-blowing?
4. What protections do I have against discrimination?
5. Do I have a right to withhold information about myself from an employer?
6. Are there laws that guarantee fringe benefits, including health insurance, pension, and family leave?
7. What are the major workplace hazards for nurses and what is the employer's responsibility?

Can I Be Fired Without Reason?

Most employment relationships are not protected by any formal contract and are for an indefinite period of time. Such an arrangement is termed *employment at will*, and either the employee or the employer may terminate the relationship at any time with cause or for no cause at all. A growing number of court decisions in such situations have recognized employee handbooks and a variety of other internal employer-generated documents as having a quasi-legal status. Thus, where an at-will dismissal violates one of these policies, the employer could be held liable. Above and beyond this presumed contractual protection, a number of states are moving forward to protect at-will employees through legislation.

Simply put, no employer is justified in an arbitrary and capricious dismissal of an employee. It is important to note what circumstances will cause a contested episode of dismissal to be adjudicated in favor of the employee if the situation goes to grievance, arbitration, or court. The most common conditions for a successful appeal on the employee's behalf are as follows:

1. The charges for the termination are not proved.
2. The severity of the consequence is inappropriate to the charge.
3. The reason for dismissal is unrelated to job performance.
4. Proper or customary disciplinary procedures were not used.

Most dismissals come as a result of growing dissatisfaction between employee and employer, not because of a single episode. The situation should have produced documentation and a series of warnings, written notices, attempts to counsel, and so on. For more details on the proper handling of grievances, refer to ANA's *What You Need to Know about Today's Workplace: A Survival Guide for Nurses*.

Is It Possible to Refuse an Assignment?

That is not an idle question today, as we deal with clinical situations that may be contrary to our personal conscience, hazardous, or require our participation in circumstances that are potentially unsafe for patients. This last situation is particularly common with reduced staffing, the substitution of less-prepared personnel in attempts to cut costs, and the perils of floating to services where you do not feel completely at ease or competent.

Nursing administration has the right to assign you where needed (providing you don't have a written contract that says otherwise), but they also have the responsibility of assigning duties appropriately. Courts have considered nurses' rights in such situations. In *Winkelman v. Beloit Memorial Hospital* (483 N.W.2d 211 WI 1992), a nurse with experience in pediatrics was ordered to float to a geriatric unit. She refused and was terminated. The court found that the hospital wrongfully discharged the nurse and offered several pertinent comments.

A nurse is not necessarily qualified or competent to practice in any area of nursing simply because the nurse has graduated from a school of nursing and has passed a licensure exam. . . . If a particular area is not a nurse's major area of employment, the nurse has a right to refuse assignment to the questionable area. If an employer wants a nurse to rotate to an area that is not the nurse's usual area of assignment, then the employer should provide for the nurse's further education and training to prepare the nurse to work in the area.[16]

In *Francis v. Memorial General Hospital* (726 P2d 852 NM 1986), a New Mexico nurse was instructed to float from the intensive care unit to the orthopedics unit. He refused and was suspended for 2 days. On his return, he informed his supervisor that he would not float if he felt incompetent. He was offered the opportunity of being oriented to all those units he might be required to cover. He declined the offer and was indefinitely suspended. The court found that the hospital was authorized to discharge the nurse, and made the following observations:

> Prior to his discharge, [the nurse] was presented with the opportunity for orientation to floors where he might "float" in the future to overcome his feeling of incompetence. This was done in deference to his ethical scruples, yet [the nurse] refused to find out whether he could ever become comfortable with "floating." Because he declined this deference to his scruples, he cannot complain now that he was fired for following them.[17]

These cases show that you have the right to refuse to float if you think you are unqualified and you can request orientation and training if the administration insists that you do. In fact, the Joint Commission requires facilities to have a systematic plan for cross-training to ensure competency. However, if orientation or training is offered and you continue to refuse, you run the risk of termination.

You also run the risk of a lawsuit and disciplinary action by the state board of nursing. Further, agreeing to float and then presumably practicing at a level lower than your license, let's say as a nurse's aide, is unacceptable. You were hired and expected to adhere to the standard of your job description.

Mandatory overtime is often co-mingled with this issue, and is becoming an increasingly difficult problem for RNs and health care facilities. Because of inadequate RN staffing, employers have used mandatory overtime as a cost-cutting strategy. Nurses are concerned about the health effects of long-term overtime and the quality of care being provided. Organized nursing has been working tirelessly for several years for the enactment of mandatory overtime legislation on both the federal and state levels. A recent study confirms that increased work hours for nurses raises the likelihood of adverse events and errors in practice, and further found the same relationship with both mandatory and voluntary overtime. Though the events toward public policy reform have targeted mandatory overtime, this seems inadequate in view of these findings.[18]

Currently, 15 states have restrictions on the use of mandatory overtime for nurses: Thirteen states have enacted restrictions in law (CT, IL, MD, MN, NJ, NH, NY, OR, PA, RI, TX, WA, and WV), while two states have provisions in regulations (CA and MO). NC (2009) has legislated the study of mandatory overtime as a staffing tool. Some of these laws protect the nurse from retaliatory action or discipline; others specify the number of hours to be worked in a week or a shift, or the number of hours between shifts.[19] Clearly, the battle is being waged on a state-by-state basis.

In some workplaces, there are labor contracts to prevent inappropriate assignment or compulsory overtime. Others have developed a form that says, in essence, that in the nurse's professional judgment, the current assignment is unsafe and places the patients at risk, but that it will be carried out under protest. The form documents the assignment, number, and condition of patients and number and type of staff. The legality of this process has not yet been tested, and there are some other concerns. If a nurse has stated that an assignment is unsafe and then takes it, she or he is vulnerable in case of a later negligence suit. And, of course, the use of the form can be abused. Conversely, if you refuse an assignment, one of the dangers is being accused of abandoning your patients. Just what that means in any specific case is not clear, but it could result in the loss of your license. You should discuss any assignment that you see as inappropriate with your supervisor to put her or him on notice about your limitations; identify your options (sharing or trading the assignment); and document the situation. In the end, it is your decision, and not an easy one, but it is almost inevitable in many institutions. It's best to think it through ahead of time.

One situation that has been gaining attention is fair treatment for nurses who cannot work on certain days for religious reasons. As might be expected, rulings have differed, but in 1985, the US Supreme Court ruled that there was no constitutional right involved; that, in fact, it was unconstitutional for a state to legislate an unqualified right not to work on the Sabbath. From a practical point of view, the nurse may be willing to accept alternatives, such as working on other holidays or on weekend days.

Are There Any Protections for Whistle-Blowers?

Whistle-blowing is a moral action of last resort and indicative of an ethical failure at the organizational level. Whistle-blowers are employees who disclose information about an organization's violation of a law, rule, or regulation; mismanagement; gross waste of funds; abuse of authority; or a substantial and specific danger to the public health or safety. The range of situations for whistle-blowing is obviously broad, and in many situations the protections are few. It is critical to have your facts straight. Because whistle-blowers must often proceed on good faith, every effort should be made to verify the correctness of the information, and to use existing channels to correct the wrong before resorting to whistle-blowing. Every state has passed legislation that offers some protection for the whistle-blower, but the devil is in the details, differing to a greater or lesser degree in each state. About 27 states specifically protect health care workers, others distinguish between public and private sector employees, and the amount for restitution to the whistle-blower differs dramatically, among other requirements and opportunities to correct the harm. Laws have been passed by the US Congress to preempt state laws and provide mandatory protection where no state laws apply. Whistle-blower protections have been included in the Homeland Security Bill of 2002, and in the new health care reform act of 2009 (the Patient Protection and Affordable Care Act of 2009).[20]

A noteworthy case occurred in 1996. Barry Adams, an RN working on a subacute care unit in a New England hospital, blew the whistle on unsafe health care practices that he observed in his work setting. Adams became increasingly concerned about the quality, safety, and dignity of patient care as the hospital implemented staffing cuts and cost-containment measures. He carefully documented unsafe practices and correlated these with inadequate staffing and a lack of adequate supervision of inexperienced nurses. There was an increased incidence of patient falls, instances where patients were left to lie in their own urine and feces, treatments not being completed, and serious medication errors. These incidents resulted from a substantial increase in the nurses' patient assignments.[21]

For 3 months, Adams and other nurses precisely followed the process outlined by the organization to communicate concerns to hospital administrators. He soon realized that the administrators were not interested in using the information he provided to correct the situation; in fact, he was harshly criticized for collecting this information. He then decided to proceed with a variation of the traditional saying, "If it's not documented, it's not done," and instead adopted the approach, "If it's not done, document it!"

Adams was threatened with the loss of his job and, in spite of previous performance reviews that were excellent, he was eventually fired. He sued and won his case. The hospital appealed and lost again.

The following are considered some necessary conditions that should be established before one undertakes whistle-blowing and it seems Adams met them all:

1. The reason the whistle-blower is blowing the whistle is because he or she sees a grave injustice or wrongdoing occurring in his or her organization that has not been resolved despite using all appropriate channels within the organization.

2. The whistle-blower morally justifies his or her course of action by appeals to ethical theories, principles, or other components of ethics, as well as relevant facts.

3. The whistle-blower thoroughly investigates the situation and is confident that the facts are as she or he understands them.

4. The whistle-blower understands that her or his primary loyalty is to client(s) unless other compelling moral reasons override this loyalty.

5. The whistle-blower ascertains that blowing the whistle most likely will cause more good than harm to client(s); that is, clients will not be retaliated against because of the whistle blowing.

6. The whistle-blower understands the seriousness of his or her actions and is ready to assume responsibility for them.

What Protections Do I Have Against Discrimination?

A host of discriminatory areas could be involved in your workplace relations. Besides the protections for race and ethnicity, gender and age are of particular interest in nursing. The discrimination against male nurses continues, especially in obstetric practice. The US District Court in Arkansas gave the opinion that "the fact that the plaintiff (male nurse) is a health care professional does not eliminate the fact that he is an unelected individual who is intruding on the obstetrical patient's right to privacy. The male nurse's situation is not analogous to that of the male doctor who has been selected by the patient."[22]

There has been significant progress through federal and state laws that protect against age discrimination in the workplace. Some laws have no upper limits; others specify protection until a certain age, perhaps 65, 70, or 75. Effective in 1994, the Age Discrimination in Employment Act covers those who work in academia, including nurse faculty (academics were excluded before 1994). The burden of proof in age discrimination is often difficult, and nurses should be vigilant; there is a growing trend to cut back on the number of nurses on staff. A typical case is reported from California, where the courts awarded damages to two nurses who sued on the basis of age discrimination. These nurses, 59 and 60 years old, were 30-year employees of the same hospital. Each had been publicly recognized for the quality of her practice. When a clinical ladder was put in place, they consciously decided to remain at a lower level of the clinical nurse category. After being told that it was mandatory for them to participate in a career advancement program and qualify for a higher status, they were both dismissed on grounds of the inability to demonstrate the competencies for the new level. Both of these nurses are now successfully employed elsewhere. There is fear that these will no longer be isolated cases in nursing. This becomes an especially significant issue with the "aging" of the nurse workforce, as described in Chapters 11 and 13.

The Americans with Disabilities Act extends protection in employment to individuals with human immunodeficiency virus and acquired immunodeficiency syndrome (HIV/AIDS) and also to people who are regarded as being infected or in close association with persons with HIV/AIDS. It should be mentioned that despite this legal means of redress against discrimination, there has been significant "under claiming" among young workers, as the segment of society that needs this protection the most. Similar protection is extended to individuals recovering from substance abuse.[23]

The issues of the HIV-infected nurse and the workplace go beyond class protection and must be detailed. The American Nurses Association (ANA) has assumed the leadership role for decades in providing policy direction to nurses and other health care professionals in dealing with HIV/AIDS. Position statements can be found at http://www.nursingworld.org, as follows:

1. Education and Barrier Use for Sexually Transmitted Diseases and HIV Infection
2. The Health Care Service System and Linkage of Primary Care, Substance Abuse, Mental Health, and HIV/AIDS-Related Services
3. AIDS/HIV Disease and Socio-Culturally Diverse Populations
4. Availability of Equipment and Safety Procedures to Prevent Transmission of Bloodborne Diseases
5. Guidelines for Disclosure to a Known Third Party About Possible HIV Infection
6. HIV-Infected Nurse, Ethical Obligations and Disclosure
7. Tuberculosis and HIV
8. HIV Disease and Correctional Inmates
9. Needle Exchange and HIV
10. Support for Confidential Notification Services and a Limited Privilege to Disclose
11. Personnel Policies and HIV in the Workplace
12. Post-Exposure Programs in the Event of Occupational Exposure to HIV/HBV
13. HIV Exposure From Rape/Sexual Assault
14. HIV Infection and Nursing Students
15. Tuberculosis and Public Health Nursing
16. HIV Infection and US Teenagers
17. HIV Testing
18. Travel Restrictions for Persons with HIV/AIDS
19. HIV Disease and Women

Nursing's continuous presence on the health care scene and commitment to comprehensive care created the need for ANA to speak out early, loudly, and often in the course of this pandemic. Certain ANA position statements are particularly important to bring to your attention and are singled out here. Issues of testing and the disclosure of HIV status are closely linked with discrimination.

> ANA opposes perpetuation of the myth that mandatory testing and mandatory disclosure of the HIV status of patients and/or nurses is a method of preventing the transmission of HIV disease, and therefore does not advocate mandatory testing or mandatory disclosure of HIV status. ANA supports the availability of voluntary anonymous or confidential HIV testing that is conducted with informed consent, and pre- and post-test counseling. ANA continues to support education regarding the transmission of HIV/AIDS, and the use and monitoring of universal precautions to prevent HIV/AIDS transmission.[24]

In every situation, the nurse's first concern is the protection of the patient. Therefore, the following policy provides direction for the HIV infected nurse:

> Nurses who know they have a transmissible bloodborne infection should voluntarily avoid exposure-prone invasive procedures that have been epidemiologically linked to HIV or other bloodborne infection transmission. The nurse has a duty to report exposure of a patient to bloodborne infection. Support and protection of the nurse with a seropositive status has been a long-standing position of ANA. The association supports the confidentiality of all information about the HIV-infected nurse.[25]

An additional dimension of the HIV-infected health care provider issue involves offers of employment. An employer may require a physical examination, including serology with HIV testing, once a conditional promise of employment has been made, but not before the promise of employment. If the anticipated employee tests HIV positive, the offer may not be withdrawn based on the positive status unless the results indicate that the employee is not qualified to perform the essential job functions. The results must be kept strictly confidential. This is consistent with the requirements of the Americans with Disabilities Act. There can often be a narrow line of interpretation here, and the possibility of frequent abuse. Some states are expanding their civil rights acts to prohibit employers from requiring HIV testing. Again, state-specific inquiries are in order.

Sexual harassment is a form of sex discrimination and a violation under Title VII of the Civil Rights Act of 1964, as affirmed by the US Supreme Court in 1986. The standard for sexual harassment has been made clearer by the Equal Employment Opportunities Commission (EEOC), defining it as unwelcome sexual advances, requests for sexual favors, and verbal or physical conduct of a sexual nature. These behaviors become *harassment* when they are a term or condition of employment or a criterion for employment decisions; when they interfere with the victim's job performance; or when they create a hostile, intimidating, or offensive work environment. Based on these definitions and circumstances, there are two categories of sexual harassment: *quid pro quo* and *hostile environment*. In the former, employment or employment conditions are contingent on submission. In the latter, the harassment creates a situation that is offensive and intimidating or seriously interferes with job performance.

Neither the high profile of this issue in recent years nor laws prohibiting sexual harassment seem to have reduced its prevalence among nurses. The following studies,

although some involve small samples, should cause us to stop and consider the true extent of this form of discrimination and the responses that are most effective in confronting this type of abuse. In a survey of critical care nurses, 46 percent of the respondents had been harassed, most frequently by offensive sexual remarks and unwanted physical contact. In 82 percent of the incidents, the harassers were physicians, and 80 percent of the nurses claimed that they had neither been trained to deal with the situation nor did policies exist to facilitate documentation or reporting. A more recent nationwide survey of hospital human resources managers reveals that, despite the actions of the courts and legislation in intervening years, allegations of sexual harassment in hospitals are increasing. Reported statistics for a 4.5-year period show that nurses continue to bring the largest number of charges. Most are hostile environment allegations, and most formal charges are levied against coworkers. When compared to data gathered in earlier surveys, these statistics show an alarming accelerating trend.

Besides some disagreement about whether a harassing incident actually occurred, nurses were generally reluctant to report these situations because of a disparity in status and power between the offender and the victim. Where incidents were reported, they were often dismissed or ignored. A good example is a case decided in 2009. Administrators at a community hospital looked the other way as a doctor sexually harassed a nurse for an 8-year period. The groping and propositioning of the nurse began shortly after she started working at the hospital. The physician's behavior was consistently bold and aggressive, and there was no attempt to hide it. Complaints to a supervisor were ignored. The plaintiff's testimony was graphic and full of allegations of both violence and sexually provocative assaults. The case brought a record-breaking payout for sexual harassment of $15 million, ordering the hospital and the physician to split the damages. Despite his behavior, the physician retained his license, though it was suspended for 2 months, and he was given 3 months of probation.[26]

In being confronted with harassment, immediate assertive action is merited. In most cases, but not all, assertiveness is effective. The suggested response is to

1. Confront the harasser and label the behavior.
2. Report and document the incident.
3. Seek support from others.

Most victims who confronted the offender put a stop to the behavior; others found themselves isolated; and still others gained nothing but additional hardship for their courage. Action offers the most hope of change; silence perpetuates the victimization.

Sexual harassment policies, procedures, and training to handle these situations effectively are necessary for a safe workplace environment. Much clarity was given to this whole area by the US Supreme Court decision of June 1998. The Court held that an employee who resists a supervisor's advances need not suffer a tangible job loss or detriment to be able to pursue a lawsuit against an employer. But such a suit cannot succeed if the company has an anti-harassment policy with an effective complaint procedure in place and the employee has unreasonably failed to use it. In other words, the employer is responsible for the development, maintenance, and dissemination of strong and fair policy, and the employee is bound to use due process.[27]

Do I Have the Right to Withhold Information About Myself From an Employer?

The degree of privacy guaranteed to an employee is directly related to the information in question and its relation to the employer's interests. The need for information is considered reasonable when it relates to the employee's competence, reliability, and honesty as a worker, or when required by the government. There are limitations both on the right to privacy and on the intrusions into that right. Some examples will help:

1. An employer can contact a former employer and check references provided by the employee about work history.
2. Employers must notify the employee about any investigation into the employee's credit or financial position and provide a copy of any investigative reports.
3. An employer can search an employee for theft of company property, but the circumstances of the detection must be reasonable (if not, the employer may be liable for false imprisonment).
4. Employees can be expected to take a lie detector test except in states where employee permission is required.
5. Many employers are subject to a law that requires mandatory drug testing of their employees under certain circumstances. (Your state nurses' association will be able to advise you on the laws that apply in your situation.)
6. An employer may only require a physical (including HIV testing) after a conditional promise of employment

has been made, and the offer of employment may not be withdrawn unless the results interfere with the ability to perform essential job functions.

Each situation is judged on the standard of reasonableness and relevance, and interpretations vary; however, more and more case law and legislation surface daily. Many privacy situations are co-mingled with protection under civil rights and the Americans with Disabilities Act. State laws are also at issue here.

Are There Laws That Guarantee Fringe Benefits, Including Health Insurance, Pension, and Family Leave?

Fringe benefits and pensions are of growing importance to nurses. Although most employers provide fringe benefit packages, there is no federal or state requirement with the exception of employer contributions to social security, workers' compensation, and unemployment insurance. However, there are a number of legislative protections that the employee should be aware of. The *Family Leave Act of 1993* requires that employees be allowed to take off a time-limited period for a new baby, adoption, or to care for a disabled family member. You are assured the right to return to a position comparable with the one you left, and your health benefits must be continued for the period of the leave, but in some cases the employee is required to reimburse the employer for these costs. In a similar fashion, you are given the right to personally pay for the continuation of your health insurance for up to 36 months after you leave a job. Over the years, pensions have also increased in their protections for the worker. Benefit plans, including pensions, must satisfy nondiscriminatory requirements, treating men and women equitably. Pension benefits have mandatory vesting schedules, guaranteeing 100 percent non-forfeiture of accrued benefits after 5 years of service or the option to phase in 100 percent vesting over 3 to 7 years. In short, no benefits or pensions are guaranteed with the exception of social security, but where these fringes are provided, there are increasing protections.

Ideally there should be a written employment contract that follows a more or less standard form and details conditions of employment, such as salary, vacation, sick leave, holidays, social security coverage, pension, and the duration of the contract. More usually, these things are shared verbally and may be found written in personnel policies. For more detail on employment contracts, refer to Chapter 22 of the sixth edition of *Dimensions*.

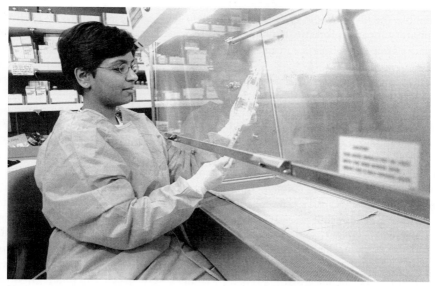

Modern diagnostics and treatment can represent workplace hazards for the nurse.
(Courtesy of Robert Wood Johnson University Hospital, New Brunswick, New Jersey)

What Are the Major Workplace Hazards for Nurses and What Is the Employer's Responsibility?

The converse of patient exposure to the HIV-infected provider is the risk of infection to the provider from the patient. This risk has been compounded by the significant incidence of tuberculosis (TB) in HIV-infected individuals. The cutback in public health funds to allow proper follow-up of TB patients, the presence of HIV-infected individuals with compromised immune systems, and the frequent use of drug therapy to treat TB have resulted in the development of multi-drug-resistant strains of TB (MDR-TB).

MDR-TB and HIV/AIDS have increased our awareness of workplace hazards. Nurses have for the most part accepted the inherent risk that comes with their practice. However, recent years have prompted a new philosophy on the part of health workers that places a high value on their own physical and psychological well-being. This has already been acted out in the US Supreme Court. In a 1998 decision (*Bragdon v. Abbott*, 66 U.S.L.W. 4601), the court held that under the Americans with Disabilities Act, patients with HIV/AIDS deserved treatment comparable to that given to other patients. Here, a dentist refused to treat an HIV/AIDS patient without extraordinary protections, and the court found this position to be discriminatory.

The obligation of the employer is to provide environmental safety, work practice controls, personal protective equipment to minimize or prevent exposure, and postexposure programs including counseling. The Centers for Disease Control and Prevention (CDC) have developed guidelines for the management of health care workers following occupational exposure to HIV. A program would include information, immediate evaluation, prophylactic intervention, counseling, and supportive care. The nurse who seroconverts should be guaranteed workers' compensation and continued health insurance coverage. Workers' compensation still presents difficulty due to probable underreporting and the burden of proving occupational transmission. Some occupational groups, such as firefighters and coal miners, have been successful in legislation that assumes occupational transmission for certain conditions and places the burden of proof on the employer to prove that the condition is not work related. The important observations for the new employee are what policies exist for postexposure management and whether adequate precautions are in place to reduce the risk of exposure. MDR-TB prevention requires a high index of suspicion for TB and early recognition of symptoms that may trigger the need for respiratory precautions. All efforts boil down to containing the infectious agent from becoming airborne.

When this is impossible, the nurse should have access to recommended respiratory apparel (protective equipment) and the ability to place a symptomatic patient in an appropriate air-managed environment.

For the protection of both patients and workers against transmission, universal precautions should be used when dealing with blood and other body fluids including semen, vaginal secretions, cerebrospinal fluid, and synovial fluid, among others. The precautions include guidelines for handling sharps and laboratory specimens, the use of gloves and gowns, hand washing, protective eyewear, disposal of linen, resuscitation procedures, and care of reusable equipment. As of December 2006, the CDC had received reports of 57 documented cases and 140 possible cases of occupationally acquired HIV infection among health care workers in the United States in the 25 years since 1981. Twenty-four of these documented cases and 35 of the possible cases were among nurses, by far the most highly exposed group (see Exhibit 30–1).[28] In addition, the risk is just as great of acquiring hepatitis B and C.

Over 1 million injuries due to sharp instruments, including needle sticks, occur in the United States annually, exposing health care workers to potentially lethal bloodborne pathogens such as HIV and hepatitis. In October 2000, the US Congress passed legislation providing needle stick protection under the Occupational Safety and Health Administration (OSHA). The Needle Stick Safety and Prevention Act requires the use of safety devices to prevent sharps injuries, input from nonmanagerial workers responsible for direct patient care in selecting work practice controls, and the maintenance of a sharps injury log to document details of any sharps injury incident.[29] This issue continues to be addressed on the state level with legislation to strengthen needle stick protections for nurses and other health care providers. Some states have introduced legislation to cover state and municipal employees who are not covered by the Needle Stick Safety and Prevention Act. Other states are pushing for protections that go beyond the federal Needle Stick Law, such as requiring workers' compensation benefits for public safety workers (including nurses) who are exposed to blood and bodily fluids during employment and contract a disease.

Ergonomic hazards, though less dramatic, are job and process design problems that are common and harmful.

■ **EXHIBIT 30–1. Health Care Personnel With Documented and Possible Occupationally Acquired AIDS/HIV Infection, by Occupation, 1981–2006**

Occupation	Documented	Possible
Nurse	24	35
Laboratory worker, clinical	16	17
Physician, nonsurgical	6	12
Laboratory technician, nonclinical	3	—
Housekeeper/maintenance worker	2	13
Technician, surgical	2	2
Embalmer/morgue technician	1	2
Health aide/attendant	1	15
Respiratory therapist	1	2
Technician, dialysis	1	3
Dental worker, including dentist	—	6
Emergency medical technician/paramedic	—	12
Physician, surgical	—	6
Other technician/therapist	—	9
Other health care occupation	—	6
Total	**57**	**140**

Source: CDC. Surveillance of Occupationally Acquired HIV/AIDS in Healthcare Personnel, as of December 2006. http://www.cdc.gov/ncidod/dhqp/bp_hcp_w_hiv.html. Retrieved June 10, 2010.

Examples are improper work methods and inadequate work and rest patterns or repetitive tasks that result in musculoskeletal damage such as back injuries and carpal tunnel syndrome. Such situations affect up to one-third of all nurses. There is no way to safely lift an average adult patient without assistive devices. Effective measures exist to perform these tasks, but few health care employers have voluntarily implemented them. Although OSHA has made little progress on this issue, the Veteran's Health Administration has begun intensive applied research in the area of ergonomic injury prevention, which may promote voluntary implementation of safe patient handling and movement programs.

Violence has been a constant threat to nursing in the workplace. Incidents have rarely been reported because of the poor public image this would create for the health care facility. We are currently caught in violent times, and the incidence of workplace violence is increasing. Such factors as weapons that are easy to obtain, deinstitutionalization of the chronically mentally ill, substance abuse, and a generally angry underclass all contribute to an increasing danger of violence and assault. Violence in the emergency department is recognized as a significant occupational hazard; however, 13 percent of incidents occur on inpatient units. According to ANA, as violence in health care escalates, nurses are the workers at greatest risk, because a high percentage of nurses are women; the nature of the work involves close physical contact, proximity, and people under stress; work is in shifts; and highly accessible worksites may not be secure. A comprehensive review of the literature identified the following factors as associated with assault in the health care workplace:

- Inexperienced health care workers are at increased risk of assault.
- The largest number of injuries occur while attempts are being made to contain patient violence.
- Short staffing and temporary staffing have been associated with increased assaults.
- Assaults seem to occur during times of high activity and high emotion on patient units.

The presence of policies that show sensitivity to these factors is necessary, as is the establishment of peer assistance and post-assault assistance programs in environments where the incidence of violence is high.

Before leaving the topic of violence, be aware that all personal threat is not from members of other disciplines, visitors, or patients and their families. Lateral violence is very real, but has had little attention. Lateral violence is disruptive, bullying, intimidating, or unsettling behavior that occurs between nurses in the workplace. For example, the perioperative setting, among others, fosters lateral violence because of the inherent stress of performing surgery, high patient acuity, shortage of experienced personnel, work demands, and the restriction and isolation of the OR, which allows negative behaviors to be concealed more easily. Lateral violence affects nurses' health and well-being and their ability to care for patients. Interventions to reduce lateral violence include the empowerment of staff members and zero tolerance for lateral violence.[30]

The most rapidly escalating workplace hazard is *latex allergy.* Latex represents a threat not only to health care workers but also to patients. There are over 40,000 latex products on the market, the majority are medical devices, and the most common is the latex glove. In 1987, the CDC introduced universal precautions, and the use of latex gloves increased dramatically. The allergic response is due to latex protein, which may differ as much as 400 percent from product to product. Allergic reactions to latex range from contact dermatitis, to asthma, to fatal anaphylaxis. About 8 to 12 percent of people exposed to latex on the job are estimated to be allergic to latex. The National Institute for Occupational Safety and Health (NIOSH) recommends that if latex gloves are worn, they should be powder free and of low allergenicity. It is possible to decrease the allergen in manufacturing, and powder predisposes to percutaneous exposure. A latex-free environment is impossible, but precautions are possible. Nonlatex, low-allergen, and powder-free gloves should be available. Employee policies should provide for latex allergy screening and education on the subject. The goal is to heighten awareness, understand your personal risk, if any, and provide options for safe practice.

The strategy has been to create a latex-safe environment through lobbying at the state level. Several state nurses' associations are working to educate legislators about the potentially tragic consequences of the use of these products and the simple remedy—eliminating the use of powdered latex products and requiring the use of only nonpowdered, low-protein latex products.

Collective Bargaining: The Process and the Issues

Some employment issues are resolved by *collective bargaining.* The process of collective bargaining, because it is set by law, is similar regardless of who the bargaining agent is; details can be found in any book on labor relations. In the context of state nurses' associations (SNAs) as collective bargaining agents, the following is presented as a brief overview:

1. The nurses (or groups of nurses) in an institution, discontented with a situation or conditions and having exhausted the usual channels for correction or improvement, ask the SNA for assistance.

2. A meeting is held outside the premises of the institution and always on off-duty time. SNA staff and the nurses explore the problem, and the nurses are given advice about reasonable, negotiable issues and how to form a unit. For instance, they are told who can be included in a unit. Administrative nurses are excluded, but the question of supervisors is still being debated in some places.

3. Authorization cards, which authorize the SNA to act as the nurses' bargaining representative, must be signed by at least 30 percent of the group to be represented. Membership forms are also suggested, because the SNA cannot provide service without funds. All collective bargaining activity must be carried out in non-work areas where the employee is protected from employer interference. (There are a series of National Labor Relations Board [NLRB] rules governing employee distribution and solicitation.)

4. If sufficient cards are signed, the SNA notifies the employer that an organizing campaign is in process, calling attention to the fact that the activity is protected. Copies of the notice are distributed to the nurses so that they know they are protected.

5. An informational meeting is held for all nurses and SNA staff.

6. If it is agreed that the SNA will represent the nurses, a bargaining unit is formed and officers are elected.

7. To seek voluntary recognition of the unit by the employer, a majority of the nurses must sign designation cards; a mutually accepted third party will probably check this.

8. If the employer chooses not to recognize the unit or if another union challenges the designation, a series of actions takes place, including an NLRB-conducted election. To petition for election, any union must have designation cards signed by 30 percent of the nurses in the proposed unit. The election is won or lost by the majority of nurses voting. They may vote for a particular union or specify none at all. The NLRB then certifies the winner as the exclusive bargaining agent. If the majority of nurses vote against any bargaining unit, the NLRB certifies this as well.

9. Assuming that the SNA wins the election, the SNA representative, at the direction of the unit, attempts to settle the problems and complaints of the nurses by negotiating with administration. There are specific rules about what is negotiable. Mandatory subjects include salaries, fringe benefits, and conditions of employment, and both sides must bargain in good faith about these issues. Voluntary subjects can be almost anything else that both sides want to discuss except for prohibited or illegal subjects, such as a requirement that all workers become members of a union before being employed for 30 days. It should be remembered that the nurse executive, both through position and under law, is an administrator. Even though this person might be in complete support of the nurses' demands, he or she cannot join them. Quite often the director has previously tried unsuccessfully to help them achieve their goals.

10. An agreement may or may not be reached, probably with some compromise on both sides. If there is agreement, a contract is voted on and signed, outlining agreed-upon conditions and the responsibilities of each group. Contracts are renegotiated at set time periods, usually of several years. If no agreement can be reached, the dispute may be referred to binding or nonbinding arbitration by an outside group, or some job action such as picketing or a strike may occur. Picketing may be merely informational, to communicate the issues to the community, or it may be intended to prevent other employees or services from entering the institution. The latter, combined with a strike, is the very last resort, to be used when all other efforts fail. If such action is decided upon, sufficient notice is given to allow planning for the maintenance of essential patient services. Even if strikes are successful, there is often a lingering, unpleasant feeling between participants and nonparticipants. However, as ANA members agreed when they gradually removed no-strike clauses from ANA and SNA policies, the strike is an ultimate weapon that may be necessary when the employer refuses any attempt to resolve the issues.

Once a labor contract is in place, there are times when individual nurses are in dispute with the employer. A *grievance procedure* is generally used to resolve the problem. A grievance may be caused by an alleged violation of a contract provision, a change in a past practice, or an employer decision that is considered arbitrary, capricious, unreasonable, unfair, or discriminatory. Simple complaints are not considered grievances. If informed discussion does not resolve the issue, a grievance procedure is followed. The steps include the following: (1) written notice of the grievance is given, with a written response within a set time; (2) if the response is not satisfactory, an appeal to the director of nursing follows; (3) the employee, SNA representative, grievance chairman, and/or delegate, director of nursing, and director of personnel meet; (4) if no resolution occurs, the final step is arbitration by a neutral third party selected by both parties involved. The technique for carrying out the process involves interpersonal and negotiating skills.

For nurses, the collective bargaining environment has always been covered with land mines. Nurses are predominantly salaried professionals. They are consequently concerned with employee–employer issues. These issues were historically settled internal to the workplace, and health care workers were of little interest to traditional trade unions in the heyday of the labor movement. With increasing government control of unions, the declining industry and manufacturing market, and the 1974 repeal of the Tyding Amendments, which since 1947 exempted the nonprofit health care industry from the requirements of the National Labor Relations Act (the right to organize for collective bargaining), health care workers were targeted for organizing. Although unionization has declined from a one-time high of over 30 percent of American labor to a current low of less than 15 percent, over 20 percent of health care workers are represented, with a significant increase in the last decade. The largest single constituency in health care is RNs. They have traditionally avoided unionization, but when forced to seek more leverage through collective bargaining, their preferred choice for representation has been the SNA (the state affiliate of the ANA). The uniqueness of nurses, their chosen representatives, and their practice patterns have given rise to a number of problems, some resolved and others still pending:

1. *Supervisory domination.* In an attempt to thwart organizing activity by the state nurses' association, employers have claimed that nurse-managers who hold office in an SNA create a situation of management intrusion into the collective bargaining activities of the association. Organizational structure, reporting relationships, and policy-making bodies have been created to insulate union activity while maintaining the program under the aegis of the professional association. The adequacy of these designs has been tested in the courts on a number of occasions.[31] This issue will continue to surface from time to time.

2. *The RN-only bargaining unit.* In April 1991, after a 17-year struggle with the hospital industry and a unanimous US Supreme Court decision, nurses were given the right to organize into bargaining units made up solely of RNs.[32] The hospital industry found it more strategic to dilute nursing issues by folding them into units with other workers. Beyond a fair wage and benefits package, the issues most compelling to RNs have always been those of patient care. This has not been the priority for other groups of employees. The unique community of interest among RNs was no longer debatable after this decision.

3. *Nurses as categorical supervisors.* The latest potential obstacle to RN organizing surfaces from a US Supreme Court decision of May 1994 and is also discussed in Chapter 25. It has been common to separate RNs as employees from their practice role as professionals, wherein they are directly accountable to the patient. Within this professional role, it is common for the RN to delegate or assign select activities to a nursing assistant while continuing to be personally responsible. Justice Ruth Bader Ginsburg, in her minority opinion, observes that it is rare that a professional does not occasionally work through someone else. In contrast, the majority opinion (which, in this case, involved licensed practical nurses) declared that the nurse was an agent of management in this relationship with subordinates. Although this case did not directly involve RNs and the incident was in a nursing home, there are still serious implications. The RN frequently works with both nursing assistants and environmental support personnel (transport, messengers). The presence of these workers is increasing with restructuring. Legislation may be necessary to set the record straight for the new millennium.

4. *Human resource techniques building cooperation between labor and management.* The last 30 years have been witness to a variety of strategies to encourage employee participation in workplace decisions. They have been called *work teams, circles, quality of work life committees,* and, in nursing, *shared governance.* The old brand of unionism built on adversarial relationships is counterproductive for the new millennium. A large number of American industries and unions have proved this point. In response, the federal government has applauded such initiatives. Meanwhile, those whose thinking is

frozen in another generation challenge these collegial efforts as "company unions" and consequently illegal. This is another example of the need for the updating of labor law to serve the twenty-first century.

■ CAREER MAPPING

You have sought the best educational preparation to enter the field of nursing. You have hopefully done so with the intent of building a career. No field offers such variety or opportunity to advance. Each decision you make can strategically build toward your long-term goal. Additionally, for the professional there is the obligation to remain current, which is no simple task, given the rate at which the science of nursing is expanding. Try to dream about where you would like to go professionally, at least in broad terms. Remember that the shortest distance between two points is a straight line.

Experience Is No Myth

You have already reviewed the process of searching and courting employment in Chapter 29. You have also been counseled to take time for a personal assessment. Identify the route in nursing you would like to take. Given today's complex clinical environment, your competence as a generalist will be short lived. You will take on the characteristics of a specialized practice area in very short order. Build your career cautiously, laying each brick in a predetermined pattern. It is a valid goal to seek out a position with the patient population that intrigues you most, resolving to provide the best possible care to those patients, growing through experience, and keeping current with a wellplanned continuing education (CE) program. It is just as acceptable to have a vision of a lateral move into education and formal schooling that stretches on for many years, and perhaps many degrees. It is also acceptable to fail, reconsider, and change courses many times. The only thing that is unacceptable is to have no goals at all.

While you are considering your lateral moves and vertical climbs, pay proper respect to the fact that nursing is a practice discipline. You definitely grow in your ability to care as you minister to patients and as you invest hours and years in your art. Experience is not a myth but one essential ingredient to bring you from novice to expert.

Maintaining Competence

Process is content today. Your educational experience is adequate only if it has taught you how to think and where

to go to find the information you need. Most of the knowledge you currently have will be outdated in 5 years. The most established professions have learned that lesson. Case material in law only provides the substance through which to cultivate analytic skills. The activities that constitute your role will be no more stable than your knowledge. During your career lifetime, the activities that are part of your practice will shift. Some will disappear and others you will delegate to less-prepared individuals. New role functions currently foreign to you will become part of your day-to-day repertoire. Beyond your own personal security and flexibility to move with the times, you need reliable sources of CE and access to information. Besides what your employers provide on their own behalf to assure your safety and currency, it is your personal obligation to maintain a curiosity and thirst for better ways to nurse.

The term *continuing education* has been interpreted in many ways. Most agree that it includes any learning activity after the basic educational program. Courses of study or programs leading to an academic degree are separated out. The basic and overriding purpose of CE in nursing is the maintenance of continued competence so that the care of the patient is safe and effective. CE is provided through your employing agency, or you may choose (or the employer may encourage you) to seek outside programs. The variety of CE programs is limitless. The secret is to be a discerning consumer and select those that are most immediately valuable to your practice. CE need not be only clinically oriented. You must also remain conversant with current issues in the discipline and with the thinking of nursing leaders. Employer funding and time off for CE is often a workplace benefit. The types of educational experiences that staff are approved to attend are often an indication of how the administration views nursing, as a technical or professional field. From another perspective, it provides insights on the staff that will be your peers. The professions have always recognized the fact that learning for practice was lifelong. Florence Nightingale was eloquent on the subject:

> Nursing is a progressive art, in which to stand still is to go back. A woman who thinks to herself, "Now I am a full nurse, a skilled nurse, I have learnt all there is to be learnt"—take my word for it, she does not know what a nurse is, and never will know; she is gone back already. Progress can never end but with a nurse's life.[33]

With CE programs proliferating (and getting more expensive), it is better to give some thought to what is worth spending time and money on. One suggested plan for diagnosing your CE needs is to develop a model of required competencies, assessing your practice in relation to the model, and identifying the gaps between your knowledge and skills and those required. Some of this preliminary testing can be done by taking some of the tests in journals and by carefully evaluating your own practice and getting feedback from peers and supervisors as well.

Other methods of CE learning, besides formal classes or conferences, are well worth investigating, although, of course, there is often the added value of interaction with other nurses in group activities. Many nursing journals offer monthly self-study programs, and Internet courses are becoming common.

Another aspect of maintaining competence is the ability to locate the information you need for your practice and access those information sources. Your educational program should have prepared you to find the information you need and impressed on you that you are responsible for the changing standard of practice. In some situations, physicians are being held liable for not conducting literature searches when appropriate; nurses are similarly at risk.

You will find your most updated indexes of the nursing and allied health literature in computerized data bases. With the technical support to review the literature in computerized form, searching becomes a highly exciting learning experience, and librarians, health care professionals, and students increasingly conduct computerized literature searches. The data bases most commonly used in nursing are the *Cumulative Index to Nursing and Allied Health Literature* (CINAHL), and MEDLINE/PUBMED. MEDLINE and CINAHL are computerized and available online.

The National Library of Medicine (NLM) provides MEDLINE free. MEDLINE is a massive, world-renowned biomedical data base, updated twice a month. Some 360,000 citations from 3500 journals are added to MEDLINE each year. It contains citations as far back as 1966. Its print counterpart is the *Index Medicus*. CINAHL is available for a fee. Its online version is updated monthly. The CINAHL collection was started in 1956 and is also available in print form. Both data bases contain abstracts of many articles.

NLM provides access to 40 additional data bases that would be of interest to nurses. Some are AIDSLINE (AIDS and related topics), AIDSDRUGS (AIDS drugs in clinical trial), BIOETHICSLINE (ethics and related public policy issues in health care), CANCERLIT (cancer topics), DIRLINE (directory of resources providing information services), Health-STAR (clinical and nonclinical issues in

health care), HISTLINE (history of medicine and related sciences), HSRPROJ (health service research including clinical practice guidelines), POPLINE (family planning, maternal/child health in developing countries, primary health care), SPACE-LINE (space life sciences), TOXLINE (toxicology), and more. All of these data bases are free, but you do need access to a computer with an Internet connection. The Internet address is

http://www.nlm.nih.gov

Formal Higher Education

Besides participating in CE programs, the graduate of a diploma or associate degree program may want to give serious consideration to formal education leading to a baccalaureate degree, and the nurse with a baccalaureate degree may want to think about getting a master's. There is no question but that educational standards for all positions in nursing are growing steadily higher. If you really want to advance professionally to positions of greater scope and challenge, you will, in the very near future, need at least a master's degree. The process of obtaining higher degrees will not only serve you well professionally, but also will add considerably to the enrichment of your personal life and interests. In fact, these are the reasons nurses give most often.

Although it would be difficult to denigrate the value of any good-quality educational program, give some thought to your future goals. The joy of exploring new fields and studying whatever you wish without the pressure of time or the need to fulfill requirements for a program may be especially tempting. If these interests are in any of the liberal arts or the social or physical sciences, which may be required or can be used as electives in many programs, a dual purpose will be accomplished in that you are also started toward a degree.

Because baccalaureate programs with a nursing major have not always been available to nurses in a particular geographic area, a number of programs have sprung up offering a degree in nursing or another field, giving credit for the lower-division nursing courses and offering no upper-division nursing. Evaluate them in relation to your career goals. These programs are not usually acceptable for future graduate studies in nursing, and you may not be able to enroll in a graduate program without having taken upper-division nursing courses. Some nurses have found it necessary to complete a second baccalaureate program, this time with a nursing major, to continue into a master's program.

As noted in Chapter 12, RNs will find that they receive varying amounts of recognition or credit for their basic nursing courses, and they may perhaps need to take challenge examinations. Nursing baccalaureate programs vary a great deal in this respect, but more and more nursing programs are offering some form of educational articulation, self-pacing, or other means of giving credit for previous learning. There are also a large number of baccalaureate programs that admit only RN students. The National League for Nursing (NLN) and American Association of Colleges of Nursing publications listing baccalaureate, master's, and doctoral programs are helpful.

Many of the same points apply to graduate education. Consider carefully what you want from a program and prepare yourself for this more competitive admissions procedure. Nurses complete graduate programs in the various sciences or education with or without any nursing input. Again, you must consider your specific career goals. Someone with a nursing major may be given preference in a position requiring a graduate degree, particularly in educational positions. Many state boards of nursing require faculty in basic nursing education programs to have a graduate degree with a major in nursing. Or if you are hired now, there is no guarantee that later, when there are more nurses with graduate nursing degrees, you may not be bypassed for promotion or may be required to take a second graduate degree in nursing to hold on to your current position. These are practical considerations presented here for information. You must still make the educational decisions you wish, but with as complete a knowledge of the pros and cons as possible.

Suppose you simply don't want a degree? Or suppose you enroll in an accredited nursing program, but then in time drop out? That's your decision. There is no reason why you can't function at an acceptable level of competence, maintaining and improving that competence through CE, and thereby making a valuable contribution to the profession and society. If, however, you withdrew because of disappointment or lack of interest in that particular program, it may well be that the program is not congruent with your philosophy. Consider a second try, taking time to determine whether a program's philosophy, objectives, approaches to teaching, and attitudes are what you want. Some of this information can be obtained from the catalog, faculty or adviser interviews, and informal contact with students, or from speaking with recent graduates (programs do change).

For RNs, going back to school is not easy, particularly if you have a family. One nurse who did it (and has a sense of humor) suggests the following:

1. Begin the course only if you're 100 percent committed.
2. Prepare yourself financially.
3. Unless you can afford days off without pay, start accumulating vacation days; you may need them for a clinical rotation.
4. If you don't type, learn; there are lots of papers to write.
5. Invest in a computer; it is critical to own.
6. Create study space for yourself that is comfortable and secluded.
7. Use your hospital library; that saves time, too.
8. Decide before beginning that you don't really need a 4.0 average to be successful; you don't need the extra stress.
9. Enlist the support of your coworkers and manager.
10. Refuse extra assignments at work.
11. Schedule something fun every week.
12. Cross off each week on a calendar.
13. Remind yourself that others completed the course and you can, too.
14. Delegate everything possible to your children.
15. Have regular study times.
16. Give yourself a mental health break by skipping a routine class occasionally.
17. Frequently visualize what you'll feel like when it's over.
18. Nourish yourself physically, spiritually, and socially, enough to feel healthy and supported.
19. When it's over, celebrate with everyone who made your dream come true.[34]

That's not bad advice for any nontraditional student, and it is still relevant and useful after more than 20 years.

Sources of Financial Aid

The problem of finances is undoubtedly the most common deterrent to advanced education for able professional nurses. First consider whether there are any educational benefits available from your workplace. Tuition reimbursement for most nurses working in acute care is still a reality. Seven in 10 full-time workers have these benefits, as do

53 percent of part timers. Although this benefit has remained relatively stable, the dollars associated with it may not have kept pace with the increasing cost of tuition. Next, review your financial resources realistically before embarking on this new venture. If you are going to request financial aid, you will need to estimate as accurately as possible your expected income and expenses. Major educational expenses will include tuition, books, educational fees, and perhaps travel. Related personal expenses depend on where and how you live. Economizing may mean enrolling in a community college for the liberal arts and later transferring to a local or state college. Economy should not include enrolling in a poor program. Graduating from a nonaccredited nursing program may create difficulties in advancing to the next higher degree. Not all nonaccredited programs are poor, but this risk does exist.

The major sources of income for a self-supporting graduate nurse in an advanced educational program are savings or other personal resources, part-time work, scholarships, and loans. If you plan to do part-time work while attending college, make reasonably sure that a position is available at a satisfactory salary and that it seems to be professionally suitable, including enough flexibility to make it possible to take courses. Consider also your mental and physical health under this double load. Can you manage?

There are a number of scholarships, fellowships, and loans earmarked for educational purposes for which professional nurses are often eligible if they seek them out and apply. The financial aid officer at the institution where you plan to enroll is an excellent source of information.

In most instances, educational scholarships, fellowships, and loans are defined as follows: (1) *scholarship*—a financial subsidy awarded for academic ability or some other quality that does not involve repayment; (2) *fellowship*—a grant for graduate study not requiring repayment, but often associated with services provided to the college; (3) *loan*— a grant for educational purposes to be repaid by the recipient either with or without interest after completion of the course or education.

Grants in aid are outright grants at both the undergraduate and graduate levels for the accomplishment of specific projects. There may also be an outright grant to meet an immediate financial emergency or a grant to a student with a claim to a restricted scholarship fund. The term *traineeship* is also used to denote federal grants with stipend and tuition costs, which need not be repaid, awarded to students in nursing programs under the Nurse Education Act and its legislative successors.

Some funds are available to members of certain organizations or religious denominations or to students who meet other special requirements. Others are offered to any deserving person who has demonstrated such qualities as good character, leadership ability, and academic achievement. In general, scholarships, loans, and grants are available from both private and governmental sources and agencies.

Financial assistance may be found at the local, state, regional, national, or international level. Where you should apply can depend on how you plan to use the money. For example, some funds are available only for advanced study in certain clinical specialties; others are designed to prepare nurses for teaching, or supervisory or administrative positions; still others have different stipulations; and many are unrestricted as long as the applicant meets the designated personal qualifications.

Local Sources

Local sources of funds include both professional and civic groups in the nursing school, community, district, and state. The alumni association of a school of nursing often has appropriations for scholarships and loans that are available to graduates of the school. The president of the association or the director of the school will have information about such sources of financial assistance. Some district and state nurses' associations and NLN constituencies have funds for advanced study and other special purposes, either as direct gifts or on a reasonable interest and repayment basis.

Other local sources of funds include chapters of national sororities, fraternities, and clubs whose memberships are not restricted to nurses, but offer financial aid to anyone who meets their qualifications. There are churches that have educational funds, as do church-affiliated groups; the Elks, Masons, Altrusa Club, American Legion, and other similar organizations; unions; corporations; and private foundations and institutes. Other good sources of information are local or state colleges or universities and the hospital associations. Your place of employment may also offer grants and loans or may pay part or all of the tuition fees.

National and International Sources

In recent years, professional nurses interested in applying for a national scholarship, fellowship, or loan would, with the assistance of the advanced nursing programs in which they were enrolled, turn to the federal government. Both general scholarships and loans, as well as some designated especially for RNs, grants, fellowships, and full-time nurse traineeships, have been of increasing and invaluable aid to the RN. Although there are never enough to meet all needs, without them a majority of RNs could not have completed advanced education. However, beginning in 1973, the federal administration became less interested in providing any financial aid to nurses, and some loans and funds were seriously reduced. Since 1975, funds for nurse traineeships have been progressively cut. Loans and special scholarships for service in underserved areas continue to be available, but there are predictions that federal money for all health professionals will gradually dry up. Much depends on the amount of pressure put on Congress to legislate funds. Such congressional action appears to fluctuate from year to year, but the trend seems to be toward fewer and more restricted funds.

The Nurses' Educational Funds, Inc. (NEF) was established in 1954 to honor nursing pioneers. It was initiated largely through the efforts of NLN, which saw the need for centralized administration of the three separate educational allocations for nurses that existed at that time: the Isabel Hampton Robb Memorial Fund, the Isabel McIsaac Loan Fund, and the Nurses' Scholarship and Fellowship Fund. Since then, other funds have been initiated and turned over to NEF for administration. Many of the awards given are in the names of nurses who contributed greatly to the nursing profession. NEF is an independent organization that grants and administers scholarships and fellowships to RNs for post-RN study. It is governed by a board of trustees, mainly leaders in nursing education, and supported by contributions from business corporations, foundations, nurses, and persons interested in nursing.

The national nursing organizations may be able to supply information about scholarships, fellowships, and loans accessible to RNs who wish to study abroad. It would be well to contact these organizations first, although the International Council of Nurses, the World Health Organization, and the US Public Health Service are also possible sources of information. As more professional nurses become interested in international nursing, governmental, professional, educational, and philanthropic groups may originate new scholarships, fellowships, and loans to assist them. The competition for available funds for international study is likely to be increasingly keen, however, because many other professional and occupational groups also are becoming more eager for education and experience in other countries.

Community Activities as a Professional

Active participation in community activities that allow you to share and utilize your professional background in full is very rewarding. Some activities are directly related to nursing, such as attending alumni and nurses' associations meetings and accepting appointments to committees and offices. Others include volunteer work on a regular or special basis, such as participating in student nurse recruitment programs or career days, soliciting donations for various health organizations, helping with the Red Cross blood program, assisting with inoculation and sessions for children, acting as adviser to a Future Nurse Club, or volunteering time at a free clinic.

The importance of nursing input into the various community, state, and national provider/consumer groups that study the means of improving the health care delivery system is obvious. Although participation at a state or national level may not be immediately feasible for a nurse who hasn't yet achieved professional recognition, just showing interest and volunteering your services will often open doors at a local level. Nurses involved in direct patient care activities are particularly welcome, because there is the feeling that they can more specifically delineate some of the problems and suggest logical, down-to-earth solutions. Participation of this kind is essential if nurses are to have a part in making policy decisions.

Consumer activism has caused the formation of other groups concerned with health delivery, and nurses offering their expertise and understanding of health care can make valuable contributions. Sometimes you need to convince these groups that you have a sincere interest in improved health care services and are willing to work cooperatively with the consumer to achieve that end. The ANA and National Consumer League have joined forces to initiate nurse/consumer partnerships at the local and state levels that will ultimately result in public policy reform. This project has been funded through the Kellogg Foundation and targets projects in Florida, Wisconsin, and Virginia. In some areas, ethnic and minority groups are especially suspicious of professional health workers outside of their own group, because unfortunate experiences have shown some of them to be more concerned with defending their own interests than the consumer's well-being. In these groups, it is even more important to listen than to talk. Such participation can lead to the development of free clinics, health fairs, health teaching classes, the recruitment of minority students for nursing programs, tutoring sessions for students, liaison activities with health care institutions, programs for the aged, and legislative activities directed toward better health care. The opportunities, challenges, and satisfactions are unlimited.

Consumer health education is being stressed more and more today, and in what better area can professional nurses offer their expertise? Classes can be held under the auspices of health care institutions, public health organizations, and public and private community groups; they may include teaching for wellness as well as teaching those with chronic and long-term illnesses. Nurses who like to teach and are skilled and enthusiastic can participate in programs already set up and, equally important, can work to develop other programs and involve others on the health team.

Keeping the public informed about nursing and the changes that have occurred in recent years in both education and practice is a contribution to the community. Offers to present programs about modern nursing are often welcome in the many community, social, business, professional, and service groups that meet frequently and are interested in community service.

Activities such as these involve you in the community and are stimulating and satisfying. They also require time, effort, and often patience. But besides the satisfaction of being of service, you will gain in self-development and growth as a professional and as an individual, a dual reward that can't be bought.

■ WRITING FOR PUBLICATION

Nurses are leaders. Leaders have things to say. Communicate your ideas in writing. Nurses who have any inclination toward writing should respond to the urge early in their career. The first requirement is to have something to say, something to share with others. Sometimes it is to react to an issue, a concern, an event, or situation in nursing or elsewhere that affects nursing. It may be in response to a newspaper article, resulting in a letter to the editor, a reaction paper, or a follow-up article. A logical reason is that there has been little if anything in the literature on that particular topic, especially if this is in the area of clinical practice. Or a nurse may be involved in the development of new techniques, the use of new equipment, or an innovative approach to caring for a particular kind of patient. Sharing such information is satisfying in itself, but it is also a contribution to the profession. The most important reason for nurses to write (always assuming, of course, that what is written has substance) is the survival of the profession.

A profession must have an adequate body of literature documenting the theoretical and philosophical base of its practice and how its practitioners operate to provide the service that is the essence of professionalism. Informational voids encourage the multiple misconceptions and stereotypes of nursing that already exist and tempt others to fill the void on the basis of their own prejudices and interests.

It is true that both the quantity and quality of the nursing literature have grown in all its dimensions. In journals alone, the increase in clinical articles attests to nurses' interest in improving their clinical practice. Many journals concentrating on a clinical specialty have sprung up, and others focus on functional roles such as education and administration. New authors are emerging. Many nurses, who were traditionally not seen as writers, have discovered that they have something to say and are learning to express it in writing.

So why don't nurses write? Or at least as much as other professionals do? Perhaps the first reason is that too many nurses think that writing is for the academician, who must function in a "publish or perish" environment, or for the researcher who, in somewhat obscure language, adds to the theory of nursing. The average nurse has a string of excuses: "I don't have anything to say"; "I don't have a degree"; "I don't have time"; or "I don't know how." All those don'ts can be overcome. A person has to start somewhere, and except for the handful that have an innate talent and inclination for writing, a little self-discipline and maybe some tutoring are needed.

It may not be easy, as shown by this litany of pains—the need for discipline, finding the time, searching out and documenting sources, having one's cherished ideas (or pet phrases) criticized, finding the right editors, even being rejected. For those who want to write but feel that they don't know how, there are various practical steps. Anyone who has graduated from a nursing program should have the basic tools of writing: a firm grasp of grammar, punctuation, spelling, and word usage. If not, there is no excuse for not remedying the situation. To go a step further, for the purpose of writing, there are three indispensable tools: a good dictionary; *Roget's Thesaurus*, a dictionary of synonyms and antonyms to turn to when you know the meaning but can't think of the word; and William Strunk, Jr., and E. B. White's *The Elements of Style*, 4th ed. (White Plains, New York: Longman Publishing, 1999), which is easily read and includes basic rules of composition, grammar, punctuation, and word usage. In addition, there is a new surge of "how to" articles and books that can be extremely helpful, some of which are directed specifically to nurses.

Here are some generally accepted guidelines to writing: the best writers write so that they are understood; there is little that cannot be said with simple words, and there is absolutely no excuse for pretentious prose or jargon. This does not mean that the technical words that may be essential to a clinical article should be omitted. It does mean that simple collections of nouns, active verbs, participles, clauses, or whatever makes sense, serve as well as, if not better than, convoluted sentences that say nothing more.

Today, the use of nonsexist gender whenever possible is also desirable. The most common writing weaknesses cited by a group of editors were overly formal and pedagogic writing, poor organization, absence of an introduction and summary, poor sentence structure (too long and "doesn't flow"), poor or fabricated documentation, and use of jargon.

A good way to break into writing is through a letter to the editor. Such letters are frequently published unless they're totally inappropriate. Editors love comments on articles, editorials, or other parts of their publication because it adds interest—sometimes controversy—or new information, or simply indicates that someone was motivated enough by what was published to write. (They don't mind compliments on how good their journal is, either.) Few journals are overwhelmed by letters, as too often people "never get around to it," even if they are especially pleased or upset by what has been written. If you choose this first step to publication, remember that it is a demonstration of your writing ability, perceptiveness, good sense, understanding of the issues, and/or knowledge about another aspect of what was published. Keep it short and to the point. It may be edited if it's too long, generally only with your approval. An emotional tirade may be published but often makes the writer look foolish. However, a difference of opinion is perfectly appropriate, and because the original author may respond in print, it can be the start of an interesting new professional relationship. If you're really good, the editor might keep you in mind to serve as a reviewer or even request an article or another response to an issue.

Don't dismiss the idea of publishing for the general public. Nurses are very consumer friendly, and the lay public is in need of much of the information that we can give. Inquire about a "health piece" for your local paper and any other publications that have a general readership. Propose writing about something that is timely and perhaps a bit controversial.

Another way to be published is to write a book review. Although someone who presents papers or has already written articles may be invited by an editor to review a book in his or her area of expertise, it's not necessary to wait to be asked. It's perfectly acceptable to write to the editors of one or more journals, in care of the book review editor, and describe your qualifications and interests, perhaps including a résumé or curriculum vitae. Most editors will follow up, and you may be asked to be on the book reviewer list. It is not appropriate to send a self-selected book review. The book and the reviewer may already have been selected, or the book may not be slated for review.

There may or may not be reimbursement for the review, and the decision on whether you may keep the reviewed book (which is sent to you) or must return it varies with the publisher. Although most reviewers develop their own style of reviewing, some journals have a general format and desired length. It's also useful to review the guidelines suggested by book review editors or at least to read reviews already published in the selected journal.

For those who are ready to write an article and have selected a topic, there are certain basic guidelines at the beginning:

1. Know as much as possible about your subject; master the literature. Research those areas you're not sure about by interviewing people involved or others who might have an opinion to offer.

2. Assemble all the ideas, arguments, facts, data, and illustrations you can think of.

3. Sort and classify them.

4. Develop an outline.

5. Write a first draft. Establish the what, where, when, why, how, and who for your beginning paragraphs.

6. Revise (a second look brings amazing insights).

7. Ask for peer review. Sometimes a friend who writes or who is an editor can be helpful in making suggestions. However, it is the writer's responsibility to see that the content is accurate and that the references and bibliography are properly cited.

8. Revise again; proofread.

Selecting the appropriate journal for submission of an article is crucial. Some editors will return an article with a suggestion that another journal might be better for that type of paper, but most do not. (Nor do most bother to critique it, in part because of the volume of mail with which they must deal.) One way to determine which journal is right is to check several recent issues of the journals that might be suitable or at least the major journals listed in respected indexes. The table of contents presents a quick overview, and several issues should give a fairly clear picture of the subject matter that is of interest to the journal. In addition, some publish authors' guidelines that include the journal's mission or purpose. It may be helpful to check the masthead for the credentials of the editors, the editorial advisory board, and the peer review panel, if any. Colleagues can also give information, or at least opinions, on the quality and reputation of the journal. It's always useful to read some of the articles; this not only gives some indication of the journal's quality, but also provides some information on its style (most journals are edited by their editorial staff). If you have a major disagreement with the style or philosophy of a journal, you should probably not send a manuscript there. Whether to choose a journal with a large circulation or a specialized journal that reaches the particular audience desired is another important decision. And remember that a refereed journal is best. (Experts who recommend whether to publish, publish pending revision, or reject the manuscript anonymously review manuscripts submitted for publication.) However, one ethical point is overriding: A manuscript should be sent to only one journal at a time. If rejected, it can then go to another. Acceptance and publication by two journals (this does not refer to reprinting by permission) is considered a serious and sometimes unforgivable embarrassment. For one thing, the author has then presumably given the copyright to two separate owners.

At times, authors, especially if they have no track record, may choose to approach an editor first to see whether there is any interest in a particular type of article. This procedure is called a *query*. Opinion is mixed as to whether this is worthwhile, especially if you are reasonably sure that the article is suitable for that journal and that a similar one has not been published within the last few years. However, should such an article already be in the editor's file for future publication, it saves the author time and money to know it.

The usual procedure is as follows:

1. Write to the editor. If you know a particular editor of that journal, address it to him or her. However, check a recent journal for accuracy. Editors do not appreciate getting mail addressed to a long-gone predecessor, and it does imply that you have not even looked at a current issue. Explain what you would like to write about, include an outline of major points, give brief autobiographical information to indicate that you are qualified to write on the subject, and list previous writings, if any. This initial correspondence may take place by e-mail or standard mail. Read the author's guidelines, and note how articles are submitted. Let this be your guide. Don't get into the issue of remuneration unless you are an established author. And besides, nursing journals are not noted for extravagant fees and may pay no cash fee at all.

2. Wait for the editor's reply. If your idea is appealing, a letter, telephone call, or e-mail will follow with instructions regarding the length of your piece and sometimes the due date, possibly also with suggestions about content, development, and style.

3. In preparing the manuscript, follow the journal's guidelines, which can usually be found online. If no details are given, it is usually appropriate to prepare the manuscript on a word processor, double-spaced, font size 12, and leaving 1-inch margins at the top, bottom, and right- and left-hand sides. Include the references or bibliography and your (brief) autobiography, as you would like to have it published with your article but using that journal's style.

4. Send a cover letter and the article in the form specified by the publication. Most use web-based online manuscript submission.

5. You should receive an acknowledgment of receipt of the manuscript and, later, word as to whether or not your article has been accepted for publication. How long that will be depends on how the article is reviewed (by one or more editors or a peer review panel), whether it appears to be a clear-cut winner, or whether it will require additional editorial conferences or reviews. You should probably allow 3 months before inquiring about the manuscript's status. It is permissible to withdraw it if you wish. Some journals return declined manuscripts with the critiques of the reviewers and/or editors. If a revision and resubmission is requested, suggestions (or directions) for revision are made.

6. If the manuscript is accepted, the editor may or may not be able to give to you a publication date, but you can ask. Much depends on the timeliness of the article, the production plans for future journal issues, and the number of articles on hand.

7. The magazine's editorial staff will edit and prepare the article for the printer. They may send the edited copy for you to check and approve, or they may send you the

galley proofs after the article is set in type. Sometimes both the edited copy and proof are sent. Read the copy promptly, request only such changes as you feel are necessary for clarity and accuracy, and return it to the editor's office right away. Delay may mean that your article will not appear in the issue it was planned for and may disrupt the magazine's production schedule.

8. One or more complimentary copies of the issue in which your article is published will be mailed to you. If you want reprints or extra copies, contact the magazine's business office for information regarding the policy for ordering and the price.

9. Much the same process occurs when an unsolicited manuscript is submitted. For those scholars who wish to publish their research, a similar approach is used, but, depending on where and how the research is to be published (as a research paper or a narrative article), the style may vary. Again, it is wise to check with potential publishers. If the research is a thesis or dissertation, it is helpful to look at strategies that make the research publishable.

Should you write with a colleague, a co-author? This may be a good idea, provided that you know your co-author and are sure that you can work together. It's possible that each of you has a particular expertise to bring to a topic that gives the reader a broader perspective, or that one of you writes better than the other, or one is willing to do most of the literature search. (Make sure he or she knows how and what to focus on.) If several of you are involved in research, two or more people frequently co-author an article. Ask these questions: Can each of us meet deadlines? Are we each willing to take the time to do this? What exactly is each of us going to do? If we both write, who puts it together? Can we agree or compromise if there have to be content or style revisions? How do we share expenses for preparation of the manuscript? Who is first author? (This becomes important in academia.) The person whose idea it was? The one who did the most work? The one who needs credit most for promotion? If you come to a parting of the ways, who has the right to publish the article? Do you have mutual respect and trust so that there is no concern about the accuracy and originality of either what is written or the activity or research it was based on? These are important issues, because if they are left to chance, you could end with no publication or, worse, a legal complication.

Suppose you followed all the rules (or didn't) and your manuscript is rejected? If the editor or reviewers gave you helpful suggestions, with which you agree, you can revise the article and send it to another suitable journal. (Usually you don't send it back to the first unless the editor specifies that a revision could make it suitable for reconsideration.) You might very well be angry, but if the suggestions sound reasonable after reflection, consider revision seriously. It may be simpler than starting with a new topic. If you don't agree with the criticism, get some other advice and send the article to another journal.

Neither reviewers nor editors are infallible, and some have hidden prejudices even they don't recognize. It's particularly difficult if you get two quite different sets of suggestions and the editor gives you no guidance. You'll then simply have to decide, perhaps with some help from reliable peers, which, if any, advice to follow. If the problem is your writing style, get some editorial help. However, the most common reason for rejection is related to content, primarily because it is found to be inaccurate, not important, undocumented, has a poor research design, or was covered recently.

One warning: Some reviewers tend to be too hasty, sarcastic, or thoughtless in wording their critiques, and the editor may not do anything about it. This is very discouraging and a blow to the writer's ego. Try not to get too upset or give up. Every author has had rejections, some not with kind words. Just try again.

The procedure for writing a book is similar to that for a journal article, but it is often more exacting and usually much more time-consuming. There is more of everything, including satisfactions and remuneration. As there is also more expense to the publisher, usually even an experienced writer has to present a book proposal to a publisher (or to more than one).

In addition to the manuscript for the main portion or body of the book, the author is usually responsible for writing the foreword or preface, sometimes for preparing the index, and for reading the galley proofs. You must also obtain written permission to use material taken or adapted from other sources, being sure that credits are included in the book as indicated to avoid any embarrassment, difficulty, or lawsuit.

The editorial staff of a book publishing company is willing to help the author in every way possible. But only in unusual instances does the staff relieve the author of the responsibility for checking data and presenting them in proper form.

It is customary for a book publisher and an author to negotiate a contract covering the main considerations in the preparation for the manuscript, responsibilities for illustrative materials, revision, and royalty rates. Because royalties, support or advances, and marketing vary among publishers, it is wise to shop around to find the one most suitable. Sometimes a lawyer or someone who has had considerable experience with publishers can be extremely helpful.

Not all nurses have writing skills, but many do have ideas that are worth sharing. There are two solutions—developing those skills through practice, study, and workshops or joining forces with someone who does write well, keeping in mind the possible pitfalls of co-authorship.

The important point is that the person who has something worthwhile to say finds a way to say it and takes the time to do it. This is a professional responsibility and a satisfying one.

■ THERE CAN NEVER BE A LAST WORD

Nursing is noble work, and you have chosen it wisely. You enter the profession in times of upheaval and paradox, but also at a point of its renaissance. This book has tried to portray faithfully the picture of a profession that is moving with the times. It is a profession that has often been the conscience of health care, speaking out on social issues with a fervor that has sometimes been self-destructive. Our past has been greatly influenced by the women's movement and the growth of modern medicine and the health care industry. Through all of the change that has characterized human affairs, nursing has remained positioned at the bedside, in the home, in the community—often the only human link between our patients and an intimidating experience in the health care delivery system.

There can never be a last word, because you will live every chapter of the profession as it unfolds and, it is hoped, contribute new, exciting episodes.

KEY POINTS

1. There has historically been an incongruity between what you expect of the nursing workplace before graduation and what you find when you get there.
2. Accepting that you hold different values from those in a bureaucracy and working out a relationship that accommodates both your values and the reality of the workplace are healthy ways to adjust to reality shock.

3. Nurses are considered a very costly resource and are being held to rigorous standards for actively managing the clinical care of their patients.
4. Burnout occurs when the various pressures of a job and dissatisfaction with the work situation seem to be impossible to cope with.
5. Being good to yourself and allowing for personal activities, as well as working with a support group, can relieve some aspects of stress and burnout.
6. Nursing is physically and psychologically dangerous work; many workplace hazards are being addressed by state and federal legislation.
7. CE for nurses may include in-service education, self-learning, and programs offered by educational institutions and professional organizations.
8. The primary purpose of CE for nurses is to ensure continued competence in practice.
9. You should proceed with care in selecting the right educational program, whether for CE or for a degree, so that you don't waste your time or money.
10. Funding for formal nursing education is available from a variety of sources, but it saves time to consult first with the financial officer of the school in which you are interested.
11. Participating in nursing and community organizations is a way to enrich your life as a nurse and as a person.
12. More nurses are successfully combining family life and a nursing career, including formal education.

REFERENCES

1. Hardy M, Conway M. *Role Theory*. Norwalk, CT: Appleton & Lange, 1988, pp 73–110.
2. Reid M. Marginal man: The identity dilemma of the academic general practitioner. *Symbolic Interaction* 5:325, February 1982.
3. Kramer M. *Reality Shock*. St. Louis, MO: Mosby, 1974.

4. Ibid, pp vi–viii, 3.

5. Ibid, pp 155–162.

6. Ibid, p 162.

7. Vance C, Bamford P. Developing caring connections: Mentorship in the academic setting. *Deans Note*s 19:1–3, March 1998.

8. Varkey P. Practical tips and strategies for designing and implementing interprofessional curricula. *Educ Prim Care* 21(1):41–44, January 2010.

9. Selye H. *Stress without Distress*. Philadelphia: Lippincott, 1974.

10. Peplau H. Peplau's theory of interpersonal relations. *Nurs Sci Q* 10:162–167, Winter 1997.

11. Kobasa S, Maddi R, Puccetti M. Effectiveness of hardiness, exercise and social support as resources against illness. *J Psychosom Res* 29:525–533, May 1985.

12. Hardy, op cit., pp 159–239.

13. Arena D, Page N. The imposter phenomenon in the clinical nurse specialist role. *Image* 24:121–125, Summer 1992.

14. Joel L. Maybe a pot watcher but never an ostrich. *Am J Nurs* 94:7, April 1994.

15. Ibid.

16. AMSF Library. Were the nurses floating? http://www.amfs.com/Syncope.html. Retrieved June 11, 2010.

17. Gobis L. The perils of floating: When nurses are directed to work outside their areas of expertise. *Am J Nurs* 101(9):78, September 2001.

18. Olds D, Clarke S. The effect of work hours on adverse events and errors in health care. *J Safety Res* 41(2): 153–162, April 2010.

19. ANA. Mandatory Overtime. November 23, 2009. http:// nursingworld.org. Retrieved June 10, 2010.

20 FindLaw. More Information on Whistleblower Laws. http://law.findlaw.com. Retrieved June 10, 2010.

21. Fletcher J, Sorrell J, Silva M: Whistleblowing as a failure of organizational ethics. Online Journal of Issues in Nursing. http://nursingworld.org/ojin/topic 8/topic 8_3.htm. Retrieved August 5, 2002.

22. Ketter J. Sex discrimination targets men in some hospitals. *Am J Nurs* 26:3, 24, April 1994.

23. US Equal Employment Opportunity Commission. The Americans with Disabilities Act. http://www.ada.gov/qandaeng.htm. Retrieved June 10, 2010.

24. ANA. Position Statements: HIV Testing. http://nursingworld. org/readroom/position/blood/bltest.htm. Retrieved June 5, 2010.

25. ANA. Position Statements: HIV Infected Nurse, Ethical Obligations and Disclosure. http://nursingworld. org/readroom/position/blood/bltest.htm. Retrieved June 5, 2010.

26. *New York Daily News*. Nurse Awarded $15 Million in Sexual Harassment Lawsuit. February 23, 2009. http://www.nydailynews.com. Retrieved June 10, 2010.

27. Court spells out rules for finding sex harassment. *The New York Times*, June 27, 1998, pp A1, 10–12.

28. CDC. Surveillance of Occupationally Acquired HIV/AIDS in Healthcare Personnel, as of December 2006. September 10, 2007. http://www.cdc.gov/ncidod/dhqp/bp_hcp_w_hiv.html. Retrieved June 0, 2010.

29. Murphy E. Needlestick safety and prevention act. *AORN J* 76(2), February 2001. http://findarticles.com/p/search/ ?qta=0&qt=needlestick+prevention%20legislation&tb=ar t&qf=all&x=0&y=0. Retrieved June 10, 2010.

30. Bigony L, Lipke T, Lundberg A, McGraw C, Pagac G, Rogers A. Lateral violence in the perioperative setting. *AORN J* 89(4):688–696, April 2009.

31. Insulation from supervisory influence. *SNA Legal Developments*, Special Issue December 22, 1989.

32. Supreme Court upholds NLRB's rulemaking in determining RN-only bargaining units: NLRB issues guidelines. *SNA Legal Developments* July 26, 1991.

33. Nightingale F. *Notes on Nursing*. New York: D. Appleton and Company, 1860 (first American Edition).

34. LeRoy A. How to survive as a non-traditional nursing student. *Imprint* 35:73–74, 79–86, April–May 1988.

Updates can be found at **www.kellysnursing.com**

HELPFUL WEBSITES FOR PART III, SECTION TWO

American Association of Colleges of Nursing: http://www.aacn.nche.edu

American Nurses Association: http://www.nursingworld.org (The above may also serve as a gateway to other nursing organizations.)

Centers for Disease Control and Prevention: http://www.cdc.gov

Global RN Website: http://nurseweb.ucsf.edu/www/globalrn.htm

Health Care Workers and HIV/AIDS: http://www.thebody.com

International Council of Nurses: http://www.icn.ch

Lippincott Publishers: http://www.nursingcenter.com (Links to endless nursing websites)

National League for Nursing: http://www.nln.org

NIOSH—Violence in the Workplace: http://www.cdc.gov/niosh/violcont.html

National Student Nurses' Association: http://www.nsna.org

NurseScribe: http://enursescribe.com/Gateway site

OSHA—Workplace: http://www.osha-slc.gov/SLTC/workplaceviolence

Sigma Theta Tau International: http://www.nursingsociety.org

University of Michigan Center for Ergonomics: http://www.engin.umich.edu/dept/ioe/C4E/

Index